BSAVA Manual of Canine and Feline Cardiorespiratory Medicine

Second edition

Editors:

Virginia Luis Fuentes
MA VetMB PhD CertVR DVC DipACVIM DipECVIM-CA (Cardiology) MRCVS

Veterinary Clinical Sciences, The Royal Veterinary College, Hawkshead Lane,
North Mymms, Hatfield, Hertfordshire AL9 7TA

Lynelle R. Johnson
DVM MS PhD DipACVIM

Department of Veterinary Medicine, University of California Davis,
1 Shields Avenue, Davis, CA 95616, USA

and

Simon Dennis
BVetMed MVM CertVC DipECVIM-CA (Cardiology) MRCVS

North Downs Specialist Referrals, The Friesian Building 3 & 4,
The Brewerstreet Dairy Business Park, Brewer Street, Bletchingley, Surrey RH1 4QP

Published by:

British Small Animal Veterinary Association
Woodrow House, 1 Telford Way, Waterwells
Business Park, Quedgeley, Gloucester GL2 2AB

A Company Limited by Guarantee in England.
Registered Company No. 2837793.
Registered as a Charity.

Printed in the UK by Severn, Gloucester GL2 5EU – a carbon neutral printer
Printed on ECF paper made from sustainable forests

17478PUBS22

Titles in the BSAVA Manuals series:

Manual of Avian Practice: A Foundation Manual
Manual of Backyard Poultry Medicine and Surgery
Manual of Canine & Feline Abdominal Imaging
Manual of Canine & Feline Abdominal Surgery
Manual of Canine & Feline Advanced Veterinary Nursing
Manual of Canine & Feline Anaesthesia and Analgesia
Manual of Canine & Feline Behavioural Medicine
Manual of Canine & Feline Cardiorespiratory Medicine
Manual of Canine & Feline Clinical Pathology
Manual of Canine & Feline Dentistry and Oral Surgery
Manual of Canine & Feline Dermatology
Manual of Canine & Feline Emergency and Critical Care
Manual of Canine & Feline Endocrinology
Manual of Canine & Feline Endoscopy and Endosurgery
Manual of Canine & Feline Fracture Repair and Management
Manual of Canine & Feline Gastroenterology
Manual of Canine & Feline Haematology and Transfusion Medicine
Manual of Canine & Feline Head, Neck and Thoracic Surgery
Manual of Canine & Feline Musculoskeletal Disorders
Manual of Canine & Feline Musculoskeletal Imaging
Manual of Canine & Feline Nephrology and Urology
Manual of Canine & Feline Neurology
Manual of Canine & Feline Oncology
Manual of Canine & Feline Ophthalmology
Manual of Canine & Feline Radiography and Radiology: A Foundation Manual
Manual of Canine & Feline Rehabilitation, Supportive and Palliative Care: Case Studies in Patient Management
Manual of Canine & Feline Reproduction and Neonatology
Manual of Canine & Feline Shelter Medicine: Principles of Health and Welfare in a Multi-animal Environment
Manual of Canine & Feline Surgical Principles: A Foundation Manual
Manual of Canine & Feline Thoracic Imaging
Manual of Canine & Feline Ultrasonography
Manual of Canine & Feline Wound Management and Reconstruction
Manual of Canine Practice: A Foundation Manual
Manual of Exotic Pet and Wildlife Nursing
Manual of Exotic Pets: A Foundation Manual
Manual of Feline Practice: A Foundation Manual
Manual of Ornamental Fish
Manual of Practical Animal Care
Manual of Practical Veterinary Nursing
Manual of Psittacine Birds
Manual of Rabbit Medicine
Manual of Rabbit Surgery, Dentistry and Imaging
Manual of Raptors, Pigeons and Passerine Birds
Manual of Reptiles
Manual of Rodents and Ferrets
Manual of Small Animal Practice Management and Development
Manual of Wildlife Casualties

For further information on these and all BSAVA publications, please visit our website: **www.bsava.com**

Contents

Contributors

Elizabeth Baines MA VetMB DVR DipECVDI MRCVS
Veterinary Clinical Sciences, The Royal Veterinary College, Hawkshead Lane, North Mymms, Hatfield, Hertfordshire AL9 7TA

Amanda Boag MA VetMB DipACVIM DipACVECC FHEA MRCVS
VetsNow, 1 Blue Central, Pitreavie Drive, Dunfermline, Fife KY11 8US

John D. Bonagura DVM DipACVIM
Veterinary Clinical Sciences, Veterinary Hospital, 601 Vernon Tharp Street, Columbus, OH 43210, USA

Adrian Boswood MA VetMB DVC DipECVIM-CA (Cardiology) MRCVS
Veterinary Clinical Sciences, The Royal Veterinary College, Hawkshead Lane, North Mymms, Hatfield, Hertfordshire AL9 7TA

Gareth Buckley MA VetMB MRCVS
Department of Clinical Sciences, Cummings School of Veterinary Medicine, Tufts University, 200 Westboro Road, North Grafton, MA 01536, USA

Brendan M. Corcoran DipPharm PhD MRCVS
Hospital for Small Animals, Easter Bush Veterinary Centre, Roslin, Midlothian EH25 9RG

Amy E. DeClue DVM MS DipACVIM (SAIM)
Department of Medicine and Surgery, College of Veterinary Medicine, University of Missouri, 900 East Campus Drive, Columbia, MO 65211, USA

Simon Dennis BVetMed MVM CertVC DipECVIM-CA (Cardiology) MRCVS
North Downs Specialist Referrals, The Friesian Building 3 & 4, The Brewerstreet Dairy Business Park, Brewer Street, Bletchingley, Surrey RH1 4QP

Joanna Dukes-McEwan BVMS MVM PhD DVC DipECVIM-CA (Cardiology) MRCVS
RCVS and European Recognised Specialist in Veterinary Cardiology
Small Animal Teaching Hospital, University of Liverpool, Leahurst Campus, Chester High Road, Neston, Cheshire CH64 7TE

Anne French MVB PhD CertSAM DVC DipECVIM-CA (Cardiology) FHEA MRCVS
RCVS and European Recognised Specialist in Veterinary Cardiology
Hospital for Small Animals, Easter Bush Veterinary Centre, Roslin, Midlothian EH25 9RG

Jennifer M. Good DVM DipACVECC
Katonah Bedford Veterinary Center, 546 North Bedford Road, Bedford Hills, NY 10507, USA

Jens Häggström DVM PhD DipECVIM-CA (Cardiology)
Department of Clinical Sciences, The Swedish University of Agricultural Sciences, Box 7037, S-75007 Uppsala, Sweden

Rosanne Jepson BVSc PhD MRCVS
Veterinary Clinical Sciences, The Royal Veterinary College, Hawkshead Lane, North Mymms, Hatfield, Hertfordshire AL9 7TA

Eric G. Johnson DVM
Department of Veterinary Medicine, University of California Davis, 1 Shields Avenue, Davis, CA 95616, USA

Lynelle R. Johnson DVM MS PhD DipACVIM
Department of Veterinary Medicine, University of California Davis, 1 Shields Avenue, Davis, CA 95616, USA

Lindsay M. Kellett-Gregory BSc(Hons) BVetMed MRCVS
School of Veterinary Medicine, University of Pennsylvania, 3900 Delancey Street, Philadelphia, PA 19104, USA

Lesley G. King MVB DipACVECC DipACVIM
School of Veterinary Medicine, University of Pennsylvania, 3900 Delancey Street, Philadelphia, PA 19104, USA

Marc S. Kraus DVM DipACVIM (Cardiology, Internal Medicine)
Department of Clinical Sciences, Cardiology College of Veterinary Medicine, Cornell University, Ithaca,
NY 14853, USA

Clarence Kvart DVM PhD DipECVIM-CA (Cardiology)
Faculty of Veterinary Medicine and Animal Science, The Swedish University of Agricultural Sciences, Box 7011,
S-75007 Uppsala, Sweden

Virginia Luis Fuentes MA VetMB PhD CertVR DVC DipACVIM DipECVIM-CA (Cardiology) MRCVS
Veterinary Clinical Sciences, The Royal Veterinary College, Hawkshead Lane, North Mymms, Hatfield,
Hertfordshire AL9 7TA

Mike Martin MVB DVC MRCVS
RCVS Recognised Specialist in Veterinary Cardiology
Martin Referrals Veterinary Cardiorespiratory Centre, 43 Waverley Road, Kenilworth, Warwickshire CV8 1JL

Catriona M. MacPhail DVM PhD DipACVS
Department of Clinical Sciences, Colorado State University, Fort Collins, CO 80523, USA

Brendan C. McKiernan DVM DipACVIM
Southern Oregon Veterinary Specialty Center, 3265 Biddle Road, Medford, OR 97504, USA

Mark A. Oyama DVM DipACVIM (Cardiology)
School of Veterinary Medicine, University of Pennsylvania, 3900 Delancey Street, Philadelphia, PA 19104, USA

Carol R. Reinero DVM PhD DipACVIM (SAIM)
Department of Medicine and Surgery, College of Veterinary Medicine, University of Missouri,
900 East Campus Drive, Columbia, MO 65211, USA

Elizabeth Rozanski DVM DipACVECC DipACVIM (SAIM)
Department of Clinical Sciences, Cummings School of Veterinary Medicine, Tufts University,
200 Westboro Road, North Grafton, MA 01536, USA

Rebecca L. Stepien DVM MS DipACVIM (Cardiology)
Department of Medical Sciences, University of Wisconsin School of Veterinary Medicine, 2015 Linden Drive,
Madison, WI 53706, USA

Harriet Syme BSc BVetMed PhD DipACVIM DipECVIM FHEA MRCVS
Veterinary Clinical Sciences, The Royal Veterinary College, Hawkshead Lane, North Mymms, Hatfield,
Hertfordshire AL9 7TA

Richard A.S. White BVetMed PhD DSAS DVR Diplomate ACVS DipECVS FRCVS
*RCVS and European Recognised Specialist in Small Animal Surgery; RCVS Recognised Specialist in
Veterinary Oncology*
Dick White Referrals, Station Farm, Six Mile Bottom, Newmarket CB8 0UH

Ruth Willis BVM&S DVC MRCVS
RCVS Recognised Specialist in Cardiology
Holter Monitoring Service, 3 Kirkland Avenue, Blanefield, Glasgow G63 9BY

Erik R. Wisner DVM
Department of Veterinary Medicine, University of California Davis, 1 Shields Avenue, Davis, CA 95616, USA

Foreword

The progression of knowledge in small animal cardiorespiratory medicine over the last 12 years since I was involved in the first edition has been truly breathtaking. Machines for echocardiography have become more complex and more affordable, new blood tests and drugs have become available, and a specific *Journal of Veterinary Cardiology* has appeared. As a result, a complete revision of the first edition became essential. The second edition encompasses these new developments and in keeping with the series of BSAVA Manuals translates the scientific advances into clinically useful applicable information.

The Surgery section in the title of the first edition has been removed and, in view of the advance of specialisation, this is a necessary change. The Manual is now divided into five sections. In keeping with the problem-oriented approach, the Manual starts with the clinical approach to common presenting signs. An expanded diagnostic techniques section now covers CT and MRI, followed by sections on mechanisms of disease and therapeutics. The final section on specific diseases is also more detailed.

The editors are to be congratulated for bringing together a talented team of international experts to contribute in their field of expertise, ensuring the Manual is as up to date as possible. The enthusiasm of the authors for their subject shines through in the writing. This Manual has a place on every clinician's shelf. It will be invaluable to dip into for specific problems but it also is a fantastic reference to be read at leisure. For a few it will kindle the enthusiasm for the subject that can take over your life!

Simon Swift MA VetMB CertSAC DipECVIM-CA (Cardiology) MRCVS
Northwest Surgeons
February 2010

Preface

It has been over 10 years since the first edition of the *BSAVA Manual of Small Animal Cardiorespiratory Medicine and Surgery*. In that time, there have been huge advances in diagnostic methods and medical therapies available for use in cardiothoracic medicine. The advent of the *BSAVA Manual of Canine and Feline Head, Neck and Thoracic Surgery* to describe surgical options has allowed us to focus more completely on medical therapies in this new edition.

The approach of the Manual has been completely remodelled to enhance the reader's access to information. Part 1 focuses on the clinical approach to the most common problems encountered in the clinic, including respiratory distress, cough, syncope, and murmurs. Part 2 centres on available diagnostic methods and starts with the essential features of history and physical examination that help differentiate cardiac from respiratory disease. This section includes detailed discussion of the use of biomarkers in cardiac disease as well as chapters on basic and advanced imaging modalities.

Part 3 concentrates on the underlying pathophysiology of disease associated with respiratory disease, heart failure and arrhythmias. Since the last edition, there has been a remarkable increase in our understanding of the mechanisms underlying heart failure, in particular. These chapters contain information essential for an understanding of the consequences of disease, as well as guidance on appropriate diagnostic tests and therapeutic management. Part 4 focuses on broad concepts of management of acute and chronic respiratory disease, as well as management of heart failure and arrhythmias. This section has been substantially updated following the findings of multiple therapeutic clinical trials, most notably in the treatment of heart failure, and is essential reading for the veterinarian who practices cardiopulmonary medicine.

In Part 5, the authors lend their experience of diagnosis and management of the disorders encountered most commonly in veterinary medicine, including valvular heart disease, feline cardiomyopathy, and canine and feline tracheobronchial disease.

This edition has a truly international flavour, with contributions from leaders in the fields of cardiology and respiratory disorders from the United Kingdom, Europe and the United States. All material has been tightly integrated to highlight global cooperation in veterinary medicine.

An update on cardiopulmonary medicine is long overdue, and this new edition has been carefully prepared to provide up-to-date information essential for the busy practitioner. We hope that it will serve as a valuable resource in the years to come. We thank all of our contributing authors for their excellent manuscripts and images. We are grateful for the assistance of the incredibly helpful staff at the BSAVA office, especially Nicola Lloyd. Special thanks are also due to Sam Elmhurst for her beautiful illustrations.

Virginia Luis Fuentes
Lynelle Johnson
Simon Dennis
February 2010

Clinical approach to respiratory distress

Jennifer M. Good and Lesley G. King

Introduction

Definitions
* *Dyspnoea* refers to a sensation of difficult or laboured breathing. As the term is used in human medicine to convey a sensation described by a person, it is technically inappropriate to apply this term to dogs and cats. However, observation of the level of distress in dogs and cats with severe respiratory disease often allows the veterinary surgeon to infer that those species are experiencing discomfort due to difficulty in breathing.
* *Tachypnoea* is defined as an increased respiratory rate and is not always associated with hyperventilation (see below). It should not be confused with panting.
* *Panting* is a method to dispel heat in the dog and does not necessarily signal distress. Panting animals are primarily increasing dead space ventilation and therefore are not usually hyperventilating. However, panting in cats is usually associated with stress, respiratory distress or cardiac arrhythmias.
* *Orthopnoea* is described as the inability to breathe unless in an upright position.

Respiratory distress is a common presentation in veterinary medicine, and prompt, effective management is paramount. Treating these animals can be challenging, as many are too distressed to be handled extensively. Excessive manipulation can result in exacerbation of respiratory distress, haemoglobin desaturation and respiratory arrest. Thus, in unstable animals, it is very important to limit diagnostic testing. Instead, initial efforts should be focused on stabilization and application of non-specific respiratory support modalities, such as oxygen supplementation. The history and signalment, observation of the pattern of respiration, and a brief physical examination are all used to make a clinical estimate of the anatomical location of disease within the respiratory tract, thereby directing effective emergency therapy to stabilize the patient prior to diagnostic testing (Figure 1.1). Depending on the cause of respiratory distress, a variety of emergency interventions may be necessary, including drug therapy, tracheostomy, thoracocentesis or thoracostomy tube placement, and positive pressure ventilation.

Physiology

Respiratory distress occurs when there is:

* An increase in arterial partial pressure of carbon dioxide (P_aCO_2)
* A decrease in arterial partial pressure of oxygen (P_aO_2)
* Significantly increased work of breathing.

In the dog, normal P_aCO_2 is 35–45 mmHg; cats have slightly lower normal values, in the range of 30–35 mmHg. *Hypercarbia* is the primary drive for respiration and is defined as a P_aCO_2 >46 mmHg. An increase in P_aCO_2 to ≥50 mmHg should trigger the central nervous system to increase tidal volume and the rate of respiration, resulting in increased minute ventilation to blow off excess CO_2. *Hypoxaemia*, or insufficient oxygen concentration in the blood, can also cause increased respiratory drive. Normal P_aO_2 is 85–100 mmHg in both dogs and cats. Respiratory distress is triggered by P_aO_2 values <60 mmHg, and significant respiratory drive is initiated at levels <50 mmHg (see Chapter 14).

The normal physiological response to either hypercarbia or hypoxaemia is to increase respiratory drive in order to improve oxygenation of the blood and expel excess carbon dioxide. It is important to keep in mind that animals with chronic respiratory disorders may have adjusted to severely abnormal arterial blood gas values over time, and therefore both hypercarbia and hypoxaemia may be far more severe than would be expected for the degree of respiratory distress exhibited.

History

The signalment of the patient and recent history can provide very important information for determining the best method of initial stabilization. For example, brachycephalic airway obstruction is likely to be an important cause of respiratory disease in an English Bulldog; a collapsing trachea should be considered a likely cause of respiratory distress in a Yorkshire

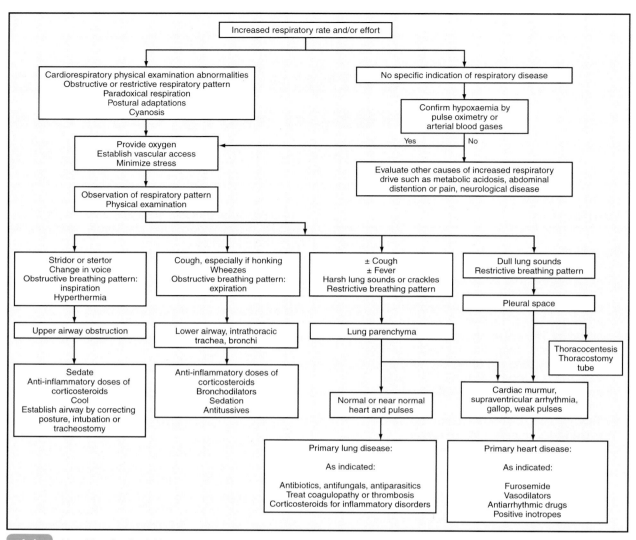

1.1 Algorithm for the initial management of animals with respiratory distress.

Terrier; and *Bordetella* pneumonia is high on the list of differential diagnoses in a puppy with respiratory difficulty that has recently been obtained from a pet shop or shelter.

Once feasible, information about the recent history should be obtained:

- Does the animal have any history of pre-existing cardiac or respiratory disease?
- Is there any history of trauma or toxin ingestion?
- Has the animal been coughing or showing exercise intolerance?
- Is there a history of syncope or seizure?
- Has the animal been previously diagnosed with any other medical conditions?
- Has there been a change in bark?
- Has the animal been coughing or sneezing?
- Has the animal been vomiting?

Initial observation

Initial observation, although it may be limited due to the animal's instability, is very important in identifying the anatomical location of respiratory disease. Observation of the animal's posture, respiratory rate and the nature of the respiratory effort is non-invasive and can be very helpful in establishing an initial therapeutic plan.

During normal quiet breathing, inspiration should involve a barely perceptible movement of the chest wall, resulting from contraction of the external intercostal muscles and diaphragm. Normal expiration is passive and results from the elastic recoil of the normal lungs. As the drive to breathe increases, secondary muscles of respiration are recruited, including the muscles of the abdominal wall, the scalenes, the sternomastoid, sternohyoid and sternothyroid muscles, and the alae nasi muscles that cause the nostrils to flare. Activation of these muscles causes a dramatic increase in movement of the chest wall, and respiratory efforts become obvious, even with cursory observation.

It is important to remember that a number of nonspecific factors can cause increased respiratory drive and recruitment of the secondary muscles of respiration, including pain, stress, metabolic, neurological and abdominal disease. Animals with true respiratory disease can be identified because they assume characteristic postural adaptations, exhibit an obstructive or restrictive respiratory pattern, or demonstrate paradoxical respiratory effort in addition to recruiting secondary muscles of respiration.

Postural adaptations

Animals with difficulty breathing often assume specific postures that optimize oxygenation and minimize resistance to air flow (Figure 1.2). Typically, they prefer to stand, sit or lie in a sternal position, thereby allowing optimal movement of both sides of the chest wall. Dogs and cats that lie in lateral recumbency are often in the terminal stages of respiratory distress and merit immediate and aggressive intervention. Abduction of the elbows is another adaptation that optimizes the animal's ability to expand the chest wall maximally. Breathing through an open mouth allows the animal to bypass the resistance to air movement offered by turbulent air flow through the nasal turbinates. Animals in respiratory distress often stretch out their head and neck in an effort to straighten the trachea and further decrease resistance to air flow.

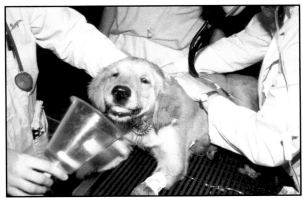

1.2 Severe respiratory distress due to neurogenic pulmonary oedema after a choking incident in a 6-month-old Golden Retriever. Note the pale mucous membranes, extended neck, abducted elbows and reluctance to have an oxygen mask placed over the face. (Courtesy of K. Drobatz and reproduced from the *BSAVA Manual of Canine and Feline Emergency and Critical Care, 2nd edition.*)

Obstructive respiratory patterns

Upper airway disease

Animals with an extrathoracic upper airway obstruction have pronounced inspiratory effort.

In animals with a dynamic upper airway obstruction, such as laryngeal paralysis, negative intrathoracic pressure that creates air flow during inspiration tends to suck the upper airway closed, narrowing the lumen and increasing resistance to air flow. Inspiration is therefore prolonged, although the respiratory rate may not be significantly elevated above normal. With an upper airway obstruction, the degree of negative pressure generated for each breath is greater than normal, causing a vicious circle of worsening airway collapse. Excitement, exercise or overheating can worsen airway obstructions because of increased respiratory drive. In animals with dynamic upper airway obstructions, expiration is often fairly normal because airway pressure blows open the upper airway. Animals with fixed upper airway obstructions tend to have problems with both inspiration and expiration.

Animals with laryngeal disease often make a noise, 'stridor', which occurs primarily during inspiration with a dynamic obstruction, and during both inspiration and expiration with a fixed obstruction. Animals with abnormalities in the pharynx (e.g. brachycephalic breeds) make a snoring noise, 'stertor', during inspiration and/or expiration.

Lower airway disease

Animals with intrathoracic obstruction of the small airways due to lower airway disease, such as dogs with chronic bronchitis or cats with asthma or bronchitis, tend to exhibit increased effort during expiration. In these patients, radial traction tends to hold the small intrathoracic airways open during inspiration. However, narrowing of the small airways due to inflammation, mucus or spasm of the smooth muscles causes early closure of the small airways during expiration, which results in air-trapping in the periphery. Recruitment and contraction of the abdominal muscles becomes evident as the animal tries to force air out of the lungs during exhalation.

Restrictive respiratory patterns

Animals with decreased lung compliance tend to adopt a 'restrictive' pattern of respiration. Lung compliance is low in animals with parenchymal, pleural or chest wall disease. Decreased lung compliance results in a significant increase in the amount of work required by the muscles of respiration to generate enough negative intrathoracic pressure for a normal tidal respiration. In order to minimize the work of breathing, tidal volume is decreased in a patient with reduced lung compliance, and minute ventilation can only be maintained by increasing the respiratory rate. Thus, animals with lung parenchymal or pleural space disease tend to have a restrictive pattern of respiration, characterized by an increased respiratory rate accompanied by increased effort, but with shallow breaths that have a low tidal volume.

Paradoxical respiration

The term 'paradoxical respiration' is applied in two different situations in small animal patients. Animals with a 'flail segment' of the ribs as a result of thoracic trauma may exhibit paradoxical respiration. In these patients, fractures in two places on one or more ribs result in a segment of the chest wall that floats independently of the rest of the chest wall. When the diaphragm contracts and the chest wall expands to generate negative intrapleural pressure, the flail segment is drawn inwards rather than expanding with the rest of the chest wall.

A second use of the term applies to patients experiencing a dramatic increase in the work of breathing (regardless of aetiology) that results in respiratory muscle fatigue and imminent respiratory failure. During normal inspiration, the ribs move cranially and laterally whilst the abdomen moves slightly outward. In animals with respiratory muscle fatigue, paradoxical breathing can be observed, whereby the intercostal spaces and the caudal ribs are drawn inward by contraction of the diaphragm during inspiration. Discordant contractions of failing respiratory muscles may also result in inward movement of the abdomen during inspiration. These conflicting motions are termed paradoxical because they oppose effective expansion of the thoracic cavity and worsen respiratory failure. Observation of discordant motion of the thoracic and abdominal walls is an ominous sign of severe disease that mandates aggressive intervention.

Physical examination

Some patients with respiratory distress require immediate stabilization prior to completion of a physical examination. The most common causes of respiratory distress are primary cardiac and primary respiratory disease, and it can be difficult to distinguish between these two aetiologies (Figure 1.3). Therefore, the initial physical examination in animals with respiratory distress should focus primarily on the cardiorespiratory systems:

1. Quickly evaluate the mucous membranes to estimate perfusion and oxygenation.
2. Palpate the thorax, including the area over the heart, and pulses and carefully auscultate the heart, lungs and upper airways.
3. For animals with suspected upper airway obstruction, measure rectal temperature as soon as possible after presentation, as severe hyperthermia may require immediate management.
4. A complete physical examination of the other body systems (abdominal, neurological, etc.) should follow as soon as possible after stabilization.

Mucous membranes
Mucous membranes of animals in respiratory distress may be normal pink, pale (suggesting anaemia or vasoconstriction), hyperaemic (suggesting hyperthermia or systemic inflammation) or cyanotic.

Cyanosis is a bluish tint to the mucous membranes (Figure 1.4), which is apparent when the level of haemoglobin in the capillaries reaches 50 g/l. In an animal with a normal packed cell volume (PCV), cyanosis occurs when haemoglobin saturation reaches 73–78% or P_aO_2 is 39–44 mmHg. Thus, cyanosis is a very late sign of severe disease. Animals with hypoxaemia and severe anaemia often have pale rather than cyanotic mucous membranes because the absolute amount of haemoglobin is so low.

- **Central cyanosis** (mucous membranes and skin) occurs when there is:
  - Arterial hypoxaemia secondary to respiratory or cardiac disease
  - Increased extraction of oxygen from capillary blood (e.g. in sepsis, with increased tissue oxygen demands)
  - An increased amount of oxygen-poor venous blood in the periphery due to congestion or blood pooling (e.g. severe hypotension or clot formation)
  - An increased concentration of abnormal haemoglobin pigments.
- **Peripheral cyanosis** occurs when there is localized hypoxaemia, as in the case of feline aortic thromboembolism at the aortic trifurcation. In these cases, circulation is cut off to the lower extremities, resulting in cyanosis of the toepads and nailbeds of the affected limbs only.

Palpation
The next part of the physical examination involves a quick palpation of the thorax, neck and pulses. Palpation of the neck and thoracic inlet may reveal obvious masses that could contribute to an airway obstruction. In cats, decreased compressibility of the cranial thorax may suggest a cranial mediastinal mass. The palm of the hand can be placed over the heart to detect whether a cardiac thrill is present, suggesting primary heart disease. Finally, the pulses should be palpated, paying attention to rate and pulse quality. Animals that are tachypnoeic and in

Parameter	Primary heart disease (congestive heart failure)	Primary airway/lung/pleural space disease
History	Coughing (dogs) Syncope	Coughing (dogs, cats) Sneezing, nasal discharge Change in bark/meow Stridor or stertor
Posture and breathing pattern	Restrictive breathing pattern Orthopnoea	Obstructive breathing pattern Stridor or stertor Restrictive breathing pattern
Physical examination	± Palpable cardiac thrill Cardiac abnormalities including murmur, arrhythmia (often supraventricular) and gallop rhythm Tachycardia is common Weak pulses and pulse deficits possible Harsh bronchovesicular sounds or fine crackles with pulmonary oedema Dull lung sounds with pleural effusion	Masses or abnormal compressibility of the thorax Normal cardiac auscultation, ventricular arrhythmias may occur Heart rate may be normal Pulse quality may be normal Harsh bronchovesicular sounds, wheezes, crackles and dull sounds Fever or hyperthermia

1.3 Clinical signs of acute congestive heart failure and primary lung disease in animals with respiratory distress.

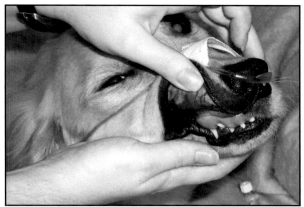

1.4 Cyanosis in a young dog secondary to methaemoglobinaemia.

distress due to congestive heart failure (CHF) often have rapid or weak pulses, whilst those with primary respiratory disease are more likely to have normal haemodynamics.

Auscultation

Further physical examination should include auscultation of the heart, lungs and upper airways. Auscultation of loud upper airway sounds over the larynx and cervical trachea suggests upper airway obstruction or disease. Palpation of the pulses at the same time as auscultation of the heart allows detection of an arrhythmia if pulse deficits are present. The presence of an arrhythmia, heart murmur or gallop rhythm can suggest underlying heart disease.

Detection of increased or harsh bronchovesicular lung sounds is a common but non-specific sign in many animals with respiratory distress. The presence of wheezes or crackles is a more specific indication of primary lung abnormalities.

- Wheezes are musical sounds caused by movement of air through narrowed small airways and usually suggest the presence of primary bronchial disease, e.g. feline asthma or chronic bronchitis.
- Soft inspiratory crackles are thought to be caused by air movement through fluid and can be noted in animals with pulmonary oedema, haemorrhage, pneumonia or severe parenchymal disorders.
- Loud crackles are loud discontinuous sounds that are likely caused by equalization of pressure as the airways snap open and closed. These are typically auscultated in animals with severe chronic bronchitis or pulmonary fibrosis.

The location of abnormal sounds can also be important in prioritizing a differential diagnosis list:

- Ventral crackles suggest pneumonia, whilst dorsal abnormalities suggest pulmonary oedema
- Unilaterally or bilaterally dull lung sounds can indicate pleural space disease – dorsal in animals with pneumothorax; ventral in those with pleural effusion.

Initial stabilization of animals with respiratory distress

Ensuring a patent airway

Severe airway obstruction is easily discernible during the initial patient evaluation: animals with complete airway obstruction make repeated, gasping respiratory efforts without air movement. This finding should prompt consideration of rapid induction of intravenous anaesthesia for immediate endotracheal intubation. Endotracheal tubes may need to be smaller than would usually be chosen for the size of the patient because of the obstructive lesion or resultant airway oedema, or a red rubber catheter may be required to pass oxygen beyond the obstruction. If an oral airway cannot be established, emergency tracheostomy may be required (see *BSAVA Manual of Canine and Feline Head, Neck and Thoracic Surgery*).

Oxygen supplementation

Most patients presenting with a respiratory emergency have sufficient airway patency that they do not require immediate intubation. Initial stabilization usually requires oxygen supplementation to optimize P_aO_2 and improve tissue oxygen delivery. Oxygen can be provided in several ways; with all methods of delivery, the gas should be humidified to avoid drying of the airways. Bubbling the oxygen through a canister containing sterile water effectively provides humidification.

Facemask

A facemask is a simple and quick method of oxygen delivery in an emergency. A high flow rate of oxygen is used and the oxygen supply is attached to an appropriately sized mask held directly to the animal's nose and mouth (Figure 1.5). The primary disadvantage of this method is the need to restrain the patient and enclose the face in a mask, which may increase stress in a patient with respiratory compromise. In addition, the fraction of inspired oxygen (F_iO_2) cannot be measured adequately without placement of a tracheal catheter for sampling.

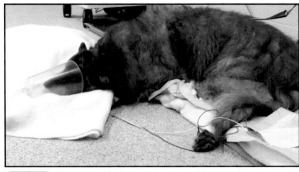

1.5 Delivery of supplementary oxygen via a facemask in an hypoxaemic dog.

Oxygen cages

Although controversial, the authors believe that oxygen cages are an excellent way of providing oxygen therapy in an emergency. Cages allow better control of F_iO_2, temperature and humidity, and permit the patient to rest quietly while protected from stressful handling, which is especially important for cats. However, examination or treatment of the patient requires that the cage door be opened, which results in a quick drop in F_iO_2 that can be dangerous for the patient. In addition, large dogs may overheat in standard oxygen cages. An *ad hoc* oxygen tent can be fashioned by placing cellophane over an Elizabethan collar and pumping in humidified oxygen, leaving a small space at the top to allow for escape of carbon dioxide and expired air.

Nasal oxygen
Nasal oxygen is a good alternative for oxygen supplementation if there is no cage available. It is suitable for patients that are too big for the cage, are able to breathe through the nose and do not have an upper airway obstruction.

- A rubber catheter can be used in one or both nostrils.
- Local anaesthetic is applied to the nose and catheter.
- The catheter is measured from the nares to the medial canthus of the eye and inserted up to that point
- The catheter is then sutured or glued in place.
- Oxygen is insufflated at a rate of 1–5 l/min.

Nasal oxygen prongs (Figure 1.6), as used in humans, are easy and quick to apply in patients that are recumbent and unlikely to move, although the efficacy of this method in veterinary patients has not been examined. Nasal prongs are undesirable in more aware patients, because they can be uncomfortable, are easily displaced and are not well tolerated.

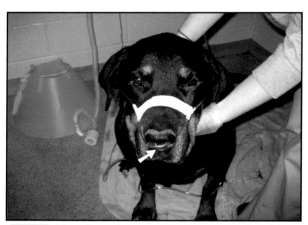

1.6 Use of nasal oxygen prongs (arrowed) to deliver supplementary oxygen to a postoperative patient.

Transtracheal oxygen
In the event that nasal oxygen is not tolerated, the patient is too large for a cage or there is a severe upper airway obstruction, transtracheal oxygen can be utilized. The ventral neck is clipped and aseptically prepared. A through-the-needle catheter is placed percutaneously between the tracheal rings in the same manner as would be used for a transtracheal

wash, and an oxygen supply is attached directly to the catheter. Transtracheal oxygen is most effective in animals that are immobilized because the narrow catheter kinks easily. When using this method, the neck region should be checked frequently for subcutaneous emphysema to ensure that the catheter has not become displaced from the airway.

Minimizing stress
A standard recommendation for any animal with respiratory compromise is to limit stress to the patient. Excessive struggling in a hypoxaemic patient leads to an increased oxygen requirement and worsened haemoglobin desaturation. In addition, restraint for diagnostic procedures, such as venepuncture or radiography, may result in an inability of the patient to assume postural adaptations (such as maintaining a sternal position or minimizing airway resistance by extending the neck and opening the mouth), further promoting haemoglobin desaturation.

Establishing vascular access
Unless the animal is so unstable that it cannot tolerate further manipulation, a peripheral intravenous catheter should be placed, usually into the cephalic vein. Obtaining vascular access is a high priority because it allows intravenous administration of emergency drugs and facilitates immediate induction of anaesthesia for intubation in a crisis if the animal's condition deteriorates. As a general rule, drugs should not be given orally to animals in respiratory distress because restraint for administration can result in worsened respiratory distress. Furthermore, if poor gastric perfusion or ileus is present, drug absorption may be compromised. If vascular access cannot be established, drugs should be administered by intramuscular injection.

Initial blood testing
When an intravenous catheter is placed, blood can be collected from the hub of the catheter to perform initial tests. When possible, an emergency database including PCV, total solids, blood smear, blood urea nitrogen dipstick, blood glucose, electrolytes and venous blood gas should be obtained. This information can give important clues as to the underlying cause of the distress and may help direct immediate therapy. For example, a venous PCO_2 >50 mmHg suggests significant hypoventilation; if this is confirmed by an arterial sample, establishing an airway (tracheostomy, intubation) or even positive pressure ventilation should be considered.

Initial management based on disease location

Once an initial physical examination has been performed, oxygen has been provided and vascular access has been established, the clinician should be able to determine the anatomical localization of the problem within the respiratory tract. At this point, specific efforts can be directed to stabilize the patient (see below) and differential diagnoses can be considered.

Extrathoracic upper airway obstruction

The extrathoracic upper airways consist of the pharynx, larynx and cervical trachea. Obstruction of the upper airways can be caused by multiple conditions (Figure 1.7). Upper airway obstruction is characterized by an obstructive pattern of respiration on inspiration, and is usually accompanied by stridor or stertor. Affected animals are often hyperthermic because of increased heat generation from muscle activity and an inability to thermoregulate by panting.

Diagnosis	Predisposing factors/clinical features
Laryngeal paralysis	Congenital in Siberian Husky, Bouvier de Flandres, Bull Terrier, Dalmatian, German Shepherd Dog, Leonberger, Pyreneen, Rottweiler Acquired: idiopathic, trauma, neuropathies Inspiratory stridor
Brachycephalic airway syndrome	English Bulldog, French Bulldog, Pug, Pekingese, Boston Terrier Features include elongated soft palate, everted laryngeal saccules, stenotic nares, laryngeal collapse, hypoplastic trachea Inspiratory and/or expiratory stertor
Collapsing trachea	Yorkshire Terrier, Maltese, Pomeranian Goose-honk cough
Tracheal foreign body	Hunting dogs are predisposed
Neoplasia	Lymphosarcoma, squamous cell carcinoma, etc.
Inflammatory laryngitis	Cats
Abscesses, pyogranulomas	Bacterial, fungal
Nasopharyngeal polyps	Cats >> dogs

1.7 Differential diagnoses for upper airway obstruction in dogs and cats.

Aggressive efforts should be made to cool the patient, accompanied by sedation and possibly an anti-inflammatory dose of a short-acting corticosteroid. Once the animal is calm, it can be positioned in sternal recumbency, with the head and neck extended, and the mouth opened with the tongue pulled forward (Figure 1.8). All of these efforts assist with minimizing airway resistance and establishing a patent airway. If these efforts are unsuccessful, short-acting intravenous anaesthetic drugs may be needed for intubation, and a temporary tracheostomy may be required.

Lower airway disease

The lower airways are made up of the bronchi, conducting airways and the lobar, segmental and terminal bronchioles. Acute tracheobronchitis can be infectious in origin in both dogs and cats; while it may result in an emergency presentation, these animals do not typically have respiratory difficulty. Most chronic diseases of the lower airways are associated with a long-standing history of coughing, which can be paroxysmal and sometimes quite severe, but does not usually result in severe respiratory distress. The most

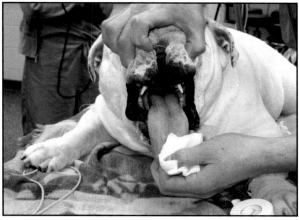

1.8 Dogs and cats with upper respiratory obstruction may benefit from sedation. To optimize oxygenation and minimize resistance to air flow, the head and neck should be stretched out in a horizontal position, with the tongue pulled forward and the mouth propped open.

common lower airway conditions that result in an emergency presentation for respiratory distress are feline asthma (cats) and end-stage chronic bronchitis, with or without airway collapse (dogs) (Figure 1.9). Affected animals usually have an expiratory obstructive respiratory pattern.

Emergency management of animals with suspected or confirmed inflammatory lower airway disease should include administration of oxygen, parenteral administration of a bronchodilator and anti-inflammatory doses of corticosteroids. Antitussive

Diagnosis	Predisposing factors/clinical features
Chronic bronchitis	Dogs and cats Idiopathic inflammatory aetiology Cough, often non-productive, but may be productive
Feline asthma	Cats only, particularly Siamese Coughing and wheezing Episodes of severe, acute respiratory distress due to smooth muscle spasm
Bronchiectasis	Congenital (rare), associated with ciliary dyskinesia Acquired due to inflammation, bronchopneumonia Productive cough Radiographic evidence of dilated, cylindrical bronchi
Neoplasia	Rare
Foreign body	Rare
Parasite	Rare Chronic cough can be a sign of dirofilariasis in cats
Bacteria/virus	*Bordetella bronchiseptica* in dogs *Mycoplasma* in dogs or cats May cause signs of bronchial disease, usually acute, usually do not cause respiratory distress

1.9 Differential diagnoses for lower airway/bronchial disease in dogs and cats.

and/or sedative drugs may also be required. If tolerated by the patient, parenteral drug administration can be supplemented by aerosol administration of inhaled medications.

Parenchymal disease

Common causes of pulmonary parenchymal disease are listed in Figure 1.10. Clinical signs can include: a restrictive pattern of breathing; orthopnoea; cough (dogs); cyanosis; open-mouthed breathing; and a paradoxical respiratory pattern. On auscultation, quiet lungs, crackles or increased bronchovesicular sounds may be appreciated. In the case of pulmonary oedema secondary to heart failure, the clinician may auscult a heart murmur or an arrhythmia. Other physical examination findings depend on the underlying cause but may include mucopurulent nasal discharge, enlarged lymph nodes, haemoptysis or increased rectal temperature.

Emergency management of animals with parenchymal lung disease includes non-specific supportive care, including stress minimization and oxygen supplementation. Ideally, thoracic radiographs should be obtained as soon as possible because identification of the location of pulmonary infiltrates, and confirmation of the size of the heart and pulmonary vessels, significantly aids in the management of these patients. However, in animals with severe respiratory distress (especially cats) it may not be possible to obtain radiographs immediately. In these cases, drug therapy directed at the most likely aetiology of respiratory distress is initiated immediately in an effort to stabilize the patient. For example, a cat with probable pulmonary oedema would be treated with furosemide, whilst a cat with suspected asthma would be administered a bronchodilator and possibly corticosteroids. Depending on the history and signalment, a dog might receive furosemide for possible pulmonary oedema,

Diagnosis	Predisposing factors/clinical features
Pneumonia	Bacterial, viral, fungal, parasitic, aspiration, foreign body Diagnosis based on clinical history and radiographs, cytology and culture, sometimes serology Treatment includes antimicrobials, nebulization, coupage, mucolytics ± bronchodilators
Cardiogenic pulmonary oedema	Congestive heart failure Physical examination evidence of heart disease: murmur, arrhythmia Radiographic evidence of cardiomegaly, distended pulmonary veins, perihilar alveolar infiltrates Treatment includes diuretics, vasodilators, antiarrhythmics, positive inotropes
Non-cardiogenic pulmonary oedema	Causes include electrocution, seizure, near drowning, head trauma, strangulation or upper airway obstruction Oedema is caused by vascular leak, therefore heart sounds normal (Drobatz *et al.*, 1995) Radiographs reveal normal heart, caudodorsal alveolar disease Supportive care, oxygen, low-dose furosemide
Acute lung injury (ALI) and Acute Respiratory Distress Syndrome (ARDS)	Systemic or focal pulmonary inflammation leads to non-cardiogenic pulmonary oedema because of vascular leak ALI is the mild form, ARDS is the severe form Heart is normal on auscultation, crackles usually evident Radiographs reveal normal heart and diffuse alveolar pulmonary infiltrates (usually bilateral) Treatment involves supportive care, elimination of underlying cause, positive pressure ventilation if severe
Pulmonary thromboembolism	Sequel of hypercoagulability associated with immune-mediated haemolytic anaemia, hyperadrenocorticism, corticosteroid use, systemic inflammatory response syndrome (SIRS)/disseminated intravascular coagulation (DIC), protein-losing nephropathy, cardiac disease, etc. Radiographs may be normal, may have dilated or truncated arteries, may have variable alveolar infiltrates or pleural effusion Treatment is supportive, elimination of underlying cause if possible, anticoagulants or thrombolytic drugs
Pulmonary haemorrhage or contusions	History of coagulopathy or trauma Auscultation may reveal dull sounds or crackles Radiographs may show patchy alveolar infiltrates, ribs should be checked for fractures Supportive care, oxygen
Neoplasia	Primary pulmonary or metastatic Auscultation findings variable Radiographs may show mass(es) or diffuse/patchy infiltrates Therapy depends on type, may include surgery or chemotherapy
Inflammatory and immune lung diseases	Pulmonary fibrosis, interstitial pneumonia, pulmonary infiltrate with eosinophils, etc. Non-specific clinical findings, signalment may help (e.g. idiopathic pulmonary fibrosis in West Highland White Terriers) Diagnosis based on imaging findings, cytology, histology Treatment may include corticosteroids, various anti-inflammatory drugs
Atelectasis	Common cause of hypoxaemia, often occurring in association with other lung diseases Diagnosis based on clinical findings, radiographs show displacement of the cardiac silhouette towards affected hemithorax Easily resolved by re-positioning, movement, encouraging increased tidal volume

1.10 Differential diagnoses for pulmonary parenchymal disease in dogs and cats.

antibiotics for pneumonia, or plasma with vitamin K for possible anticoagulant exposure. When the animal is sufficiently stabilized, radiography and additional testing can be performed to establish a diagnosis. If the animal does not become more stable, anaesthesia, intubation and positive pressure ventilation may be required to alleviate respiratory distress and facilitate diagnostic testing.

Pleural space disease

The pleural space is lined by two pleural membranes: the parietal pleura lining the thoracic wall; and the visceral pleura, which covers the lungs. The parietal pleura contains multiple lymphatic vessels that drain the pleural cavity. Normally, a small amount of fluid is present in the pleural space. If a large volume of fluid, air or soft tissue accumulates in the pleural space (Figure 1.11), elastic recoil causes the lungs to collapse. Clinical signs of pleural space disease include a restrictive breathing pattern, respiratory distress and open-mouthed breathing. On auscultation, lung and heart sounds are often dull: ventrally in the case of fluid accumulation, and dorsally with accumulation of air.

Diagnosis	Predisposing factors/clinical features
Modified transudate	Congestive heart failure, neoplasia, pancreatitis, pulmonary thromboembolism
Pure transudate	Hypoproteinaemia
Haemorrhage	Trauma, coagulopathy, neoplasia
Haemorrhagic effusion	Lung lobe torsion, neoplasia
Chylothorax	Ruptured thoracic duct, neoplasia, congestive heart failure, lung lobe torsion
Pyothorax	Bacterial or fungal infection, foreign body
Pneumothorax	Traumatic Spontaneous due to bullae, other pulmonary lesions such as neoplasia
Diaphragmatic hernia	Traumatic, acute or chronic
Neoplasia	Mediastinal, thoracic wall, pulmonary

1.11 Differential diagnoses for pleural space disease in dogs and cats.

Initial therapy should include oxygen supplementation and thoracocentesis (see below), which is performed before any other diagnostic tests unless the risk for a coagulopathy is high. Once the patient is more stable following thoracocentesis, further diagnostic tests such as radiography or echocardiography can be attempted. Worsened respiratory distress following thoracocentesis suggests development of an iatrogenic pneumothorax or re-expansion pulmonary oedema, which is a rare sequel of evacuation of the pleural cavity. Lungs that have been chronically compressed have reduced blood flow because of pulmonary hypoxaemic vasoconstriction. When the lungs re-expand, the return of both blood flow and oxygen results in ischaemia–reperfusion injury and non-cardiogenic pulmonary oedema (Neustein, 2007).

Chest wall and diaphragmatic disease

The chest wall may not function normally because of trauma, such as rib fractures or penetrating chest wounds. Alternatively, interruption of the innervation of the intercostal muscles or diaphragm may result in an inability to ventilate. Disorders that result in ventilatory failure include spinal cord injury in the C1–C6 region, hypokalaemia and neuromuscular disorders such as myasthenia gravis, botulism or polyradiculoneuritis. Clinical signs can include decreased movement of the chest wall, lack of movement of the abdomen or diaphragm, and respiratory distress. Initial management of severely affected animals should include intubation and positive pressure ventilation.

Initial diagnostic tests

After the animal has been assessed and initially stabilized, diagnostic tests can be carefully considered. Emergency diagnostic testing should be limited to those tests that can be performed safely without exacerbating respiratory distress. Low doses of sedatives may help calm the animal so that tests can be performed, but the clinician should be ready to intubate any patient that decompensates following sedation. If the animal cannot tolerate manipulation whilst breathing spontaneously, it may be safer to anaesthetize the patient and complete tests whilst a high concentration of oxygen can be administered through a controlled airway. The client should be warned that intubated patients with respiratory disease may require ongoing positive pressure ventilation if the underlying problem cannot be treated quickly.

Thoracocentesis

Thoracocentesis should be quickly performed in an animal with a restrictive breathing pattern that has dull lung sounds and dampened heart sounds.

- A small-gauge needle is inserted between ribs 7 and 9, in either the ventral third (in the case of fluid) or the dorsal third (in the case of air) of the thoracic wall (Figure 1.12).
- The needle should enter the chest off the cranial aspect of the rib to avoid the vessels and nerves that run along the caudal aspect of the ribs.
- Fluid should be submitted for cytology and culture (aerobic and anaerobic).

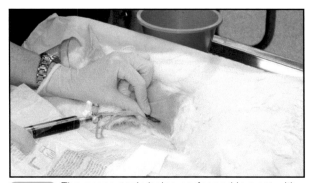

1.12 Thoracocentesis being performed in a cat with pleural effusion.

If the pleural space refills rapidly, if multiple thoracocentesis attempts are required, or if negative pressure cannot be achieved during the initial thoracocentesis, a thoracostomy tube should be placed to allow easy access for repeated or continuous evacuation of the pleural space.

Imaging

Radiographs of the thorax (see Chapter 6) are required for any animal presented for evaluation of respiratory difficulty, but **should not be obtained at the expense of an unstable animal's safety**. Often, radiography is delayed whilst initial treatment is administered to stabilize the animal. If radiographs are deemed vital for the management of an unstable patient, the number of views obtained should be minimized. The first view should be obtained with the animal in sternal recumbency.

> **WARNING**
> **Avoid placing the animal in dorsal recumbency. In severe cases, lateral recumbency can also result in worsened respiratory distress.**

Oxygen should be provided and the procedure should be accomplished as rapidly as possible. Radiographs of the neck should be included in animals with upper airway obstruction.

Other imaging techniques occasionally needed in animals with respiratory distress include fluoroscopy in cases of suspected tracheal collapse or ultrasonography for those with pleural or cardiac disease. When stable for anaesthesia, computed tomography (CT), endoscopy or surgery may be required in animals with interstitial lung disease or suspected neoplasia.

Cardiac diagnostic tests

Animals suspected to have CHF may require electrocardiography and an echocardiogram (see Chapters 9 and 11). These tests allow the clinician to rule out heart disease as a cause of respiratory distress.

Respiratory diagnostic tests

Laryngoscopy, tracheoscopy and bronchoscopy (see Chapter 10) are often required to define the underlying aetiology of respiratory distress. Great care should be taken during anaesthesia to support oxygenation and ventilation because the endoscope provides additional obstruction of air flow. Samples should be obtained from the airways for cytology and appropriate cultures.

References and further reading

Drobatz KJ, Saunders M, Pugh CR and Hendricks J (1995) Non-cardiogenic pulmonary edema in dogs and cats: 26 cases (1987–1993). *Journal of the American Veterinary Medical Association* **206**, 1732–1736

Lee J and Drobatz K (2004) Respiratory distress and cyanosis in dogs. In: *Textbook of Respiratory Disease in Dogs and Cats*, ed. LG King, pp. 1–11. WB Saunders, St Louis

Marino PL (1998) Hypoxemia and hypercapnea. In: *The ICU Book, 2nd edn*, ed. PL Marino, pp. 339–354. Lippincott Williams and Wilkins, Philadelphia

Neustein SM (2007) Re-expansion pulmonary edema. *Journal of Cardiothoracic and Vascular Anesthesia* **21(6)**, 887–891

Petrie JP (2005) Cyanosis. In: *Textbook of Veterinary Internal Medicine 6th edn*, ed. SJ Ettinger and EC Feldman, pp. 219–222. Elsevier, St Louis

Waddell LS and King LG (2007) General approach to dyspnoea. In: *BSAVA Manual of Canine and Feline Emergency and Critical Care, 2nd edn*, ed. LG King and A Boag, pp. 85–113. BSAVA Publications, Gloucester

West JB (2005) *Respiratory Physiology: the Essentials, 7th edn*. Lippincott Williams and Wilkins, Baltimore

2

Clinical approach to coughing

Brendan M. Corcoran

Introduction

Coughing is a normal function that serves to expel secretions from the airways, prevent inhalation of material into the airways and delay entry of material deeper into the lungs. It is therefore an extremely important mechanism in the protection of the respiratory system. This raises the issue of control of coughing in disease situations, where the benefits of coughing might outweigh the benefits of suppressing the cough. In fact, in some situations, such as chronic bronchitis, stimulating coughing by chest coupage is believed to be therapeutically beneficial.

Mechanism

Coughing relies mainly on the mucociliary escalator to move airway secretions rostrally to contact cough receptors concentrated at airway bifurcations. This stimulates the cough reflex and the material is expectorated. The reflex instigates a deep inspiration and then a forceful expiration against a closed glottis, resulting in high airway pressure. The glottis is opened suddenly and the marked pressure difference between the airways and the oral cavity forces material out. In the majority of cases, expectorated material is immediately swallowed. In some cases, there is retching at the end of a paroxysm of coughing and the patient may expectorate white frothy material. Cough receptors are concentrated in the larger airways and at the point where the airways divide, and coughing is relatively ineffectual in diseases affecting the distal airways and the alveoli. In such cases, rostral movement of material will eventually elicit the cough reflex but local clearance mechanisms, such as lymphatic drainage and macrophage activity, provide the major contribution for removing inflammatory material.

The cough reflex is fundamentally autonomic in nature but is also under a degree of conscious control; therefore, it may be possible that some dogs cough as they have 'learnt' that coughing attracts attention (conditioned behaviour). A further important consideration is determining whether the patient is genuinely coughing and that the owner is not reporting gagging, choking or retching. Being able to elicit coughing in the consulting room, typically by compressing the trachea at the thoracic inlet, and asking the owner to confirm that this is what they have heard can be useful.

Causes

Coughing is caused by activation of the cough receptors due to:

- Airway inflammation
- Airway secretions
- Airway compression.

Some diseases elicit coughing using just one of these methods, whilst others may use two or three.

Airway inflammation
Diseases causing airway inflammation include acute tracheobronchitis, parasitic tracheobronchitis and chronic bronchitis. In the case of chronic bronchitis, excess airway secretions are implicated in coughing, and in more advanced forms of the disease (where there may be secondary lung changes or airway collapse) airway wall compression might also contribute to coughing.

Airway secretions
Bacterial bronchopneumonia is a good example of a disease where airway secretions are likely to be the sole reason for coughing. Coughing in pneumonia cases is due to secretions travelling up the larger airways to activate the cough receptors. Coughing in bronchopneumonia cases is often soft and ineffectual, reflecting the low number of cough receptors in the distal airways.

Airway compression
For a primary lung tumour to cause coughing, it must be of sufficient mass to compress a large airway at end-expiration (Figure 2.1), which suggests that the presence of coughing is indicative of relatively long-standing disease.

Collapse of the airways as a cause of coughing can be associated with tracheal collapse or idiopathic pulmonary fibrosis (IPF). In IPF, increased lung elasticity results in expiratory airway collapse and in addition to coughing, pronounced expiratory effort may be noted. In tracheal collapse, the cough is often described as a 'goose-honking' sound and is associated with expiratory collapse of the intrathoracic trachea or

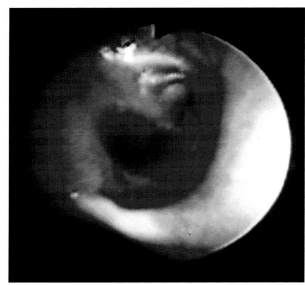

2.1 Dynamic collapse of the left mainstem bronchus at end-expiration by an extraluminal mass (primary lung tumour).

mainstem bronchi. Cervical tracheal collapse is more likely to result in inspiratory difficulty. If a dog with tracheal collapse has only expiratory flow limitation, this may generate an expiratory honking sound or grunt, but technically speaking it is not coughing. Tracheal collapse is seen in small breeds of dog and reflects an inherent compressibility of the airways in such dogs, something not seen in larger breeds of dog.

One of the best examples of airway collapse causing coughing is that seen with compression of the left mainstem bronchus by an enlarged left atrium (LA) in the dog (Figure 2.2). This is seen in dogs with cardiac disease, with or without left-sided congestive heart failure (CHF), and it is more likely to occur in smaller breeds of dog where the mainstem bronchi are more easily compressed. Larger breeds of dog with CHF might not cough, even though they may have significant pulmonary oedema. The role of

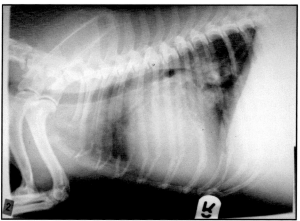

2.2 Lateral thoracic radiograph of a dog with CHF due to myxomatous mitral valve disease. Note the marked cardiomegaly, displacement of the caudal trachea, carina and mainstem bronchi by the enlarged LA, and the partial compression of the left mainstem bronchus. This is a major contributing cause to the dog's coughing.

cardiogenic and non-cardiogenic pulmonary oedema (bronchial and alveolar) in eliciting coughing is not clear cut. Cats with severe pulmonary oedema typically have severe tachypnoea and respiratory distress, but do not cough; and in the dog, it is left mainstem bronchus compression that is probably the main cause of coughing. When oedema alone causes coughing, it is likely due to the presence of fluid in the larger communicating airways activating the cough receptors.

Differentiation between cardiac and respiratory origin

Certain useful clinical features, such as the presence of a murmur or arrhythmia, increase the likelihood that coughing in a dog is cardiac in origin. The nature of the cough is proposed by some to be of benefit in differentiating cardiac from respiratory disease, but such interpretation should be made with caution. In many cases with coughing due to cardiac or respiratory disease, the cough is exacerbated by exercise, excitement, lead pulling or when the dog moves position, so accurate differentiation using these features alone is not possible. The breed and size of the dog can be a useful discriminator because smaller dogs are more likely to cough with heart disease than larger breeds, and small dogs are also more likely to have tracheal collapse.

A respiratory cause of coughing in a dog showing evidence of cardiac disease should be considered in the appropriate circumstances, such as when the dog has been recently kennelled and may have encountered bordetellosis, or if the dog has a history of vomiting or regurgitation, raising the suspicion for inhalation pneumonia. The presence of sinus arrhythmia would suggest that the cough is respiratory and not cardiac in origin. Alternately, if there is an arrhythmia, particularly sinus tachycardia or atrial fibrillation, the cough should be considered of cardiac origin until proven otherwise. The presence of a loud left apical heart murmur (indicating mitral valve disease) should also raise suspicion that the cough is cardiac in origin, although if the dog has a sinus arrhythmia, the murmur is more likely to represent compensated endocardiosis and the cough is probably respiratory in origin. When an arrhythmia, murmur and other signs of left-sided CHF are present, the cough is most likely to be cardiac and appropriate therapy for CHF should be considered. If the cough subsides, this would support a cardiac cause. Persistence of the cough does not exclude a cardiac cause; however, it indicates that concurrent respiratory disease should be considered.

Thoracic radiography (see Chapter 6) is of immense value in determining whether a cough is of cardiac origin. Right lateral recumbent and dorsoventral (DV) views should be inspected for evidence of left ventricular and left atrial enlargement. This includes measuring the vertebral heart score (VHS) for evidence of cardiomegaly, identifying straightening of the caudal border of the heart, loss of the caudal waist, elevation of the distal portion of the trachea and the mainstem bronchi, splitting and/or compression of the mainstem bronchi, elevation of the caudal vena cava (on the right lateral recumbent view), and visualizing an auricular bulge at the 2–3 o'clock position and displacement of the left mainstem bronchus (on the DV view). Confirmation of left atrial enlargement and auricular bulging can be made on two-dimensional (2D) echocardiography using the right side short-axis view (see Chapter 11). This involves comparing the size of the LA to the aorta at the time of closure of the aortic valve leaflets (typically <1.7) and visualizing the blood-filled auricular appendage.

Occasionally, 2D echocardiograms suggest left atrial enlargement when this is not clearly apparent on thoracic radiographs. If there is enough evidence to suggest CHF (particularly visibly distended pulmonary veins on radiography), then treatment is warranted and any improvement in coughing can be presumed evidence that the cough was cardiac in origin. However, if there is radiographic evidence of significant respiratory disease, this has to be considered a likely cause of the coughing. In cats, the presence of a heart murmur and coughing suggests concurrent cardiac and respiratory disease, with bronchial disease being a common explanation for the coughing.

Differential diagnoses for respiratory causes

The differential diagnoses for respiratory causes of coughing require consideration of the signalment, history, physical findings and the results of diagnostic tests.

Signalment and history

Breed and age, but not gender, can be useful in the diagnosis of respiratory disease. Breed is particularly useful in recognizing diseases causing respiratory difficulty, such as anatomical deformities seen with brachycephalic airway syndrome. Such deformities might make these dogs more predisposed to developing bronchopneumonia or aspiration pneumonia, which can be associated with coughing. These problems tend to arise in young animals rather than adults, and may be implicated in puppy mortality.

Tracheal collapse is commonly seen in smaller and toy breed dogs and is a particular problem in the Yorkshire Terrier and Pomeranian. Chronic bronchitis appears to be more prevalent in terrier breeds, but can affect any breed, whilst IPF is more commonly seen in the West Highland White Terrier and other related terrier breeds such as the Cairn and Border Terrier. Laryngeal paralysis, which secondarily can result in airway and lung disease because of chronic aspiration injury, is common in the ageing Labrador Retriever and other large breeds of dog. Large-breed dogs may have a greater predilection for bacterial or aspiration bronchopneumonia, in part due to a higher incidence of swallowing disorders, laryngeal paralysis and megaoesophagus, and possible inherited immunodeficiency states (Irish Wolfhound). There may be geographical variations in breed association for several respiratory diseases; the examples cited here are the author's own experience in the UK.

Some diseases, such as acquired idiopathic laryngeal paralysis, IPF and pulmonary neoplasia, are exclusively diseases of middle- to old-aged dogs. A diagnosis of these diseases in young dogs, apart from the rare form of congenital laryngeal paralysis, is probably an error. Chronic bronchitis is more likely to be seen in adult dogs, and young animals are expected to be more susceptible, although not exclusively so, to acute tracheobronchitis. Parasitic tracheobronchitis (*Oslerus osleri*) is a disease of young adults, but *Crenosoma vulpis* infection is unlikely to have an age predilection.

Physical examination

Physical examination of the coughing dog is directed in the first instance at deciding whether the cough is likely to be cardiac or respiratory in origin. This is important as it will determine the appropriate selection of diagnostic tests in order to achieve a definitive diagnosis. For the respiratory patient, the presence or absence of tachypnoea and/or respiratory distress, cyanosis and pyrexia are important in determining the severity of disease. Patients have not died from coughing, but increased respiratory effort or obvious difficulty breathing is a worrying finding. Pyrexia in conjunction with coughing and tachypnoea is very suspicious for severe acute bacterial bronchopneumonia, and with supporting radiographic findings can be sufficient to make a presumptive diagnosis. The presence of cachexia is a worrying sign and is often found with advanced pulmonary neoplasia or chronic bronchitis of long standing. The presence of obesity can contribute to the respiratory signs seen with many disorders, but in itself is not diagnostic of any particular disease.

Thoracic auscultation will identify the presence of abnormal respiratory sounds; however, respiratory sounds are normal in many coughing cases. A diffuse increase in respiratory sounds tends to reflect the severity of disease and not the actual diagnosis, but there are exceptions. Wheezing heard in cats is highly suggestive of bronchial disease, and the wheezing may be subtle, localized and intermittent. Inspiratory crackles are associated with pulmonary oedema, chronic bronchitis and IPF. Regional differences in respiratory sounds can be helpful in identifying the location of disease and are most likely to be found with lobar pneumonia and neoplasia, which generate focal pulmonary infiltrates and thus focal alterations in lung sounds. Obvious end-expiratory effort is suggestive of air-trapping or fixed/dynamic obstruction of airflow during expiration. Good examples of conditions with this finding are intrathoracic tracheal collapse, feline bronchial disease, IPF and neoplasia.

Using a combination of signalment, history and physical findings, a reasonable tentative diagnosis may be made, which can then be confirmed through radiography and ancillary diagnostic tests. Definitive diagnosis of some diseases requires pathological confirmation, but as this is rarely obtained *ante mortem*, the best possible diagnosis is achieved using a combination of haematology, radiography, bronchoscopy, airway and transthoracic sampling. The latter technique most closely approximates pathological confirmation, but is usually only effective in pulmonary neoplasia cases. Thus, radiography is still the most important diagnostic tool in the evaluation of the respiratory patient.

Radiography

Thoracic radiography is crucial for the diagnosis of coughing associated with respiratory disease, although its sensitivity is somewhat limited. The importance of thoracic radiography in identifying a cardiac cause of coughing cannot be overstated, and coughing cases should not undergo further investigative tests without first having had radiographs taken. The utility of radiography in respiratory disease is very dependent on radiographic quality. This is covered in detail in Chapter 6, but it is important to state that subtle pattern changes will be missed or over-interpreted with poor quality radiographs, thereby compromising diagnostic accuracy. Radiography will be more convincing if the changes seen are obvious and extensive. However, radiographic changes that are mild or equivocal can also aid diagnosis through a process of exclusion. For example, a geriatric dog with a history of chronic coughing that has normal thoracic radiographs should not have pulmonary neoplasia as a differential diagnosis.

Tracheal collapse can sometimes be identified on radiography; inclusion of the neck on the lateral view is needed. However, there can be many false-negative and false-positive findings, particularly with the widespread adoption of sedation during radiographic procedures in the UK (the stress of restraint often elicits visible tracheal collapse). A subtle disparity in tracheal lumen size when comparing intra- and extrathoracic portions of the trachea can be suggestive of tracheal collapse, and detection may be augmented by obtaining inspiratory and expiratory lateral views. However, confirmation of tracheal collapse requires fluoroscopy or bronchoscopy.

An alveolar pattern, consisting of fluffy coalescent densities with air bronchograms, is suggestive of bronchopneumonia and typically has a cranioventral distribution. Often the presence of air bronchograms can be difficult to appreciate and may be best seen close to the ventral edge of the lung on the lateral view. Increased bronchial markings have to be interpreted with caution. Some increase in bronchial or interstitial markings can be expected in normal dogs as an ageing change or may represent previous disease that has resolved. Abnormal bronchial markings can be identified as 'doughnut'-shaped rings and are readily seen in the dorsocaudal lung field. With lateral views, bronchial walls tend to have a blurred outline, which contrasts with the sharply delineated walls of normal calcified airways and the larger central airways. Bronchial wall thickening can also be appreciated as 'tramlines' on ventrodorsal (VD)/DV views. While bronchial markings would logically equate with bronchial disease, this is not necessarily the case, and confirmation of significant bronchial disease requires bronchoscopy with lavage for cytological and microbiological assessment. Bronchial markings associated with feline bronchial disease can appear nodular or interstitial, and only with close inspection (preferably with a magnifying glass) can it be appreciated these 'nodules' are in fact airways.

An interstitial pattern may be present and associated with diseases causing coughing. The diseases that show the most obvious interstitial pattern are pulmonary infiltration with eosinophilia and IPF, with severe changes often noted with the latter. An interstitial pattern can be linear, reticular or nodular and it obscures the normal vascular pattern of the lung. The absence of an alveolar pattern or of increased bronchial markings supports the conclusion that the pattern is interstitial, but the presence of a mixed pattern can also be found. Poor radiographic technique can markedly affect the appearance of interstitial patterns, and it is generally accepted that this is the hardest pattern to identify with confidence. Lastly, well defined soft tissue densities may be seen and typically these are associated with pulmonary neoplasia. For primary neoplasia, the density can be localized to a single lobe and coughing will be due to compression of bronchi at that site. For secondary pulmonary neoplasia, the changes more typically spread throughout the lung.

As with any diagnostic test, the interpretation of radiographic findings should be taken in the context of all the other evidence of disease; the temptation to over-interpret radiographic findings to fit the presumed diagnosis should be avoided. The absence of cardinal changes on radiography can be used to exclude likely differential diagnoses, but the failure to identify any radiographic abnormality does not exclude respiratory disease as the cause of coughing. (See also Chapters 6 and 10.)

References and further reading

Foster D (1998) Diagnosis and management of chronic coughing in cats. *In Practice* **20,** 261–267
McCarthy G (1999) Investigation of lower respiratory tract disease in the dog. *In Practice* **21,** 521–527

3

Clinical approach to syncope

Marc S. Kraus

Introduction

Syncope is a sudden loss of consciousness associated with loss of postural tone (collapse) from which recovery is spontaneous. The evaluation of syncope in animals is often challenging. Difficulties arise from the very nature of syncope: episodes are usually unpredictably sporadic, sometimes infrequent, and intersyncopal periods are often unremarkable. The common denominator leading to all forms of syncope is decreased or brief cessation of cerebral blood flow.

Pre-syncope is a term used to describe episodic hindlimb or generalized weakness, ataxia, or altered (but not complete loss of) consciousness. Compared with syncope, pre-syncope is associated with a less severe or more transient insult that leads to less severe cerebral hypoxia.

Severe heart rhythm disturbances are probably the most common cause of syncope in dogs and cats.

Is it syncope?

Distinguishing syncope from seizure can be difficult. Clues for differential diagnosis include situational triggers, prodromal signs, behaviour during the episode, and the events that follow (Figure 3.1).

- Collapse episodes that are precipitated by exercise, stress, cough, gag, emesis, micturition, defecation and pain are most likely syncope rather than seizure.

- Disorientation after the event with slow recovery of normal consciousness is common with seizure; but protracted cerebral hypoxia resulting from cardiac arrhythmia may also be followed by relatively slow recovery.
- Differentiating seizure from syncope can be confounded by the possibility of *hypoxaemic convulsive syncope*, where prolonged cerebral hypoperfusion results from profound cardiac arrhythmia.
- Syncope or pre-syncope without prodromal signs, without violent tonic–clonic activity, and with quick recovery suggests a heart rhythm disturbance.
- Although usually associated with flaccid collapse, syncope due to arrhythmia can be associated with extensor rigidity and spontaneous urination or defecation.
- Hypersalivation is rarely associated with syncope due to heart rhythm disturbances.
- Other causes of transient loss of consciousness include syncope-like episodes caused by hypoxaemia or hypoglycaemia.

Neurally mediated syncope

Neurally mediated syncope is the development of arterial vasodilatation in the setting of relative or absolute bradycardia. Numerous terms have been used to identify neurally mediated syncope, including neurocardiogenic syncope, vasodepressor syncope, vasovagal syncope, situational syncope and reflex syncope. Typically, bradycardia is

Clinical features	Syncope	Seizure	Neuromuscular [a]
Mentation before episode	Normal	May be abnormal	Normal
Gait between episodes	Normal	Normal	Often abnormal
Alteration of consciousness	Yes	Frequently yes [b]	No
Precipitating events (e.g. excitement, stress, cough, gag)	Yes	Usually none	Variable depending on specific disease
Duration of episode	Brief but can be longer	Seconds to minutes	Varies
Abnormal mentation after the event	Uncommon	Frequent	No
Urination/defecation during the event	Uncommon	Frequent	No

3.1 Differential diagnosis for syncope. [a] Neurological causes of collapse include polymyositis, polyneuropathy, myasthenia gravis, narcolepsy, botulism, tick paralysis, hepatic encephalopathy, paraneoplastic syndromes and central nervous system lesions. [b] Some seizures (e.g. simple focal/partial seizures) are not associated with alteration of consciousness.

expected, but vasodepressor syncope (i.e. carotid sinus hypersensitivity) is defined as a pure vaso-depressor reaction.

These mediated syndromes are the result of an incompletely understood autonomic reflex mechanism. Some theories have been proposed:

- Baroreflex dysfunction:
  - Inability to sense or compensate for changes in gravitational forces
  - Paradoxical activation of the baroreceptors.
- Neurohormonal imbalances (e.g. adrenaline (epinephrine), serotonin, renin, vasopressin, nitric oxide)
- Cerebral blood flow imbalances (impaired cerebral autoregulation).

Sympathetic stimulation normally leads to vaso-constriction, increased heart rate and increased cardiac contractility. In susceptible humans, increased ventricular contractility stimulates afferent vagal traffic from the ventricular mechanoreceptors to the brainstem. This is particularly likely with volume underloading of the left ventricle (LV) in the presence of dehydration or venodilatation, and is usually precipitated by orthostasis ('empty ventricle syndrome'). The next step in the reflex is sympathetic withdrawal, which results in vasodilatation and sometimes an increase in vagal efferent traffic resulting in bradycardia.

In dogs, neurocardiogenic bradycardia is usually precipitated by fight, flight, fright or startle situations. Furthermore, it is not evident that ventricular under-filling is a predisposing factor. In fact, in the most common scenario (the elderly small dog with advanced mitral valve disease) the patient is generally volume expanded. Nonetheless, the hyper-dynamic LV of the patient with advanced mitral regurgitation may, under the influence of a sympathetic surge, simulate 'empty ventricle syndrome' because of a further increase in contractility and massive regurgitation. Also, vagal afferent receptors at the left atrium/pulmonary vein junction may trigger the reflex when suddenly stretched further by a sympathetically mediated increase in right ventricular output.

The common denominator of all neurally mediated syncope is vagal input to the cardiovascular centre of the brainstem with subsequent sympathetic withdrawal, often accompanied by vagal outflow.

In the clinical setting, the most easily recognized sign in dogs is bradycardia. However, the author has observed 'apparent' neurally mediated syncope in the absence of bradycardia. Lethargy persists in some patients after bradycardia has resolved and these patients may be hypotensive from vasodilatation. Other cardiac conditions that may be associated with neurally mediated syncope include other causes of pulmonary hypertension and left ventricular outflow tract (LVOT) obstruction.

The 'broad' diagnosis of neurally mediated syncope is usually presumptive and based upon the triggering situation, underlying disorder, signalment and absence of identifiable other cause.

Situational syncope

A specific variant of neurally mediated syncope is *situational syncope*, which is named after the specific situation that is associated with the syncopal episode. Both neurally mediated and situational syncope are also referred to under the term 'reflex-mediated syncope'. Coughing, emesis, micturition, defecation and exertion are all possible triggers for situational syncope. In dogs, very often the precipitating situations are exertion with excitement, abrupt change from inactivity to sudden 'normal' activity, being startled, climbing stairs, physical restraint, bathing, grooming, or barking/jumping with excitement. An electrocardiogram (ECG) or auscultation is required for documentation of bradycardia. A 24–48-hour ambulatory ECG (Holter) and even a 5–7-day event recording are somewhat insensitive since the episodes are often infrequent.

Causes of syncope

Many disorders can result in transient loss of consciousness (Figure 3.2), including seizures and syncope-like episodes caused by respiratory disease or metabolic abnormalities.

Cardiac

The most common cause of syncope is disturbance of the heart rhythm (arrhythmias). Advanced atrioventricular (AV) block is one of the most common causes of bradycardia and syncope, though sick sinus syndrome is the most common cause in middle-aged and older West Highland White Terriers, Miniature Schnauzers and American Cocker Spaniels. Situational bradycardia and syncope can occur in small-breed dogs of all ages, but are more frequently seen in older patients. Paroxysmal tachyarrhythmias can also cause syncope, in particular ventricular tachycardia, which may be suspected in certain breeds prone to cardiomyopathy (Boxers and Dobermanns) (Figure 3.3).

Mechanical/structural cardiac disease is another important cause of syncope, with obstruction to filling, outflow and myocardial failure potential mechanisms for decreased cardiac output. Pericardial effusion, resulting in cardiac tamponade, may also cause poor cardiac output via decreased filling.

Neurally mediated

Dogs with advanced mitral valve disease

So-called neurocardiogenic bradycardia is a variant of the neurally mediated syncope that often occurs in elderly small-breed dogs with advanced mitral regurgitation and, commonly, pulmonary hypertension. Respiratory arrest, pale mucous membranes or cyanosis can be observed during severe and protracted bradycardia. Most episodes persist for only seconds to minutes, but bradycardia can persist for as long as 30 minutes in patients with pulmonary oedema. As with all reflex-mediated syncope in elderly small-breed dogs, neurocardiogenic bradycardia is seldom fatal in isolation. However, it is a warning of advanced disease and often of pulmonary hypertension.

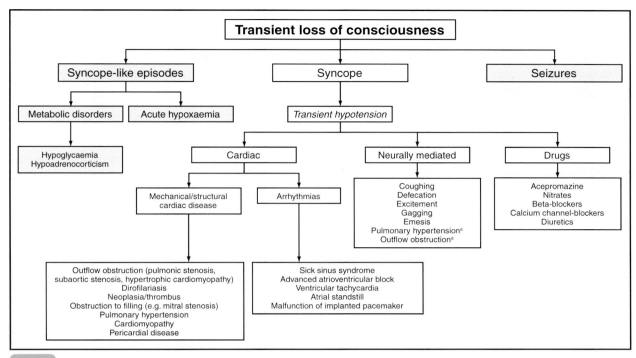

Transient loss of consciousness

- Syncope-like episodes
  - Metabolic disorders
    - Hypoglycaemia
    - Hypoadrenocorticism
  - Acute hypoxaemia
- Syncope
  - *Transient hypotension*
    - Cardiac
      - Mechanical/structural cardiac disease
        - Outflow obstruction (pulmonic stenosis, subaortic stenosis, hypertrophic cardiomyopathy)
        - Dirofilariasis
        - Neoplasia/thrombus
        - Obstruction to filling (e.g. mitral stenosis)
        - Pulmonary hypertension
        - Cardiomyopathy
        - Pericardial disease
      - Arrhythmias
        - Sick sinus syndrome
        - Advanced atrioventricular block
        - Ventricular tachycardia
        - Atrial standstill
        - Malfunction of implanted pacemaker
    - Neurally mediated
      - Coughing
      - Defecation
      - Excitement
      - Gagging
      - Emesis
      - Pulmonary hypertension[a]
      - Outflow obstruction[a]
    - Drugs
      - Acepromazine
      - Nitrates
      - Beta-blockers
      - Calcium channel-blockers
      - Diuretics
- Seizures

3.2 Causes of transient loss of consciousness. [a] Conditions with multiple possible mechanisms.

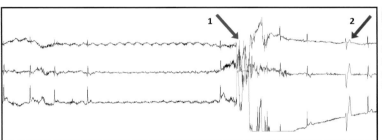

3.3 ECG from a Holter recording of a Boxer with abrupt onset of bradycardia followed by a period of sinoatrial arrest for approximately 6 seconds followed by a ventricular escape beat (arrow 2). There is an artefact after the long pause as the patient fell over due to syncope (arrow 1).

Dogs without structural cardiac disease

Neurocardiogenic bradycardia can also occur in otherwise healthy dogs, particularly in Boxers, Golden Retrievers and working dogs, and with strenuous activity. In Boxers, in the author's experience, neurocardiogenic bradycardia seems to have a bimodal age of first occurrence: 6–24 months and 7–10 years. It is usually triggered by either exertion coupled with excitement or startle, and can occur without evidence of cardiomyopathy (absence of ventricular arrhythmias, cardiac enlargement and decreased contractility). However, since both conditions are common, both can occur in the same dog, usually the older patient.

Holter or event recording is necessary in these patients to help differentiate these conditions. Holter recordings in Boxers and Dobermanns performed within 48 hours following syncope due to ventricular tachycardia usually reveal thousands of ventricular premature beats with couplets, triplets and non-sustained ventricular tachycardia. There is also a subset of Dobermanns and Boxers that collapse from bradyarrhythmias (Calvert *et al.*, 1996; Thomason *et al.*, 2008).

Neurocardiogenic bradycardia and syncope in Dobermanns and Boxers can coexist with cardiomyopathy. Often there is intermittent bradycardia with ventricular tachyarrhythmias of variable severity. Cardiomyopathic patients may have a subtle autonomic dysfunction that predisposes to neurocardiogenic bradycardia.

Situational syncope

Situational syncope is most common in small-breed, middle-aged to old dogs wherein it is often associated with cough (tussive syncope) caused by tracheal or bronchial disease and/or advanced mitral valve disease leading to atrial enlargement and compression of a mainstem bronchus. In addition to tussive syncope, other situational triggers include gag-retch, emesis, micturition and defecation. Hence, the situation defines the trigger (i.e. tussive syncope, emesis syncope, micturition syncope or defecation syncope).

In the author's opinion, advanced mitral valve disease in elderly small-breed dogs predisposes to all situational syncope. Although sometimes controversial, when the heart rate is documented during situational syncope, it is almost always slow. More difficult to document is the systemic blood pressure at the time of syncope.

Situational syncope in affected dogs is not consistently precipitated by any given situation. Patients are variably affected and so cough, emesis, exertion/excitement, micturition and defecation do not inevitably cause syncope.

Drugs

Syncope can result from drug-induced hypotension caused by vasodilation (e.g. acepromazine, nitrates), decreased inotropy (beta-blockers, calcium channel-blockers), excessive preload reduction (diuretics) or changes in heart rate and/or rhythm (any antiarrhythmics).

Diagnostic approach

The patient history, physical examination, situational activity and the clinical signs that occur during and after the event are crucial to establishing the cause of syncope. Another important diagnostic goal is to document the heart rhythm at the time of the event. Figure 3.4 details the presenting signs and causes of syncope. In some cases, no underlying cause of syncope can be identified. If the description of the episode is strongly suggestive of syncope, then the cause is generally assumed to be neurally mediated.

General diagnostic tests

When the history and physical examination suggest metabolic disorders, serum chemistry profiles should be evaluated for electrolyte abnormalities, renal function, and to rule out hypoglycaemia. In addition, a complete blood count is used to detect anaemia/polycythaemia or white blood cell abnormalities. However, generally these are uncommon in diseases causing syncope.

Imaging

Echocardiography should be performed in patients with a heart murmur and/or arrhythmias to assess cardiac structure and function. If a seizure is suspected, brain imaging may be indicated.

Testing for arrhythmias

The only certain way to confirm an arrhythmia as the cause of syncope is to document the rate and rhythm during an episode. A 24-hour Holter recording is the gold standard to document an intermittent arrhythmia such as supraventricular tachycardia, ventricular tachycardia or bradyarrhythmias. For longer-term monitoring an implantable loop recorder can be utilized.

Real-time auscultation (by the owner or veterinary surgeon) during the episode of collapse is useful since it documents the associated heart rate as fast, slow or normal. Caution is advised with real-time auscultation because with very rapid arrhythmias an accurate assessment of heart rate can be difficult to ascertain, or the arrhythmia responsible may have already terminated by the time the animal becomes syncopal.

Presumptive diagnosis is sometimes legitimate when faced with selected breeds, clinical disorders, precipitating situations, or if an arrhythmia is observed on an ECG when the patient is not showing clinical signs. Ventricular tachycardia can be presumed as the most likely cause of syncope in Dobermanns and Boxers, even when subsequent ECGs contain only frequent ventricular premature beats (see Figure 3.4). If the arrhythmia is episodic, 24–48-hour Holter monitoring or 5–7-day event recording is useful.

Treatment

Treatment varies depending on the cause and is aimed at managing the underlying disorder. If an arrhythmic cause is identified, antiarrhythmic medication or a pacemaker is indicated (see Chapter 20).

Treatment of neurocardiogenic bradycardia and syncope in Boxers and Dobermanns is problematic. Usually, the episodes are infrequent and treatment is not required. The administration of beta-blockers can

Presentation	ECG findings	Type/cause of syncope
Syncope following coughing, gagging, retching, swallowing, vomiting, micturition or defecation	Normal (± bradycardia immediately preceding event)	Neurally mediated (situational) syncope
Older small-breed dog with loud systolic murmur	Normal (± bradycardia immediately preceding event)	Neurally mediated syncope (? Pulmonary hypertension)
Young dog with loud systolic basilar murmur	Normal (± bradycardia immediately preceding event) Ventricular arrhythmias	Consider subaortic or pulmonic stenosis (neurally mediated or arrhythmic cause of syncope)
Older West Highland White Terrier/Miniature Schnauzer/American Cocker Spaniel	Sick sinus syndrome: sinus arrest; sinus bradycardia; junctional or ventricular escape beats and brief rhythm; atrial or junctional premature contractions; atrial or junctional tachycardia; ventricular premature contractions (occasional)	Bradyarrhythmia
Boxer/Dobermann	Ventricular tachycardia	Tachyarrhythmia
Dog of any age/breed with slow heart rate	Advanced second- or third-degree atrioventricular block	Bradyarrhythmia

3.4 Presenting signs and causes of syncope.

precipitate bradycardia-related syncope in cardiomyopathic Dobermanns. Boxers with ventricular tachyarrhythmias that are treated with sotalol and then experience new or more frequent syncopal episodes may be suffering from neurocardiogenic bradycardia. The author recommends pacemaker implantation if a bradyarrhythmia is documented during the event. However, if hypotension occurs in conjunction with the bradyarrhythmia, pacemaker implantation may not solve the collapsing episodes. Unfortunately, it is difficult to predict which patients experience hypotension as a component of the syncopal event. In humans, a table tilt test (to test for orthostatic hypotension) can be useful, but for practical reasons this is not performed in veterinary medicine.

Neurally mediated syncope due to high preload and pulmonary hypertension usually responds favourably to cardiac unloading therapy.

Exertion/excitement-related syncope in elderly small-breed dogs with loud mitral regurgitation murmurs may be a warning of impending congestive heart failure. Potentially beneficial treatment includes furosemide, pimobendan, angiotensin-converting enzyme (ACE) inhibitors and perhaps spironolactone. The author uses furosemide and ACE inhibitors, even if pulmonary oedema is not present on thoracic radiographs. After 1–2 weeks, the author adds amlodipine to the treatment regimen to further reduce afterload. The addition of digoxin may decrease the number of syncopal episodes. Although the exact mechanism is unknown, digoxin modulates baroreceptor function and inhibits sympathetic nerve discharge (the trigger for this type of neurally mediated syncope).

Neurally mediated syncope, particularly in elderly small-breed dogs with mitral regurgitation, is best 'treated' by avoiding the instigating situations. Anticholinergic therapy can be attempted if behaviour modification does not decrease the syncopal episodes. The response to the type of preventive medical therapy is variable, and is therefore only recommended when episodes are predicable (i.e. scheduled exertion that might precipitate an event).

Beta-blockade has been recommended for treatment of humans with neurocardiogenic syncope precipitated by a sympathetic surge, but the overall evidence in favour is weak (Sheldon *et al.*, 2006). In the author's experience beta-blockade exacerbates neurally mediated syncope in dogs. This relates to the fact that, when documented, episodes are almost always associated with bradycardia.

A randomized clinical trial of fludrocortisone for the prevention of neurally mediated syncope in humans is in progress (Raj *et al.*, 2006). To date, the author has not used this drug in veterinary patients experiencing neurally mediated syncope. In the future, drugs such as fludrocortisone, midodrine and selective serotonin reuptake inhibitors may be used for the treatment of neurally mediated syncope (Medow *et al.*, 2008).

Syncope in cats

Syncope in cats is usually the result of an arrhythmia. Neurally mediated bradycardia is rare. In old cats, intermittent and high-grade second- or third-degree (complete) AV heart block is the most common arrhythmic cause of syncope and episodic weakness. Hyperthyroidism should be ruled out as a primary cause for these arrhythmias. Young to middle-aged cats with cardiomyopathy may have rapid ventricular tachycardia causing syncope (or sudden death). Sick sinus syndrome is rare.

Cats with hypertrophic cardiomyopathy and loud apical systolic heart murmurs may also experience exertional syncope or pre-syncope as a result of LVOT obstruction. These patients usually respond favourably to beta-blocker treatment.

Metabolic causes of apparent syncope in cats are uncommon. Occasionally, hypoglycaemia can occur as a result of insulin treatment in diabetic cats. Profound anaemia can result in exertional syncope or pre-syncope.

References and further reading

Abboud FM (1993) Neurocardiogenic syncope. *New England Journal of Medicine* 15, 1117–1120

Bright JM and Cali JV (2000) Clinical usefulness of cardiac event recording in dogs and cats examined because of syncope, episodic collapse, or intermittent weakness: 60 cases (1997–1999). *Journal of the American Veterinary Medical Association* 216, 1110–1114

Calvert CA, Jacobs GJ and Pickus CW (1996) Bradycardia-associated episodic weakness, syncope, and aborted sudden death in cardiomyopathic Doberman Pinschers. *Journal of Veterinary Internal Medicine* 10, 88–93

Davidow EB, Proulx J and Woodfield JA (2001) Syncope: pathophysiology and differential diagnosis. *Compendium on Continuing Education for the Practicing Veterinarian* 23, 608–619

Fogoros RN (1999) The evaluation of syncope. In: *Electrophysiologic Testing, 3rd edn*, pp. 241–252. Blackwell Science, Oxford

Kapoor WN (2000) Syncope. *New England Journal of Medicine* 343, 1856–1862

Kittleson MD (1998) Syncope. In: *Small Animal Cardiovascular Medicine*, ed. MD Kittleson and RD Kienle, pp. 495–501. Mosby, St Louis, Missouri

Medow MS, Stewart JM, Sanyal S *et al.* (2008) Pathophysiology, diagnosis, and treatment of orthostatic hypotension and vasovagal syncope. *Cardiology Review* 16, 4–20

Mosqueda-Garcia R, Furlan R, Tank J *et al.* (2000) The elusive pathophysiology of neurally mediated syncope. *Circulation* 102, 2898–2906

Oberg B and Thoren P (1972) Increased activity in left ventricular receptors during hemorrhage or occlusion of caval veins in the cat. A possible cause of the vaso-vagal reaction. *Acta Veterinaria Scandinavica* 85, 164–173

Raj SR, Rose S, Ritchie D *et al.* (2006) The Second Prevention of Syncope Trial (POST II) – a randomized clinical trial of fludrocortisone for the prevention of neurally mediated syncope: rationale and study design. *American Heart Journal* 151, 1131–1386

Rush JE (1999) Syncope and episodic weakness. In: *Textbook of Canine and Feline Cardiology*, ed. PR Fox, D Sisson and NS Moise, pp. 446–454. WB Saunders, Philadelphia

Sheldon R, Connolly S, Rose S *et al.* (2006) Prevention of Syncope Trial (POST): a randomized, placebo-controlled study of metoprolol in the prevention of vasovagal syncope. *Circulation* 113, 1164–1170

Thomason J, Kraus M, Surdyk K *et al.* (2008) Bradycardia-associated syncope in 7 boxers with ventricular tachycardia (2002–2005). *Journal of Veterinary Internal Medicine* 22, 931–936

4

Clinical approach to cardiac murmurs

Clarence Kvart

Introduction

The practice of cardiac auscultation remains one of the most widely used diagnostic techniques in veterinary medicine. Technical considerations of cardiac auscultation and interpretation of heart sounds and murmurs are therefore of wide interest to the veterinary practitioner. Although it may not be possible to establish the diagnosis of a specific heart disease with the sole use of a stethoscope, or in combination with a phonocardiogram (PCG), optimal use can narrow down the list of differential diagnoses substantially. A gentle approach and a quiet environment are essential for the animal to relax and for the auscultator to be undisturbed. It is also essential to auscultate all cardiac areas to detect local murmurs and, in the case of a heart murmur, the point of maximum intensity (PMI).

Stethoscopes

There are a number of different types of stethoscope commercially available. Most of the better quality standard stethoscopes are adequate for use in veterinary practice, but paediatric stethoscopes are not recommended for most auscultation as a larger bell is often needed for optimal amplification. It is essential for the veterinary surgeon to become familiar with the stethoscope, and how normal and abnormal heart and lung sounds are perceived using this particular instrument. It is also important to obtain a stethoscope with earpieces that fit snugly. This helps to avoid discomfort during prolonged auscultation and to reduce the 'leakage' of sound around the earpieces. For most veterinary surgeons, it is useful to angle the earpieces to better fit the ear canal. Sound 'leakage' is one cause of problems in the auscultation of abnormally low-intensity heart sounds or failure to detect murmurs.

It is useful to have a stethoscope with bells and diaphragms of different sizes. A small-sized bell can be used to localize the PMI of murmurs, especially in small dogs and cats. A larger diaphragm can be used to determine whether or not the patient has normal heart sounds. An open bell is sometimes useful to detect low-frequency sounds (such as an S3 sound) that may be inaudible using a diaphragm bell. Many standard stethoscopes have unnecessarily long tubing for use with small animals, and this may lead to dampening of sounds. Fortunately, tubes can always be shortened to an appropriate length of 36–46 cm (14–18 inches). A

sensor-based (non-microphone) stethoscope is also available (Meditron™). This stethoscope can be connected to a computer to store and filter the sounds as PCGs with simultaneous electrocardiogram (ECG) recordings. The ability to record, filter and analyse digital PCGs offers substantial advantages.

Origin of murmurs

Blood flow in normal vessels and the heart is usually laminar with minimal turbulence, and consequently does not result in a heart murmur. Heart murmurs all arise due to vibrations created within the cardiovascular system, which may originate from turbulent blood flow. However, not all animals with heart murmurs have heart disease, as some individuals with normal cardiovascular anatomy may have audible murmurs in early systole. These murmurs may be caused by high-velocity flow or low fluid viscosity (e.g. in severe anaemia). Murmurs in small animals that have a long duration in systole (more than 50%) are often caused by pathological conditions such as valvular regurgitation, shunting or obstruction of blood flow.

Situations that can cause turbulent flow (and therefore murmurs) include increased flow velocity in a normal vessel (such as the aorta), or more commonly, obstruction to blood flow or valvular incompetence. Murmurs from shunts and valvular incompetence are created by the combination of high-velocity flow through a narrow orifice combined with flow entering a cardiac structure of increased diameter.

Evaluation of the timing of murmurs is helpful in the interpretation of the significance of a murmur. A general rule is that holosystolic/diastolic murmurs are often significant, meaning that they indicate heart disease. Conversely, low-intensity early systolic murmurs tend to be associated with insignificant flow murmurs. Murmurs which have a duration of more than early systole are usually indicative of a cardiac abnormality.

Systole is defined as the time period between the onset of S1 and the onset of S2. Diastole is defined as the time period between the onset of S2 and the onset of S1 (Figure 4.1). Systolic and diastolic murmurs can also be characterized as early, mid or late, depending on their location in systole or diastole. Holosystolic murmurs fill the whole systolic period, and holodiastolic murmurs fill all of the diastolic period.

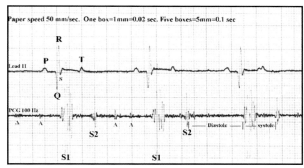

Paper speed 50 mm/sec. One box=1mm=0.02 sec. Five boxes=5mm=0.1 sec

4.1 ECG lead II and PCG from a healthy large dog, recorded at the mitral area. The PCG was recorded with the dog standing on the examination table. Notice the timing between the ECG and the PCG. Artefacts (noise) will also be recorded on the PCG, but appear differently timed to S1, S2 and the ECG (artefacts are marked A). Undulations of the baseline can be caused by noise from the surroundings, muscle tension and respiration. If respiratory sounds cause PCG deflections, limit interpretation to expiratory phases only, or occlude the mouth and nostrils of the patient while recording the PCG.

Auscultation and the point of maximum intensity

General advice for cardiac auscultation

- It is important to minimize background noise. If a quiet environment is impossible to achieve, an electronic stethoscope with the option to amplify heart sounds is useful. Clients often take the opportunity to talk when the veterinary surgeon is quiet; therefore, it is a good idea to explain the need for a quiet environment before auscultation and that only fragments of the information that a client is trying to impart will be heard.
- Small animals should preferably be in a standing position on all four limbs during cardiac auscultation. If the animal is sitting, the forelimbs will cover the different PMIs and the diaphragm of the animal will be positioned in a more cranial direction, compressing the thorax, which may leave the heart sounds less audible. If the animal is in right or left lateral recumbency, the heart will move towards the dependent side, leaving the heart sounds less distinct on the non-dependent side.
- Dogs often pant, and auscultation should be carefully interpreted in these patients because panting generates disturbing sounds, and breathing sounds may be mistaken for murmurs. Warm examination rooms should be avoided and if the animal is panting, the client should be asked to manually close the mouth of the dog for brief periods of time. If this is not sufficient, manual occlusion of both the ▶

mouth and nostrils can allow a few seconds of undisturbed auscultation or PCG recording.

- Cats may purr, which often makes evaluation of heart sounds impossible. Blowing short bursts of expired air into the face of the cat or exposing the animal to visual stimuli, such as another animal, can be tried to stop the purring. Short occlusion of one or both nostrils can also be attempted or holding an alcohol-soaked cotton-wool ball near the cat's nose. Holding the cat near a sink with running water often works.

All valve areas (and the sternum in cats) should be auscultated in order to detect local murmurs (Figure 4.2). One approach to performing this is to move the left leg of the animal forward so that the third intercostal space (pulmonic valve) is accessible. Some murmurs associated with common congenital malformations (such as patent ductus arteriosus (PDA) and pulmonic stenosis) have maximum intensity

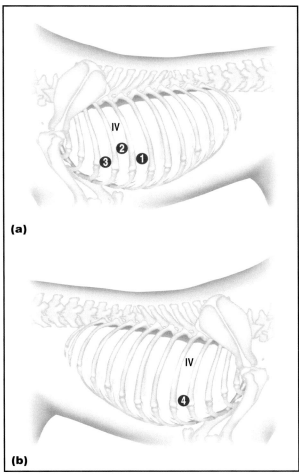

4.2 Points of maximum intensity. **(a)** Left side of the thorax. 1 = Mitral area; 2 = Aortic area; 3 = Pulmonic area. **(b)** Right side of the thorax. 4 = Tricuspid area. IV = 4th intercostal space.

over this area. The bell is then moved to the fourth and fifth intercostal spaces on the left side, just below the level of the point of the shoulder. The aortic area is located at this site. The examination is continued by auscultation a little lower at the level of the costochondral junctions at the fifth intercostal space, and thereafter proceeds to the sixth and seventh intercostal spaces over the apex of the heart until the intensity of the heart sounds decreases. The stethoscope is then placed on the right side of the thorax and moved forward and backwards over the third to fifth intercostal spaces at the level of the costochondral junctions, which is approximately midway between the point of the shoulder and olecranon in standing animals.

Auscultation of the tricuspid area may detect murmurs originating from the right side of the heart (such as ventricular septal defects, VSDs) or left-sided heart murmurs that are radiating over to the right side of the thorax (so called 'referred murmurs'). If abnormal sounds are detected, the PMI can be located by counting the intercostal spaces. Important diagnostic information can be obtained by localization of the PMI because this may serve as a guide to the origin of the murmur. For example, a physiological flow murmur always has a PMI over the outflow tracts (aortic and pulmonic areas). If a murmur has a PMI over the apex of the heart (mitral area), heart disease may be suspected. In cats and small dogs, identification of the PMI may require a stethoscope that can be changed to a smaller bell or the use of a paediatric stethoscope. Distinction between the pulmonic and the aortic areas may be difficult, but it is usually not difficult to establish whether the PMI is over the base (pulmonic or aortic area – outflow tracts) or the apex (mitral area – left ventricle, LV) of the heart. Details on the presence and direction of murmur radiation will add further information to support a specific diagnosis. Detection of S3, S4 or gallops in dogs may require auscultation with an open bell or sensor-based (digital) stethoscope, but almost all other abnormal heart sounds in cats and dogs can be detected with diaphragm stethoscopes.

Grading of murmurs
Murmurs are graded on a scale of 1 to 6.

Low-intensity murmurs
- Grade 1 – a low-intensity murmur heard in a quiet environment only after careful auscultation over a localized cardiac area.
- Grade 2 – a low-intensity murmur heard immediately when the stethoscope is placed over the PMI.

Moderate-intensity murmurs
- Grade 3 – a murmur of moderate intensity.
- Grade 4 – a high-intensity murmur that can be auscultated over several areas without any palpable precordial thrill.

High-intensity murmurs
- Grade 5 – a high-intensity murmur with a palpable precordial thrill.
- Grade 6 – a high-intensity murmur with a palpable precordial thrill that may even be heard when the stethoscope is slightly lifted off the chest wall.

Grading of murmurs may serve as a guide to roughly estimate the severity of heart disease for some conditions, such as aortic/pulmonic stenosis and mitral regurgitation, but is less reliable in other conditions, such as myocardial disease. High-intensity murmurs often, but not always, indicate more severe forms of heart disease. Exceptions include small VSDs, which can generate very loud murmurs. Rarely, degenerative mitral valve disease may generate very strong vibrations of the valvular apparatus, causing musical murmurs despite comparatively modest mitral regurgitation. Other exceptions are low-intensity murmurs that may be present in cases of myocardial failure caused by dilated cardiomyopathy (DCM), end-stage degenerative mitral valve disease with multiple small infarcts, and myocardial disease in cats.

Differential diagnoses for different cardiac murmurs
The general guidelines for the most common differential diagnoses based on the intensity and PMI of murmurs are presented in Figure 4.3.

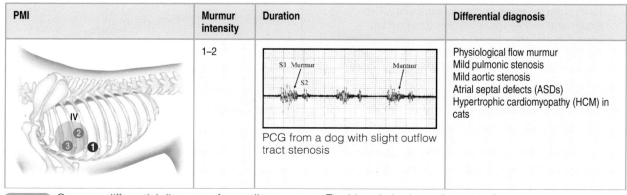

PMI	Murmur intensity	Duration	Differential diagnosis
IV ② ③ ①	1–2	PCG from a dog with slight outflow tract stenosis	Physiological flow murmur Mild pulmonic stenosis Mild aortic stenosis Atrial septal defects (ASDs) Hypertrophic cardiomyopathy (HCM) in cats

4.3 Common differential diagnoses for cardiac murmurs. The blue circle shows the point of maximum intensity. IV = 4th intercostal space. (continues) ▶

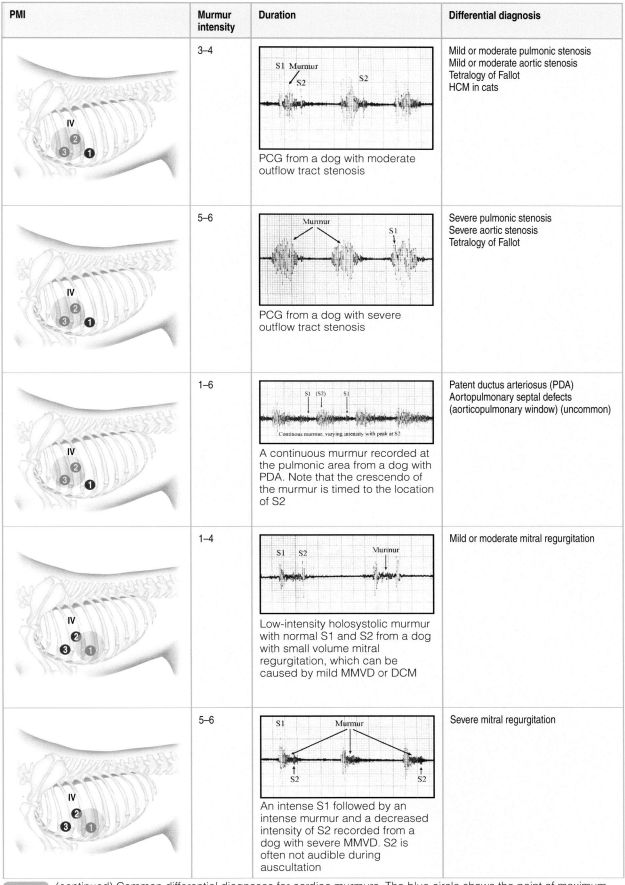

PMI	Murmur intensity	Duration	Differential diagnosis
	3–4	PCG from a dog with moderate outflow tract stenosis	Mild or moderate pulmonic stenosis Mild or moderate aortic stenosis Tetralogy of Fallot HCM in cats
	5–6	PCG from a dog with severe outflow tract stenosis	Severe pulmonic stenosis Severe aortic stenosis Tetralogy of Fallot
	1–6	A continuous murmur recorded at the pulmonic area from a dog with PDA. Note that the crescendo of the murmur is timed to the location of S2	Patent ductus arteriosus (PDA) Aortopulmonary septal defects (aorticopulmonary window) (uncommon)
	1–4	Low-intensity holosystolic murmur with normal S1 and S2 from a dog with small volume mitral regurgitation, which can be caused by mild MMVD or DCM	Mild or moderate mitral regurgitation
	5–6	An intense S1 followed by an intense murmur and a decreased intensity of S2 recorded from a dog with severe MMVD. S2 is often not audible during auscultation	Severe mitral regurgitation

4.3 (continued) Common differential diagnoses for cardiac murmurs. The blue circle shows the point of maximum intensity. IV = 4th intercostal space. (continues)

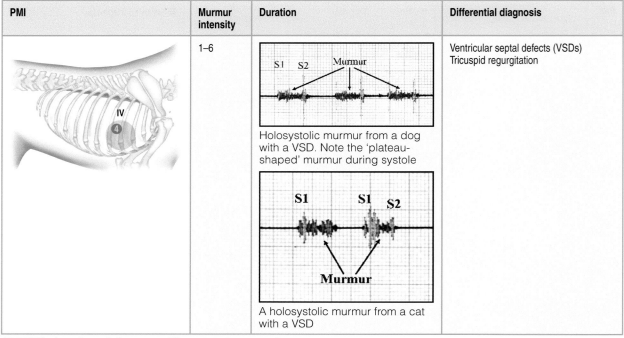

PMI	Murmur intensity	Duration	Differential diagnosis
IV ④	1–6	Holosystolic murmur from a dog with a VSD. Note the 'plateau-shaped' murmur during systole A holosystolic murmur from a cat with a VSD	Ventricular septal defects (VSDs) Tricuspid regurgitation

4.3 (continued) Common differential diagnoses for cardiac murmurs. The blue circle shows the point of maximum intensity. IV = 4th intercostal space.

Heart disease without murmurs

Fortunately, the majority of canine cardiac patients have a murmur. However, some conditions are not associated with heart murmurs. In a few of these cases, altered heart sounds may be present (e.g. gallop sounds), especially in advanced cases of heart disease.

Examples of heart disease without murmurs include: pericardial effusions; DCM; atrial septal defects (ASDs, murmurs originating from a relative pulmonic stenosis and which may be the result of larger shunts, especially after exercise); and right-to-left shunting with VSDs or PDA with pulmonary hypertension. Cats with myocardial disease may have no murmur at all.

Physiological flow murmurs in systole

Physiological flow murmurs are low-intensity, soft murmurs caused by turbulent flow in the aorta or pulmonary artery during early systole (Figure 4.4). The PMI is over the outflow tracts (aortic/pulmonic area). These murmurs do not indicate any underlying cardiac disorder that may be identified by thoracic radiography, echocardiography or post-mortem findings. A large stroke volume in relation to the size of the outflow vessels of a normal heart may cause turbulent flow and murmurs in young animals. These murmurs can disappear within a few weeks, more commonly within 4 to 5 months, or sometimes later during adolescence. In some individuals (especially athletes) these murmurs may remain in the adult animal.

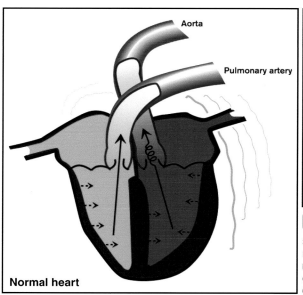

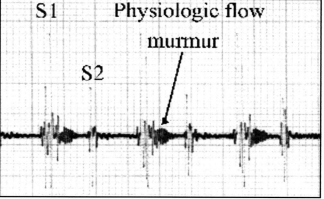

4.4 Physiological flow murmurs are caused by turbulent flow in the aorta or pulmonary artery during early systole with a duration of less than half of systole. The PCG recorded in a puppy showed that murmur intensity was low/moderate at the aortic/pulmonic area. The murmur had disappeared when the dog was re-examined as a 1-year-old. (Left image © C. Kvart.)

These murmurs are usually of low intensity (grade 1–2) and comprise high-frequency sounds, sometimes with medium-frequency sounds. They are early systolic murmurs, meaning that they end before the middle of systole and are usually of a decrescendo, but sometimes of a crescendo–decrescendo, character.

Differential diagnosis

- Athletic heart.
- Severe anaemia.
- Low-grade aortic or pulmonic stenosis.
- Fever.
- Hyperthyroidism.
- Any condition leading to increased cardiac output (e.g. pregnancy).
- Low-grade mitral regurgitation is sometimes associated with early to mid-systolic murmurs. PMI is over the mitral area in these dogs, in contrast to physiological flow murmurs where the PMI is over the aortic area.

Outflow tract stenosis in dogs

Pulmonic stenosis and aortic stenosis are two of the most common congenital malformations in dogs. Pulmonic stenosis is more common in small-breed dogs and aortic stenosis in large-breed dogs. These lesions are characterized by obstruction of the subvalvular, valvular or supravalvular area, causing turbulent blood flow. In contrast with aortic stenosis, the valvular form with fused cusps is more common in pulmonic stenosis. Supravalvular stenosis is less common. Acquired aortic stenosis may develop in association with bacterial endocarditis. Differentiation between aortic stenosis and pulmonic stenosis is best performed with echocardiography. The PMI is the pulmonic or aortic area at the left side of thorax (see Figure 4.3).

Cases of low-grade stenosis often have a low-intensity murmur (grade 2–3). Cases of moderate stenosis often have a moderate-intensity murmur (grade 3–4). Cases with a severe degree of stenosis usually have a high-intensity murmur (grade 4–6). The murmurs are often of a crescendo–decrescendo character and occupy from 50–100% of the systole, with longer durations for severe obstructions.

Outflow tract obstruction murmurs in cats

Congenital pulmonic and aortic stenoses occur in cats but are much less common than in dogs. The most common cause of outflow tract obstruction murmurs in cats is hypertrophic cardiomyopathy (HCM). The PMI may be on either side of the thorax, or even sternal.

Ejection murmurs can develop in cats with HCM if hypertrophy obstructs blood flow through the aortic or pulmonic outflow tracts (Figure 4.5). Dynamic *left* ventricular outflow tract obstruction is often caused by septal hypertrophy and systolic anterior motion of the mitral valve; dynamic *right* ventricular outflow tract obstruction may occur in cats with HCM or normal cats. Concurrent mitral regurgitation may complicate accurate identification of outflow tract murmurs.

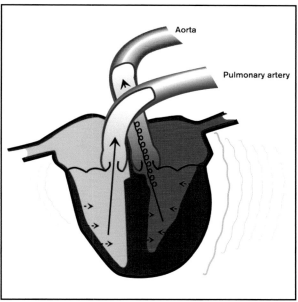

4.5 Hypertrophy of the upper portion of the interventricular septum may cause obstruction and turbulent blood flow. (© C. Kvart.)

Hyperthyroidism or renal disease with hypertension may cause secondary cardiac hypertrophy accompanied by obstruction to blood flow, creating low-intensity murmurs. Cats with more than two heart sounds (i.e. gallop rhythms) should always be examined with echocardiography as the majority of cases will have myocardial disease.

Tetralogy of Fallot

The audible murmur from tetralogy of Fallot is usually caused by pulmonic stenosis, which is associated with this complicated and uncommon congenital heart disease. The polycythaemia that accompanies tetralogy of Fallot causes hyperviscosity, which tends to reduce the murmur intensity.

Patent ductus arteriosus

PDA occurs when the fetal ductus between the aorta and the pulmonary artery fails to close *post partum*. The ductus can close to different degrees, and consequently the shunting of blood can range from insignificant to very severe. The pressure in the aorta is normally higher than the pressure in the pulmonary artery, during both systole and diastole. Therefore, blood is shunted through the ductus during the entire cardiac cycle, causing a continuous murmur (Figure 4.6). In some cases, pulmonary hypertension may develop, leading to reduced or even reversed shunting during diastole and, if severe, in systole as well.

PDA is associated with a continuous heart murmur (see Figure 4.3) with maximum intensity timed to the peak pressure gradient between the aorta and the pulmonary artery, which is at the end of systole. The intensity of the murmur decreases during diastole, as the pressure gradient decreases. The intensity and radiation of the murmur also varies with the size of the ductus. Small shunts have local low-intensity murmurs; moderate shunts often have murmurs of moderate-

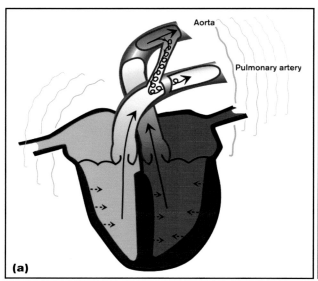 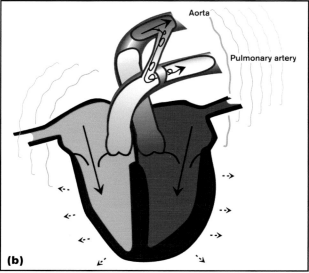

4.6 PDA is characterized by turbulent flow from the aorta to the pulmonary artery both during **(a)** systole and **(b)** diastole, with greater flow at the end of systole and beginning of diastole. (© C. Kvart.)

intensity with some radiation; and severe shunts are associated with intense murmurs that radiate widely. If pulmonary hypertension develops, the murmur can become systolic only and may even disappear as pulmonary hypertension increases and polycythaemia develops. Depending on the size and degree of shunting, exercise intolerance and left-sided heart failure may occur if surgical correction is not attempted.

Murmurs with the PMI at the apex of the heart

Differential diagnosis

- Mitral regurgitation.
  - Myxomatous mitral valve disease (MMVD).
  - Congenital mitral dysplasia.
  - DCM.
  - Endocarditis affecting the mitral valve.
  - Other causes of mitral regurgitation.
- (VSDs or tricuspid regurgitation may radiate to the left side of the thorax but the PMI is usually at the tricuspid area.)

MMVD is the most common cardiovascular lesion causing murmurs in middle-aged or older small-breed dogs. Progressive pathological changes of the atrio-ventricular (AV) valves will, at some point, cause the valves to become incompetent (Figure 4.7). Initially, mitral regurgitation may cause intermittent, soft murmurs. Over time, the murmur becomes holosystolic and persistent (Figure 4.8), with increasing intensity as the severity of the mitral regurgitation progresses. The holosystolic 'plateau' shape of the murmur can be explained by a similar degree of regurgitation throughout systole.

The low-intensity of the murmur indicates that only a small proportion of the stroke volume is regurgitated during the early stages of the disease (see Figure 4.3). As the disease progresses, forward stroke volume is reduced as the regurgitant fraction increases. However, this is counteracted by eccentric

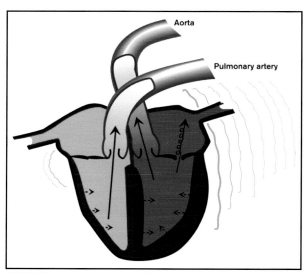

4.7 Incompetence of the mitral valve causes mitral regurgitation with turbulent blood flow, usually throughout systole. This causes a holosystolic murmur. (© C. Kvart.)

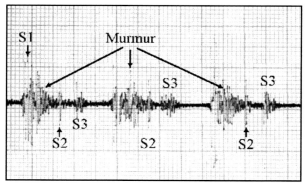

4.8 A moderate-intensity systolic murmur from a dog with moderate MMVD. This patient was still asymptomatic and not in need of therapy. Note that the second heart sound is of decreased intensity but still visible. A low-intensity (often inaudible) third heart sound (S3) is sometimes present, as in this case.

hypertrophy and increased ventricular filling, leading to increased force of contraction according to the Frank-Starling mechanism (see Chapter 15). Eccentric hypertrophy in combination with hyperkinesis maintains cardiac output despite an increasing degree of mitral regurgitation, and the intensity of the murmur and first heart sound increases. With further increase in the severity of the disease, the second heart sound decreases in intensity as forward stroke volume is reduced (see Figure 4.3).

Congenital dysplasia of the AV valves can also cause different degrees of mitral regurgitation. Many dogs with DCM have no murmurs, but dilatation of the mitral valve annulus and papillary muscle dysfunction may cause mitral regurgitation with a systolic murmur over the apex of the heart (mitral area). An audible diastolic gallop (usually S3) may also be present. In cases of DCM, heart sounds and murmurs are often of a lower intensity than in animals with MMVD. This is because reduced myocardial contractility prevents the heart from generating forceful mitral regurgitation jets and strong vibrations.

Murmurs with the PMI on the right side of thorax

Differential diagnosis

- VSDs.
- Tricuspid regurgitation caused by dysplasia, degeneration or pulmonary hypertension.
- Aortic stenosis.

Ventricular septal defect

Although VSDs may occasionally be located in the muscular portion of the septum, most commonly they are found in the upper (perimembranous) portion of the septum, just below the aortic valve. VSDs may cause shunting of blood during systole from the LV to the right ventricle (RV) because the systolic pressure within the LV is normally considerably higher than in the RV (Figure 4.9). The PMI is usually over the cranioventral right hemithorax, but the murmur may radiate to the left side of the thorax. Animals with a VSD usually have a holosystolic murmur of low- or moderate-intensity (see Figure 4.3). The intensity of the murmur cannot be used to estimate the size or the degree of shunting, as pulmonary hypertension may reduce shunting in severe cases.

Tricuspid regurgitation

Acquired or congenital lesions of the tricuspid valve or right ventricular dilatation can cause valve insufficiency during all or part of systole (Figure 4.10). Dogs with tricuspid regurgitation commonly have holosystolic murmurs, usually of low- to moderate-

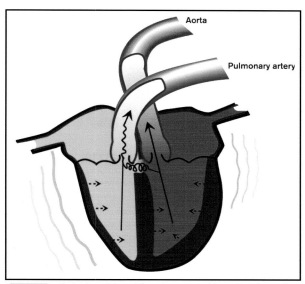

4.9 Turbulent blood flow is caused by shunting of blood from the LV to the RV throughout systole. This is due to a significant difference in blood pressure during systole, a difference that disappears during diastole. (© C. Kvart.)

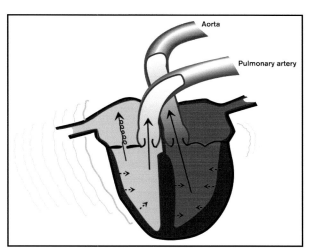

4.10 Incompetence of the tricuspid valve causes tricuspid regurgitation with turbulent blood flow, usually throughout systole, causing a holosystolic murmur. (© C. Kvart.)

intensity. With tricuspid regurgitation, the murmur may vary in intensity with respiration more than is the case with murmurs caused by mitral regurgitation.

References and further reading

Kvart C and Häggström J (2002) *Cardiac Auscultation and Phonocardiography in Dogs, Horses and Cats*. Uppsala, Sweden (www.cardiacauscultation.com)

5

History and physical examination

Lynelle R. Johnson and Virginia Luis Fuentes

History

Successful management of the animal with cardio-respiratory disease depends on accurate anatomical localization of disease and efficient diagnostic planning. Determination of the history of the complaint, assessment of the pattern of breathing, and careful examination and auscultation will assist in determining the site responsible for generation of cardiorespiratory complaints.

Respiratory distress

Causes of respiratory distress to be considered include acute congestive heart failure (CHF), broncho-constrictive crisis in feline asthma, acute or chronic pleural effusion, and pulmonary thromboembolism. The approach to the patient in respiratory distress is covered in more detail in Chapter 1.

Coughing

Chronicity can give some indication of the underlying cause and may be as helpful as character of the cough. Chronic coughing is most commonly associated with an airway disorder, whilst acute onset of coughing is more likely due to CHF or pneumonia. Coughing is covered in more detail in Chapter 2.

Syncope

Syncope may be a presenting clinical sign with both respiratory and cardiac disease. Syncope is a relatively common clinical complaint for patients with pulmonary hypertension but can be encountered in animals with cardiac arrhythmias or airway obstruction. Chapter 3 covers the approach to syncope in more detail.

Exercise intolerance

Exercise intolerance is often quoted as a presenting sign in heart disease, although other obvious signs are often evident by the time exercise capacity is limited. This may be because exercise intolerance is hard to detect in sedentary animals and cats, or it may be because dogs compensate for a decrease in their ability to exercise. Even in athletic dogs, it is unusual for valve disease or myocardial disease to present as exercise intolerance. In contrast, dogs with cyanotic heart disease or heartworm disease may have exercise intolerance as the main presenting sign. The ability to exercise can also be reduced with upper or lower airway disease and parenchymal disease.

Limb paresis

Cats with myocardial disease are at risk of systemic thromboembolism and may present with limb paresis. This may affect one or both pelvic limbs, or sometimes affects a single forelimb. These cats are distressed and in pain, and may be mistaken for victims of trauma. Lower motor neuron signs with absence of a palpable pulse should raise suspicion for systemic thromboembolic disease.

Breathing patterns

Patient assessment begins with a visual appraisal of the respiratory pattern before the patient is stressed by an examination. Restrictive respiratory diseases, such as pleural effusion and parenchymal disorders (pneumonia or oedema), cause rapid and shallow respiratory motions; whilst obstructive disorders, such as bronchitis, result in slow, deep breathing. Increased expiratory effort, prolonged expiratory time and abdominal effort on expiration should be considered suggestive of lower airway disease. However, some cats with inflammatory airway disease will exhibit both hyperpnoea and tachypnoea. Upper airway obstruction can lead to incessant panting, although prolonged and laboured inspiration would be the classic finding. Interpretation of breathing patterns is a vital part of the physical examination and is covered in more detail in Chapter 1.

General physical examination

General health and demeanour are helpful in determining both the underlying cause of presenting signs as well as the severity of illness. In general, animals with airway-oriented diseases (tracheal collapse, chronic bronchitis, feline bronchial disease) are in excellent systemic health, have a normal body temperature and have a stable (or often increased) body condition score. In contrast, animals with parenchymal, pleural or cardiac disease with failure are more likely to be systemically debilitated or cachexic. Animals with pneumonia may have an increased body temperature.

Mucous membranes

Mucous membranes are inspected for pallor, cyanosis and rubor in relation to cardiac or respiratory disease. Pallor can indicate anaemia, but can also be associated with severe peripheral vasoconstriction in low output states or conditions of elevated sympathetic tone. Profound vasoconstriction also tends to result in prolonged capillary refill time. Cyanosis indicates an increased concentration of desaturated haemoglobin and imparts a mucous membrane colour ranging from slightly 'dusky' in mild cases to nearly navy blue in patients with severe hypoxaemia. Cyanosis is most often seen with severe hypoxaemia resulting from respiratory disease (including pulmonary oedema or pleural effusion with CHF) but can also be seen with a right-to-left congenital shunt. With right-to-left shunts (sometimes termed 'cyanotic heart disease') detection of the bluish colour of cyanosis can be hampered by coexisting polycythaemia, which itself gives a dark red colour to the mucous membranes. The resulting colour may be closer to maroon than blue.

Jugular veins
Inspection of the jugular veins is an often neglected part of the physical examination; however, the jugular veins allow evaluation of systemic venous pressure. In the absence of a cranial mediastinal mass or obstruction of the cranial vena cava, distension of the jugular veins above the level of the right atrium (RA) indicates elevation of right atrial pressures (Figure 5.1). In long-haired animals, it is possible to get an impression of jugular venous distension without clipping the hair if the coat is instead wetted with spirit. For milder degrees of elevation of right-sided pressures, pressure on the cranial abdomen may increase venous return to the right heart sufficiently to cause temporary jugular distension ('hepatojugular reflux'). The distension resolves when the abdominal pressure is released. Jugular pulsation may be prominent with tricuspid regurgitation or when atrial contraction occurs against a closed tricuspid valve.

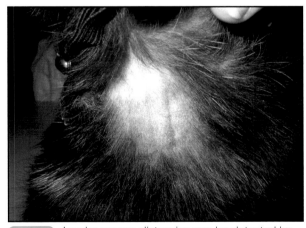

5.1 Jugular venous distension can be detected by palpation or observation, which is facilitated by soaking the neck with alcohol or shaving the jugular furrow.

Femoral pulses
The arterial pulse reflects the difference between diastolic and systolic arterial pressure. This pulse pressure is determined by stroke volume, but conditions that lower diastolic pressure (e.g. patent ductus arteriosus or aortic insufficiency) will also have a profound effect on pulse quality, causing a 'bounding' pulse. Weak pulses may reflect poor stroke volume.

Pulses may be absent with systemic thromboembolism, although blood flow may return within a few hours to a few days following acute embolization.

Abdominal palpation
Liver enlargement will accompany right-sided heart failure in dogs. The liver may be more palpable than normal in some cats with severe hyperpnoea and air-trapping, when it extends beyond the costal arch. Small, scarred kidneys may be associated with systemic hypertension, and should prompt blood pressure measurement. Small abdominal effusions may be appreciated as 'slipperiness' of the small intestines. Larger ascitic effusions are unmistakable on percussion of a fluid thrill.

Cardiac auscultation

Auscultation of heart sounds is a very important part of the physical examination. Auscultation allows assessment of heart rate and rhythm, intensity of heart sounds, presence of additional heart sounds, and presence of abnormal sounds such as murmurs and clicks. The approach to evaluation of cardiac murmurs is covered in detail in Chapter 4.

Heart rate
Heart rate can be helpful in differentiating cardiac from respiratory disease in those dogs where respiratory disease is associated with elevated vagal tone, leading to an exaggerated respiratory sinus arrhythmia. Dogs with CHF are more likely to have increased sympathetic tone and an increased heart rate, although the degree of tachycardia may be modest. Care should be taken not to place too much reliance on heart rate in brachycephalic dogs with suspected heart failure, as concurrent airway obstruction may cause sufficient elevation in vagal tone that sinus arrhythmia persists despite overt heart failure. Although it is often said that large dogs have slow heart rates and small dogs have fast heart rates, there are many exceptions. The most important determinant of heart rate in dogs is autonomic tone. Cats do not appear to develop a consistent tachycardia with heart failure, and may be more likely than dogs to develop sinus bradycardia with life-threatening CHF.

Heart rhythm
Normal dogs will have either a regular heart rhythm, or a sinus arrhythmia where the heart rate speeds up with inspiration and then slows with expiration. Cats normally have a regular heart rhythm. Bradyarrhythmias can be recognized by the slow heart rate, but it can be difficult to distinguish sinus arrest from high-grade atrioventricular block solely on auscultation, unless the S4 sounds of unconducted P waves can be heard. Atrial fibrillation sounds characteristically 'chaotic' on auscultation, but can still be confused with frequent atrial or ventricular premature beats.

Intensity of heart sounds
Two heart sounds (S1 and S2) are normally heard in dogs and cats (Figure 5.2). S1 is heard loudest at the

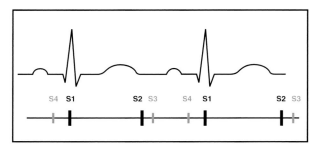

5.2 Timing of heart sounds in relation to the electrical activity of the heart. Normal heart sounds in the dog and cat consist of S1, which occurs after closure of the atrioventricular valves, and S2, which occurs after closure of the aortic and pulmonic valves.

apex, and S2 is heard loudest at the base. High cardiac output states, cardiac enlargement, thin body condition and increased sympathetic tone can increase the intensity of heart sounds; whereas pericardial effusion, severe myocardial failure, obesity, space-occupying lesions and pleural effusion may decrease heart sound intensity. The intensity of heart sounds may vary from beat to beat with atrial fibrillation and ventricular tachycardia. Variation in the PR interval will alter the intensity of S1.

Additional heart sounds

Additional heart sounds (S3 and S4) are associated with diastolic ventricular filling. These sounds are called *gallop sounds* and should not be audible in the normal dog or cat. When atrial pressures are increased, the blood flow velocity of rapid ventricular filling increases and may result in an audible gallop sound. With myocardial disease, blood flow may decelerate more rapidly in a stiff left ventricle (LV), again producing an audible gallop sound. Delayed ventricular relaxation can also cause an audible gallop, and may account for the presence of a gallop in some geriatric cats in the absence of obvious structural heart disease. In all other groups of cats and dogs, a gallop sound can be considered to be an indication of myocardial disease or heart failure.

Murmurs and clicks

Murmurs are produced when blood flow becomes turbulent. This is more likely with increased velocity of blood flow (e.g. with valve stenosis/insufficiency or increased sympathetic tone). The approach to identification of murmurs is discussed in depth in Chapter 4. Systolic clicks are transient heart sounds associated with myxomatous mitral valve disease. They may be mistaken for diastolic gallop sounds, but actually occur in systole. They may be present at an earlier stage of mitral valve disease than a systolic murmur, and may be masked by the systolic murmur itself later on in the course of the disease.

Thoracic auscultation and percussion

Auscultation should include the larynx, trachea and all lung fields. Over the larynx and trachea, loud, hollow sounds are heard on inspiration and expiration

with a noticeable pause between the two phases. The larynx is evaluated first to establish normal upper airway noises for the individual (Figure 5.3). Upper airway obstructive disease can cause a multitude of abnormal sounds (primarily on inspiration), and these sounds radiate into the thorax.

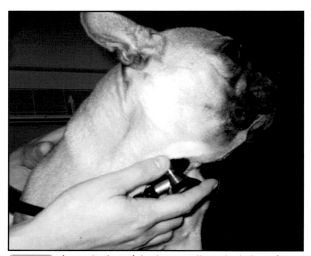

5.3 Auscultation of the larynx allows isolation of upper airway sounds in dogs and cats. This can be particularly helpful when auscultating a brachycephalic dog to provide differentiation of stertorous upper airway sounds from normal lung sounds.

Normal respiratory sounds

Normal sounds are termed bronchial, vesicular or bronchovesicular. Bronchial sounds are loud, high-pitched sounds heard best over the large airways near the hilum of the lung, and they are louder and longer during expiration than inspiration. Bronchial sounds should not be heard in the lung periphery unless disease is present, causing referral of sounds to distant regions. Vesicular lung sounds are heard over most of the chest in normal individuals. These are heard best on inspiration and the sounds are subtle, resembling a breeze passing through trees. Inspiration and expiration produce bronchovesicular sounds (a mixture of bronchial and vesicular harmonics) of similar duration and quality.

Adventitious lung sounds

Crackles and wheezes are examples of abnormal noises produced in diseased lungs. Detection of abnormal lung sounds can be enhanced by inducing a cough or deep breath in the animal, or by exercising the patient. Determining the specific phase of the respiratory cycle in which abnormal lung sounds occur is important in categorizing the sound and determining the most likely pathology present. Wheezes are musical, continuous sounds heard on expiration as air flows out of mucus-filled airways or airways narrowed by bronchoconstriction or remodelling, and are most commonly detected in dogs or cats with chronic bronchial disease. Crackles can be heard at any point during inspiration or may be heard on expiration. Crackles are discontinuous, non-musical sounds produced when air pressures fluctuate within the airways during respiration, or when air rushes through fluid- or mucus-filled alveoli. Absence of lung sounds is also an important finding and typically reflects disease of the pleural space, although consolidation of a lung segment can also lead to an absence of lung sounds. Loss of lung sounds dorsally generally indicates air accumulation. If pleural effusion is present due to pulmonary, cardiac or systemic causes, heart and lung sounds will be dampened ventrally whilst lung sounds are heard in the dorsal lung regions.

The presence, type and location of abnormal lung sounds can be important in determining the underlying cause of clinical signs. Crackles on inspiration are often heard diffusely in dogs and cats with interstitial pneumonia, and they may be soft or coarse. The crackles detected in animals with bronchial disease are generally harsher than those heard in dogs and cats with pulmonary oedema or interstitial pneumonia. Expiratory wheezes would be anticipated in the dog or cat with inflammatory airway disease because obstruction of the small airways results in difficulty during the expiratory phase. Crackles detected in animals with pneumonia are often softer than those heard with bronchial disease and may be localized to certain lung regions. In an animal with aspiration pneumonia, abnormal lung sounds may be localized to the cranioventral lung regions or the middle lung lobes. In animals with heart failure, lung sounds can be relatively normal if pulmonary oedema is mainly interstitial, although soft crackles will be heard with alveolar oedema. Loss of lung sounds in one hemithorax is suggestive of unilateral pleural effusion, which occurs most commonly with pyothorax or chylothorax. Herniation of organ contents through one side of the diaphragm can also lead to unilateral loss of lung sounds.

Tracheal sensitivity
Tracheal sensitivity is a non-specific sign of airway irritation and is usually present in airway or parenchymal disease. Some dogs with alveolar pulmonary oedema will also cough, although coughing is not usually a feature of CHF in cats. Pleural disease should not result in coughing, unless concurrent pulmonary disease or airway compression stimulates the intra-airway cough receptors. The character of the cough is different in airway disorders in comparison with heart disease. In dogs and cats with chronic bronchitis, airway collapse or pneumonia, a harsh cough is usually elicited with tracheal palpation, while a soft cough is more typical in dogs with severe pulmonary oedema.

Thoracic percussion
Percussion causes vibration of the chest and intrathoracic structures, and the pitch reflects the underlying air:tissue ratio within the thorax. To perform percussion:

1. The fingers of one hand are placed flat against the thoracic cage.
2. The fingers of the other hand are curved gently and held rigid.
3. The fingers of the free hand sharply strike the fingers on the chest wall (Figure 5.4), causing production of sounds.

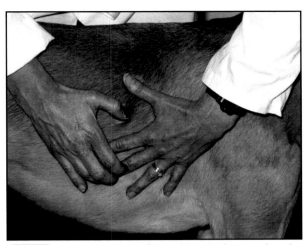

5.4 Percussion is performed by placing one hand on the thoracic wall and rapping the fingers with the other hand to detect differences in pitch caused by accumulation of air or fluid in the pleural space or lung.

Percussion is initiated in one site, then all lung fields are examined to detect localized differences in the transmission of sound. Over the heart, a dull percussive sound is heard because of the presence of soft tissue that dampens the transmission of sound. When the chest cavity is filled with fluid, or the lung is consolidated by disease, dull sounds are noted in the affected areas; whilst over air-filled lung structures, more resonant sounds are heard. In an animal with pneumothorax or air-trapping, sounds have increased resonance. Percussion is usually most useful in larger dogs.

Clinical signs of heart failure

Low output failure
It is uncommon for dogs or cats to present with obvious weakness due to cardiac disease, which usually reflects acute deterioration without time for the compensatory responses of sodium and water retention. Rarely, cardiac patients may be depressed or have abnormal mentation. They are usually hypothermic with cold extremities. Mucous membranes are pale with prolonged capillary refill time. Cats, particularly, may be bradycardic. Congestive signs may or may not accompany the low output signs.

Left-sided congestive heart failure
Pulmonary oedema causes an increase in respiratory rate and effort. No other abnormalities may be detected with mild interstitial oedema. More severe cases with alveolar oedema will have soft end-inspiration crackles on auscultation of the lung fields, and in the worst cases this may even be audible without a stethoscope when the examiner's ear is placed close to the dog's nose or mouth. This category of patient may also expectorate pink blood-tinged foam or have pink froth coming from the nostrils. Mucous membranes in these cases will be severely cyanosed. Some cats will develop pleural effusion with left-sided heart disease.

Right-sided congestive heart failure

Dogs with right-sided failure will usually have distended jugular veins with varying degrees of abdominal effusion. Milder or treated cases may only have hepatojugular reflux, although hepatomegaly is usually appreciable. Some dogs will develop pleural effusion, although this is more common with biventricular failure. It is unusual for subcutaneous oedema to develop with right-sided failure in small animals, but oedema of the distal limbs and prepuce may be observed in severe cases. It is unusual for cats to develop ascites with heart failure, but this may reflect the rarity of pure right-sided problems. Cats with right ventricular cardiomyopathy, right-sided congenital defects and refractory biventricular congestive failure may ultimately develop ascites.

6

Radiology

Elizabeth Baines

Larynx and trachea

Indications for imaging
The indications for imaging the larynx and trachea include:

- Stridor or stertorous respiration
- Inspiratory distress
- Palpable cervical mass
- Suspected tracheal collapse
- Suspected laryngeal paralysis or collapse
- Pain on palpation of the laryngeal region.

Upper airway

- **The upper airway comprises the larynx and trachea.**
- **The most useful radiographic views are: the extended lateral view of the neck for the larynx and extrathoracic trachea; and the lateral view of the thorax for the thoracic trachea (see below).**
- **The extended lateral view of the neck is best achieved under general anaesthesia, to avoid the need for restraining aids being placed over the neck, thus restricting visualization of the area of interest!**
- **Removal of the endotracheal tube during exposure maximizes the information available on the radiograph.**
- **For extrathoracic structures, the orthogonal view is usually of little value due to superimposition by the cervical vertebrae. Within the thorax, the dorsoventral (DV) or ventrodorsal (VD) view may be useful for assessing tracheal displacement.**
- **Both inspiratory and expiratory radiographs should be taken to show dynamic changes within the trachea.**
- **Ultrasonography of the larynx may provide functional information, and computed tomography (CT) can also be used for assessment of the trachea.**

Normal appearance
The hyoid apparatus and soft tissues of the larynx are visible on a well exposed radiograph, and the tubular air lucency of the trachea can be seen coursing craniocaudally in the ventral part of the neck towards the thoracic inlet. Mineralization of the laryngeal cartilages and tracheal rings may occur as a normal ageing change. The epiglottis may be seen contacting the caudal border of the soft palate, but commonly, following extubation, it will remain in close contact with the base of the tongue and not be visible radiographically. The air-filled nasopharynx, oropharynx and laryngopharynx are usually visible, although less so in brachycephalic breeds. The trachea should be very slightly narrower than the larynx cranially, and at the thoracic inlet, the width of the trachea should be 20% the height of the thoracic inlet in non-brachycephalic breeds.

Diseases
Diseases of the larynx and trachea include:

- Laryngeal masses
- Functional abnormalities
- Tracheal displacement
- Tracheal mass
- Tracheal hypoplasia
- Tracheal collapse
- Tracheal rupture
- Tracheal inflammation and haemorrhage.

Laryngeal masses
Laryngeal masses are uncommon. If small, they can be difficult to differentiate from normal soft tissue structures and if large, they may obliterate air-filled cavities. They can be particularly difficult to detect in brachycephalic breeds, where the air-filled spaces are smaller. Carcinoma is the most common neoplastic lesion in dogs, lymphosarcoma in cats. Other differential diagnoses include foreign bodies, polyps and abscesses.

Functional abnormalities
Functional abnormalities are best assessed by direct visualization, although ultrasonography may also be useful.

Tracheal displacement
Tracheal displacement may be created artefactually by overextension or flexion of the neck during radiography, thus a functional erect neck position should be maintained during the exposure. If there is tracheal displacement which cannot be explained by breed variation or positioning, a mass should be searched for in the region of the displacement. Causes of tracheal displacement include tumour, lymphadenomegaly, abscess, oesophageal enlargement,

great vessel enlargement and cardiomegaly. CT and/or ultrasonography will often be useful to determine the cause of the displacement.

Tracheal mass
Tracheal tumours are uncommon, with osteochondroma in the dog and carcinoma in the cat, respectively, being the most common types. Other causes of mass lesions within the trachea include: abscess; polyp; foreign body; and nodules of *Oslerus osleri* infection.

Tracheal hypoplasia
Tracheal hypoplasia is a condition predominantly of brachycephalic breeds, particularly the Bulldog, and affected dogs may or may not show clinical signs of airway obstruction. Measurements at the thoracic inlet can be made on well positioned lateral radiographs. In most breeds, the ratio between the trachea and the thoracic inlet should be 0.20; in non-Bulldog brachycephalic breeds the ratio is 0.16; and in Bulldogs is 0.13.

Tracheal collapse
If the trachea is abnormal, its diameter may vary according to the respiratory cycle. Tracheal collapse is a dynamic condition with cervical tracheal collapse occurring on inspiration and thoracic tracheal collapse occurring on expiration. The abnormal trachea may also 'balloon' during the opposite phase of respiration. Lateral radiographs (Figure 6.1) of the whole trachea should be taken during expiration and inspiration. Fluoroscopy is also useful to appreciate the dynamic nature of the condition.

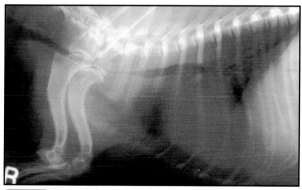

6.1 Lateral thoracic radiograph of a 7-year-old Jack Russell Terrier with tracheal collapse.

Tracheal rupture
Tracheal rupture is an unusual condition, more common in the cat, secondary either to trauma or to iatrogenic damage following intubation for general anaesthesia. Loss of continuity of the air shadow of the tracheal lumen may be seen, leading to pneumomediastinum and eventually pneumothorax. Tracheal rupture may be chronic or acutely severe and life-threatening.

Tracheal inflammation or haemorrhage
Rarely, inflammation of the tracheal wall can lead to radiographically visible narrowing of the lumen. Submucosal haemorrhage secondary to clotting defects has also been reported.

Thorax

Indications for imaging
The indications for imaging the thorax are many and varied and include:

- Investigation of coughing and/or respiratory distress
- Severe acute upper or lower respiratory tract disease
- Chronic respiratory disease
- Recurrent respiratory disease
- Moderate to severe thoracic trauma
- Prior to anaesthesia induction in cases with thoracic trauma
- Prior to anaesthesia induction in cases with severe extrathoracic trauma
- Prior to anaesthesia induction in cases with suspected respiratory or cardiac problems
- Heart disease
- Thoracic wall abnormalities
- Swallowing problems or regurgitation for which no extrathoracic cause can be found
- Electric shock or toxin ingestion with cardiorespiratory signs
- Postoperative complications of thoracic surgery
- Screening for metastases in cases of neoplasia.

Radiographic technique
Good technique is paramount, with movement blur (usually due to respiratory or cardiac motion) being the most common technical fault.

Equipment
- The maximum mA available should be used to keep exposure time to the minimum possible (ideally <0.05 seconds).
- Scattered radiation is not often a problem in the thorax and a grid should only be used if the patient's thorax is thicker than 15 cm. However, use of a grid requires an increased mAs, and with a low fixed mA machine, the exposure time must be increased. Thus, it is preferable not to use a grid in most instances.
- Fast film–screen combinations should be used to keep exposure time to a minimum.

Exposure factors
- The air-filled lungs within the osseous thoracic wall result in a body region of high inherent contrast. Thus, a high kV, low mAs technique is preferred.
- This results in a long greyscale radiograph being produced, which enables better interpretation of intrathoracic structures.
- High contrast black and white radiographs should be avoided.
- Using a high kV also allows a low mAs to be used, potentially reducing the exposure time further.

Positioning
In lateral recumbency the dependent lung will partially collapse, which may result in a lack of visualization of lesions within that lung. This is particularly true in

animals under general anaesthesia. The DV or VD view should be obtained first, before the animal is placed in lateral recumbency. Good positioning is of paramount importance. Rotation of the animal should be avoided, as should excessive flexion or extension of the neck.

- Two orthogonal views should be taken; right lateral recumbent and DV views are taken routinely.
- For the right lateral recumbent view, the forelimbs should be extended cranially to reduce superimposition of the brachial musculature on the cranioventral thorax. A foam wedge is often required under the sternum to elevate the sternum and spine into the same horizontal plane. Collimation should include the cranial border of the scapulohumeral joint and the last rib.
- An additional left lateral recumbent view is useful, particularly when investigating right hemithoracic disease or during a metastases screen.
- For the DV or VD view, the sternum and spine should be superimposed. The forelimbs may be extended cranially or allowed to abduct comfortably. A radiolucent trough or cradle may be used to reduce axial rotation. A VD view may be preferred for assessment of the accessory lung lobe and caudal mediastinum. However, VD views should be avoided in animals with respiratory distress that appear to have pleural space disease and in animals with cardiac or mainstem bronchial disease because compression of these regions during dorsal recumbency could worsen clinical signs.
- Additional positional or gravitational views may be taken, utilizing a horizontal primary beam, in certain situations:
  - *Decubitus lateral view:* This is useful in cases with small volumes of pleural fluid or air. The animal is placed in lateral recumbency and the X-ray beam centred at the lower (for fluid) or upper (for air) lateral margin of the thoracic wall. Fluid will drain dependently, and air will rise to the highest point of the thorax, just under the curve of the ribs. This view can also be used for patients with suspected air-trapping: the animal is placed in lateral recumbency (on the affected side in the case of unilateral disease) and a normally centred VD radiograph is taken using a horizontal beam. In animals with air-trapping, the heart will remain on the midline, whilst in unaffected animals positional atelectasis and collapse of the dependent lung will result in a mediastinal shift towards the tabletop
  - *Standing/sitting lateral view:* This is useful in large breeds of dog (e.g. Great Dane), particularly when lateral recumbency is resented and sternal recumbency difficult to achieve (Figure 6.2). Superimposition of the brachial musculature on the cranioventral thorax will reduce information. Cats that are in respiratory distress can be confined to a box and a horizontal beam lateral thoracic

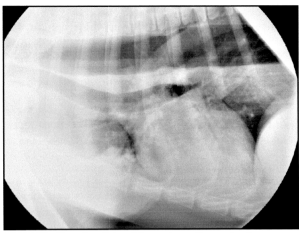

6.2 Standing lateral thoracic radiograph of a 5-year-old Great Dane with suspected megaoesophagus and aspiration pneumonia. A dilated partially fluid-filled oesophagus can be seen dorsally, causing ventral deviation of the trachea. There is an alveolar pattern in the ventral part of the cranial and middle lung lobes. The brachial musculature can be appreciated overlying the cranioventral part of the thorax.

radiograph obtained if lateral recumbency is not possible. Again the information gained will be incomplete, but may be better than nothing!
  - *Decubitus DV/VD view:* This is rarely used, but may be useful to detect a mediastinal mass in the presence of a moderate volume of pleural fluid.
- Ultrasonography greatly assists in determining the presence of pleural fluid or a mediastinal mass.

Restraint
Manual restraint for radiography is not permitted in the UK under the current Ionising Radiations Regulations 1999 (IRR99), unless the radiograph is essential at that time and restraint cannot be achieved in any other way. Judicious use of sandbags and limb ties will often obviate the need for manual restraint and appropriate doses of sedatives may relieve some degree of anxiety-associated tachypnoea. However, general anaesthesia with its additional airway protection may be preferred, particularly if further diagnostic procedures (such as bronchoscopy) are to be performed.

Timing of exposure
Ideally, a radiograph should be taken at full inspiration to provide optimal detail and contrast within the lungs, as expiratory radiographs are considerably less informative than those taken at or near the height of inspiration. In rapidly breathing or panting animals, it may be preferable to take the radiograph during the expiratory pause in order to minimize movement blur due to respiratory motion, but these radiographs will be inferior to the ones taken at full inspiration. In such cases, sedation or (if the patient has non-cardiac disease and is sufficiently stable) general anaesthesia may be preferred to achieve a radiograph of diagnostic quality, and fully inflated views should be obtained. On occasion, it can be difficult to differentiate emphysema from air-trapping on inflated views and in that instance, radiographs taken during expiration can be useful.

Film development
Development should be of optimal quality to provide the maximum range of contrast on the radiograph. If manual processing is used, radiographs may be briefly viewed wet, just to ensure that the study is of diagnostic quality, but should be thoroughly reviewed when dry to ensure best interpretation.

Serial radiographs
Serial radiographs may be taken:

• To assess progression of a disease
• To assess response or lack thereof to treatment
• To reinvestigate if initial findings were equivocal.

Consistency of technique is very important, particularly when repeating radiographs: exposure factors should be the same. In addition, due to the great difference in the appearance of normal lungs between inspiration and expiration, it is pointless to try to compare initial and follow-up films if the degree of lung inflation is different.

Viewing
Viewing should be carried out in an appropriately darkened room, and a spotlight or bright light should be available to allow full assessment of relatively overexposed regions of the radiograph. Sufficient X-ray viewers should be available to enable all radiographs to be displayed at one time; however, uncovered regions of the X-ray viewers should be masked off to provide optimal viewing conditions.

Radiological interpretation
A thoracic radiograph can be daunting to look at due to the wealth of information available. Interpretation should be systematic and thorough to ensure that all structures are assessed.

Normal appearance

• In dogs, there is a wide range of normal variation in the appearance of the thorax, depending on breed, age, body condition, phase of respiration and exposure factors. Thus, interpretation of thoracic radiographs can be very challenging. Normal ageing changes include mineralization of the bronchial walls and development of pulmonary osteomas (osseous metaplasia, calcified pleural plaques), which should not be confused with genuine pathological change, such as metastases.
• The thorax is defined by the thoracic inlet cranially, the diaphragm caudally, the ribs and intercostal muscles laterally, the thoracic vertebrae dorsally and the sternebrae ventrally.
• The thoracic cavity is lined with the pleura and divided into two approximate halves by the mediastinum. The mediastinum contains the heart, trachea, origins of the bronchi, great vessels, oesophagus, thoracic duct, vagus nerves, lymph nodes, venae cavae, azygos vein, thymus (in the developing animal) and several other smaller vessels and nerves.

• The rest of the thoracic cavity comprises the pleural space, which is very small in the normal animal, containing just a small volume of serous fluid to reduce friction during respiration, and the lungs.

Thoracic wall
The thoracic wall comprises the thoracic vertebrae, sternum, ribs, costal cartilages, subcutaneous and intercostal muscles, parietal pleura, fat, skin, lymphatics and blood vessels. There is quite a lot of breed variation in the shape of the thorax, particularly caudally. Mineralization of the costal cartilages occurs very commonly. In cats, mineralization is often interrupted or fragmented, mimicking the appearance of cartilage fracture. In dogs, there can be marked irregular mineralization around the costochondral junctions. Superimposition of these regions on the radiograph can lead to misinterpretation of pulmonary parenchymal disease.

Conditions: Thoracic wall conditions include:

• Congenital and developmental abnormalities
• Trauma
• Rib tumours and infection
• Sternebral tumours and infection
• Soft tissue tumours and infection.

Congenital and developmental abnormalities: Deformities of the sternum, such as sternebral fusion or pectus excavatum ('funnel chest'), are relatively common and alone rarely cause clinical signs. Pectus excavatum and sternal dysraphism may be associated with peritoneal–pericardial–diaphragmatic hernia (PPDH).

Trauma: Radiological signs of minor soft tissue trauma may include focal soft tissue swelling or subcutaneous emphysema. More major trauma can result in tearing of the intercostal muscles and rib fractures. These can be difficult to detect on lateral views due to superimposition.

Rib tumours and infection: Thoracic wall masses are often described as 'iceberg' lesions because the size of the external component of a mass is often much less than its intrathoracic component. A thoracic wall mass which invades the thoracic cavity creates an extrapleural sign. This is a soft tissue opacity associated with the thoracic wall, which has a well defined convex margin facing the lung. The extrapleural sign will only be visible on a radiograph if it is tangential to the primary beam of the X-ray. Identification of an extrapleural sign greatly assists in the diagnosis of thoracic wall masses. Lysis of a rib is common and may be associated with ill defined new bone, with or without a periosteal reaction on adjacent ribs. Focal destruction of a rib is most likely due to neoplastic invasion because rib infections are rare; however, a biopsy is required to confirm the diagnosis. Osteosarcoma and chondrosarcoma (Figure 6.3) are the most common rib tumours. Pleural effusion often occurs in advanced cases; this may obscure the primary lesion, impeding correct diagnosis (Figure 6.4).

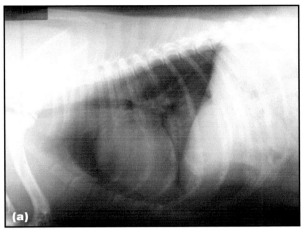

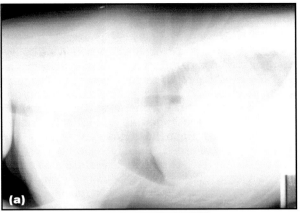

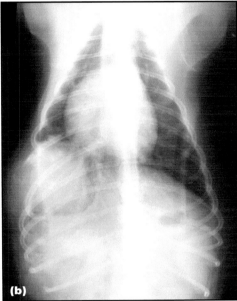

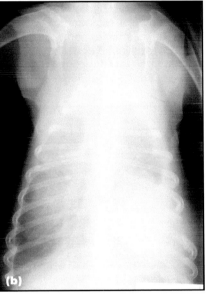

6.3 **(a)** Lateral and **(b)** DV thoracic radiographs of a 7-year-old Labrador with a thoracic wall chondrosarcoma. A large mixed opacity mass is visible on the right 7th rib, causing medial deviation of the right caudal lobe.

6.4 **(a)** Lateral and **(b)** DV thoracic radiographs of a 9-year-old Staffordshire Bull Terrier with a malignant thoracic wall mass. There is a poorly defined increase in soft tissue opacity over the caudal part of the left hemithorax, with destruction of the distal part of the 8th rib. Pleural fissures can be seen on the right side at the sixth and ninth intercostal spaces.

Sternebral tumours and infection: These are uncommon. Sternebral infections may result from external trauma, such as bites or migrating foreign bodies, or following sternotomy.

Soft tissue tumours and infection: Lipoma is the most common soft tissue tumour affecting the thoracic wall, although other mesenchymal tumours can arise, as can tumours of mammary or other skin adnexal origin. Cellulitis is uncommon.

Diaphragm
The diaphragm comprises a thin musculotendinous sheet dividing the thorax and abdomen. It is identified radiographically by virtue of the surrounding structures. It can be seen as a cranially oriented convex curvilinear structure, highlighted by the air-filled lungs on the cranial aspect and silhouetting with the liver on the caudal aspect. Falciform fat often highlights the caudoventral aspect of the diaphragm. Centrally and

ventrally is the cupula, and the two crura extend back dorsally and laterally to insert on the ventral aspect of the third (right) and fourth (left) lumbar vertebrae. The shape of the diaphragm on the DV/VD view varies according to the centring of the X-ray beam.

If diaphragmatic rupture is suspected, a DV view should be obtained first to determine the affected side. The animal should then be positioned on that side to obtain the orthogonal view, thus minimizing respiratory compromise.

Conditions: Diaphragmatic conditions include:

- Hernia
- Rupture.

Hernia: This is defined as herniation of abdominal contents into the thoracic cavity through a congenital defect or pre-existing hole in the diaphragm. Included in this group are PPDH, hiatal hernia, gastro-oesophageal intussusception and peritoneopleural hernia (rare and often associated with umbilical hernia).

PPDH is a congenital disorder in which a defect in the diaphragm results in continuity between the peritoneum and pericardium. Abdominal viscera are displaced into the pericardial sac, resulting in gastrointestinal and/or respiratory signs. These signs may occur at any age, or the condition may remain silent and only be detected as an incidental finding. The liver is most frequently herniated, although the stomach, omentum and small intestine may also be present within the hernia sac. Radiological signs include a large round cardiac silhouette (Figure 6.5) of inhomogenous opacity, with tubular gas lucencies, and dorsal displacement of the trachea. The cardiac silhouette is continuous with the diaphragm; the dorsal peritoneopericardial mesothelial remnant is a valuable aid to diagnosis in the cat. Sternal abnormalities such as dysraphism or pectus excavatum and umbilical hernia may be present. Gastrointestinal contrast studies or echocardiography can confirm the diagnosis.

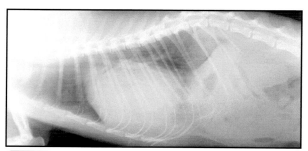

6.5 Lateral thoracic radiograph of a 2-year-old Domestic Shorthaired cat with a PPDH. The cardiac silhouette is enlarged and is confluent with the ventral half of the diaphragm. Within the abdomen, the stomach and transverse colon are displaced cranially.

Hiatal hernia and gastro-oesophageal intussusception have similar radiological signs: soft tissue opacity in the caudodorsal thorax in the position of the oesophagus, adjacent to the left crus; cranial displacement of the cardia and abnormal gastric shape; and a dilated oesophagus. Oesophagography allows differentiation of these two conditions.

Rupture: Traumatic diaphragmatic rupture results in a tear in the diaphragm, usually involving the muscular portion of the diaphragm. The most frequently herniated organs are the liver, small intestine, stomach, spleen and omentum. Radiologically, abdominal organs may be seen within the thorax (most easily seen if the small intestine or stomach have herniated), there is cranial displacement of the remaining organs within the abdomen, loss (partial or complete) of the diaphragmatic outline, and within the thorax, there may be cranial or lateral displacement of the heart and mediastinal structures and pleural fluid (Figure 6.6). Oral administration of barium may allow the identification of displaced gastrointestinal structures. The use of positive contrast peritoneography to identify the break in the parietal peritoneal surface has been superseded by the use of ultrasonography to identify abdominal organs within the thorax.

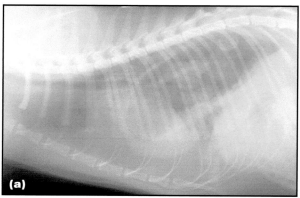

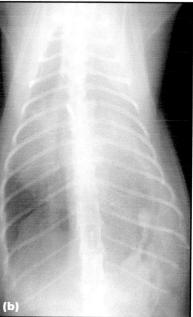

6.6 **(a)** Lateral and **(b)** DV thoracic radiographs of a 2-year-old Domestic Shorthaired cat with diaphragmatic rupture. The outline of the left side of the diaphragm has been lost and the left hemithorax contains mixed opacities, consistent with abdominal contents. The transverse colon is displaced cranially within the abdomen.

Mediastinum

Mediastinal disease is difficult to evaluate clinically, and diagnostic imaging is vital in its detection and assessment. The mediastinum is most easily seen on the DV/VD view as it is a midline structure that divides the thorax into right and left sides. It is continuous with the fascial planes of the neck and the retroperitoneal space in the abdomen. The cranial mediastinum should be no wider than twice the width of the thoracic spine, although it may be wider in obese patients. Ultrasonography or CT may be required to differentiate deposition of fat in the mediastinum from a mass lesion.

Conditions: Mediastinal conditions include:

- Mediastinal shift
- Mediastinal mass
- Mediastinal fluid
- Pneumomediastinum.

Mediastinal shift: This occurs secondary to a change in the volume of one hemithorax. It can only be appreciated on the DV/VD view, and poor positioning and rotation of the patient may result in over or under-detection of mediastinal shift. Decrease in lung volume results in an ipsilateral shift, whereas an increase in lung volume (e.g. unilateral lobar emphysema) or an intrathoracic mass result in a contralateral shift. Mediastinal shift can be a useful sign to differentiate pathological (contralateral shift) from non-pathological (ipsilateral shift) increases in lung opacity.

Mediastinal mass: Causes of a mediastinal mass include neoplasia, abscess, cyst, haematoma, granuloma and lymphadenomegaly. A mediastinal mass may be identified radiologically when it alters the width or shape of the mediastinum, or if it displaces the intrathoracic trachea or cardiac silhouette. Both lateral and DV/VD views should be taken; any soft tissue opacity seen is likely to be mediastinal if it is on or near the midline, if it is in the position of one of the mediastinal reflections, or if it deviates a mediastinal structure (Figure 6.7). Ultrasonography is very useful in determining the nature of a mediastinal mass if there is an appropriate acoustic window, and ultrasound-guided aspiration or biopsy of the mass should allow definitive diagnosis. CT is an excellent tool for assessing the mediastinum, allowing identification of the site of origin of the mass and determining the relationship between the mediastinal mass and the normal mediastinal structures such as vessels.

Mediastinal fluid: Mediastinal fluid (Figure 6.8) alone is uncommon. Causes include trauma, coagulopathy and mediastinal masses. It is most easily seen radiologically on a DV/VD view. The mediastinum appears diffusely widened with a homogenous soft tissue opacity, and reverse fissures may be seen. These are triangular soft tissue opacities extending away from the midline towards the periphery, giving the mediastinum a 'Christmas tree' or 'rose thorn' like appearance (Figure 6.9).

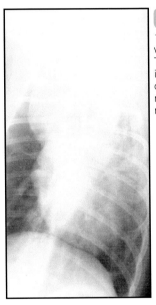

6.8 DV thoracic radiograph of a 1-year-old Golden Retriever with a history of trauma. There is a massive increase in homogenous soft tissue opacity in the cranial mediastinum due to mediastinal fluid.

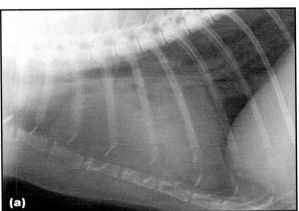

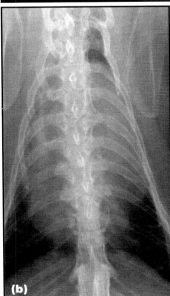

6.7 **(a)** Lateral and **(b)** DV thoracic radiographs of a 6-year-old Domestic Longhaired cat with lymphoma. There is increased soft tissue opacity within the cranial mediastinum, with border effacement of the cranial cardiac silhouette.

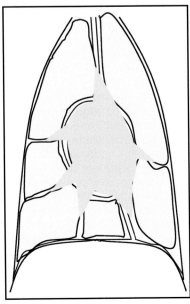

6.9 Position of reverse fissures in patients with a small volume of mediastinal fluid.

Pneumomediastinum: This is free gas within the mediastinum and provides excellent radiographic contrast. Causes include pulmonary trauma without damage to the visceral pleura, extension of gas in the fascial planes of the neck or in the retroperitoneal space into the mediastinum, tracheal or oesophageal perforation, and mediastinal infection with a gas-producing organism. Pneumomediastinum is best seen on a lateral radiograph and appears as an increased radiolucency within the mediastinum, highlighting the serosal surfaces of the mediastinal structures; in particular, the tracheal wall can be appreciated as both luminal and serosal surfaces can be seen. Small volumes of free gas are more difficult to detect and may appear as patchy regions of radiolucency. Clinical signs are uncommon with pneumomediastinum alone, but if it progresses to pneumothorax, respiratory distress is likely. CT is useful in the detection of pneumomediastinum but is rarely required.

Pleural space

The pleural space is a potential space, containing only a small volume of free fluid, between the visceral pleura (covering the pulmonary parenchyma) and the parietal pleura (covering the diaphragm, mediastinum and thoracic wall). Pleural space disease usually results in respiratory difficulty, and both clinical signs and physical examination findings will strongly suggest pleural space disease. Diagnostic imaging with radiography, ultrasonography and/or CT is extremely useful in the investigation of pleural space disease. Normal pleura is not visible radiographically as it is so thin that it does not absorb sufficient X-rays to produce a detectable radiographic opacity.

Conditions: Pleural space conditions include:

- Pleural thickening
- Pleural effusion
- Pneumothorax.

Pleural thickening: In older dogs, the pleura may become thickened perhaps due to fibrosis or previous pleural disease. This may result in it becoming visible radiologically as fine curvilinear radiopacities arcing from the hilus towards the periphery in the position of the interlobar divisions. This thickening is unlikely to be clinically significant.

Pleural effusion: This may be transudate (hydrothorax), chyle (chylothorax), haemorrhage (haemothorax), septic exudates (pyothorax) and non-septic exudates (Figure 6.10). Causes include congestive heart failure (CHF), infection, neoplasia, trauma, hypoproteinaemia, bleeding disorders and inflammatory conditions. Both orthogonal views should be taken, with the DV view being taken first to assess the degree of pleural space disease. If necessary, the orthogonal view should be taken using a horizontal beam in order to avoid having to place the animal in lateral recumbency, which may lead to a deterioration in its condition. Radiological changes include retraction of the lungs from the periphery of the thorax, increased radiopacity around the lungs, widened

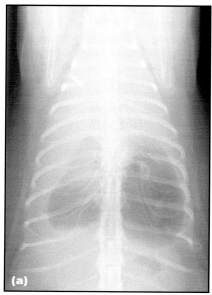

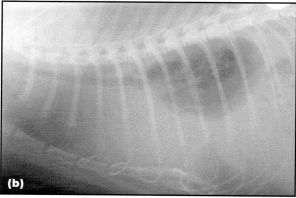

6.10 **(a)** DV and **(b)** lateral thoracic radiographs of a 7-year-old Ragdoll with chylothorax. The lungs are retracted from the periphery of the thorax and there is an overall increase in opacity. The cardiac silhouette and ventral part of the diaphragm are obscured due to the pleural effusion.

and more prominent pleural/interlobar fissures, and border effacement of the cardiac silhouette and diaphragm.

Effusions are usually bilateral and symmetrical but may be unilateral in an animal with an intact mediastinum. Inflammatory effusions, such as pus or chyle, may become localized or unilateral due to occlusion of the mediastinal fenestrations, which may also become occluded by a mass. Chronic or inflammatory effusions often result in extensive fibrosis of the pleura. This can result in marked 'scalloping' or rounding of the lung margins. Small volume effusions are more difficult to identify radiographically and may be more easily identified using ultrasonography. Ultrasonography allows assessment of the pleurae, mediastinum, thoracic wall and diaphragm, and thoracocentesis can be performed under ultrasonographic guidance. In the absence of ultrasonography, radiography can be repeated following thoracocentesis to try to determine the underlying cause of the effusion.

Pneumothorax: The causes of free gas within the pleural space include trauma (both to the thoracic wall and/or to the pulmonary parenchyma, resulting in damage to the visceral pleura), extension of pneumo-mediastinum, and rupture of cavitary lung lesions. Radiological signs of pneumothorax include retraction of the lungs from the periphery of the thorax (surrounded by radiolucency), increased opacity of the lungs due to collapse and apparent elevation of the

cardiac silhouette from the sternum (Figure 6.11). Occasionally, it can be difficult to determine whether the lungs are retracted from the periphery when they are surrounded by radiolucency. In these cases, the radiograph should be examined using a bright light to look for the absence of vascular lung markings extending to the periphery of the thorax. Pneumothorax is usually bilateral and symmetrical but may be unilateral or localized for the same reasons as pleural effusion (see above). The DV view is the most valuable to take initially.

Tension pneumothorax results if there is a one-way valve effect at the site of ingress of pleural space gas, resulting in pleural space pressure exceeding atmospheric pressure during both stages of respiration. This leads to extensive lung collapse, which is potentially fatal without immediate thoracocentesis. Unilateral tension pneumothorax can be recognized on a DV view by the presence of a contralateral mediastinal shift. Bilateral tension pneumothorax may be more difficult to detect due to the absence of mediastinal shift. Caudal displacement or flattening of the diaphragm may be detected to the extent that the costal attachments may be seen.

Pulmonary parenchyma

The pulmonary parenchyma comprises the lobes of the lungs and, apart from air within the alveoli, contains three structures which are normally seen on thoracic radiographs: the walls of the larger bronchi, the pulmonary arteries and veins, and the lung interstitium. In the normal lung, the ratio of air to soft tissue should be high; however, increased soft tissue density may be due to physiological or technical factors rather than pathological change. Underexposure, underdevelopment, underinflation, sedation, prolonged recumbency, obesity and age will all result in increased pulmonary opacification, which may be misinterpreted as pathological change.

The right lung is divided into cranial, middle, caudal and accessory lobes and the left lung is divided into cranial (cranial and caudal parts) and caudal lobes

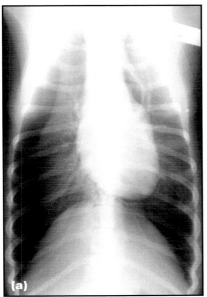

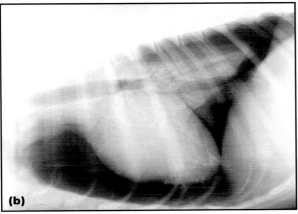

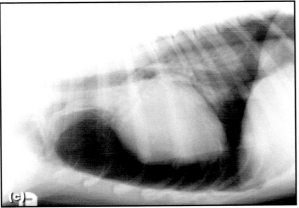

6.11 **(a)** DV, **(b)** right lateral recumbent and **(c)** left lateral recumbent thoracic radiographs of a 10-month-old Rottweiler with bilateral pneumothorax. There is also a small pneumomediastinum. The thymic sail can be seen in the DV view as a triangular soft tissue opacity extending from the midline into the left hemithorax.

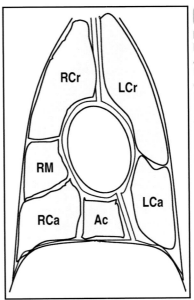

6.12

Position of the lobar divisions. Ac = Accessory lobe; LCa = Left caudal lobe; LCr = Left cranial lobe; RCa = Right caudal lobe; RCr = Right cranial lobe; RM = Right middle lobe.

(Figure 6.12). The pulmonary arteries and veins can be seen on both views. On a well exposed radiograph, the branching, tapering pulmonary vessels should be visible to the periphery of the lung fields. They run parallel to and on either side of the bronchi. On the lateral view, the cranial lobar veins are ventral and the arteries are dorsal to the bronchi; on the DV view, the veins are medial and the arteries are lateral to the bronchi. The vessels should be of equal diameter and should not exceed the width of the proximal part of the 4th rib on the lateral view and of the 9th rib at the level of intersection on the DV view (Figure 6.13).

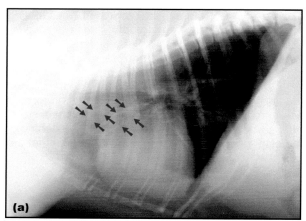

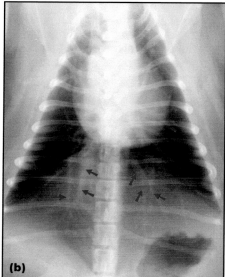

6.13 **(a)** Lateral and **(b)** DV thoracic radiographs demonstrating the normal pulmonary vessels. The veins (blue arrows) are ventral and medial, and the arteries (red arrows) are dorsal and lateral to the corresponding lobar bronchus.

Principles of interpretation: The pulmonary parenchyma must be assessed and interpreted in a consistent and thorough manner. Pattern recognition is frequently used for interpreting changes within the pulmonary parenchyma. The patterns described are alveolar, bronchial, interstitial and vascular. Commonly, more than one pattern is present, but deciding which patterns are present and which is the predominant pattern is useful in determining the cause of the changes (Figure 6.14).

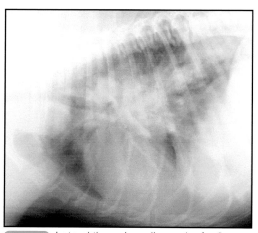

6.14 Lateral thoracic radiograph of a 2-year-old Boxer with a pulmonary infiltrate with eosinophils. There is a marked alveolar pattern, particularly in the perihilar region and the caudal lobes with a lobar sign between the middle and caudal lobes, overlying the cardiac silhouette. There are also bronchial infiltrates and a craniodorsal soft tissue opacity, which most likely represents lymphadenomegaly in the mediastinum.

Alveolar pattern: This term is used to describe radiological changes (Figure 6.15) occurring within the terminal airspaces or alveolar lumina of the lungs when air is replaced by fluid (such as exudate, oedema or haemorrhage) or cells. Loss of air within the alveoli results in a fluffy, ill defined increase in homogenous soft tissue opacity, resulting in border effacement of the pulmonary vessels and bronchial walls. Areas of alveolar pattern may coalesce. Alveolar patterns may be focal, multifocal, restricted to one lobe or generalized. A lobar sign is seen when one lobe is affected and the adjacent lobe is unaffected, resulting in a sharp demarcation between the two lobes. Air bronchograms may be seen when the homogenous soft tissue opacity of the alveolar pattern is interrupted by a tapering, branching, air lucency, consistent with air within the lumen of the bronchi. The differential diagnoses for alveolar patterns are summarized in Figure 6.16.

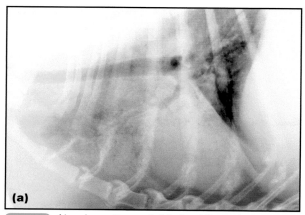

6.15 Alveolar patterns. **(a)** Lateral thoracic radiograph of a 9-year-old Labrador following a road traffic accident. There is a widespread alveolar pattern in the cranial and middle lobes, with air bronchograms clearly visible over the cardiac silhouette. A lobar sign can be appreciated between the middle and caudal lobes. The alveolar pattern is likely to be due to haemorrhage. (continues) ▶

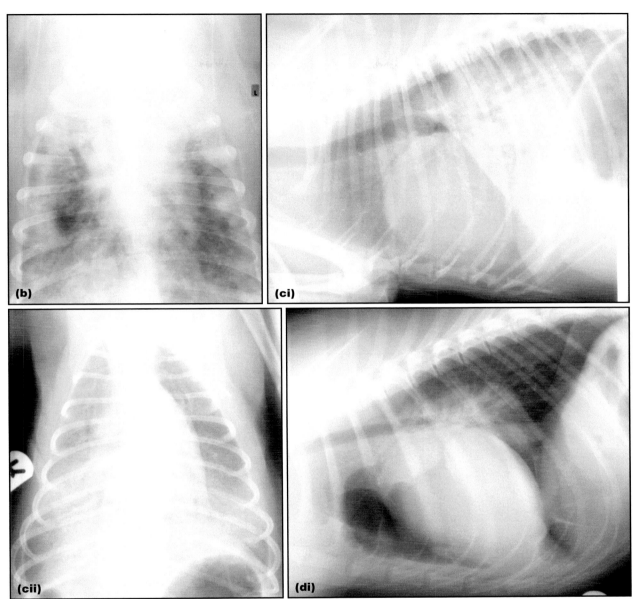

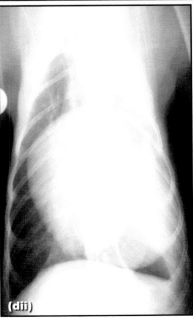

6.15 (continued) Alveolar patterns. **(b)** DV thoracic radiograph of a 3-year-old Mastiff with angiostrongylosis. There is a widespread alveolar pattern throughout the lobes with air bronchograms visible. The cardiac silhouette is partially obscured and there is a lobar sign between the cranial and caudal parts of the left cranial lobe. The alveolar pattern is likely to be due to haemorrhage.
(ci) Lateral and **(cii)** DV thoracic radiographs of an 11-year-old Cavalier King Charles Spaniel with acute CHF. There is a widespread alveolar pattern, particularly in the right caudal lobe with a lobar sign between the middle and caudal lobes. The cardiac silhouette is partially obscured but there is some elevation of the carina. The alveolar pattern is likely due to pulmonary oedema. **(di)** Lateral and **(dii)** DV thoracic radiographs of a 4-year-old Whippet with lung lobe torsion. There is a homogenous increase in soft tissue opacity in the position of the caudal part of the left cranial lobe, with some localized pleural fluid. On the lateral view, the left bronchus cannot be seen over the heart and the lobar shape is abnormally triangular and displaced dorsally. The left crus of the diaphragm is displaced cranially, suggesting some decrease in volume of the left hemithorax.

Cause		Ancillary radiological signs
Bronchopneumonia		Usually localized
Aspiration pneumonia		Usually cranioventral or ventral distribution
Oedema	Cardiogenic	Often perihilar distribution (less so in cats), may be generalized and patchy, responds to diuretic therapy, labile, left atrial enlargement
	Upper respiratory tract obstruction	
	Neurogenic, near-drowning, smoke inhalation, toxic	Usually generalized and patchy
Haemorrhage		Signs of trauma (e.g. fractures) should be looked for
Neoplasia		Lobar distribution
Lobar collapse or atelectasis		Ipsilateral mediastinal shift
Lobar torsion		Usually right middle lobe, pleural fluid, abnormal orientation of bronchus

6.16 Differential diagnoses for alveolar patterns.

Bronchial pattern: This term is used to describe enhancement of the normal bronchial wall pattern seen in the lungs (Figure 6.17). The enhancement may be due to increased thickness or increased opacity of the bronchial walls, resulting in more prominent bronchial wall markings and perhaps extending further into the periphery of the lungs. There may also be changes in shape of the bronchi, for example, in bronchiectasis. The differential diagnoses for bronchial patterns are summarized in Figure 6.18.

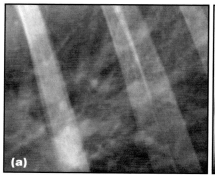
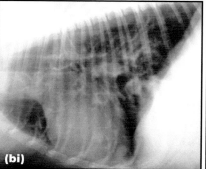
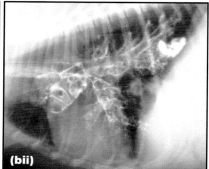
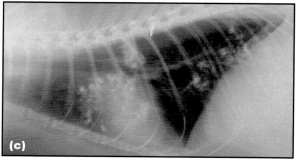

6.17 Bronchial patterns. **(a)** Close up of a lateral thoracic radiograph of a 10-year-old Poodle with a pulmonary infiltrate with eosinophils. There is enhancement and thickening of the bronchial walls. Lateral **(bi)** survey radiograph and **(bii)** bronchogram of a mature Cocker Spaniel with chronic bronchial disease and bronchiectasis. There is marked dilatation and sacculation of the bronchi in all lobes, especially the cranial and middle lobes. Some of the bronchi appear truncated, possibly secondary to mucus plugging. **(c)** Lateral thoracic radiograph of an 8-year-old Domestic Longhaired cat with chronic bronchial disease. There are multiple small, coalescing mineral foci throughout the lungs, consistent with mineralization of the peribronchial mucus glands.

Radiological finding	Cause	Ancillary radiological signs
Bronchial thickening (may be peribronchial infiltrate)	Chronic bronchitis Pulmonary infiltrate with eosinophils Aelurostrongylosis Bronchopneumonia Cardiogenic oedema Neoplasia	
Bronchial mineralization	Age Broncholithiasis (cats) Hyperadrenocorticism	Increased opacity but not thickness
Bronchiectasis	Congenital Chronic bronchitis Chronic pneumonia	Saccular or cylindrical non-tapering bronchial markings

6.18 Differential diagnoses for bronchial patterns.

Interstitial pattern: This can be subdivided into unstructured and nodular interstitial patterns. In both types of pattern, air is still present within the alveoli and it is the interstitium that becomes more prominent. In an unstructured interstitial pattern there is a coarse, diffuse, ill defined increase in fine reticular/linear soft tissue opacities throughout the lungs, superimposed on the normally visible vascular structures (Figure 6.19). A nodular interstitial pattern comprises pulmonary nodules of different sizes and different opacities within the lung (Figure 6.20). Nodules may be solid or cavitated. The centre of a cavitated nodule will only be visible if it contains gas, due to either a necrotic centre or communication with an airway. Air is present within the alveoli, but it may be compressed by the interstitial nodules. The differential diagnoses for interstitial patterns are summarized in Figure 6.21.

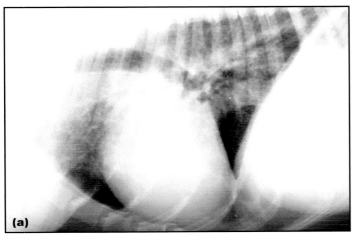
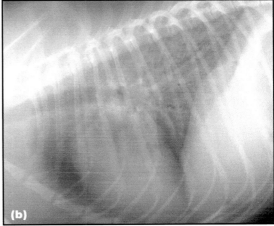

6.19 Unstructured interstitial patterns. **(a)** Lateral thoracic radiograph of a 9-year-old Labrador with lymphosarcoma. There is a diffuse unstructured, honeycomb interstitial pattern throughout the lobes. Fine-needle aspiration confirmed the diagnosis. **(b)** Lateral thoracic radiograph of a 2-year-old Cavalier King Charles Spaniel with *Pneumocystis carinii* infection. There is a marked hazy, unstructured interstitial pattern throughout the lungs. This appearance may be confused with an alveolar pattern as it may be thought that air bronchograms are visible, but the abaxial margins of the lobar vessels are still visible, indicating that the alveoli remain aerated.

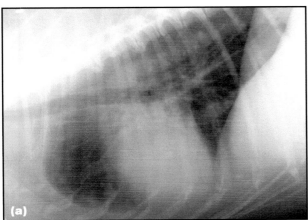
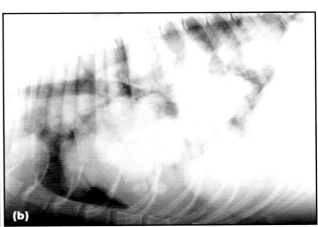
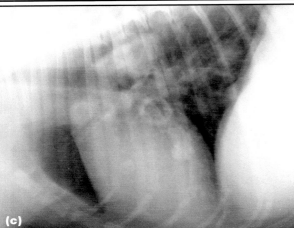

6.20 Nodular interstitial patterns. **(a)** Lateral thoracic radiograph of a 12-year-old Rough Collie bitch with nasal adenocarcinoma. There are multiple, poorly defined soft tissue nodules throughout the lungs, consistent with pulmonary metastases. **(b)** Lateral thoracic radiograph of an 8-year-old Rottweiler with a primary malignant bone tumour. There are multiple, large, soft tissue opacity nodules which summate with one another. In the cranial lobe there is also an alveolar pattern; this may be due to accumulation of secretions, secondary to bronchial obstruction by a perihilar nodule. **(c)** Lateral thoracic radiograph of a 9-year-old Border Terrier with prostatic carcinoma. There are multiple nodules of various sizes and mixed opacities throughout the lung fields, consistent with pulmonary metastases. Some nodules appear solid and others have radiolucent centres.

Unstructured pattern	Nodular pattern	
	Radiopaque	*Radiolucent*
Artefact Interstitial oedema Inflammation Haemorrhage Diffuse neoplasia Disease in transition Chronic respiratory disease Pulmonary thromboembolism Paraquat toxicity Idiopathic pulmonary fibrosis	Neoplasia (primary or secondary) Abscess Granuloma Cyst Haematoma Foreign body	Bulla/bleb Cavitated nodule (neoplasia, abscess, granuloma)

6.21 Differential diagnoses for interstitial patterns.

Vascular pattern: The causes and radiological signs of vascular patterns are summarized in Figure 6.22. Vascular patterns may be hypervascular (enhancement, enlargement or increased tortuosity of the normal vascular pattern; Figure 6.23) or hypovascular (attenuation of the normal vascular pattern; Figure 6.24).

Having identified an abnormality within the pulmonary parenchyma on a thoracic radiograph, steps must be taken to determine its nature, location and severity (Figure 6.25). A differential diagnosis list can then be devised.

Pattern	Vessels affected	Causes	Additional radiological signs
Hypervascular	Both	Left-to-right shunt (VSD, PDA)	Enlarged LA, LV, MPA ± RV
		Iatrogenic fluid overload	Generalized cardiomegaly
	Veins >> arteries	Cardiac disease: mitral regurgitation	Enlarged LA ± LV
		Cardiac disease: primary myocardial dysfunction	Enlarged LA ± LV
		Non-cardiac disease: left atrial obstruction	
	Arteries >> veins	Dirofilariasis	Enlarged MPA ± RV and RA; PA truncation
		Pulmonary thromboembolism	PA truncation and pruning
		Pulmonary hypertension secondary to severe chronic lung disease	Enlarged MPA, RV ± RA
Hypovascular Differential diagnoses include air-trapping, overinflation and overexposure	Both	Right-to-left shunt (ToF, reverse PDA)	Enlarged RV ± RA
		Pulmonic stenosis	Enlarged RV ± RA and MPA bulge
		Hypovolaemia	Microcardia

6.22 Abnormal pulmonary vessel patterns. LA = Left atrium; LV = Left ventricle; MPA = Main pulmonary artery; PA = Pulmonary artery; PDA = Patent ductus arteriosus; RA = Right atrium; RV = Right ventricle; ToF = Tetralogy of Fallot; VSD = Ventricular septal defect.

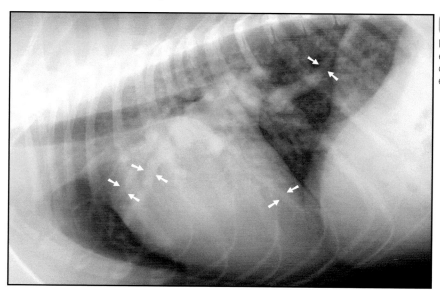

6.23 Lateral thoracic radiograph of a 3-year-old Standard Poodle with PDA. All lobar vessels are enlarged (arrowed) due to over-circulation of the lungs. There is an enlarged LA.

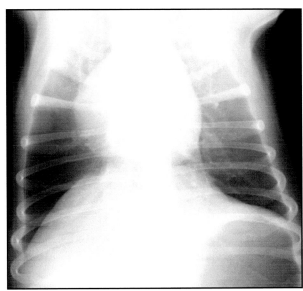

6.24 DV thoracic radiograph of a 6-year-old Shar Pei with pulmonary thromboembolism secondary to renal disease. The right caudal lung lobe is hyperlucent with only thready vessels visible within it.

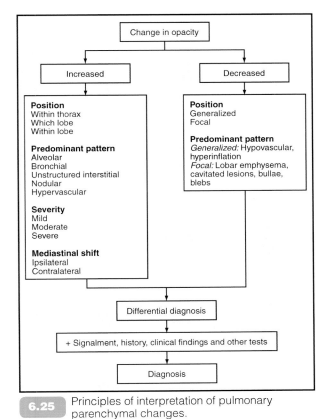

```
                    Change in opacity
                          |
         +----------------+----------------+
         |                                 |
     Increased                         Decreased
         |                                 |
+----------------+              +---------------------+
| Position       |              | Position            |
| Within thorax  |              | Generalized         |
| Which lobe     |              | Focal               |
| Within lobe    |              |                     |
|                |              | Predominant pattern |
| Predominant    |              | Generalized: Hypo-  |
| pattern        |              | vascular,           |
| Alveolar       |              | hyperinflation      |
| Bronchial      |              | Focal: Lobar        |
| Unstructured   |              | emphysema,          |
| interstitial   |              | cavitated lesions,  |
| Nodular        |              | bullae,             |
| Hypervascular  |              | blebs               |
|                |              +---------------------+
| Severity       |
| Mild           |
| Moderate       |
| Severe         |
|                |
| Mediastinal    |
| shift          |
| Ipsilateral    |
| Contralateral  |
+----------------+
         |                                 |
         +----------------+----------------+
                          |
                 Differential diagnosis
                          |
   + Signalment, history, clinical findings and other tests
                          |
                      Diagnosis
```

6.25 Principles of interpretation of pulmonary parenchymal changes.

Cardiovascular system

Although echocardiography is the most important imaging modality for diagnosing primary cardiac disease, radiography remains a vital complementary tool for assessing the cardiac silhouette. Ideally both right lateral recumbent and DV thoracic radiographs should be taken. Radiography is also useful for assessing the development of CHF and monitoring the progression of disease or response to treatment.

Normal radiological anatomy: The borders of the cardiac silhouette comprise the different chambers of the heart and great vessels. On the DV view, the cardiac silhouette can be visualized as a clock face (Figure 6.26). There is quite a wide range of heart shapes and sizes, depending on breed. Barrel-chested breeds, such as spaniels, have hearts with more sternal contact which appear oval on the DV view; narrow, deep-chested breeds, such as Dobermanns, have

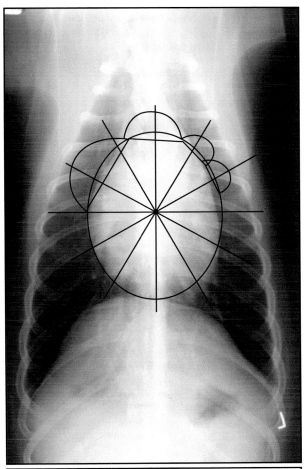

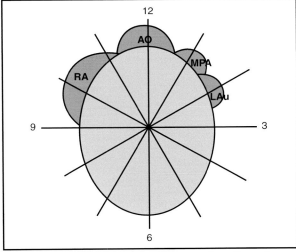

6.26 Clock face analogy of the cardiac silhouette on a DV or VD view. The location of dilatation of the left auricular appendage (LAu), main pulmonary artery (MPA), aorta (AO) and right atrium (RA) are shown.

47

upright hearts which appear relatively small and circular on the DV view. The cardiac silhouette is more uniform in the cat and occupies relatively less of the thoracic cavity. In older cats the angle between the long axis of the heart and the sternum reduces, which can lead to errors in measurement.

Cardiac size

Dogs:
Lateral view: the heart should occupy two-thirds the height of the thorax and its width should be 2.5–3.5 intercostal spaces.
DV view: the heart should occupy two-thirds the width of the thorax at its widest point.

Cats:
Lateral view: the heart should occupy half to two-thirds the height of the thorax and its width (perpendicular to the long axis) should be 2–2.5 intercostal spaces.

Vertebral heart scale system
The maximal dimensions of the long and short axes of the heart are measured against the mid-thoracic vertebrae, starting at the cranial edge of the fourth vertebra. The sum of the long and short axes is 9.7 ± 0.5 for normal adult dogs and 7.5 ± 0.3 for normal adult cats (Figure 6.27). Some breed specific ranges have been determined.

Cardiac measurement is most useful if performed on serial radiographs of a single animal, as it allows appreciation of changes over time; it is a fairly coarse method for assessing and drawing any conclusions about the heart in a single study.

- The global heart size and shape should be assessed in combination with the great vessels and pulmonary circulation.
- The caudal vena cava varies in size markedly according to the phase of the respiratory or cardiac cycle. In the normal animal, it should be parallel to or taper towards the diaphragm, and its diameter should not exceed the height of the body of the fifth or sixth thoracic vertebra.
- The aorta and caudal vena cava are approximately equal in diameter and the caudal vena cava should never exceed 1.5 times the diameter of the aorta.
- The main pulmonary artery is not normally visible as a separate structure. If enlarged, it may be identified as a focal bulge at the 1–2 o'clock position on a DV radiograph (see Figure 6.26).

Increased cardiac size: An increase in cardiac silhouette size may be due to:

- Specific chamber enlargement
- Generalized cardiomegaly
- Pericardial effusion.

Specific chamber enlargement:

- *Left atrium (LA):* This is the most frequent cardiac abnormality identified. Enlargement is almost exclusively due to dilatation. Causes include mitral regurgitation, patent ductus arteriosis (PDA), ventricular septal defect (VSD), dilated cardiomyopathy (DCM) and hypertrophic cardiomyopathy (HCM). On the lateral view there is straightening of the caudal cardiac border, increased height of the heart, elevation of the carina and splitting of the mainstem bronchi. On the DV view, the mainstem bronchi are separated at a greater angle and there may be increased opacity of the cardiac silhouette in the midline. The left auricular appendage (LAu) may be visible as a focal bulge at the 2–3 o'clock position (Figure 6.28).
- *Left ventricle (LV):* Eccentric hypertrophy and dilatation of the LV, usually due to increased preload, may lead to radiologically detectable enlargement. Causes include mitral regurgitation, PDA and DCM. The cardiac silhouette appears taller, with elevation of the trachea on the lateral view, and the left heart border and apex may be more rounded on the DV view (Figure 6.29).

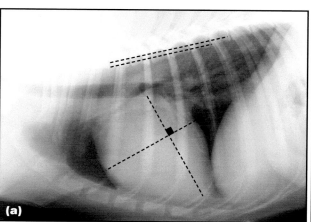 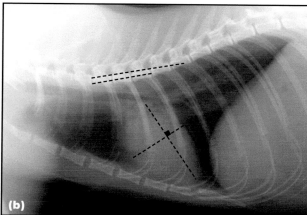

6.27 Vertebral heart scale. **(a)** Canine. **(b)** Feline.

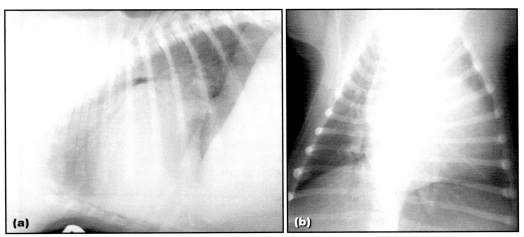

6.28 **(a)** Lateral and **(b)** DV thoracic radiographs of a 19-week-old Bulldog with mitral dysplasia. There is marked elevation of the carina, straightening of the caudal cardiac border and tenting of the LA. On the DV view there is a bulge at the 2–3 o'clock position in the location of the LAu, and splitting of the mainstem bronchi. There is an increased opacity overlying the cupula of the diaphragm, consistent with a massively enlarged LA.

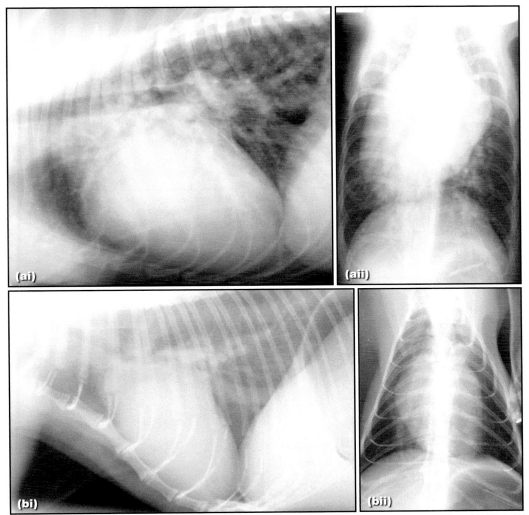

6.29 **(ai)** Lateral and **(aii)** DV thoracic radiographs of a 3-year-old Standard Poodle with PDA. There is an increase in height of the cardiac silhouette with elevation of the caudal trachea and carina, increased sternal contact, straightening of the caudal cardiac border and some tenting of the LA. The apex is displaced markedly to the right on the DV view and there is a bulge at the 2–3 o'clock position, consistent with an enlarged LAu. The lungs have a hypervascular pattern. **(bi)** Lateral and **(bii)** DV thoracic radiographs of a 17-year-old Domestic Shorthaired cat with HCM. The cardiac silhouette is more rectangular and less egg-shaped than normal. On the DV view, the heart is wider than normal and has bulges on its cranial border consistent with atrial enlargement. There is a diffuse unstructured interstitial pattern, which could be consistent with mild pulmonary oedema.

- *Right atrium (RA):* Enlargement of the RA to the degree that it is radiologically detectable is unusual. The most frequent cause is tricuspid dysplasia, although pulmonic stenosis and pulmonary hypertension may lead to right atrial enlargement if severe enough. On the lateral view a bulge may be identified on the craniodorsal aspect of the cardiac silhouette, and on the DV view there may be a bulge from the 9–11 o'clock position.
- *Right ventricle (RV):* The commonest causes of right ventricular enlargement are pulmonic stenosis, pulmonary hypertension and dirofilariasis, although other congenital defects

(especially tricuspid dysplasia) may cause enlargement of the RV. On the lateral view there is increased sternal contact and rounding of the cranial cardiac border, and on the DV view there is rounding of the right cardiac border (giving the heart a reverse 'D' shaped appearance) and an apex shift to the left (Figure 6.30).

Generalized cardiomegaly: Different combinations of chamber enlargement or even enlargement of all four chambers may develop as a result of myocardial disease or due to progression of any cardiac disease (Figure 6.31).

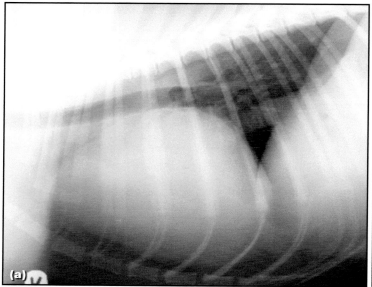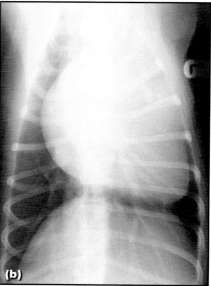

6.30 **(a)** Lateral and **(b)** DV thoracic radiographs of a 1-year-old Golden Retriever with tricuspid dysplasia and atrial septal defect. The cardiac silhouette is enlarged with markedly increased sternal contact, rounding of the cranial cardiac border and elevation of the trachea cranial to the carina. The craniocaudal width of the heart is five intercostal spaces. On the DV view, the apex of the heart is displaced to the left and the heart has a reverse 'D' shaped appearance. The caudal vena cava is widened and tapers towards the cardiac silhouette, suggesting increased systemic venous pressures.

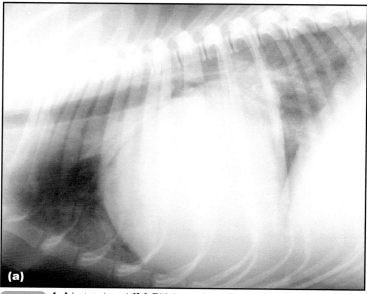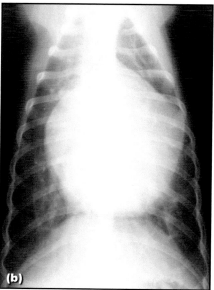

6.31 **(a)** Lateral and **(b)** DV thoracic radiographs of a 3-year-old German Shepherd Dog with DCM. The cardiac silhouette is of increased height and width, with elevation of the trachea and carina, straightening of the caudal and rounding of the cranial cardiac borders. On the DV view, the right lateral border is rounded and there is a bulge at the 2–3 o'clock position, consistent with enlargement of the LAu.

Pericardial effusion: Causes of pericardial effusion include neoplasia, idiopathic, left atrial rupture, haemorrhage, infection, right-sided heart failure and chronic uraemia. In cats, cardiomyopathy and feline infectious peritonitis (FIP) are the most common causes. There is enlargement of the cardiac silhouette with rounding and loss of the normal cardiac margins. The cardiac silhouette appears globular on both views and will often appear distinct as there is no motion artefact (Figure 6.32). Cardiac tamponade may develop, leading to signs associated with right-sided heart failure.

Survey radiography is a fairly insensitive and non-specific modality for evaluation of the heart unless abnormalities are pronounced, and the cardiac silhouette may be normal in the presence of profound cardiac disease. Concentric hypertrophy and mild chamber enlargement will not be detected.

Congestive heart failure: Increased filling pressures in the left side of the heart leading to left-sided heart failure results in pulmonary venous hypertension. This may progress to transudation of fluid into the interstitium and then into the alveoli. These changes present a continuum of radiological changes: initially a pulmonary venous hypervascular pattern will be seen, then a hazy interstitial pattern, progressing to an alveolar pattern, which is frequently generalized but patchy (Figure 6.33). Radiological signs of right-sided heart failure include pleural effusion, caudal vena cava dilatation and abdominal changes such as ascites and hepatosplenomegaly (see Figures 6.30 and 6.32).

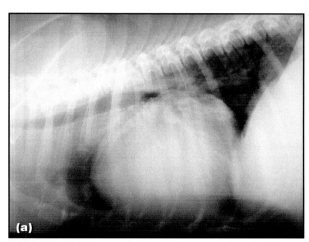

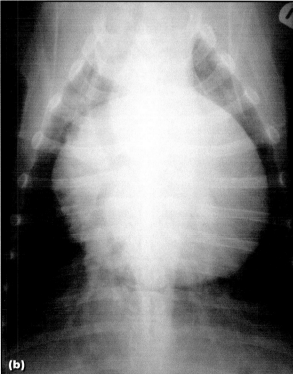

6.32 **(a)** Lateral and **(b)** DV radiographs of a 10-year-old Rottweiler with a haemorrhagic pericardial effusion secondary to a right atrial mass. The cardiac silhouette is enlarged with a globoid appearance. There is rounding of all borders with no discrete bulges. The caudal vena cava is enlarged and ascites is present. A splenic mass was detected on abdominal ultrasonography and a presumptive diagnosis of haemangiosarcoma was made. (Courtesy of S. Dennis.)

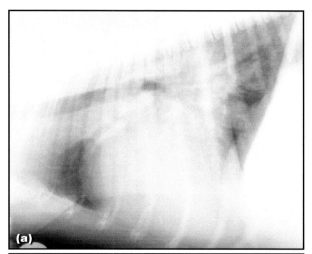

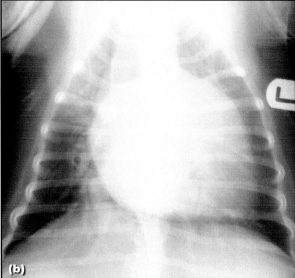

6.33 **(a)** Lateral and **(b)** DV thoracic radiographs of an 11-year-old Jack Russell Terrier with mitral insufficiency in CHF. There is gross generalized cardiomegaly with an ill defined fluffy increase in opacity in the perihilar region. The pulmonary veins are enlarged relative to the arteries; this is particularly visible in the right caudal lobe.

Microcardia: Overall reduction in cardiac size is seen in hypovolaemic states as a consequence of reduced venous return. The cardiac silhouette appears more pointed and there is a hypovascular pulmonary pattern (Figure 6.34).

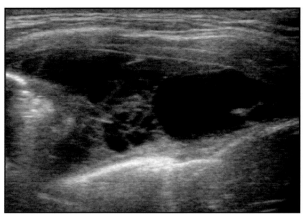

6.35 Transverse plane ultrasonogram of the thorax in a 12-year-old Domestic Shorthaired cat with pleural effusion secondary to neoplasia. The effusion is anechoic and loculated. The hyperechoic interfaces indicate the pleural surfaces of the collapsed lung.

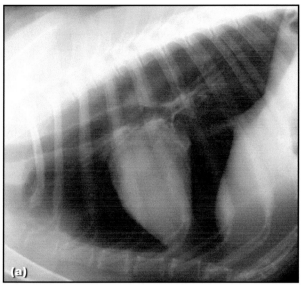
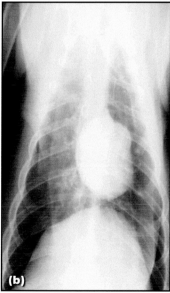

6.34 **(a)** Lateral and **(b)** DV thoracic radiographs of a 6-year-old German Shepherd Dog with hypoadrenocorticism. The cardiac silhouette is greatly reduced in size with the apex just contacting the sternum, and has an abnormal pointed shape. The lung fields appear relatively hyperlucent and the pulmonary vessels are thready.

Indications for advanced imaging

Thoracic radiography is an important first choice when imaging the small animal with respiratory signs, but other imaging modalities may be required. Ultrasonography is invaluable in cases with pleural fluid (Figure 6.35) for assessing consolidated lung that is in contact with the parietal pleura. It is also useful for interventional techniques such as fine-needle aspiration or biopsy. CT is also highly useful for investigation of intrathoracic disease (see Chapter 7).

References and further reading

Bahr RJ (2007) Heart and pulmonary vessels. In: *Textbook of Veterinary Diagnostic Radiology, 5th edn*, ed. DE Thrall, pp. 568–590. WB Saunders, Philadelphia
Bavegems V, Val Caelenberg A, Duchateau L, Sys SU, Van Bree H and De Rick A (2005) Vertebral heart size ranges specific for whippets. *Veterinary Radiology and Ultrasound* **46**, 400–403
Berry CR, Graham JP and Thrall DE (2007) Interpretation paradigms for the small animal thorax. In: *Textbook of Veterinary Diagnostic Radiology, 5th edn*, ed. DE Thrall, pp. 462–485. WB Saunders, Philadelphia
Buchanan JW and Bucheler J (1995) Vertebral scale system to measure canine heart size in radiographs. *Journal of the American Veterinary Medical Association* **206**, 194–199
Kneller SK (2007) Larynx pharynx and trachea. In: *Textbook of Veterinary Diagnostic Radiology, 5th edn*, ed. DE Thrall, pp. 486–489. WB Saunders, Philadelphia
Kraetschmer S, Ludwig K, Meneses F, Nolte I and Simon D (2008) Vertebral heart scale in the beagle dog. *Journal of Small Animal Practice* **49**, 540–543
Lamb CR (2007) The canine and feline lung. In: *Textbook of Veterinary Diagnostic Radiology, 5th edn*, ed. DE Thrall, pp. 591–608. WB Saunders, Philadelphia
Lamb CR, Wikeley H, Boswood A and Pfeiffer DU (2001) Use of breed-specific ranges for the vertebral heart scale as an aid to the radiographic diagnosis of cardiac disease in dogs. *Veterinary Record* **148**, 707–711
Litster AL and Buchanan JW (2000) Vertebral scale system to measure heart size in radiographs of cats. *Journal of the American Veterinary Medical Association* **216**, 210–214
Park RD (2007) The diaphragm. In: *Textbook of Veterinary Diagnostic Radiology, 5th edn*, ed. DE Thrall, pp. 525–540. WB Saunders, Philadelphia
Prather AB, Berry CA and Thrall DE (2005) Use of radiography in combination with computed tomography for the assessment of non-thoracic disease in the dog and cat. *Veterinary Radiology and Ultrasound* **46**, 114–122
Samii VF (2007) The thoracic wall. In: *Textbook of Veterinary Diagnostic Radiology, 5th edn*, ed. DE Thrall, pp. 512–524. WB Saunders, Philadelphia
Schwarz T and Johnson V (2008) *BSAVA Manual of Canine and Feline Thoracic Imaging.* BSAVA Publications, Gloucester
Smallwood JE and Spaulding KA (2007) Radiographic anatomy of the cardiopulmonary system. In: *Textbook of Veterinary Diagnostic Radiology, 5th edn*, ed. DE Thrall, pp. 486–488. WB Saunders, Philadelphia
Thrall DE (2007) The mediastinum and the pleural space. In: *Textbook of Veterinary Diagnostic Radiology, 5th edn*, ed. DE Thrall, pp. 541–554, pp. 555–567. WB Saunders, Philadelphia

7

Advanced imaging

Erik R. Wisner and Eric G. Johnson

Introduction

Although conventional radiographic examination continues to play a central role in the initial diagnostic imaging evaluation of cardiorespiratory disorders, newer imaging modalities including ultrasonography, computed tomography (CT) and magnetic resonance imaging (MRI) are becoming increasingly important for more enhanced documentation of disease and for improved therapeutic planning and monitoring. Although these advanced imaging technologies are often not directly accessible to the general practitioner, it is important to have an understanding of the clinical uses for these imaging modalities and to recognize when referral for such studies is indicated.

Fluoroscopy

The basis of X-ray fluoroscopic image production is similar to that of conventional radiography; however, fluoroscopy employs an image intensifier or a digital flat panel detector to produce a dynamic radiographic image of the patient. Although the spatial resolution (as defined by the size of the smallest structure unequivocally recognized on an image) is typically inferior to that of conventional radiographs, fluoroscopy provides superior functional information in addition to anatomical diagnostic information.

Applications

Tracheobronchial collapse

A common use of fluoroscopy is to confirm tracheobronchial collapse in the dog (Macready *et al.*, 2007). Historically, fluoroscopy was considered superior to inspiratory and expiratory radiographs for diagnosis of this disorder because the dynamic nature of fluoroscopy afforded an opportunity to capture transient collapse during the induction of a cough or rapid forced expiration (Figure 7.1). However, with the recent introduction of digital radiographic equipment into many veterinary hospitals, the comparative value of fluoroscopy for this purpose has diminished since digital radiography allows near instantaneous image production.

Functional diaphragmatic disorders

Diaphragmatic dysfunction in the form of hemiplegia or paralysis can occur due to injury or disease of the phrenic nerve. In affected patients, stasis of one or

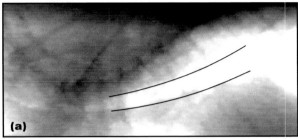

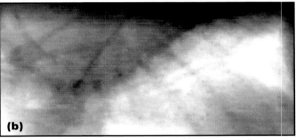

7.1 **(a)** Fluoroscopic image of the thorax of a dog in lateral recumbency during end-inspiration. The head is to the left of the image. The curvilinear black lines define the dorsal and ventral margins of the intrathoracic trachea. **(b)** Fluoroscopic image at end-expiration during induction of a cough, revealing complete collapse of the intrathoracic trachea.

both diaphragmatic crura may be evident on fluoroscopic examination during normal resting respiration. To evaluate both sides of the diaphragm adequately, diaphragmatic motion should be observed fluoroscopically with the patient positioned in both left and right lateral recumbency. The affected crus will demonstrate paradoxical movement, shifting cranially on inspiration and caudally on expiration, due to the relative decrease or increase in intrathoracic pressure, respectively, during the respiratory cycle. In addition, due to the loss of muscular tone, the affected crus will generally be displaced cranially by the abdominal viscera.

Localization of thoracic masses

Fluoroscopy can be used to distinguish between a peripheral pulmonary and a thoracic wall mass when findings from thoracic radiographs are not definitive. Pulmonary masses that are not adherent to the parietal pleura will move independently of the thoracic wall during normal respiration when viewed fluoroscopically.

Guidance for invasive procedures

Fluoroscopy can be used for image guidance during aspiration or biopsy of a pulmonary mass or thoracic wall mass. Such procedures require particular skill and experience, and are not without risk to the patient. Fluoroscopy is also used to guide more complex minimally invasive therapeutic procedures, for example, tracheal stent placement in patients with a collapsing trachea or coil embolization in patients with patent ductus arteriosus.

Computed tomography and magnetic resonance imaging

Computed tomography

For a CT scan, the patient is placed on a scanning bed that is drawn through the CT gantry whilst an X-ray tube and a series of electronic X-ray detectors rotate around the patient. A series of cross-sectional images is generated based on tissue density differences: dense bone appears white; gas appears black; and soft tissues, fluid and fat have intermediate shades of grey. The cross-sectional nature of CT images eliminates ambiguity due to anatomical superimposition and provides superior contrast resolution compared with conventional radiography. Depending on the sophistication of the CT scanner, imaging data can also be reformatted into any anatomical plane.

CT is particularly useful for evaluation of upper and lower respiratory tract disorders, pulmonary vascular disorders and for lesions of the mediastinum, thoracic wall and diaphragm. Although CT can also be used for examination of the heart, cardiac motion limits its utility and other imaging modalities such as echocardiography are often more diagnostically useful.

The anaesthetized patient is placed in sternal recumbency with the head positioned toward the CT gantry. Time should be taken to position the patient symmetrically, since even minor patient obliquity can result in diagnostic ambiguity. For imaging of the thorax, 3–7 mm collimated axial images are obtained from the thoracic inlet through the cranial abdomen using a single forced breath-hold technique. The patient is hyperventilated to suspend voluntary respiration during the acquisition. The patient is manually maintained in full inspiration at a pressure of approximately 15 cmH$_2$0 throughout the acquisition. All studies are acquired in 60 seconds or less. Additional thinly collimated images are acquired as needed through selected areas of interest, and contrast-enhanced CT is used on a case-by-case basis.

Magnetic resonance imaging

Unlike conventional radiography and CT, MRI relies on differences in the chemical properties of the soft tissues for image formation. Important practical factors to be aware of in regard to cardiorespiratory imaging are that air and dense bone contribute very little to the image formation and, in fact, can induce artefacts that degrade image quality. In addition, physiological motion (such as cardiac contractions or respiration) markedly degrades image quality and can lead to non-diagnostic studies.

There are few reports of the use of MRI for cardiopulmonary diagnostic evaluation in veterinary medicine. It can be used for the evaluation of mediastinal masses and for pulmonary thromboembolism detection; however, these studies are not routinely performed in veterinary medicine. The impediments of cardiac and respiratory motion, the interference of intrapulmonary air with image formation, and the readily available alternatives of radiography, ultrasonography and CT, limit the practical use of MRI for cardiopulmonary diagnostics at this time.

Applications

Lower respiratory tract disorders

A large body of literature is devoted to the characterization of pulmonary disease using high-resolution, thin-section CT in human medicine. It is tempting to adopt this terminology to describe characteristic lung patterns of specific diseases seen on CT images from veterinary patients. However, because the sub-gross anatomy of the dog and cat differs from that of humans, specifically in regard to the absence of well formed interlobular septa and the greater degree of alveolar collateral ventilation, some patterns described for humans may appear different or may not exist in veterinary patients, and caution should be used in applying these terms.

Bronchial disease in dogs: Radiographic findings of uncomplicated infectious and non-infectious bronchitis in dogs can be subtle; however, CT findings of bronchial wall thickening due to inflammatory airway disease are often more evident due to the inherent cross-sectional nature of the images (Figure 7.2). Often even small peripheral airways can be seen due to the lack of tissue superimposition.

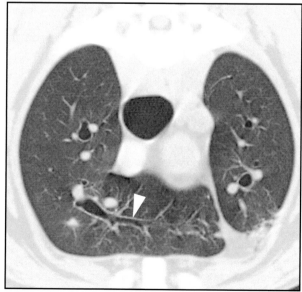

7.2 Transverse CT image of a dog with bronchitis acquired at the level of the cranial lung lobes. The bronchial walls are thickened (arrowhead) and are easily followed out to the lung periphery. There is a focal alveolar pattern present in the dependent region of the left cranial lung lobe indicative of focal bronchopneumonia.

Feline airway disease: Cats with chronic inflammatory airway disease can show radiographic evidence of hyperinflation from expiratory air-trapping, bronchial wall thickening with bronchial lumen narrowing or occlusion from consolidated bronchial wall secretions, and increased interstitial lung density. Other findings may include lobar collapse and occasionally bronchiectasis. These findings are more clearly delineated on CT images and the extent of disease is more readily apparent (Figure 7.3).

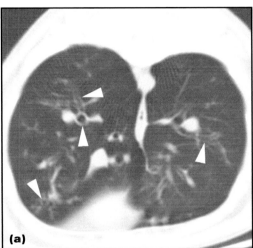

(a)

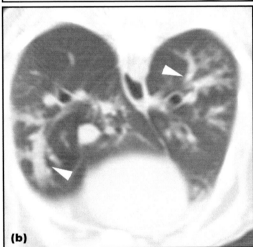

(b)

7.3 **(a)** Transverse CT image of a cat with chronic airway disease acquired at the level of the caudal lung lobes. The airways are prominent and the walls are uniformly thickened (arrowheads).
(b) Transverse CT image of another cat with chronic inflammatory airway disease acquired at the level of the caudal lung lobes. The branching linear opacities (arrowheads) represent bronchi occluded with inspissated bronchial secretions.

Bronchiectasis: This is the irreversible dilatation of airways secondary to loss of support in the bronchial wall. Bronchiectasis is more easily recognized on CT images than on conventional radiographs. In humans, bronchiectasis is recognized on CT images by a ratio of bronchial lumen to pulmonary artery diameter that exceeds 1:1. In normal dogs, it appears that the ratio of bronchial lumen to pulmonary artery diameter should not exceed 2.0. Bronchiectasis appears on CT

images as dilatation of the bronchi (Figure 7.4), often associated with sacculation and tortuosity. Smaller airways in the peripheral subpleural lung regions, which are not normally visible, can also be seen due to increased luminal diameter. Architectural alterations in the bronchi are often associated with pulmonary consolidation due to overlying bronchopneumonia.

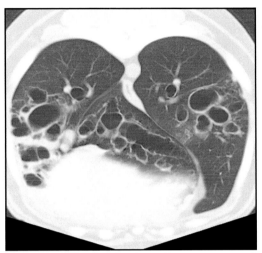

7.4 CT image of a dog with severe generalized bronchiectasis acquired at the level of the caudal and accessory lung lobes. The large circular thick-walled lucencies in the caudal lobes represent markedly dilated bronchi in cross-section. Centrally a large bronchus is seen in long axis. This bronchus is markedly enlarged and sacculated.

Interstitial disorders: The list of disorders producing interstitial infiltrates is long, and in many instances CT may not provide any additional information beyond what is gleaned from conventional thoracic radiographs. Diffuse interstitial disease can result in a 'ground-glass' pattern on CT images (Figure 7.5),

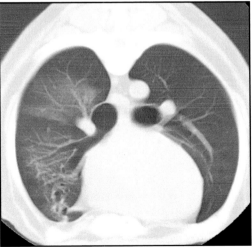

7.5 CT image of a dog with a large primary lung tumour involving the right caudal lung lobe. The mass is not seen in this CT slice but there is a regional increase in pulmonary opacity in the right caudal lobe (dorsally) and right middle lobe (ventrally) due to peritumoral oedema. This is typical of an interstitial 'ground-glass' opacity that results in an increase in pulmonary density but does not obscure vascular and bronchial wall margins.

which is loosely defined as an increased interstitial opacity that fails to obscure the underlying vascular anatomy. Common causes include oedema and inflammatory interstitial infiltrates. Pulmonary fibrosis can also produce an increased interstitial pulmonary opacity that may be regionally diffuse or focal (Johnson *et al.*, 2005). The specific appearance on CT images depends on the cause and extent of the fibrosis.

Alveolar disorders: Alveolar infiltrates can be the result of fulminant oedema, inflammatory disease involving the bronchoalveolar compartment, haemorrhage or neoplasia, and must be differentiated from simple atelectasis. Although alveolar infiltrates can usually be identified on conventional radiographs, CT provides a better understanding of the extent and distribution of disease and can be useful in identifying other relevant abnormalities such as bronchial foreign bodies. Distribution of alveolar infiltrates depends on the inciting disorder.

Cardiogenic oedema will typically be centred on the hilar region in dogs but is often asymmetrically distributed in cats. Non-cardiogenic oedema is also variable in distribution but is often most prominent in the caudodorsal lung fields. Alveolar infiltrates from bronchopneumonia are typically most pronounced in the dependent regions of the lung (Figure 7.6).

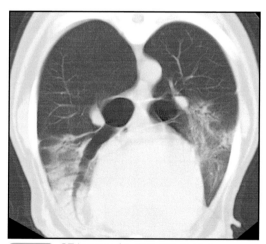

7.6 CT image of a dog with bronchopneumonia. The prominent increased opacity in the right ventral thorax represents an alveolar pattern due to consolidation within the right middle lung lobe. Branching air bronchograms can be seen. A similar but less defined pattern is also present ventrally in the caudal segment of the left cranial lung lobe.

The distribution of pulmonary haemorrhage is also unpredictable but can be asymmetrical and, when due to anticoagulant toxicity, may be associated with mediastinal haemorrhage. Although lung tumours usually appear as a discrete mass, primary lung carcinomas and invasive secondary neoplasms (such as haemangiosarcomas) may infiltrate the bronchoalveolar compartment, resulting in alveolar infiltrates peripheral to the tumour. Neoplastic infiltrates due to histiocytic sarcoma can be very ambiguous and often appear as ill defined alveolar infiltrates on conventional radiographs. These infiltrates can be mistaken

for simple bronchopneumonia with conventional radiography; however, mass lesions are more readily identified using CT.

Focal and multifocal pulmonary lesions: CT is of diagnostic value for identifying focal mass lesions including cysts, granulomas, abscesses or neoplasms that might not be clearly differentiated using conventional radiography or other imaging techniques. Bullae and abscesses can contain both gas and fluid and typically appear as a thin- to thick-walled cavitary lesion on contrast-enhanced CT images (Figure 7.7).

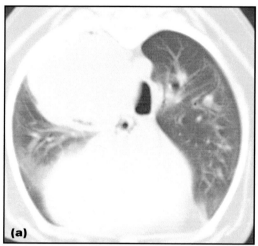

(a)

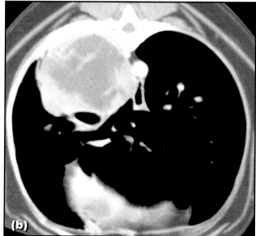

(b)

7.7 Contrast-enhanced CT images of a large spherical mass in the right caudal lung lobe viewed using soft tissue settings. **(a)** A small volume of gas was seen along the dorsal and ventral rim of this mass when viewed using standard settings for lung evaluation. **(b)** The mass has a hypodense (fluid) core surrounded by an irregular, contrast-enhancing rim. Findings are consistent with a diagnosis of pulmonary abscess, which was confirmed surgically.

Granulomas and pulmonary neoplasms can appear as solid, contrast-enhancing masses. Bronchogenic carcinoma, the most common primary lung tumour in the dog, usually appears as a well delineated, smoothly marginated, spherical mass, most often arising from one of the caudal lung lobes (Figure 7.8). A granuloma, because of the inflammatory nature of the lesion, may have a less

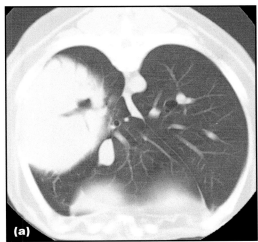

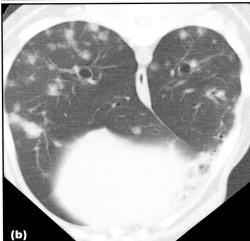

7.8 **(a)** CT image of a large moderately well marginated soft tissue mass in the right caudal lung lobe. The lucency evident centrally represents a bronchus preserved within the expansile mass. The mass was confirmed to be a bronchoalveolar carcinoma. **(b)** CT image of a dog with a previously diagnosed malignant nerve sheath tumour. Multiple irregularly margined soft tissue nodules are present in all lung lobes. The nodules were confirmed to represent widespread pulmonary metastasis.

well defined margin and is often associated with other imaging findings such as hilar lymphadenopathy or bronchopneumonia. However, needle aspiration or tissue core biopsy is necessary to distinguish between these two causes of mass lesions. CT is far superior to conventional radiography for detection of pulmonary metastatic lesions (Johnson *et al.*, 2004; Figure 7.8). A recent study revealed that CT detected approximately 10 times the number of metastatic nodules that radiography found, and that the lower limit for consistent lesion detection was approximately 1–2 mm, compared with 7–9 mm for radiography (Nemanic *et al.*, 2006).

Pleural effusion: CT does not provide an advantage over conventional radiography for detecting pleural effusion, but it is useful for determining underlying causative lesions. These lesions include masses that might be obscured by overlying fluid and lung lobe torsion, which can be the primary cause of the pleural

effusion or may occur secondary to the effusion. In addition, idiopathic chylothorax can be more confidently diagnosed when CT is negative for other causes of chylous effusion such as a mediastinal mass.

Pneumothorax: CT is highly sensitive for detection of pulmonary bullae in fully inflated lungs and has been shown to be an effective diagnostic tool for identifying bullae in dogs with spontaneous pneumothorax (Lipscomb *et al.*, 2004; Au *et al.*, 2006) (Figure 7.9). However, a word of caution is advised: in patients with moderate to marked pneumothorax, atelectasis can obscure ruptured bullae. Even in those patients in which the lungs have been re-inflated by placement of an indwelling chest tube, underlying lesions of pulmonary bullae or emphysematous disease can be difficult to identify due to residual atelectasis or adjacent alveolar infiltrates.

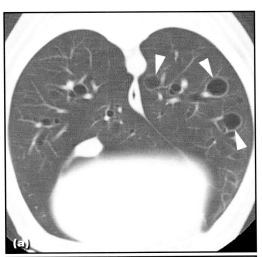

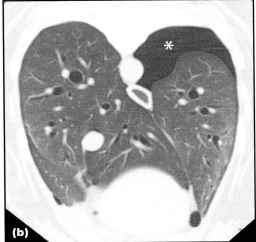

7.9 **(a)** CT image of a dog with multiple pulmonary bullae (arrowheads). The bullae are differentiated from bronchi in cross-section due to size, lack of associated pulmonary arteries and veins, and a spherical rather than cylindrical shape when multiple consecutive images are viewed. **(b)** CT image of a dog with spontaneous pneumothorax. Free pleural air is present in the non-dependent region of the left pleural space (*). As it is not fully expanded, the remainder of the lung is denser than normal and could obscure concurrent pulmonary pathology.

Mediastinal disease: CT can also be used to evaluate the cranial mediastinum and hilar region, and is particularly illuminating when these structures are obscured by pleural effusion, heavy pulmonary infiltrates or mediastinal fat. Sensitivity for detecting mediastinal or hilar lymphadenopathy or other mediastinal masses (Figure 7.10) is far greater than that of conventional radiography. Although ultrasonography can also be used to evaluate the cranial mediastinal region, the imaging window is often limited and evaluation can be incomplete compared with CT (Prather *et al.*, 2005).

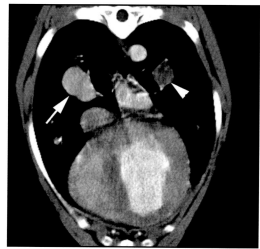

7.11 Contrast-enhanced CT image of the thorax of a dog with pulmonary thromboembolism. The right pulmonary artery (arrowed) is distended, has irregular margins and a non-uniform density, indicative of intraluminal filling defects. The left pulmonary artery (arrowhead) is smaller and shows no evidence of intraluminal contrast enhancement, indicating a loss of flow. (Courtesy of T. Schwarz.)

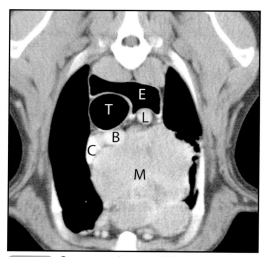

7.10 Contrast-enhanced CT image of the thorax of a dog with a mediastinal mass acquired at the level of the cranial mediastinum, immediately cranial to the heart. Histopathology confirmed a thymoma. B = Brachiocephalic trunk; C = Cranial vena cava; E = Air-dilated oesophageal lumen; L = Left subclavian artery; M = Cranial mediastinal mass; T = Tracheal lumen.

Cardiovascular disorders

Alterations in pulmonary perfusion: Pulmonary thromboembolism occurs as a sequel to severe systemic disorders that induce hypercoagulability, stasis of blood flow and endothelial damage. Conventional radiographic findings can include truncation of the pulmonary arteries, reduction in the pulmonary vein diameter and hyperlucency in affected lung lobes due to decreased lung perfusion; however, normal chest radiographs are commonly encountered. Pulmonary perfusion scintigraphy is helpful in defining regions of decreased perfusion, but this test is non-specific for determining the underlying cause of the perfusion deficit.

Contrast-enhanced CT angiography can be used to detect luminal filling defects and truncation in the pulmonary arteries. The thorax is scanned immediately following administration of a rapid bolus of iodinated contrast medium, when the contrast material is still predominantly intravascular. Thromboemboli appear as relatively hypodense filling defects in relation to the contrast-enhanced blood (Figure 7.11). Magnetic resonance angiography, using pulse sequences that employ both non-contrast and contrast medium, can also be used for the

same purpose. Clinical investigations have revealed similar sensitivity and specificity for detection using both methods. A limitation of using CT or MRI is the need for heavy sedation or anaesthesia, which is often contraindicated in pulmonary thromboembolism patients.

Cardiac disease: CT and MRI have not been widely used for the diagnosis of primary cardiac disease in veterinary patients because of the widespread availability of radiography and echocardiography, as well as the need for anaesthesia with advanced imaging modalities. The sophistication of CT and MRI technology has improved with the development of sub-second volumetric cardiac image acquisitions, and these modalities may be more commonly exploited for cardiac imaging in the future (Figure 7.12).

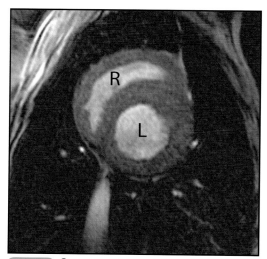

7.12 Contrast-enhanced T1-weighted transverse image of a canine heart at the level of the ventricles. L = Left ventricle; R = Right ventricle.

Quantitative assessment of cardiac parameters:
A limited number of reports in the veterinary literature describe the use of MRI for quantification of myocardial masses, estimation of myocardial fibrosis in cats with cardiomyopathy, and assessment of ventricular chamber volume. Some multi-slice helical CT scanners are capable of allowing calculation of similar volumetric data. However, with either modality, the availability of appropriate scanner hardware and software is still limited, calculations are tedious and the clinical utility is questionable (MacDonald *et al.*, 2005, 2006).

Developmental anomalies: Cardiac anomalies are most often diagnosed using a combination of conventional radiography and echocardiography; however, some lesions, particularly vascular ring anomalies, can be detected using CT. It is likely that intra- and extracardiac shunting lesions could also be detected using appropriately timed image acquisitions, following bolus injection of contrast medium, although this has not been reported in veterinary medicine.

Cardiac masses: CT can be used to detect and characterize the origin and extent of cardiac associated masses, which may not be fully described using other imaging approaches (Figure 7.13). Administration of contrast medium is important in these patients to delineate the mass from adjacent myocardium, and to define the mass margins in relation to invasion of the cardiac chambers as may occur in patients with haemangiosarcoma of the right atrium.

References and further reading

Au JJ, Weisman DL, Stefanacci JD and Palmisano MP (2006) Use of computed tomography for evaluation of lung lesions associated with spontaneous pneumothorax in dogs: 12 cases (1999–2002). *Journal of the American Veterinary Medical Association* **228**, 733–737
Johnson VS, Corcoran BM, Wotton PR, Schwarz T and Sullivan M (2005) Thoracic high-resolution computed tomographic findings in dogs with canine idiopathic pulmonary fibrosis. *Journal of Small Animal Practice* **46**, 381–388
Johnson VS, Ramsey IK, Thompson H *et al.* (2004) Thoracic high-

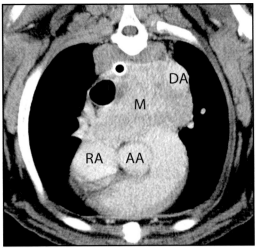

7.13 Delayed contrast-enhanced CT image of a dog with a chemodectoma located at the heart base. This is a solid soft tissue mass with a mildly heterogenous pattern of contrast enhancement. AA = Ascending aorta; DA = Descending aorta; M = Mass; RA = Right atrium.

resolution computed tomography in the diagnosis of metastatic carcinoma. *Journal of Small Animal Practice* **45**, 134–143
Lipscomb V, Brockman D, Gregory S, Baines S and Lamb CR (2004) CT scanning of dogs with spontaneous pneumothorax. *Veterinary Record* **154**, 344
MacDonald KA, Kittleson MD, Garcia-Nolen T, Larson RF and Wisner ER (2006) Tissue Doppler imaging and gradient echo cardiac magnetic resonance imaging in normal cats and cats with hypertrophic cardiomyopathy. *Journal of Veterinary Internal Medicine* **20**, 627–634
MacDonald KA, Kittleson MD, Reed T *et al.* (2005) Quantification of left ventricular mass using cardiac magnetic resonance imaging compared with echocardiography in domestic cats. *Veterinary Radiology and Ultrasound* **46**, 192–199
Macready DM, Johnson LR and Pollard RE (2007) Fluoroscopic and radiographic evaluation of tracheal collapse in dogs: 62 cases (2001–2006). *Journal of the American Veterinary Medical Association* **230**, 1870–1876
Nemanic S, London CA and Wisner ER (2006) Comparison of thoracic radiographs and single breath-hold helical CT for detection of pulmonary nodules in dogs with metastatic neoplasia. *Journal of Veterinary Internal Medicine* **20**, 508–515
Prather AB, Berry CR and Thrall DE (2005) Use of radiography in combination with computed tomography for the assessment of non-cardiac thoracic disease in the dog and cat. *Veterinary Radiology and Ultrasound* **46**, 114–121

59

8

Laboratory tests

Adrian Boswood

Introduction

Laboratory tests are frequently used in the investigation and monitoring of patients with cardiac disease and failure. These can broadly be divided into general laboratory tests that may be affected by the presence of heart disease or failure, and specific laboratory tests that provide information directly pertinent to the heart. This chapter will consider the following tests and the impact of cardiac disease and failure on the results obtained:

- General tests:
  - Serum biochemistry profile
  - Haematology profile
  - Urine analysis
  - Analysis of effusions
  - Blood cultures.
- Specific tests:
  - Cardiac troponins I and T
  - Natriuretic peptides.

General tests

Broadly, there are three motives for the performance of general tests and particularly biochemical, haematological and urine analyses in patients undergoing investigation for cardiovascular disease. The first is to allow the clinician to rule in or out significant concurrent disease that might be responsible for the clinical signs observed; thus the tests aid in the differential diagnosis of the case. The second is to assist in the identification of underlying systemic diseases that may contribute to the development or exacerbation of the cardiovascular disease identified; examples of this would be in helping to rule in or out renal disease in elderly cats with evidence of cardiovascular abnormalities, or endocrine disease in older patients with evidence of cardiovascular dysfunction. Finally, and perhaps most importantly, the performance of biochemical analysis allows evaluation of the impact of cardiovascular disease and its treatment on the function of other organ systems. It is for the latter reason that biochemical analysis is most frequently undertaken in patients with cardiovascular disease and the following section will mainly focus on these points. It should be realized that in these circumstances the tests are not being performed in order to make the diagnosis; rather they are being performed to assess the impact of a disease that the patient is already known to have.

Serum biochemistry profile

Cardiovascular disease, congestive heart failure (CHF) and their treatment have profound effects on perfusion, volume homeostasis and maintenance of the integrity of normal body fluid compartments. These lead to effects on substances measured in the biochemistry profile through underperfusion of body systems, congestion of body systems, dilution of normal substances and loss into effusions.

- Effects of underperfusion:
  - Development of pre-renal azotaemia, particularly elevation of the blood urea concentration.
- Effects of congestion:
  - Hepatic congestion may lead to the elevation of certain liver enzymes, including alkaline phosphatase.
- Dilution of normal substances by fluid retention:
  - Rapid development of right-sided heart failure may be associated with hypoproteinaemia
  - Severe CHF may be associated with the development of hyponatraemia.
- Loss into effusions:
  - The rapid development or redevelopment (following drainage) of body cavity effusions may be associated with the development of hypoproteinaemia.

In the interpretation of biochemical abnormalities it is important to realize that none of the changes is specific to heart disease; thus azotaemia, elevation of liver enzymes, hypoproteinaemia and hyponatraemia are all commonly caused by other disease states. Therefore, a *diagnosis* of heart disease or CHF can not be made on the basis of a biochemical profile alone. These changes, when found in a patient with typical clinical signs of CHF, can help to corroborate the diagnosis, but differential diagnoses should always be considered. For instance, a patient with elevated liver enzymes, ascites and hypoproteinaemia is more likely to have primary hepatic disease than hepatic dysfunction secondary to CHF.

As previously stated, the most important reason for performing and monitoring the results of biochemical analysis in animals with CHF is to evaluate the impact of the cardiac disease and its treatment on other organ systems, and particularly on renal function and electrolyte status. For this reason the author routinely performs at least a limited biochemical analysis on patients when embarking on treatment of cardiac disease, or when treatment has recently been altered. The variables most likely to be altered and therefore most worthy of measurement are the urea, creatinine, sodium and potassium concentrations. These all provide slightly different but important information.

Urea

Urea is a by-product of protein metabolism. It is produced at a fairly consistent rate and is excreted via the renal system. Elevations in urea concentration (Figure 8.1) can be brought about by increased production in animals that are highly catabolic or have recently ingested a high-protein meal, but it is more likely that an elevation on the blood profile is as a consequence of decreased renal excretion.

Clinical finding	Cause
↓ Circulating fluid volume	**Pre-renal azotaemia (e.g. dehydration, hypovolaemia)** **Over-diuresis**
↓ Renal excretion of urea	**↓ GFR**
	Pre-renal azotaemia (↓ renal perfusion) **ACE inhibitor therapy (efferent arteriolar dilatation causing ↓ glomerular capillary hydrostatic pressure)** Renal disease (glomerular or tubular disease) Post-renal obstruction (↑ hydrostatic pressure in Bowman's capsule)
	↑ Urea resorption
	Pre-renal azotaemia (↓ renal tubular flow)
↑ Production of urea	Recent high-protein meal Increased catabolism Gastrointestinal haemorrhage

8.1 Causes of increased urea concentration (causes most likely linked with cardiovascular disease are in **bold**).

Within the kidney, urea is filtered at the glomerulus but can be reabsorbed from the renal tubule, particularly in states of low flow. In heart failure, as in other states where renal blood flow may be reduced, several mechanisms are activated that tend to reabsorb fluid from the renal tubule. The resorption of fluid tends to be accompanied by resorption of urea. The resulting increase in urea concentration is disproportionate compared with the increase in creatinine concentration (i.e. the creatinine concentration may be 50% greater than the top of the normal range, but the urea concentration may be 100% greater). Animals with heart disease sufficient to result in signs of congestive failure are often found to have an elevated urea concentration (Boswood and Murphy, 2006).

It is frequently difficult to judge whether elevation of urea and/or creatinine in patients with heart disease is due to intrinsic renal disease or pre-renal azotaemia. Urine specific gravity (SG) cannot be used in many patients to distinguish between these two conditions because they are receiving diuretics. A disproportionate elevation of urea would tend to suggest that the azotaemia may be pre-renal rather than renal in origin.

The administration of diuretics, although leading to a contraction in circulating fluid volume and potentially worsening of renal underperfusion, may result in an increase in tubular flow (due to the increased volume of urine being produced) and therefore there may be either no effect on urea or, if the volume contraction is sufficiently marked, an increase in urea.

Creatinine

Creatinine is produced in skeletal muscle at a relatively constant rate and excreted via the kidneys. Creatinine is an inert molecule in the renal tubule and is neither excreted nor reabsorbed. There is a fairly consistent and predictable inverse relationship between creatinine concentration and glomerular filtration rate (GFR). In heart disease and states of low renal blood flow, glomerular filtration may be maintained at normal levels via many intra-renal mechanisms; and the creatinine concentration, although it may increase, does not seem to rise to the same extent as urea (Boswood and Murphy, 2006). An elevation of creatinine following the introduction or modification of treatment could be due to a combination of factors, such as reduction of the circulating fluid volume (Figure 8.2). For example: with loop diuretics, the creatinine concentration will increase relative to a decrease in plasma fluid volume, as it is produced and excreted at a constant rate. The creatinine concentration may also increase with a reduction in GFR, e.g. with the use of angiotensin-converting enzyme (ACE) inhibitors.

Clinical finding	Cause
↓ Circulating fluid volume	**Pre-renal azotaemia (e.g. dehydration, hypovolaemia)** **Over-diuresis**
↓ Renal excretion of creatinine	**↓ GFR**
	Pre-renal azotaemia (↓ renal perfusion) **ACE inhibitor therapy (efferent arteriolar dilatation causing ↓ glomerular capillary hydrostatic pressure)** Renal disease (glomerular or tubular disease) Post-renal obstruction (↑ hydrostatic pressure in Bowman's capsule)

8.2 Causes of increased creatinine concentration (causes most likely linked with cardiovascular disease are in **bold**).

An elevated creatinine concentration found in a patient prior to the introduction of treatment should generate concern about the possibility of pre-existing intrinsic renal disease as well as reduced cardiac output. Several studies in humans have demonstrated that an elevated creatinine concentration confers a worse outcome in patients with heart failure (Nohria *et al.*, 2008). The opposite was found in dogs in the QUEST study, where higher concentrations seemed to be associated with a lower risk of a poor outcome (Haggstrom *et al.*, 2008). The latter result may be a consequence of the study not enrolling animals with significant renal dysfunction, but may also indicate the effects of cachexia and volume expansion in tending to lower creatinine concentrations.

A large increase in creatinine following the introduction of treatment should raise concern that the treatment has compromised glomerular filtration. This is particularly common in cats, as they are more likely to be dependent upon elevated preload to be able to maintain a normal cardiac output.

Sodium

Sodium concentration is usually tightly regulated and seems to be maintained in the normal range until heart failure is advanced. Although the development of CHF is brought about by mechanisms resulting in the retention of sodium, this sodium is usually retained along with water, leading to maintenance of a normal sodium concentration. When the need to retain fluid overwhelms the normal volume-expanding mechanism, 'non-osmotic' release of anti-diuretic hormone (ADH/arginine vasopressin) occurs (Figure 8.3).

Clinical finding	Cause
↑ ADH production (↑ H_2O retention)	↓ **Arterial pressures (e.g. poor cardiac output)** ↓ **Venous pressures (e.g. over-diuresis)** ↑ **Angiotensin II production (e.g. CHF)** Nausea/vomiting Stress (e.g. post-surgery)
↑ Na⁺ loss	**Third-space loss (e.g. ascites, pleural effusion, particularly following repeated drainage)** **Thiazide diuretics (also through inhibition of free water excretion)** Gastrointestinal loss (vomiting, diarrhoea) Hypoadrenocorticism
↓ Na⁺ intake	Dietary Na⁺ restriction (may exacerbate electrolyte abnormality in conjunction with other causes)
Dilution of Na⁺	↑ H_2O intake Iatrogenic (e.g. hypotonic i.v. fluids)

8.3 Causes of hyponatraemia (causes most likely linked with cardiovascular disease are in **bold**).

ADH is normally involved in the regulation of osmolality; increased concentrations lead to retention of free water and therefore reduce osmolality. When ADH is released in response to a non-osmotic stimulus and free water is retained, this dilutes the serum sodium resulting in hyponatraemia. This has been seen to develop in dogs with advanced heart failure (Boswood and Murphy, 2006); in humans lower sodium concentrations have been associated

with a worse prognosis (Gheorghiade *et al.*, 2007). Thus, hyponatraemia in patients with heart disease may indicate more advanced disease and possibly a worse prognosis.

Diuretics and ACE inhibitor treatment in patients with heart disease and heart failure will lead to the loss of sodium. This is usually accompanied by a loss of water, leading to volume contraction without the development of hyponatraemia. The development of hyponatraemia can occur after diuresis, particularly where multiple diuretics are used. This may be due to the volume contraction being so marked as to result in non-osmotic release of ADH, rather than simply sodium loss.

Potassium

Increases or decreases in potassium concentration can have significant effects on cardiac rhythm. Electrolyte concentrations should always be checked in any patient with a newly identified cardiac rhythm disturbance. Hyperkalaemia may cause brady-arrhythmias, and hypokalaemia may predispose to atrial and ventricular tachyarrhythmias.

Hypokalaemia can develop secondary to significant cardiac disease for many reasons, including translocation across the cell membrane brought about by sympathetic stimulation and renal loss secondary to high aldosterone concentrations (Figure 8.4). The latter reason is particularly common secondary to the treatment of heart failure with diuretics (Boswood and Murphy, 2006). The use of ACE inhibitors and potassium-sparing diuretics may ameliorate this effect.

Clinical finding	Cause
↑ K⁺ loss	**Loop or thiazide diuretics** **Renin-angiotensin-aldosterone system (RAAS) stimulation (e.g. CHF)** **Alkalosis (secondary to loop diuretics)** Gastrointestinal loss (vomiting, diarrhoea) Chronic renal failure High dietary Na⁺ intake (may exacerbate electrolyte abnormality in conjunction with other causes)
↑ K⁺ translocation into cells	**Catecholamines (e.g. CHF, dobutamine)** **Alkalosis** Insulin-glucose therapy
↓ K⁺ intake	**Anorexia (especially cats)**
Dilution of K⁺	Iatrogenic (e.g. K⁺-free/deficient i.v. fluids)

8.4 Causes of hypokalaemia (causes most likely linked with cardiovascular disease are in **bold**).

Given the potentially significant and deleterious interaction of heart failure, high sympathetic tone, diuretic use and arrhythmias, it is worth monitoring potassium concentrations routinely in patients receiving treatment for heart failure, and intervening with modification of therapy or potassium supplementation when hypokalaemia is discovered. Causes of hyperkalaemia and hypochloraemia are given in Figures 8.5 and 8.6.

Clinical finding	Cause
↓ K+ loss	**ACE inhibitor therapy** **Spironolactone therapy** **Acidosis** **Low dietary Na+ intake** (may exacerbate electrolyte abnormality in conjunction with other causes) Acute renal failure Post-renal obstruction Hypoadrenocorticism
↑ K+ translocation from cells	**Reperfusion injury (e.g. aortic thromboembolism)** Acidosis Beta adrenergic blocker therapy (may exacerbate electrolyte abnormality in conjunction with other causes) Digoxin therapy (may exacerbate electrolyte abnormality in conjunction with other causes)
↑ K+ intake	Iatrogenic (excessive infusion of K+-containing fluids)

8.5 Causes of hyperkalaemia (causes most likely linked with cardiovascular disease are in **bold**).

Clinical finding	Cause
↑ Cl- loss	**Loop or thiazide diuretics** Gastric loss (vomiting)

8.6 Causes of hypochloraemia (causes most likely linked with cardiovascular disease are in **bold**).

When to check biochemical profiles
There are three time points in the investigation and treatment of cases with cardiovascular disease when the evaluation of a biochemical profile, and particularly the analytes discussed above, is advised.

1. When the patient is undergoing an initial evaluation to determine the presence of any concurrent disease and the impact that this might be having on the cardiovascular system.
2. Prior to the introduction of any treatment.
3. After the introduction of treatment or dose modification.

Patients will typically have developed a new equilibrium approximately 10 days after any change in medications (Rose, 1989) and therefore any change in electrolyte concentration or renal function will probably have occurred by that time.

Haematology profile
Relatively few cardiovascular diseases result in significant changes in the haematology profile. An association between heart failure, anaemia and a poor prognosis has been recognized in human patients with heart disease and failure (Mitchell, 2007) but has not been described in veterinary patients. Conversely, anaemia can be a cause of volume overload and precipitate congestive signs, particularly in cats.

Changes in white blood cell type and number may be seen in inflammatory cardiovascular disease. The most common of these, although rare by comparison

with other cardiovascular diseases of dogs and cats, is bacterial endocarditis. Bacterial endocarditis is typically associated with a leucocytosis with a monocytosis, neutrophilia and a left shift. Leucocytosis has been reported to be present in nearly 90% of patients in one case series (Sykes *et al.*, 2006a). Anaemia and thrombocytopenia may also be present with this disease, and the latter may be associated with a worse outcome (Sykes *et al.*, 2006a).

In the majority of cases the haematology profile is useful during the initial investigation to rule in or out concurrent or underlying diseases. Other than in rare cases of thromboembolic or inflammatory disease, it rarely contributes to the diagnosis.

Urine analysis
Urine analysis is rarely useful in the investigation of patients with cardiovascular disease, but it may be helpful under specific circumstances. Urine SG in azotaemic patients with cardiovascular disease not receiving treatment may help to differentiate concurrent (or underlying) primary renal disease from pre-renal azotaemia. In thromboembolic disease there may be casts in the urine, indicating the presence of recent renal tubular damage.

In cats, microalbuminuria has been shown to be associated with renal disease and raised systolic blood pressure (i.e. cats with higher blood pressure were more likely to have elevated urinary albumin concentrations; Syme *et al.*, 2006). Urine culture may be useful in patients where bacterial endocarditis is suspected, because in some patients the causative organism may be cultured from the urine.

The relatively limited value of urine analysis in patients with common cardiac diseases means that, although this is a simple and relatively inexpensive test, it is not recommended for routine use other than at the initial examination of patients not on medication.

Analysis of effusions
In canine and feline patients, heart failure can result in the development of pleural, abdominal and in some cases pericardial effusions. These are typically modified transudates, although chylothorax can develop secondary to cardiac disease in both species.

Pericardial effusions can be the cause of or secondary to heart failure. Typically, where they develop secondary to heart failure they have the characteristics of a modified transudate. Primary haemorrhagic pericardial effusions occur most commonly in dogs and are often secondary to neoplastic disease or idiopathic in origin. Occasionally, septic pericardial effusions can occur in dogs, and non-septic exudates can develop in cats secondary to feline infectious peritonitis.

Different types of fluid can be distinguished on the basis of: the protein, triglyceride and cholesterol concentrations; cell count and characterization of the population of cells present; and, where appropriate, culture (Figure 8.7). Samples of effusions should routinely be taken for analysis. They should be collected into plain tubes (for biochemical analyses) and tubes containing EDTA (for cytological analysis).

Type of effusion	Gross appearance	Protein (g/l)	Nucleated cells (x10⁹/l)	Cytology/other features	Cause
Transudate, protein-poor	Clear; colourless	<20	<1.0	Variable	Hypoproteinaemia Fluid overload
Transudate, protein-rich	Clear to moderately turbid; slightly red, orange or yellow	>20	<5.0	Neutrophils; macrophages	CHF Lung lobe torsion (Neoplasia)
Non-septic exudate	Yellow, tan, cream; hazy	>20	<5.0		Feline infectious peritonitis
Septic exudate	Turbid; purulent; yellow, tan, cream	>20	>5.0	Degenerate neutrophils; macrophages; bacteria	Bacteria
Chylothorax	Grossly milky	>20	<10.0	Lymphocytes (acute); neutrophils; macrophages with lipid vacuoles (chronic); triglyceride concentrations > plasma	High systemic venous pressures Neoplasia Thrombosis of cranial vena cava Lymphangiectasia Idiopathic
Haemorrhagic effusions	Haemorrhagic in appearance, should not clot when left to stand	40–60	>2.0	Neutrophils; lymphocytes; (platelets if very recent haemorrhage); macrophages; erythrophages; siderophages if chronic	Neoplasia Trauma Coagulopathy Lung lobe torsion
Neoplastic effusions	Pale yellow, orange; clear to cloudy	>20	Variable	Cells with malignant features	Lymphoma Mesothelioma Carcinoma

8.7 Types of effusions.

Neoplastic and idiopathic pericardial effusions are commonly haemorrhagic in appearance. Determination of the underlying causes of a pericardial effusion on the basis of fluid analysis is notoriously unreliable (Sisson *et al.*, 1984) and it is better not to form a judgement on the basis of cytology alone, except where the effusion has formed secondary to less common causes such as a septic effusion or lymphoma. Similarly, pH of pericardial fluid is an unreliable indicator of cause.

Blood cultures

Bacteriological culture of blood from patients suspected to be suffering from bacteraemia or bacterial endocarditis may allow isolation of the organism responsible for the clinical signs. For a detailed description of one technique for carrying out blood cultures in dogs and cats, see Greiner *et al.*, 2008.

In order to avoid contamination of the sample with commensal organisms from the skin of the patient during collection, the site must be prepared aseptically. Blood must be taken into special enhancement media and only after isolation of the same organism from at least two separately collected samples would the result be considered to be definitely positive. Even with optimal sample collection and handling, blood cultures may be negative in patients very strongly suspected of being bacteraemic or having bacterial endocarditis. In a retrospective study the causative organism was identified in only 58% of patients with endocarditis (Sykes *et al.*, 2006b). One reason often cited for the failure to isolate organisms in some cases is the frequency with which many animals have received antibiotics prior to sample collection.

Specific tests

There has been a plethora of articles on various different cardiac biomarkers in recent years (Boswood, 2009). An editorial regarding the use of biomarkers in human patients outlined three questions that must be answered before a test can be considered to be useful (Morrow and de Lemos, 2007):

1. Can the clinician measure it?
2. Does it add new information?
3. Does it help the clinician to manage patients?

The two markers, or types of marker, that come closest to answering at least the first two of these questions affirmatively are troponins and natriuretic peptides. The extent to which the knowledge of the concentration of these peptides will help in managing patients is only beginning to be explored.

Troponins

The troponin complex is a group of proteins (I, T and C) that regulate the interaction between actin and myosin. They have distinct myocardial isoforms. Troponins are intracellular proteins and thus increased concentrations of these proteins are only found in the circulation when a significant number of myocardial cells are compromised or die simultaneously. Markers that must necessarily be released from dead or dying cells are sometimes referred to as 'leakage' markers.

In human patients, troponins have become the preferred indicators of ischaemia and infarction due to their excellent sensitivity and specificity.

Troponins I and T have been evaluated in a number of different circumstances in veterinary patients, and their circulating concentrations are found to be elevated in association with many cardiac diseases in both cats and dogs (Connolly *et al.*, 2003, 2005; Oyama *et al.*, 2003). At first glance this would therefore appear to make them excellent tests, but what about their genuine value?

The problem with troponin concentrations lies in their lack of specificity. They increase in response to numerous cardiac diseases, yet their concentration does not correlate predictably with the severity of the cardiac disease or failure in dogs. Thus, if it is already known that the patient has heart disease, the test simply confirms that the patient has heart disease; it does not give any further information. Although one study suggested that troponin concentrations may have some value in the diagnosis of heart failure in dogs (Spratt *et al.*, 2005), this conclusion was not supported by a larger study (Oyama and Sisson, 2004). Their greatest clinical value is in cases where a diagnosis of infarction or myocarditis is suspected, both of which are rare diagnoses in small animals. In such cases dramatic elevations of troponin can be seen – in contrast to the relatively modest elevations seen in most animals with cardiomyopathy or valvular heart disease.

As well as having diagnostic value, it has been suggested that troponin concentrations may have value in prognostication (Oyama and Sisson, 2004). In this respect they may provide more information than is already known, thus fulfilling criterion 2 outlined above. It is possible that patients with more rapidly progressive disease may tend to have higher concentrations of these proteins.

Natriuretic peptides

Natriuretic peptides are hormones manufactured in and released from the ventricular and atrial myocardium. Their manufacture is increased in response to myocardial stretch and increased end-diastolic wall stress.

The heart releases two peptides: atrial natriuretic peptide (ANP) and B-type natriuretic peptide (BNP). Both these peptides are manufactured as larger pro-peptides and the active peptide is cleaved from the C-terminal end of the molecule. This means that equimolar quantities of the *N*-terminal pro-peptide are manufactured and released into the circulation. Concentrations of either the active peptides or their *N*-terminal pro-peptides can be measured in the circulation.

Assays are available for ANP, NTproANP, BNP and NTproBNP. Their concentrations have all been shown to increase in response to cardiac disease in small animals. A genuine superiority of one assay or one molecule over the others has yet to be demonstrated, but there are hypothetical reasons why NTproBNP may be a more stable marker of disease, and recent attention has tended to focus on the measurement of this polypeptide in both dogs and cats.

Studies conducted to demonstrate the clinical utility of NTproBNP have shown it to be superior to NTproANP in dogs (Boswood *et al.*, 2008). Sensitivity and specificity have been shown to be in the region of 80–85% for the discrimination of dogs with heart disease from dogs with respiratory disease. Other authors have shown similarly promising results for natriuretic peptides using different assays (Prosek *et al.*, 2007).

Several studies have demonstrated the clinical value of using species-specific assays to measure NTproBNP in both cats and dogs (Boswood *et al.*, 2008; Connolly *et al.*, 2008; Fine *et al.*, 2008; Oyama *et al.*, 2008). These have shown accurate discrimination between canine and feline patients with and without heart disease, and between individuals with and without heart failure. The test also shows reasonable accuracy for the detection of patients with cardiomegaly secondary to heart disease (Oyama *et al.*, 2008).

Different canine studies have generated apparently conflicting cut-off values (Boswood *et al.*, 2008; Fine *et al.*, 2008; Oyama *et al.*, 2008), but the cut-offs have been generated with differing sample handling and to differentiate between different patient populations. In order to provide optimal accuracy, samples should probably be taken and cells separated from plasma or serum within a few hours. Ideally the plasma or serum should then be frozen if there is going to be a significant delay before processing. Summarizing published values, it would appear that patients with NTproBNP concentrations below about 450 pmol/l are unlikely to have clinically significant cardiac disease. Patients with overt signs of heart failure are likely to have concentrations above 800 pmol/l, with most severely affected patients having values well over 1000 pmol/l.

NTproBNP has been shown to be highly discriminatory in distinguishing normal cats from those with heart disease and heart failure (Connolly *et al.*, 2008). Cats are a species in which the diagnosis of cardiac disease can be very challenging. They tend to demonstrate fewer outward clinical signs and often present only when they have progressed to the point of development of overt signs of heart failure. The potential for a blood test to assist in the detection of heart disease prior to the development of overt signs in this population is an exciting development.

If natriuretic peptide concentrations prove to be as useful in veterinary patients as they have been shown to be in human patients further developments might be anticipated, including the ability to prognosticate and possibly treat patients on the basis of NTproBNP concentrations. For instance, preliminary data from studies in dogs with mitral valve disease would suggest that dogs with an NTproBNP concentration greater than about 750 pmol/l are much more likely to succumb to heart disease in the near future than dogs with lower concentrations.

Further avenues that have been explored in human patients, but have yet to be explored in veterinary patients, are the potential to use natriuretic peptide concentrations as a basis for introducing or modifying therapy in heart failure. At least two studies in human patients have demonstrated an improved outcome compared with conventional therapy when treatment has been targeted specifically at modifying concentrations of the peptides (Troughton et al., 2000; Jourdain et al., 2007).

If natriuretic peptides are to become widely used in the management of heart disease and failure in veterinary patients, it will require the development of a more sophisticated approach to the interpretation of test results. These tests are unlikely to provide unequivocal yes/no answers in many of the patients in which they are performed. They will need to be interpreted in conjunction with other clinical and diagnostic information, and the clinician will then need to consider whether or not the result increases or decreases the likelihood of the abnormality in question being present. There are also a number of confounding factors that affect the interpretation of these tests in human patients, including sample handling, concurrent renal disease, body condition score, age and sex. NTproBNP concentrations have been shown to be significantly increased in dogs with azotaemia and no cardiac disease (Raffan et al., 2009; Schmidt et al., 2009), although the magnitude of increase is typically not as great as that seen associated with heart failure. Knowledge of a patient's serum creatinine concentration is therefore likely to be important for accurate interpretation of concentrations of this biomarker. Other factors are only beginning to be explored in veterinary patients.

References and further reading

Boswood A (2009) Biomarkers in cardiovascular disease: beyond natriuretic peptides. *Journal of Veterinary Cardiology* **11** (Suppl. 1), S23–S32

Boswood A, Dukes-McEwan J, Loureiro J *et al.* (2008) The diagnostic accuracy of different natriuretic peptides in the investigation of canine cardiac disease. *Journal of Small Animal Practice* **49**, 26–32

Boswood A and Murphy A (2006) The effect of heart disease, heart failure and diuresis on selected laboratory and electrocardiographic parameters in dogs. *Journal of Veterinary Cardiology* **8**, 1–9

Connolly DJ, Cannata J, Boswood A *et al.* (2003) Cardiac troponin I in cats with hypertrophic cardiomyopathy. *Journal of Feline Medicine and Surgery* **5**, 209–216

Connolly DJ, Guitian J, Boswood A and Neiger R (2005) Serum troponin I levels in hyperthyroid cats before and after treatment with radioactive iodine. *Journal of Feline Medicine and Surgery* **7**, 289–300

Connolly DJ, Soares Magalhaes RJ, Syme HM *et al.* (2008) Circulating natriuretic peptides in cats with heart disease. *Journal of Veterinary Internal Medicine* **22**, 96–105

Fine DM, Declue AE and Reinero CR (2008) Evaluation of circulating amino terminal-pro-B-type natriuretic peptide concentration in dogs with respiratory distress attributable to congestive heart failure or primary pulmonary disease. *Journal of the American Veterinary Medical Association* **232**, 1674–1679

Gheorghiade M, Abraham WT, Albert NM *et al.* (2007) Relationship between admission serum sodium concentration and clinical outcomes in patients hospitalized for heart failure: an analysis from the OPTIMIZE-HF registry. *European Heart Journal* **28**, 980–988

Greiner M, Wolf G and Hartmann K (2008) A retrospective study of the clinical presentation of 140 dogs and 39 cats with bacteraemia. *Journal of Small Animal Practice* **49**, 378–383

Haggstrom J, Boswood A, O'Grady M *et al.* (2008) Effect of pimobendan or benazepril hydrochloride on survival times in dogs with congestive heart failure caused by naturally occurring myxomatous mitral valve disease: the QUEST study. *Journal of Veterinary Internal Medicine* **22**, 1124–1135

Jourdain P, Jondeau G, Funck F *et al.* (2007) Plasma brain natriuretic peptide-guided therapy to improve outcome in heart failure: the STARS-BNP Multicenter Study. *Journal of the American College of Cardiology* **49**, 1733–1739

Mitchell JE (2007) Emerging role of anemia in heart failure. *American Journal of Cardiology* **99**, 15D–20D

Morrow DA and de Lemos JA (2007) Benchmarks for the assessment of novel cardiovascular biomarkers. *Circulation* **115**, 949–952

Nohria A, Hasselblad V, Stebbins A *et al.* (2008) Cardiorenal interactions: insights from the ESCAPE trial. *Journal of the American College of Cardiology* **51**, 1268–1274

Oyama MA, Fox PR, Rush JE, Rozanski EA and Lesser M (2008) Clinical utility of serum N-terminal pro-B-type natriuretic peptide concentration for identifying cardiac disease in dogs and assessing disease severity. *Journal of the American Veterinary Medical Association* **232**, 1496–1503

Oyama MA and Sisson DD (2004) Cardiac troponin-I concentration in dogs with cardiac disease. *Journal of Veterinary Internal Medicine* **18**, 831–839

Oyama MA, Solter P, Prosek R, Ostapkowicz R and Sisson D (2003) Cardiac troponin-I levels in dogs and cats with cardiac disease. *Journal of Veterinary Internal Medicine* **17**, 400

Prosek R, Sisson DD, Oyama MA and Solter PF (2007) Distinguishing cardiac and noncardiac dyspnea in 48 dogs using plasma atrial natriuretic factor, B-type natriuretic factor, endothelin, and cardiac troponin-I. *Journal of Veterinary Internal Medicine* **21**, 238–242

Raffan E, Loureiro J, Dukes-McEwan J *et al.* (2009) The cardiac biomarker NT-proBNP is increased in dogs with azotaemia. *Journal of Veterinary Internal Medicine* **23**(6), 1184–1189

Rose BD (1989) Clinical use of diuretics. In: *Clinical Physiology of Acid–Base and Electrolyte Disorders, 3rd edn*, ed. BD Rose, pp. 389–415. McGraw-Hill, New York

Schmidt MK, Reynolds CA, Estrada AH *et al.* (2009) Effect of azotaemia on serum N-terminal proBNP concentration in dogs with normal cardiac function: a pilot study. *Journal of Veterinary Cardiology* **11**(Suppl. 1), S81–S86

Sisson D, Thomas WP, Ruehl W and Zinkl JG (1984) Diagnostic value of pericardial fluid analysis in the dog. *Journal of the American Veterinary Medical Associaton* **184**, 51–55

Spratt DP, Mellanby RJ, Drury N and Archer J (2005) Cardiac troponin I: evaluation of a biomarker for the diagnosis of heart disease in the dog. *Journal of Small Animal Practice* **46**, 139–145

Sykes JE, Kittleson MD, Chomel BB, Macdonald KA and Pesavento PA (2006a) Clinicopathologic findings and outcome in dogs with infective endocarditis: 71 cases (1992–2005). *Journal of the American Veterinary Medical Association* **228**, 1735–1747

Sykes JE, Kittleson MD, Pesavento PA *et al.* (2006b) Evaluation of the relationship between causative organisms and clinical characteristics of infective endocarditis in dogs: 71 cases (1992–2005). *Journal of the American Veterinary Medical Association* **228**, 1723–1734

Syme HM, Markwell PJ, Pfeiffer D and Elliott J (2006) Survival of cats with naturally occurring chronic renal failure is related to severity of proteinuria. *Journal of Veterinary Internal Medicine* **20**, 528–535

Troughton RW, Frampton CM, Yandle TG *et al.* (2000) Treatment of heart failure guided by plasma aminoterminal brain natriuretic peptide (N-BNP) concentrations. *The Lancet* **355**, 1126–1130

9

Electrocardiography and ambulatory monitoring

Ruth Willis

Electrocardiography

An *electrocardiograph* is a device for measuring electrical activity at the body surface. The electrical activity is generated by neuromuscular and cardiac tissue activity but, as the objective is to document cardiac muscle activity, precautions should be taken to minimize skeletal muscle movement. The *electrocardiogram* (ECG) produced is a record of the potential difference (in mV) between electrodes plotted on the vertical axis against time (in seconds) plotted on the horizontal axis.

Electrical activity is generated in cardiac tissue by changes in the transmembrane electrical potentials as a result of ion movement. This electrical activity then triggers myocardial cell contraction and is therefore essential for normal cardiac function. In the heart, pacemaker cells are located in the sinoatrial (SA) node and also in the atrioventricular (AV) node, Bundle of His, bundle branches and Purkinje fibres (Figure 9.1). These pacemaker cells have the ability to depolarize spontaneously (automaticity). The SA node depolarizes spontaneously at the fastest rate and is therefore the dominant pacemaker under normal conditions. The rate of discharge of the SA node can be influenced by numerous external factors, primarily sympathetic and parasympathetic tone.

Formation of the normal electrocardiogram

Figure 9.2 illustrates normal ECG waveforms and intervals.

- The impulse starts at the SA node and the depolarization spreads across the atria. The small potential difference between depolarized cells and cells that have not yet been stimulated is shown on the ECG as a deflection known as the *P wave*.
- When all the atrial cells are depolarized the ECG trace returns to baseline, which is also known as the *isoelectric point*.
- The atria are electrically insulated from the ventricles by a fibrous ring around the AV junction and therefore the electrical impulse cannot pass from the atrial cells to the ventricular cells other than via the AV node. The electrical impulse is delayed at the AV node, which allows time for the atria to contract and complete filling of the ventricles. This delay is shown on the ECG as the *PR interval* (though strictly it is the PQ interval when a Q wave is present).

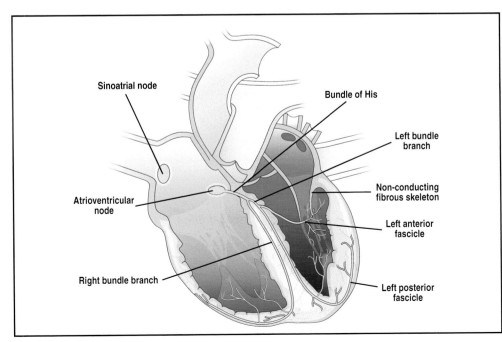

9.1

The electrical conduction system. Note that the tricuspid valve leaflets have been removed to more accurately show the position of the AV node in the right atrial endocardium. The AV node lies directly above the septal leaflet of the tricuspid valve.

Sinoatrial node

Bundle of His

Left bundle branch

Non-conducting fibrous skeleton

Left anterior fascicle

Atrioventricular node

Right bundle branch

Left posterior fascicle

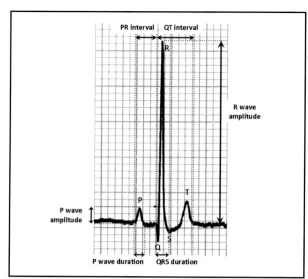

9.2 Normal ECG waveforms and intervals from a dog (lead II shown; paper speed 25 mm/s; gain 1 cm/mV).

- The electrical impulse then passes rapidly through into the Bundle of His, which after a short distance divides into the left and right bundle branches; the left bundle divides again into the posterior and anterior fascicles (see Figure 9.1). Distally the bundle branches subdivide to form the Purkinje network, which transmits the electrical impulse to the ventricular myocytes. The depolarization of this relatively large mass of tissue creates a large deflection on the ECG known as the *QRS complex*.
  - The *Q wave* is defined as the first negative deflection of the QRS complex.
  - The *R wave* is defined as the first positive deflection and is normally a large positive deflection in lead II (see 'Lead systems' below).
  - The *S wave* is defined as the first negative deflection following the R wave.
- Ventricular repolarization results in a lower amplitude deflection known as the *T wave*, which may be positive, negative or biphasic.

Indications

The indications for performing an ECG include:

- History of collapse
- History of exercise intolerance
- Detection of an arrhythmia during clinical examination
- As part of the investigation of heart disease
- Suspected electrolyte abnormality, particularly hyperkalaemia
- Pericardial disease
- Suspected drug toxicity (e.g. digoxin)
- Monitoring during anaesthesia or in a critical care setting.

Equipment

Many machines are available, including systems that are targeted specifically at the veterinary market.

Features that are advantageous in small animal patients include the following:

- Six-lead system with at least three leads displayed simultaneously to assist in distinguishing artefact from genuine cardiac electrical activity
- Good quality hard copy of the trace with clear grid lines
- Different paper speeds such as 50 mm/s and 25 mm/s
- A filter that can be turned off, as otherwise it may filter out P waves, particularly in cats
- Variable amplification gain (sensitivity), so that complex amplitude can be adjusted
- LCD screen, so that the quality of the recording can be checked prior to printing and also for monitoring patients
- A lead II rhythm strip recorded over 3–5 minutes without using large quantities of paper (useful but not essential).

Lead systems

Electrodes are placed on the limbs of the patient and the ECG works as a galvanometer, measuring the potential difference between electrodes in different locations. The standard lead configuration used in small animal patients is three bipolar leads – I, II and III – which have the following positions (Figure 9.3):

- *Lead I*: Left forelimb is the positive electrode; right forelimb is the negative electrode
- *Lead II*: Left hindlimb is the positive electrode; right forelimb is the negative electrode
- *Lead III*: Left hindlimb is the positive electrode; left forelimb is the negative electrode
- *Earth electrode*: attached to right hindlimb.

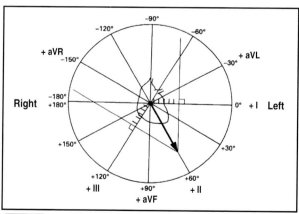

9.3 Lead systems.

There are also three augmented unipolar leads – aVR, aVL and aVF – which combine the results from two limbs and compare this to a third point as follows:

- Lead aVR: The right forelimb forms the positive electrode and the combined left forelimb and left hindlimb leads form the negative electrode
- *Lead aVL*: The left forelimb is the positive electrode and the combination of the right forelimb

and left hindlimb form the negative electrode

- *Lead aVF*: The left hindlimb is the positive electrode and the combined left forelimb and right forelimb form the negative electrode.

Recordings can also be made using unipolar chest (precordial) leads, which are primarily used in humans to detect ST segment change suggestive of myocardial hypoxia. In cats and dogs these leads are more useful for helping to visualize low-amplitude P waves. Recording of chest leads requires electrodes to be attached both around the chest wall and on the limbs.

Recording a good quality electrocardiogram

Positioning

The animal should be calm and relaxed before being placed on a surface that is electrically insulated, such as a rubber mat or thick blanket. Ideally dogs should be placed in right lateral recumbency (Figure 9.4), but in uncooperative patients or those in respiratory distress this may not be possible and recordings in sternal recumbency, sitting or standing are sufficient to gain most information regarding heart rhythm. A caveat to this is that complex amplitude and orientation will be more variable in non-standard patient positions.

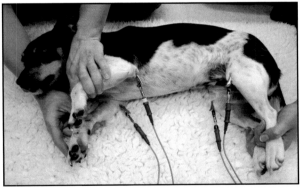

9.4 Patient positioning and restraint for a resting ECG. (Courtesy of S. Dennis.)

In cats, body position appears to be less important. Ideally cats should be gently restrained in right lateral recumbency, but other positions may result in improved patient compliance and a better quality trace with less artefact.

Preparation

Sedative and anaesthetic drugs may affect heart rate and rhythm via their effects on autonomic tone and also some drugs are potentially proarrhythmic. Therefore, the ECG should ideally be recorded prior to the administration of these agents.

ECG electrode clips are generally placed on the skin overlying bony protuberances to minimize the effect of muscle interference. Standard electrode placement for limb leads are shown in Figures 9.4 and 9.5. Some clinicians prefer to use the skin on the cranial surface of the elbow and hock, which may be useful

Electrode	Colour UK	Colour US	Position
Right forelimb	Red	White	On skin over right olecranon
Left forelimb	Yellow	Black	On skin over left olecranon
Left hindlimb	Green	Red	On skin over left patellar tendon
Right hindlimb	Black	Green	On skin over right patellar tendon

9.5 Standard electrode placement for limb leads.

particularly in giant-breed dogs that often have thick skin calluses over the caudolateral area of the elbow.

Crocodile clips should have their inner surfaces ('teeth') filed down to minimize skin trauma. When a more prolonged ECG is required, such as during echocardiography or critical care monitoring, self-adhesive electrodes may be attached to the footpads and the clips attached to these (Figure 9.6) to minimize patient discomfort and also eliminate the possibility of skin necrosis as a result of chronic compression by a crocodile clip. Electrodes attached to footpads are reported to result in lower amplitude R waves in cats (Ferasin *et al.*, 2006).

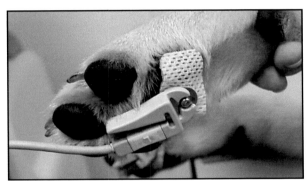

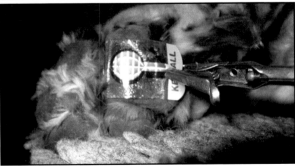

9.6 Clips attached by adhesive pads to prevent skin trauma.

The clips are then sprayed with surgical spirit (*caution: flammable!*) or covered in ECG gel to achieve good electrical conductance. There is no need to remove hair from these areas prior to clip attachment.

Procedure

Normally at least three good quality complexes should be recorded in all six leads at 50 mm/s. Before doing this it is important to ensure that the gain/sensitivity (vertical axis scale) is set to optimize complex size to a height that is clearly seen without the overlapping of different leads or the complex being too big and not fitting on to the paper. The filter should be turned off. After obtaining good quality examples of all six limb leads, a 25 mm/s rhythm strip is recorded for 1–5 minutes.

Electrocardiogram storage

Most systems will provide a hard copy of the trace on thermal paper. Note that recordings on thermal paper may fade with time, or on contact with plastics. Newer systems may allow electronic storage with the patient's record. It is useful if the name of the animal and the date and time of the recording are printed on the trace. Many machines will automatically label the leads and print the paper speed and gain/sensitivity on the header or footer of the page, which facilitates later analysis.

Approach to interpretation

To interpret an ECG, the clinician should:

1. *Assess the trace for presence of artefacts.*
2. Calculate the heart rate.
3. Assess heart rhythm.
4. Evaluate P:QRS relationship.
5. Assess QRS complex morphology.
6. Measure size of complexes and interval durations.
7. Calculate the mean electrical axis.

Assess the trace for presence of artefacts

Electrical interference: Electrical interference appears as regular sharp undulations of the ECG trace, which in the UK occur with a frequency of 50 Hz (Figure 9.7). To correct this problem:

- Ensure that there is good electrode contact with the patient
- Ensure that the patient is on an insulated surface (e.g. a thick blanket)
- Ensure that the ECG machine is earthed
- Turn off unnecessary electrical equipment in the room.

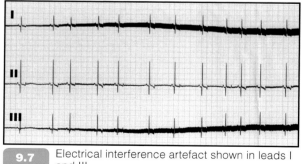

9.7 Electrical interference artefact shown in leads I and III.

Muscle tremor or movement: Muscle tremor or movement artefact is common in animals and results in random baseline deflections generally associated with patient movement, panting, trembling or purring. This artefact can be minimized by gently restraining the patient in a position that it finds comfortable.

Chemical restraint should be avoided as this is likely to alter heart rate and rhythm, for example alpha-2 agonist drugs may elicit bradyarrhythmias. Muscle tremor artefacts on an ambulatory ECG (see Figure 9.10) appear similar to movement artefacts of a resting ECG.

Calculate the heart rate

By knowing the paper speed, 1-second intervals can be calculated. A quick way of calculating heart rate is to measure a 6-second interval (15 cm at 25 mm/s, 30 cm at 50 mm/s), count the number of QRS complexes within this period, and multiple by 10 to obtain the heart rate in beats per minute. An alternative method is to use the RR intervals to calculate heart rate. At a paper speed of 25 mm/s, the heart rate is calculated by dividing 1500 by the RR interval in millimetres (or 3000/RR interval with a paper speed of 50 mm/s).

Normal heart rates are shown in Figure 9.8 but should always be interpreted in light of patient temperament and the level of anxiety during the recording.

Parameter	Dogs	Cats
Heart rate (beats/min)	Adult: 70–160 Puppy: 70–220	Adult: 140–240
P wave duration (seconds)	Adult: <0.04 Giant-breed: <0.05	<0.04
P wave amplitude (mV)	<0.4	<0.2
PR interval (seconds)	0.06–0.13	0.05–0.09
QRS duration (seconds)	<0.06	<0.04
R wave amplitude (mV)	<3.0	<0.9
T wave	<25% of R wave amplitude	
QT interval (seconds)	0.15–0.25	0.12–0.18

9.8 Normal ECG measurements in dogs and cats.

Assess heart rhythm

Sinus rhythm is a normal heart rhythm in cats and dogs characterized by a consistent RR interval with complexes of normal P–QRS–T morphology. Sinus arrhythmia is commonly seen in normal dogs – particularly in the brachycephalic breeds, which tend to have a higher resting vagal tone. Sinus arrhythmia results in a rhythmic change in the RR interval, which approximately follows respiratory movements but is also influenced by other factors affecting vagal tone. Abnormalities of rhythm include premature beats and prolonged pauses (see Chapter 16).

Evaluate P:QRS relationship

In a normal small animal ECG, every P wave should be followed by a normal QRS complex, with a consistent relationship between the two deflections; therefore, the ratio of P waves to QRS complexes should be 1:1. The trace should be closely examined to ensure that this is the case. Wandering pacemaker is caused by changes in vagal tone influencing the exact site of impulse generation within the SA node, and this may result in cyclical changes in P wave morphology, although the P wave will generally always by visible in at least one lead (see Chapter 16). Baseline artefacts can make distinguishing each individual P wave more challenging.

Assess QRS complex morphology

Normal QRS complexes are upright and narrow, whereas complexes originating from the ventricles (also known as ectopic or ventricular beats) have a wide, bizarre appearance. These complexes are wide and bizarre because they are not conducted through the myocardium via the normal conducting tissue, but instead are conducted from myocardial cell to myocardial cell, which takes longer. As the wave of depolarization has an abnormal route, this results in a change in QRS–T morphology.

QRS complex morphology can also be affected by patient and limb position, which can cause changes in R wave amplitude. Q waves (if present) may also be more pronounced in young animals and this is usually not a clinically significant finding.

QRS complex abnormalities: Conduction abnormalities can result in changes in ECG interval measurements and also changes in complex morphology.

• *Left bundle branch block* describes a block of conduction down the left bundle branch: there is normal depolarization of the right ventricle (RV) but a delay in depolarization of the left ventricle (LV), resulting in a tall wide (>0.07 seconds in cats and toy breeds, >0.08 seconds in all other dog breeds), positive QRS complex in leads I, II, III and aVF and negative QRS complex in leads aVR and aVL. This conduction deficit can be difficult to distinguish from a left ventricular enlargement pattern.
• *Right bundle branch block* results from a delay or failure of impulse conduction down the right bundle branch: there is normal depolarization of the LV but a delay in depolarization of the RV, resulting in a prolonged QRS complex (>0.07 seconds in cats and toy breeds, >0.08 seconds in all other dog breeds). The QRS complex is negative in leads I, II, III and aVF and positive in leads aVR and aVL.
• *Left anterior fascicular block* describes a failure of conduction through the anterior fascicle of the left bundle branch (see Figure 9.1). This conduction deficit is more common in cats with heart disease and usually results in a QRS complex of normal duration but tall R waves in leads I and aVL and deep S waves in leads II, III and aVF. The mean electrical axis tends to be shifted to the left, resulting in R wave amplitude being greatest in lead aVL.
• *Splintered or notched QRS complexes* can be seen commonly in small animals with heart disease, but the clinical significance is debatable. Notching of the QRS complex can be seen in dogs with tricuspid valve dysplasia and pre-excitation of the ventricles via an accessory pathway. This change may also be associated with microscopic intramural myocardial infarction(s) or fibrosis of the ventricle.

• *Low voltage QRS complexes* are most commonly associated with poor contact caused by insufficient conduction medium, broad chest conformation and thick hair coat. However, low voltage QRS complexes can also be associated with pleural effusion, pericardial effusion, intrathoracic masses, obesity and hypothyroidism.
• *Electrical alternans* is a regular alternation in QRS amplitude usually occurring on every other beat. Electrical alternans can be seen in panting dogs, in dogs with pericardial effusion (presumably associated with the heart swinging within the effusion), with some supraventricular tachycardias and also occasionally in normal animals.

Measure size of complexes

For normal measurements, see Figure 9.8. Changes in these measurements may reflect conduction abnormalities and/or chamber enlargement. It is important to remember that the ECG is an indirect indicator of chamber size and that echocardiography is far superior for assessment of cardiac chamber dimensions.

Changes suggestive of chamber enlargement

• *Left atrial enlargement* can result in prolongation of the P wave and sometimes notching of the P wave, which is known as 'P mitrale'.
• *Right atrial enlargement* may result in an increase in P wave amplitude, particularly in leads II, III and aVF (also known as 'P pulmonale').
• *Left ventricular enlargement* may result in tall R waves in leads II, III and aVF, and occasionally, when severe, prolongation of the QRS complex.
• *Right ventricular enlargement* may result in S waves in leads I, II, III and aVF, and a QRS axis deviation to the right (>100 degrees).

Calculate the mean electrical axis

The mean electrical axis describes the net vector of depolarization across the heart muscle. It is approximately in the direction of the lead with the highest amplitude R wave. In dogs it will usually be between +40 and +100 degrees (leads II and aVF) and in cats between 0 and +160 degrees. The assigned configuration of the scale for measuring the angle is shown in Figure 9.3, and this measurement can be used to determine whether there is an intraventricular conduction abnormality such as left anterior fascicular block.

Ambulatory monitoring

Indications

Ambulatory electrocardiographs are monitors worn by the patient that can record heart rate and rhythm over a longer period than is possible using static electrocardiography equipment. The advantage of obtaining an ambulatory ECG is that the patient can leave the clinic with the monitor attached and therefore perform normal activities such as rest and exercise, which may allow documentation of the heart rate and rhythm whilst the patient is showing clinical signs. There are several indications for obtaining an ambulatory recording, including:

- Intermittent collapse
- Exercise intolerance
- Screening breeds at risk of arrhythmias (such as Boxers and Dobermanns)
- If an arrhythmia is detected or suspected
- Assessing the severity of an arrhythmia
- Deciding whether antiarrhythmic treatment is indicated
- Monitoring the efficacy of antiarrhythmic treatment.

Equipment

There are many systems available for recording an ambulatory ECG and they can be classified into event (or loop) recorders, telemetry systems and Holter monitors.

Loop recorders

Loop recorders are used commonly in human patients but are less useful in veterinary patients, as the monitor needs to be carried on the patient for a long period; they are usually activated during an episode of collapse. Loop recorders may be external, but in cases where collapse is only very occasional it may be better to implant the loop recording device subcutaneously. These devices may be activated remotely by the owner, or some newer devices may be activated automatically. The auto-activation settings should be carefully programmed for small animal patients, as the algorithms that determine activation are devised for detection of arrhythmias in humans. As a consequence, some physiological arrhythmias such as sinus arrhythmia and sinus pauses at rest can trigger auto-activation settings, resulting in the memory filling with material that is physiological rather than pathological. The battery life in these devices is generally about 9 months (or up to 2 years in newer models); after this time, the monitor should be removed under sedation or a general anaesthetic. One such implantable device, known as a 'Reveal™', has been used to investigate the cause of collapse in small animals (Willis *et al.*, 2003).

The advantages of the implantable system are the long recording time and the ability to download information with the device still *in situ*. The disadvantages are:

- That general anaesthesia or sedation is required to implant the device
- That owner activation is required on some systems, obliging the owner to carry a remote control at all times
- The high cost of the device
- Problems with programming algorithms designed for humans, not animals.

Telemetry systems

Telemetry systems allow close-range transmission of an ECG to a receiver. In small animals these are best suited to a critical care setting, where the patient is stationary.

Holter monitoring

Holter monitoring is a non-invasive means of continuously recording an ECG over a period of up to 7 days and is a useful, readily available and non-invasive means for the detection of intermittent arrhythmias. Modern lightweight digital monitors weigh about 150 g and are fastened to the dog using a harness and three electrodes (Figure 9.9).

The key to obtaining a successful recording is good electrode contact with the skin; therefore hair should be clipped and surgical spirit used to remove grease from the skin. The electrodes should be attached carefully, and adhered to the skin using adhesive tape or even tissue glue.

The digital recorders are reliable and usually well tolerated by dogs as they are able to perform all normal activities, but cats sometimes need to be hospitalized during the recording with the monitor placed next to them within the kennel. The monitor does not require remote activation during an episode and may document significant arrhythmias even if the patient does not exhibit clinical signs during the recording.

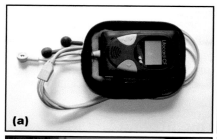
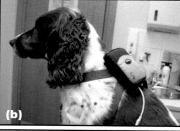
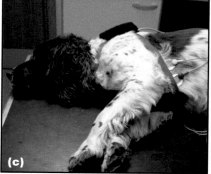
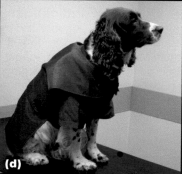

9.9 Holter monitor set up. **(a)** Lightweight digital Holter monitor. **(b)** Monitor inside padded case positioned in dorsal midline using harness. **(c)** Position of adhesive electrodes on the left side of the chest. The third electrode is placed over the apex beat on the right side of the thorax. **(d)** A small T-shirt is used to prevent the hindlegs becoming tangled in the leads running from the monitor to the electrodes. A waterproof jacket is used to protect the monitor if the dog is exercising in the rain.

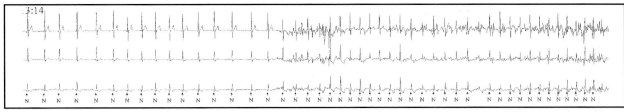

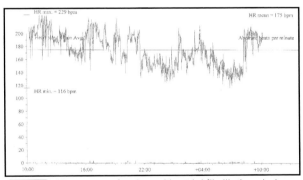

9.10 Excerpt from a Holter recording from a dog during an episode of collapse. The trace shows sinus rhythm with a normal rate and baseline artefact, suggesting vigorous muscle activity. This implies that an arrhythmia is not the cause of the signs seen.

Reasons for using a Holter monitor

Distinguishing atypical seizures from syncope

Classically seizures will occur at rest; there may be a prodromal phase; there is tonic–clonic movement during the episode; urination or defecation may occur; and recovery tends to be gradual. Some dogs do not exhibit these classic signs (e.g. they show signs during exercise) and also some arrhythmias may elicit hypoxic seizures. Therefore, a Holter recording to document heart rate and rhythm during an episode can be useful in determining the course of further investigation and treatment (Figure 9.10). The characteristic features of syncope are described in Chapter 3.

Screening breeds at risk of cardiovascular disease

Dobermanns and Boxers have an increased prevalence of arrhythmias compared with other dog breeds, particularly ventricular arrhythmias that have the potential to be life-threatening. These arrhythmias may affect an animal's suitability for breeding and also prompt intervention with antiarrhythmic drugs. These arrhythmias are intermittent and there can be considerable day-to-day variability (up to 80–85% in Boxers). Holter monitoring is a useful modality for detecting them.

Detecting intermittent arrhythmias

Collapse is a common presenting sign in small animal practice and it is understandably of concern to owners. The investigation of collapse can be challenging, due to the intermittent nature of clinical signs and also the wide-ranging differential diagnosis list (see Chapter 3). Animals rarely exhibit signs in the surgery and therefore a Holter monitor recording can be useful if an intermittent arrhythmia is suspected. Brachycephalic breeds have an increased prevalence of vasovagal (neurally mediated) syncope (see Chapter 3), and Holter monitoring is useful in distinguishing this relatively benign abnormality from potentially life-threatening arrhythmias such as ventricular tachycardia (see Figure 16.16).

Determining antiarrhythmic drug efficacy

In cases with atrial fibrillation, monitoring the ventricular rate whilst the dog is in the consulting room may not be representative of heart rate at home or during exercise, due to patient anxiety. Sustained tachycardia may result in worsening of systolic failure and therefore good heart rate control is important to preserve ventricular function. Holter monitoring is a useful means of determining whether there is adequate ventricular rate control in cases with atrial fibrillation (Figure 9.11). Mean heart rate over 24 hours in normal dogs is usually 80–90 beats/minute.

Assessing for proarrhythmia

The treatment of arrhythmias is challenging and some cases may continue to show signs (e.g. collapse) after treatment has started, raising the possibility of proarrhythmia. Proarrhythmia implies that the antiarrhythmic drug has actually caused another arrhythmia, which may be identified on Holter recordings.

9.11 Heart rate of a dog with atrial fibrillation during a 24-hour Holter recording. Heart rate is shown on the vertical axis and time on the horizontal axis. The mean heart rate is 175 beats/minute, suggesting suboptimal heart rate control.

References and further reading

Ferasin L, Amiodo A and Murray JK (2006) Validation of two techniques for electrocardiographic recording in dogs and cats. *Journal of Veterinary Internal Medicine* **20**, 873–876

Martin M and Corcoran B (2006) Electrocardiography. In: *Notes on Cardiorespiratory Diseases of the Dog and Cat, 2nd edn,* ed. M Martin and B Corcoran, pp. 24–38. Blackwell Publishing, Oxford

Tilley LP (1992) General principles of electrocardiography. In: *Essentials of Canine and Feline Electrocardiography, 3rd edn*, ed. LP Tilley, pp. 21–55. Lea and Febiger, Philadelphia

Willis R, McLeod K, Cusack J and Wotton P (2003) Use of an implantable loop device to investigate syncope in a cat. *Journal of Small Animal Practice* **44**, 181–183

10

Airway sampling and introduction to bronchoscopy

Brendan M. Corcoran

Tracheal wash and bronchoalveolar lavage

Indications

Airway sampling is a very important component of the diagnostic work up of respiratory cases, and in many instances it is the method that will give a definitive diagnosis since the results of such tests will reflect lung and airway pathology. Until routine lung biopsy is adopted in companion animal medicine, airway sampling will remain one of most important diagnostic tests in respiratory medicine.

The main use of airway sampling is to obtain samples for cytological analysis. In addition, airway sampling can allow identification of significant bacterial infections and can identify respiratory parasites. However, culture might not always be successful and the veterinary surgeon has to be wary of false-negative results or erroneous positive results (i.e. culturing organisms that are of no concern).

Techniques

Airway samples can be obtained by transtracheal wash (TTW), blind sampling via an endotracheal tube or bronchoalveolar lavage (BAL) using a bronchoscope. The latter technique is preferable as it will give the best return and allows samples to be collected from specific sites. A TTW can give a variable return and is usually reserved for those patients where there is a high anaesthetic risk. Blind sampling via an endotracheal tube can be reasonably effective, is the usual method used in cats, and is a valuable technique if bronchoscopy is not available. Whichever technique is used, the collected material should be separated for cytological analysis and culture. For cytological analysis, assessment needs to be undertaken as soon as possible. If the sample has to be sent to an external laboratory, it should by spun and air-dried smears made from the pelleted sample. This will preserve the cells and greatly improve the quality of the sample. Seeking advice and guidance from the laboratory and the cytopathologist is also worthwhile. For specific culture requirements, the proper containers and transport media have to be used, and again advice and guidance should be obtained from the laboratory.

Tracheal wash

A TTW should be carried out, preferably, without sedation so as to encourage coughing and thereby improve yield. A jugular catheter system can be used.

- The ventral neck should be clipped and aseptically prepared.
- The dog can be restrained in a sitting position with the head extended and elevated, and the junction of the cricoid cartilage and the trachea identified.
- A small amount of lidocaine should be injected at this site, a small stab incision made and the needle inserted at an angle of about 45 degrees.
- Once the needle is in place the catheter can be threaded through the needle. This will often induce coughing. The needle is withdrawn and a needle guard placed around it to avoid inadvertent severing of the catheter.
- Between 3 ml and 20 ml (depending on the size of the dog) of warmed sterile saline can be instilled and slowly aspirated, at the same time applying coupage to the chest to stimulate coughing.

The return can be disappointing, but the procedure can be repeated two or three times without adverse effects, and the combined return may be sufficient for analysis. It is likely that a TTW will collect material representative of the trachea only. If there is active inflammation of the lower airways or lungs and material has been moved rostrally by mucociliary clearance and coughing, a TTW can result in a diagnostic sample. However, of the three techniques available, a TTW is the least sensitive.

Endotracheal tube wash

The advantage of an endotracheal tube wash (ETW) over a TTW is the greater chance of obtaining a more representative sample from the lower airways and lungs. However, it is still a blind sampling technique and can give a variable return. It is a particularly useful technique in cats, and when there is significant active inflammatory disease an ETW usually provides a representative sample. The only difference from a TTW is that the patient is anaesthetized and the catheter is placed via a sterile endotracheal tube. A longer catheter can be used, such as one designed for a bronchoscope biopsy channel, which gives access to more distal parts of the lungs. A rough guide as to how far to insert the catheter should be determined by measuring the catheter against the patient. To reach the carina, the long catheter should extend to approximately the fourth intercostal space. Similar volumes to those used for a TTW of warmed sterile saline can be instilled and retrieved using either the same syringe or a suction pump connected to a sample trap. The one potential complication of an ETW is inadvertent pushing of the catheter tip through the airway wall or lung, resulting in pneumomediastinum or pneumothorax. The catheter should be advanced gently and with caution. If it feels as though there is an obstruction, the catheter should be repositioned rather than forced.

Bronchoalveolar lavage

The advantage of BAL over a TTW or an ETW is that it allows more complete and accurate sampling by targeting the site of disease and is more likely to obtain a true alveolar sample. The limitation is that it requires bronchoscopic guidance and so is restricted to those practices with the appropriate facilities (see below).

- With the bronchoscope in the airway of interest, the catheter should be advanced through the biopsy channel as far as possible into the airway.
- The bronchoscope should be withdrawn a short distance to allow the operator to visualize the sample being collected.
- Warmed sterile saline (3 ml to 20 ml) should be instilled and suction immediately applied, either with the same syringe or by attaching a suction pump connected to a sample trap (preferred).
- The catheter position should be adjusted gently and the fluid observed travelling inside the catheter. The operator then knows a good representative sample will be obtained.
- The position of the catheter should continued to be adjusted until there is no further fluid moving inside the catheter. The catheter should then be withdrawn.

If there has been reasonable return (40–50%), this is usually sufficient for diagnostic purposes and the sample should be processed. Using suction and a sample trap greatly improves the quantity of fluid retrieved, and the procedure can be repeated up to three times if needed. The presence of particulate matter in a cloudy/frothy sample is ideal, but the sample may be visibly clear in normal animals.

Complications

The complications of airway sampling are limited if the procedures are carried out cautiously. The effect of restraint or anaesthesia on patients with respiratory compromise needs to be appreciated and the potential value of the procedure measured against the potential risk. Excessive instillation of saline into the airways can compromise respiratory function, but when recommended volumes are used there should be no problems. Placement of catheters with excessive force can damage the lungs and airways and in the worst case scenario result in pneumothorax.

Bronchoscopy

While in recent years bronchoscopy has tended to be the preserve of specialist centres, the greater availability of affordable fibreoptic endoscopes has meant its wider adoption in general practice.

Indications

In specialist referral practice, bronchoscopy is fundamental to the investigation of respiratory cases, particularly chronic respiratory disease. Its use in the investigation of acute respiratory cases (such as bacterial bronchopneumonia) where a reasonably confident diagnosis can be made by other means, or conditions that are likely to be self-limiting (such as acute tracheobronchitis), is questionable, although if foreign body aspiration is suspected as the cause for acute coughing, bronchoscopy is indicated. The main value of bronchoscopy is that it allows direct inspection of the tracheobronchial tree, which improves diagnostic accuracy, and it also allows the clinician to better understand underlying disease processes. An additional diagnostic value of bronchoscopy is its use in disease exclusion. Under all circumstances, bronchoscopy is used in conjunction with standard diagnostic procedures, most importantly thoracic radiography.

Technique

Bronchoscopy is carried out under general anaesthesia. Prior to bronchoscopy, thoracic radiography should be performed to provide some guidance as to what might be seen on the endoscopic examination. This should include standard right lateral recumbent and ventrodorsal (VD) views and if indicated a left lateral recumbent view. If the dog is anaesthetized at this time, a lateral view of the cervical region and thoracic inlet should be obtained with the endotracheal tube removed. The radiographs should be reviewed to determine whether there are any visible abnormalities and also to clarify the locality of such changes. An additional reason for carrying out radiography first is that BAL, which is undertaken during bronchoscopy, results in radiographic artefacts (alveolar pattern).

Anaesthetic monitoring

High-quality anaesthetic monitoring is required for safe bronchoscopy, and the endoscopist should have confidence in the quality of monitoring. The main danger is hypoxaemia as a result of airway obstruction by the bronchoscope. Throughout the procedure, the anaesthetist should have complete authority and should stop the procedure as soon as they are concerned for the safety of the patient. This usually means stopping for a short period until the hypoxaemia has been reversed, but it can also mean abandoning the procedure if the hypoxaemia persists or if other complications such as arrhythmias arise. To reduce the risk of hypoxaemia, an additional oxygen supply can be delivered via a side catheter and the bronchoscope can be introduced to the endotracheal tube via a two-way attachment (Cobb piece). This also allows continual delivery of anaesthetic gases. The anaesthetist will also need to inflate the patient's lungs periodically to reverse positional atelectasis. For very short procedures or where intubation is not possible as it will prevent introduction of the bronchoscope (small dogs and cats), continuous or intermittent total intravenous anaesthesia is required. Propofol is commonly used for this purpose. In medium- to large-breed dogs, the bronchoscope causes minimal occlusion of the endotracheal tube and the risk of hypoxaemia is greatly reduced, thus increasing the margin of safety throughout the duration of the procedure. Nevertheless, the endoscopist should aim to keep the procedure as short as possible. For those with limited experience the best way to learn is to endoscope repeatedly for short periods, as this gives time to interpret what is being seen.

Equipment

Prior to initiating the endoscopic procedure, it is also useful to have ready the materials for BAL, including:

- Syringes
- Sterile normal saline
- Containers (x2)
- Fluid trap if pump suction is available (preferred)
- Sampling catheter and appropriate sampling forms (cytology and culture).

The preferred bronchoscope is a 3.5–6.0 mm diameter fibreoptic endoscope with a working length of at least 55 cm. These are the typical dimensions for human bronchoscopes and an endoscope of 5 mm diameter will be perfectly adequate for most sizes of dogs. For endoscopy of cats a narrower broncho-scope is needed. Endoscopes of 55 cm working length can be too short to adequately inspect the lobar bronchi of large breeds of dogs. Longer veteri-nary endoscopes are available to overcome this prob-lem, but an alternative approach is to use a gastroduodenoscope. While such endoscopes are up to 8 mm in diameter, occlusion of the airway is relative as the dog is also larger. One problem of using an endoscope longer than 55 cm and <6 mm in diameter, or an endoscope of even narrower dimensions, is that the image tends to be less clear because fewer fibres transmit less light. The latest advance is the develop-ment of videobronchoscopes. Such technology is cur-rently expensive but is likely to become less so in coming years and may replace fibreoptic endoscopes in due course.

The image from the endoscope can be viewed directly through the lens aperture (although this facil-ity has been removed from many modern endo-scopes). This is the least expensive set up; however, visualizing the image on a video monitor is preferable, not least in terms of operator comfort. Being able to display and capture the image also allows recording of images for subsequent interpretation, comparison with repeated examinations, obtaining opinions from colleagues, teaching, and explaining findings with greater clarity to the client.

Positioning

Positioning of the patient depends on operator preference. Sternal recumbency would appear to be the logical position; however, handling, introducing and operating the endoscope can be less difficult if the patient is in lateral recumbency (personal preference). If the latter position is chosen, intermittent inflation of the lungs by the anaesthetist will overcome any problems with positional atelectasis.

Procedure

- The endoscope is introduced into the endotracheal tube, with lubricant applied to the distal end if necessary, and passed into the trachea. The C-shaped cartilage rings and the dorsal membrane can be clearly seen. In some dogs, the dorsal membrane will divide at the carina and continue down both mainstem bronchi. The carina is used to provide accurate identification of the entrance to the right and left mainstem bronchi (Figure 10.1). The right mainstem bronchus can be clearly seen on the operator's left and appears to be a direct extension of the trachea.
- The endoscope is advanced beyond the carina into the right mainstem bronchus, and the entrance to the right cranial lung lobe bronchus is immediately seen on the operator's left. A short distance beyond that point is the entrance to the right middle lung lobe bronchus, on the same side and usually at the same level. At that point, the entrance to the accessory lung lobe bronchus can be seen to the operator's right. Beyond that point is the entrance to the right caudal lung lobe bronchus and at intervals along its length, dorsal and ventral side-bronchi can be seen.
- Returning to the carina, the entrance to the left mainstem bronchus is seen (the endoscope should be reoriented using the tracheal dorsal membrane if necessary); often the endoscope has to be twisted to the operator's right to get a clear view. The entrance to the left cranial lung lobe bronchus is seen immediately and if the endoscope is placed just beyond its entrance, the cranial (dorsal) and caudal (ventral) divisions of the left cranial lobar bronchus are seen. The left caudal lung lobe bronchus continues on from the left mainstem bronchus and has side branches at set intervals, as with the right mainstem bronchus.

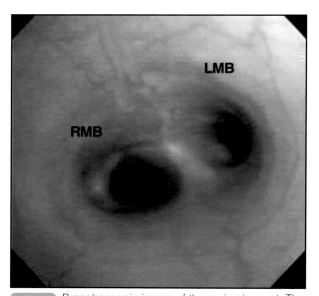

10.1 Bronchoscopic image of the carina in a cat. The opening to the left mainstem bronchus (LMB) and right mainstem bronchus (RMB) are valuable landmarks for performing bronchoscopy. (Courtesy of L. Johnson.)

Beyond this simple identification of the tracheo-bronchial tree, further identification of bronchial sub-divisions can be difficult, partly due to accessibility but also due to disorientation caused by the operator having to manipulate the endoscope to get into the airways. Depending on the size of the animal and the diameter of the endoscope being used, some bronchi are inaccessible using standard diameter endoscopes.

For a more detailed inspection of the trachea the endotracheal tube has to be removed. This allows endoscopic examination of the larynx, the glottis and the cricoid-tracheal junction, but is mainly undertaken to assess the degree of tracheal collapse along its entire length. Gaining entrance to the glottis can be difficult, particularly in small dogs. By straightening and extending the head and neck of the animal, pulling the tongue forward and displacing the soft palate and epiglottis with a probe, entering the glottis can be made much easier.

Normal appearance

The normal bronchoscopic appearance of the canine airway is best described as salmon-pink, smooth and lacking in secretions; the feline airway is much paler. In the trachea, the tracheal rings and inter-ring gaps give a striking striped appearance. The subepithelial blood vessels can be clearly seen and form a rich plexus overlying the whole tracheal surface. This is often still distinct at the level of the carina, and it is important the operator does not misinterpret this as an abnormal finding. The dorsal membrane may be relatively broad to span the distance between the two arms of the car-tilage rings, or it may be a narrow ridge. This variation in the appearance of the dorsal membrane might reflect differences in breed or size of dog.

Abnormal appearance

Abnormal bronchoscopic findings include:

- Mucosal hyperaemia
- Pallor or erosions
- Roughening of the mucosal surface
- Bronchial dilatation and thinning/distortion of the bronchial wall at the point of bronchial division
- Increased bronchial secretions including: clear gelatinous mucus; viscid, discoloured and occasionally caseous purulent/inflammatory material; blood-tinged mucus/pus; and frank blood.

Tracheal collapse can be identified (confirmed) and is typically seen at the thoracic inlet, the intrathoracic trachea and the carina and mainstem bronchi. Dynamic expiratory bronchial collapse can be seen, typically associated with primary lung neoplasia. Foreign bodies might also be identified, typically on the right side, and can be readily retrieved endoscopically. Secretions can also be localized to a specific side of the lung or to a specific lung lobe, and can be seen to accumulate at sites of airway division or form narrow bands adherent to the mucosal surface. These findings are usually typical of broncho-pneumonia. Intramural masses are very rare in dogs and cats, but are occasionally seen and can

significantly occlude the airway lumen. More detail on the interpretation of bronchoscopic findings is included in specific disease chapters.

Complications

The complications with bronchoscopy are few, and with proper care and attention can be easily avoided. The main consideration is hypoxaemia induced by the endoscope occluding the airway. Simple monitoring of oxygen saturation with a pulse oximeter and allowing the anaesthetist to make decisions on proceeding will avoid potentially catastrophic outcomes. Even the most severely compromised respiratory patient can undergo bronchoscopy safely. Keeping the procedure as short as possible will also reduce anaesthetic complications. Other complications can be related to operator inexperience and overzealous attempts to introduce the endoscope into the distal airways. In the worst case, this can result in life-threatening tension pneumothorax. Complications following bronchoscopy are also extremely rare, but one particular problem can be recovering dogs from anaesthesia that have severe tracheal collapse, where the excitement of recovery itself causes severe collapse.

Cytology and culture

Airway samples need to be handled and processed as described above. In many instances culture may be unsuccessful or, more importantly, organisms typically found in the normal airway may be grown.

Cytology

Normal canine and feline airway cytological samples contain small to moderate numbers of cells and typically include epithelial cells, a predominance of macrophages, a small number of neutrophils, and even smaller numbers of lymphocytes and eosinophils. Some erythrocytes might be present, but this is presumed to be iatrogenic. In some normal cats, and to a lesser extent dogs, there may be more than expected numbers of eosinophils. Quantifying cell numbers in BAL fluid samples is of little value as there are too many variables in the collection process to make comparison between animals valid. Measure-ment of cell numbers is qualitative and typically cytopathologists refer to numbers as small, moderate or high. This in itself can be subjective and dependent on the pathologist's definitions of these descriptors as well as their own experience in examining BAL fluid samples. Some cytopathologists will report the relative percentage of particular cells in a sample, but this is only of value if the cellularity is moderate or high.

Abnormal samples typical of a non-specific inflammatory process may have the same cellular profile as normal samples, but usually contain many more cells, particularly neutrophils (Figure 10.2). There may also be rafts of hyperplastic or metaplastic epithelium in the sample. In addition, neutrophils and macrophages may demonstrate evidence of activation, differentiation and degeneration typical of an ongoing infectious reaction. The presence of phagocytosed debris and intracellular bacteria is characteristic of bacterial bronchopneumonia (Figure 10.3).

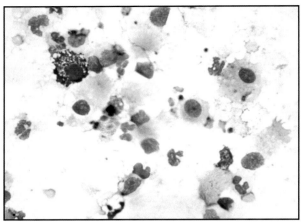

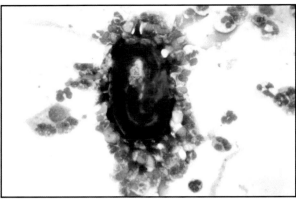

10.2 BAL sample illustrating non-specific inflammatory reaction. This sample was collected from a dog with chronic bronchitis and shows a mixed inflammatory profile dominated by neutrophils and macrophages.

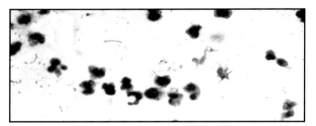

10.3 BAL sample illustrating a mixed inflammatory reaction associated with bacterial infection. This sample was collected from a dog with lobar bronchopneumonia and shows a mixed inflammatory profile with extra- and intracellular bacteria.

Increased numbers of eosinophils suggest an allergic (hypersensitivity) disorder or pulmonary parasitism. A concurrent but not inevitable circulating eosinophilia is often found in such cases. In the cat, airway eosinophilia is a typical clinical sign of asthma (but it should be borne in mind this might be normal in some cats); however, in some asthmatic/bronchitic cats a pronounced airway neutrophilia may be present and the predominant cell type can even vary between repeated samples from the same cat. In the dog, a diagnosis of pulmonary infiltration with eosinophilia (eosinophilic bronchopneumopathy) is usually made when a high percentage of eosinophils is found in the BAL fluid. If there is direct or indirect evidence of respiratory parasitism, airway eosinophilia can be used to support the diagnosis (Figure 10.4). Mast cells and basophils are rarely found in canine and feline airway samples, but their presence also supports a hypersensitivity or parasitism diagnosis. The presence of neoplastic cells or parasitic larvae is definitively diagnostic for these diseases, but false-negative results are a common occurrence with both of these conditions. Lastly, the identification of a normal airway sample is not conclusive evidence of normality as this may be due to the sampling technique, operator skill or experience, and the fact that some respiratory diseases do not affect airway cytology profiles.

10.4 BAL sample illustrating an inflammatory reaction with increased numbers of eosinophils surrounding an airway parasite (*Crenosoma*). (Courtesy of E. Milne.)

Culture

The airways of dogs and cats have a normal bacterial flora, usually Gram-negative organisms. Typical isolates from the airways of healthy cats and dogs include *Klebsiella*, *Pasteurella*, *Acinetobacter*, *Enterobacter*, *Eschericha coli*, *Staphylococcus* and *Streptococcus*. Therefore, the presence of such organisms in an airway sample has to be interpreted with caution. Heavy growth of bacteria can be viewed as significant and this is particularly so if intracellular organisms are also seen on cytology. The presence of *Bordetella bronchiseptica* is significant in all cases, but may represent persistent infection in a dog that has already recovered from kennel cough. If the dog is still coughing, appropriate antibacterial therapy based on sensitivity profiles should be instituted with the presumption that the organism is implicated in the disease. It may prove difficult to culture certain organisms, such as *Mycoplasma* and anaerobic or microaerophilic organisms such as *Actinomyces* and *Nocardia*, unless the sample is submitted in a specific medium and appropriate culture methods are used.

The time delay in obtaining culture and sensitivity data is problematic in dogs and cats with severe bronchopneumonia, and conventionally empirical broad-spectrum and intensive antibacterial therapy is instituted based on what is known about the organisms likely to be present in the respiratory tract.

References and further reading

Andreason CB (2003) Bronchoalveolar lavage. *Veterinary Clinics of North America: Small Animal Practice* **33**, 69–88
Johnson LR and Drazenovich TL (2007) Flexible bronchoscopy and bronchoalveolar lavage in 68 cats (2001–2006). *Journal of Veterinary Internal Medicine* **21**, 219–225
Norris CR, Griffey SM, Samii VF, Christopher MM and Mellema MS (2002) Thoracic radiography, bronchoalveolar lavage cytopathology and pulmonary parenchymal histopathology: a comparison of diagnostic results in 11 cats. *Journal of the American Animal Hospital Association* **38**, 337–345
Peeters DE, McKiernan BC, Weisiger RM, Schaeffer DJ and Clercx C (2000) Quantitative bacterial cultures and cytological examination of bronchoalveolar lavage specimens in dogs. *Journal of Veterinary Internal Medicine* **14**, 534–541
Rha YJ and Mahoney O (1999) Bronchoscopy in small animal medicine: indications, instrumentation, and techniques. *Clinical Techniques in Small Animal Practice* **14**, 207–212

11

Echocardiography

Virginia Luis Fuentes

Introduction

Echocardiography is probably the single most useful tool available for assessment of cardiac disease, with the possible exception of physical examination (Boon, 1998). Echocardiography is safe and versatile, giving information about both cardiac structure and function. Nevertheless, echocardiography findings should always be interpreted in the context of other clinical findings and all echocardiography results should be integrated to produce a plausible 'story'. In other words, physical examination findings, chamber enlargement and Doppler echocardiography findings should all be consistent with one another.

The echocardiographer needs to be more than just a good ultrasonographer. In addition to possessing the technical skills to record standard imaging planes in a variety of patients, the echocardiographer should have a good understanding of cardiac pathophysiology and of the haemodynamic effect of different diseases and lesions. Although a standardized protocol should form the basis of every echocardiography study, some ability to 'think on one's feet' enables additional questions to be answered during the course of the examination.

Types of echocardiography

The different types of echocardiography are shown in Figure 11.1.

- *M-mode echocardiography* depicts linear dimension plotted against time.
- *Two-dimensional (2D) echocardiography* usually takes the form of a sector scan that produces tomographic slices through the heart.
- *Three-dimensional (3D) echocardiography* is also now available with some machines.
- *Doppler echocardiography* can be used to record the velocity of blood flow (*spectral Doppler*). The direction and timing of blood flow can also be depicted in colour (*colour Doppler*) superimposed on 2D black-and-white echocardiographic images. Myocardium velocity can also be recorded (*tissue Doppler imaging, TDI*).

M-mode echocardiography

M-mode echocardiography is limited to providing information in one plane only. The cursor is aligned using a 2D image, and the action of the anatomical structures of the heart crossed by the cursor are plotted against time. The advantage of M-mode echocardiography is the excellent time resolution for measurement of cardiac dimensions at precise time points. The main disadvantage is that the sampling area is very limited. M-mode echocardiography gives little information about changes in cardiac size or shape in other dimensions, or about specific lesions. It is also quite technically demanding, which is often under-appreciated. M-mode echocardiography remains widely used for measuring left ventricular diameters.

M-mode

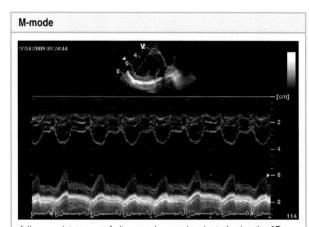

A linear point-source of ultrasound waves is oriented using the 2D image (see cursor in small image) to produce a graph of depth against time

2D

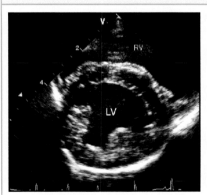

A wedge-shaped sector of ultrasound waves is used to produce a tomographic image of the heart
LV = Left ventricle; RV = Right ventricle

11.1 Types of echocardiography. (continues) ▶

Spectral Doppler

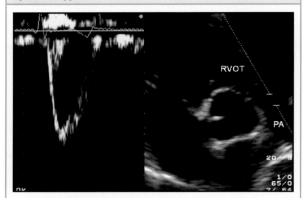

Velocity–time graph of blood flow
The cursor is aligned on the 2D image, parallel with flow
Blood flow velocity is recorded within the 'region of interest' (pulsed wave, PW) or along the length of the cursor (continuous wave, CW)
PA = Pulmonary artery; RVOT = Right ventricular outflow tract

Colour flow Doppler

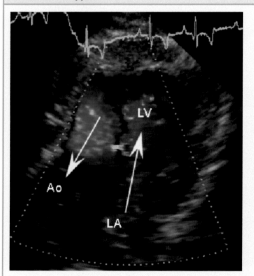

Blood flow is 'coded' in colour and superimposed on a 2D image. Red shows blood flow towards the transducer. Blue shows blood flow away from the transducer
Ao = Aorta; LA = Left atrium; LV = Left ventricle

Tissue Doppler imaging (TDI)

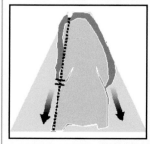 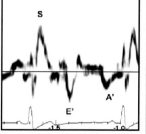

Velocity–time graph of myocardial motion
The cursor is aligned parallel to myocardial motion, and velocities are recorded within a 'region of interest' (PW-TDI)
A' = Atrial TDI mitral annular velocity; E' = Early diastolic TDI mitral annular velocity; S = Systolic TDI mitral annular velocity

11.1 (continued) Types of echocardiography.

2D echocardiography

2D echocardiography is very versatile, as many different slices can be made through the heart to provide numerous different imaging planes. In this way, 2D echocardiography can demonstrate abnormalities of cardiac size and shape, as well as lesions. 2D frame rates are now sufficiently good on many machines that there is little advantage to using M-mode echocardiography, and many quantitative measurements are made directly from 2D images (see Figures 11.8, 11.9 and 11.11). More importantly, there is much qualitative information available in 2D echocardiography.

Doppler echocardiography

Doppler echocardiography gives information about the *direction* and *velocity* of blood flow, utilizing the Doppler principle whereby the frequency of reflected ultrasound waves is changed if the reflecting target is moving towards or away from the source. It is critically angle-dependent: the beam of ultrasound waves *must* be parallel with the direction of the moving target (i.e. blood flow).

Spectral Doppler

With spectral Doppler, the velocity is displayed as a velocity–time graph (Figure 11.2), with blood flow away from the transducer displayed below the baseline and blood flow towards the transducer displayed above the baseline.

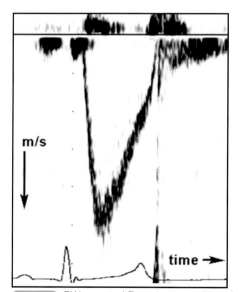

11.2 PW spectral Doppler recording of aortic blood flow. Velocity (m/s) is displayed along the y axis and time is displayed along the x axis. An ECG is shown for reference.

For all forms of spectral Doppler, the most important consideration is to *align the cursor parallel with flow*, or peak velocity will be underestimated. Spectral Doppler varies according to the sampling area:

- In *pulsed wave (PW) Doppler echocardiography*, a very limited area of blood flow is sampled. A user-defined 'region of interest' (or 'sample volume') samples velocities in a specific site, using a 2D image for guidance. This allows precise localization of blood flow velocities, but this restricts the maximum velocity that can be displayed unambiguously. High velocity flow cannot be recorded accurately, as it results in '*aliasing*', where the velocity 'wraps around the baseline' (Figure 11.3)

- In *continuous wave (CW) Doppler echocardiography*, blood flow is sampled along the entire length of the cursor. This allows much higher velocities to be displayed, but there is 'range ambiguity' as the exact location of the high velocity flow along the cursor cannot be determined from the spectral signal.

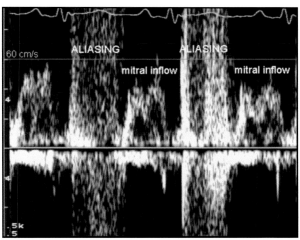

11.3 PW spectral Doppler recording of mitral valve inflow (above the baseline during diastole) with an aliased signal during systole caused by high velocity mitral regurgitation.

The velocity of blood flow primarily depends on the driving pressure (pressure gradient), and can be estimated using the simplified Bernoulli equation:

$$\text{Pressure gradient (mmHg)} = 4 \times \text{velocity}^2$$

This equation allows estimation of pressure gradients (not absolute pressures) and so knowledge of normal intracardiac pressures is necessary (Figure 11.4).

Colour Doppler

Colour Doppler can resolve some of the problems of range ambiguity found with CW Doppler, as high velocity or turbulent flow can be displayed as a different colour superimposed on the 2D black-and-white image. Flow towards the transducer is coded as red, and flow away from the transducer is coded as blue. *Aliasing will still occur with high velocities* and is displayed as reversal of colour (red to blue, or blue to red). *Variance* occurs with turbulent flow (usually displayed as green).

Technique

Most dogs can be scanned without sedation, but handling must be particularly sensitive when scanning non-sedated cats. Sedation with an opiate

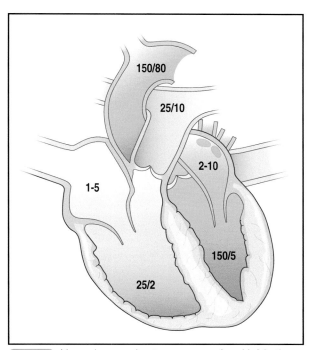

11.4 Normal approximate pressures (mmHg) in the cardiac chambers and great vessels. Right-sided heart chambers are blue, left-sided heart chambers are red.

such as butorphanol is often sufficient to improve patient cooperation. Clipping of the haircoat improves contact between the probe and the skin, but is not always essential. Sufficient use of acoustic gel is vital for good image quality.

Most echocardiographers scan small animal patients in lateral recumbency, using a table with a cut-out area to enable scanning from underneath. It is also possible to scan the patient in a standing position. A simultaneous *electrocardiogram (ECG)* allows accurate timing of events within the cardiac cycle and concurrent screening for arrhythmias, and facilitates acquisition of digital image loops.

A standard protocol should be adopted so that a set sequence of views is recorded. Some views are more difficult than others and it may not be possible to obtain all views in all patients. Sometimes additional non-standard views may be needed, as it is important that any abnormalities are followed up during the study, acquiring additional views or velocity flow patterns as needed.

2D views

The standard right-sided views are shown in Figure 11.5 and the standard left-sided views are shown in Figure 11.6, together with common applications of each view.

Doppler views

Flow through each valve should be interrogated at multiple locations for the best alignment (Figure 11.7). *Fast or turbulent blood flow* is always of interest, as it usually results in a murmur and may occur as a result of valvular regurgitation, valvular stenosis or a shunt.

View	Probe position	Image	Uses
Right parasternal long-axis four chamber			2D: Excellent overview of all four chambers LA dimensions LV dimensions Mitral valve morphology and motion Colour Doppler: Mitral regurgitation Tricuspid regurgitation
Right parasternal long-axis five chamber			2D: LVOT abnormalities LV wall thickness Ventricular septal defects Systolic anterior motion of the mitral valve Colour Doppler: LVOT obstruction Aortic regurgitation Mitral regurgitation
Right parasternal short-axis (papillary muscle level)			2D: LV dimensions Relationship between LV and RV pressures M-mode: LV dimensions
Right parasternal short-axis (mitral valve level)			2D: Mitral valve morphology M-mode: E-point to septal separation Colour Doppler: Mitral regurgitation
Right parasternal short-axis (aortic valve level)			2D: LA dimensions Aortic valve morphology Interatrial septum abnormalities 2D/Colour Doppler: Ventricular septal defects Tricuspid valve abnormalities
Right parasternal short-axis (pulmonary artery level)			2D: RVOT/pulmonic valve morphology Colour Doppler: Tricuspid regurgitation Pulmonary artery blood flow Patent ductus arteriosus Spectral Doppler: Pulmonary artery blood flow velocities

11.5 Standard right-sided echocardiographic views. Ao = Aorta; AoV = Aortic valve; LA = Left atrium; LV = Left ventricle; LVOT = Left ventricular outflow tract; MV = Mitral valve; PA = Pulmonary artery; RA = Right atrium; RV = Right ventricle; RVOT = Right ventricular outflow tract.

View	Probe position	Image	Uses
Left apical four chamber			2D: Overview of all four chambers Mitral valve morphology and function Colour Doppler: Mitral regurgitation Tricuspid regurgitation Spectral Doppler: Mitral valve inflow
Left apical five chamber			2D: LVOT Colour Doppler: LVOT obstruction Aortic regurgitation Spectral Doppler: Aortic flow velocity
Left apical two chamber			2D: LAur Colour Doppler: Mitral regurgitation Spectral Doppler: Mitral valve inflow
Left cranial tricuspid valve			2D: Tricuspid valve morphology and function RAur Colour Doppler: Tricuspid regurgitation Spectral Doppler: Tricuspid inflow Tricuspid regurgitation
Left cranial aorta			2D: Aortic valve morphology Ascending aorta Colour Doppler: Aortic regurgitation

11.6 Standard left-sided echocardiographic views. Ao = Aorta; LA = Left atrium; LAur = Left auricular appendage; LV = Left ventricle; LVOT = Left ventricular outflow tract; RA = Right atrium; RAur = Right auricular appendage; RV = Right ventricle. (continues)

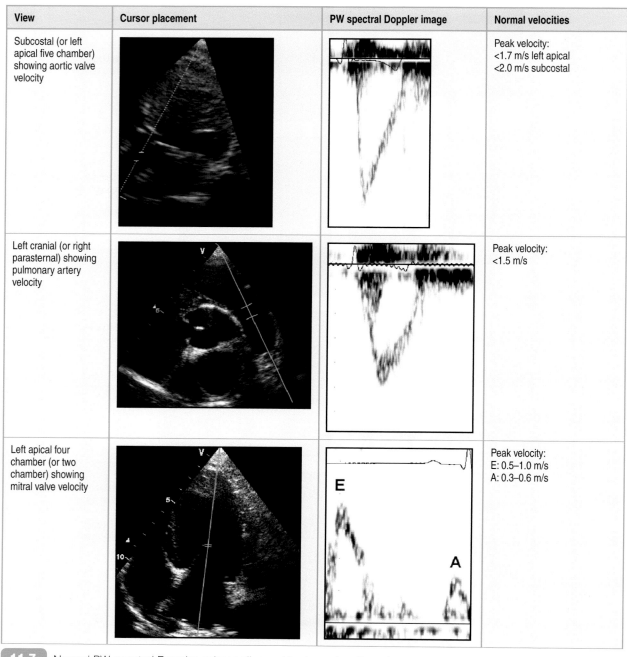

View	Probe position	Image	Uses
Left cranial pulmonary artery			2D: Pulmonic valve morphology Colour Doppler: Pulmonary artery blood flow Patent ductus arteriosus flow

11.6 (continued) Standard left-sided echocardiographic views. PA = Pulmonary artery; RVOT = Right ventricular outflow tract.

View	Cursor placement	PW spectral Doppler image	Normal velocities
Subcostal (or left apical five chamber) showing aortic valve velocity			Peak velocity: <1.7 m/s left apical <2.0 m/s subcostal
Left cranial (or right parasternal) showing pulmonary artery velocity			Peak velocity: <1.5 m/s
Left apical four chamber (or two chamber) showing mitral valve velocity			Peak velocity: E: 0.5–1.0 m/s A: 0.3–0.6 m/s

11.7 Normal PW spectral Doppler echocardiographic views. (continues)

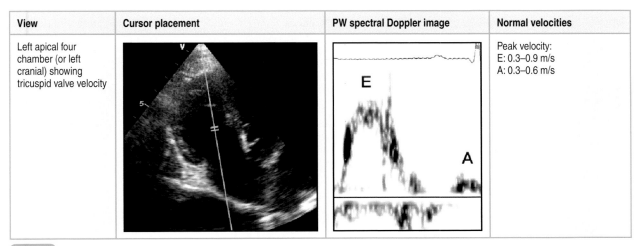

View	Cursor placement	PW spectral Doppler image	Normal velocities
Left apical four chamber (or left cranial) showing tricuspid valve velocity		E A	Peak velocity: E: 0.3–0.9 m/s A: 0.3–0.6 m/s

11.7 (continued) Normal PW spectral Doppler echocardiographic views.

Chamber measurements

Echocardiography is ideally suited to identification of structural lesions, but quantitative assessment of cardiac dimensions and function is also important. Estimates of chamber dimensions should always be interpreted in the context of qualitative information.

Measurements are most important when assessing left heart dimensions, partly because the left heart is an easier shape to quantify than the right, and partly because the most important acquired diseases primarily affect the left heart. As a general rule, measurements should be taken from at least three cardiac cycles and averaged.

Left atrium
Quantification of left atrium (LA) size is an extremely important application of cardiac imaging, as it strongly relates to risk of pulmonary oedema and clinical signs. Although M-mode echocardiography is still sometimes used for measurement of LA size (particularly in cats), it has largely been superseded by 2D techniques (Hansson *et al.*, 2002). A summary of methods for LA size evaluation is given in Figure 11.8.

Left ventricle
Methods of assessing left ventricle (LV) size are listed in Figure 11.9.

Diameter: M-mode echocardiography is still the most commonly used method for quantifying LV diameter. There are inherent pitfalls with M-mode, as it can be difficult to recognize oblique or off-centre views. The diameter measured differs according to whether a short-axis or long-axis 2D view has been used to acquire the M-mode (Schober and Baade, 2000). *M-mode should not be used to derive LV volumes.* Normal canine reference intervals are problematic because of the range in bodyweight and conformation. Methods used to compensate for the range of sizes include:

- Ratio indices
- 'Cornell' method
- Breed-specific values.

Image	Technique	Normal values
M-mode (LA:Ao$_{M-mode}$)		
	Timing: Aorta measured at the start of the QRS complex LA measured at end-systole Measure: Leading edge to leading edge	LA:Ao$_{M-mode}$ Dogs and cats: <1.3

11.8 Measurement of LA dimensions. Ao = Aorta; LA = Left atrium. (continues) ▶

Image	Technique	Normal values
Short axis (LA:Ao_{SAX})		
	Timing: Early diastole (when the aortic valve leaflets are closed) **Measure:** Aorta from middle of right coronary cusp to commissures between the left and non-coronary cusps LA from line extending from aortic measurement out to wall of LA, trying to avoid the pulmonary vein Inside edge to inside edge	$LA:Ao_{SAX}$ Dogs: <1.6 Cats: <1.5
Long axis (LA_{LAX} and Ao_{LAX})		
	Timing: End-systole **Measure:** LA from the interatrial septum to the epicardial surface of the LA free wall, bisecting the LA Inside edge to inside edge	LA_{LAX} Cats: <1.6 cm
	Timing: Systole **Measure:** Between the open aortic leaflets Inside edge to inside edge	$LA_{LAX}:Ao_{LAX}$ Dogs: <2.5

11.8 (continued) Measurement of LA dimensions. Ao = Aorta; LA = Left atrium; LV = Left ventricle.

View	Image	Technique	Normal values
M-mode LV diameter		Timing: End-diastole: at start of the QRS complex (this is not necessarily maximum LV diameter) End-systole: at peak septal motion (this is not necessarily the same time as peak free wall motion) Leading edge to leading edge	Dogs: Varies with size and breed Consider Cornell method (see Figure 11.10) Cats: LVDd: 11–20 mm LVDs: 6–15 mm
2D LV volumes		Timing: End-diastole: at first frame after the mitral valve closes before systole End-systole: at smallest LV dimensions before the mitral valve opens Trace endocardial border from septal mitral valve annulus to lateral wall mitral valve annulus **Vital to obtain true apex**	Dogs: Varies with size and breed Normal reference intervals not established
Sphericity index		Timing: End-diastole Length: measured from line across mitral valve annulus to apex Diameter: taken at chordal level or from M-mode LVDd	Dogs: Length/diameter: ≥1.7 (may be higher in narrow-chested dogs)

11.9 Measurement of LV dimensions. LV = Left ventricle; LVDd = Left ventricular diameter in diastole; LVDs = Left ventricular diameter in systole.

Ratio indices: These can be used for LV diameters just as they can for the LA (Brown *et al.*, 2003). In some ways this technique mimics subjective assessment of LV diameters, as experienced observers often 'eyeball' changes in chamber dimensions by noting differences in size relative to other chambers or vessels. The ratio of the LV diameter to the actual (or predicted) aortic diameter is relatively consistent.

Cornell method: The Cornell method uses a similar calculation, acknowledging that the relationship between bodyweight and LV diameter is not linear (Cornell *et al.*, 2004). LV diameters are predicted based on normalizing the diameter to approximately the cube root of the bodyweight (Figure 11.10):

- Predicted LVDd = LVDd × 1.53 × $BW^{0.294}$
- Predicted LVDs = LVDs × 0.95 × $BW^{0.315}$

Where: BW = Bodyweight; LVDd = Left ventricular diameter in diastole; and LVDs = Left ventricular diameter in systole.

Bodyweight (kg)	LVDd (cm)	LVDs (cm)	LVFWd (cm)	IVSd (cm)
3	2.1 (1.8–2.6)	1.3 (1.0–1.8)	0.5 (0.4–0.8)	0.5 (0.4–0.8)
4	2.3 (1.9–2.8)	1.5 (1.1–1.9)	0.6 (0.4–0.8)	0.6 (0.4–0.8)
6	2.6 (2.2–3.1)	1.7 (1.2–2.2)	0.6 (0.4–0.9)	0.6 (0.4–0.9)
9	2.9 (2.4–3.4)	1.9 (1.4–2.5)	0.7 (0.5–1.0)	0.7 (0.5–1.0)
11	3.1 (2.6–3.7)	2.0 (1.5–2.7)	0.7 (0.5–1.0)	0.7 (0.5–1.1)
15	3.4 (2.8–4.1)	2.2 (1.7–3.0)	0.8 (0.5–1.1)	0.8 (0.6–1.1)
20	3.7 (3.1–4.5)	2.4 (1.8–3.2)	0.8 (0.6–1.2)	0.8 (0.6–1.2)
25	3.9 (3.3–4.8)	2.6 (2.0–3.5)	0.9 (0.6–1.3)	0.9 (0.6–1.3)
30	4.2 (3.5–5.0)	2.8 (2.1–3.7)	0.9 (0.6–1.3)	0.9 (0.7–1.3)
35	4.4 (3.6–5.3)	2.9 (2.2–3.9)	1.0 (0.7–1.4)	1.0 (0.7–1.4)
40	4.5 (3.8–5.5)	3.0 (2.3–4.0)	1.0 (0.7–1.4)	1.0 (0.7–1.4)
50	4.8 (4.0–5.8)	3.3 (2.4–4.3)	1.0 (0.7–1.5)	1.1 (0.7–1.5)
60	5.1 (4.2–6.2)	3.5 (2.6–4.6)	1.1 (0.7–1.6)	1.1 (0.8–1.6)
70	5.3 (4.4–6.5)	3.6 (2.7–4.8)	1.1 (0.8–1.6)	1.1 (0.8–1.6)

11.10 Predicting canine LV M-mode measurements based on allometric scaling. (Data from Cornell *et al.*, 2004).

Breed-specific values: These are the ideal source for reference intervals and are preferred when available.

Volumes: 2D echocardiography can be used to record LV volumes, which should *not* be calculated using M-mode measurements. The right parasternal view is normally used, but great care must be taken to include the true apex of the LV (this requires practice). The endocardial borders of the LV are traced, ignoring the papillary muscles and drawing a straight line across the mitral valve annulus. The LV volume is calculated using either a modified Simpson's technique (method of discs) or an area–length formula.

The normal LV end-systolic volume (ESV) and end-diastolic volume (EDV) will vary according to size and breed. The LV volumes can be normalized by dividing by body surface area to produce an end-diastolic volume index (EDVI) or an end-systolic volume index (ESVI).

Sphericity index: Rather than measuring absolute diameter, an alternative way to identify increased LV dimensions is to look for a change in LV geometry, or LV 'remodelling'. This can be done by noting an increase in LV diameter in relation to LV length. The LV long axis/short axis ratio is called the sphericity index, and reduced values indicate a more spherical LV. Short axis dimensions can be obtained by M-mode echocardiography, and long axis dimensions from 2D views. Diastolic dimensions are normally used. Ideally, normal values for each breed should be derived. Deep-chested dogs have more elongated hearts, and the normal sphericity index may be greater than the figure of ≥1.7 in general use.

Left ventricular wall thickness

Cats: Measurement of LV wall thickness is much more important in cats than in dogs (Figure 11.11). The criteria used to determine LV hypertrophy vary, but whichever technique is used it is *crucial to measure the end-diastolic frame*, as measurement at any other time point will result in over-estimation of wall thickness. It is also important to avoid including extraneous echoes from LV 'false tendons'.

M-mode measurement is restricted to one area of the septum and free wall. This means that regions of LV hypertrophy in other areas may be missed. Therefore, many practitioners use a cut-off value of <5.5 mm as normal, reflecting the decreased sensitivity of M-mode echocardiography for detection of LV hypertrophy. It is also difficult to avoid papillary muscles, which can lead to falsely increased free wall measurements.

2D echocardiography allows measurement of hypertrophy in other areas. The maximal wall thickness is measured in up to three views. It is easier to avoid including false tendons and papillary muscles using 2D images (Figure 11.12).

Dogs: There are fewer indications for measuring wall thickness in dogs, although aortic stenosis and systemic hypertension may result in LV hypertrophy. The Cornell method is probably the best method for identifying hypertrophy:

- Predicted IVSd = IVSd × 0.41 × BW$^{0.241}$
- Predicted LVFWd = LVFWd × 0.42 × BW$^{0.232}$

Where: BW = Bodyweight; IVSd = Interventricular septal thickness in diastole; and LVFWd = Left ventricular free wall thickness in diastole (see Figure 11.10).

View	Image	Technique	Normal values
M-mode LV wall thickness		Timing: End-diastole: at start of QRS complex Leading edge to leading edge	Cats: IVSd, LVFWd: ≤5.5 mm Dogs: Varies with size and breed Consider Cornell method
2D LV wall thickness		Timing: End-diastole: wall thickness at first frame after mitral valve closes before systole Measure in right parasternal long-axis four chamber view, right parasternal long-axis five chamber view and short-axis view (see Figure 11.5). **Avoid papillary muscles and false tendons**	Cats: Maximal diastolic thickness: <6 mm in any view

11.11 Measurement of left ventricular wall thickness. IVSd = Interventricular septal thickness in diastole; LV = Left ventricle; LVFWd = Left ventricular free wall thickness in diastole.

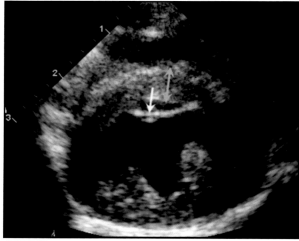

11.12 2D right parasternal short-axis view at the level of the papillary muscle in a cat. The interventricular septal thickness is shown by the green arrow. The white arrow indicates a false tendon, which can easily be mistaken for the endocardial surface of the LV (falsely increasing wall thickness).

Systolic function

Measurement of systolic function is particularly important for diagnosis of dilated cardiomyopathy (DCM), but systolic function may also be abnormal in other conditions. Most echocardiographic methods of measuring systolic function (Figure 11.13) are profoundly affected by loading conditions. *LV wall motion is increased with increased preload and decreased afterload.* This is particularly important with mitral regurgitation, where the effects of the regurgitation itself on preload and afterload result in a hyperdynamic LV, thus potentially masking any underlying systolic dysfunction. Particular care should be taken in the setting of moderate to severe mitral regurgitation when echocardiography measurements of systolic function are in the low normal range, as this is likely to indicate reduced systolic function.

Fractional shortening

The percentage change in LV diameter in systole is called the LV fractional shortening (FS). This is usually

View	Image	Technique	Normal values
M-mode fractional shortening (FS%)		Timing: LVDd: measured at end-diastole at the start of the QRS complex LVDs: measured at peak septal motion Leading edge to leading edge FS% = (LVDd – LVDs)/LVDd x 100	Dogs: 25–50% Cats: 30–50%
M-mode E-point to septal separation (EPSS)		Timing: Peak opening of mitral valve in early systole From leading edge of septal LV endocardial surface to leading edge of anterior mitral valve leaflet	Dogs: <7 mm in large dogs

11.13 Measurement of left ventricular systolic function. LV = Left ventricle; LVDd = Left ventricular diameter in diastole; LVDs = Left ventricular diameter in systole. (continues) ▶

View	Image	Technique	Normal values
LV end-systolic volume index (ESVI)		Timing: End-systolic volume (ESV) at smallest LV dimensions before mitral valve opens Trace endocardial border from septal mitral valve annulus to lateral wall mitral valve annulus **Vital to obtain true apex**	ESVI: ESV/body surface area ≤ 30 ml/m^2
2D ejection fraction (EF%)		Timing: End-diastolic volume (EDV) at first frame after mitral valve closes before systole ESV at smallest LV dimensions before mitral valve opens EF% = (EDV − ESV)/EDV x 100	Dogs: 50–65%
LV systolic time intervals		Aortic spectral Doppler Timing: Pre-ejection period (PEP): from start of QRS complex to onset of aortic ejection (green) Ejection time (ET): duration of aortic spectral Doppler flow signal (blue)	Dogs: PEP/ET: 0.24–0.38

11.13 (continued) Measurement of left ventricular systolic function. LV = Left ventricle.

measured from an M-mode image obtained from a short-axis view. FS is the most commonly used measurement of systolic function, but should not be used as the sole measurement if values are below the normal reference intervals. Other indicators of systolic function should always be measured in addition to FS before diagnosing systolic dysfunction (see Chapter 23). LV dilatation also increases suspicion that systolic dysfunction is genuine (Dukes-McEwan *et al.*, 2003).

Mitral E-point to septal separation

M-mode images can also be used to measure the maximal opening of the mitral valve in diastole, by measuring the distance between the septum and early opening (E-point) of the anterior mitral valve leaflet (EPSS). This distance is increased with systolic dysfunction, but care should be taken to avoid oblique views. EPSS is used far less than FS.

Left ventricle end-systolic volume index

The end-systolic volume (ESV) can be normalized to body surface area. Although normal values of 30 ml/m^2 are often quoted, it should be noted that this may not be valid for smaller breeds of dog.

2D left ventricle ejection fraction

The percentage change in LV volume during systole can be calculated from the volumes measured from a right parasternal long-axis view. Generally, LV wall definition in left apical views is less good, and the maximal length of the LV can be more easily derived from right-sided views. *Ejection fraction* (EF) *should not be derived from volumes estimated from M-mode measurements.* When calculated from 2D images, EF more accurately assesses global systolic function (rather than systolic function at one level and in one plane as with M-mode images).

Systolic time intervals

A different method of assessing systolic function uses the timing of ejection with respect to electrical activation. The interval between the beginning of the Q wave on the ECG and the onset of ejection of blood into the aorta (the *pre-ejection period,* PEP) can be divided by the duration of aortic ejection (the *ejection time,* ET) to give the systolic time interval PEP/ET. This ratio is increased with systolic dysfunction and can be measured from the spectral Doppler flow signal with a concurrent ECG. As with other echocardiographic indices of systolic function, PEP/ET should be interpreted in the light of concurrent cardiac abnormalities, since systolic time intervals can still be affecting by loading conditions or heart rate (Boon, 1998).

Valve function

Echocardiography allows assessment of valve function in a number of different ways:

- Valve lesions can be assessed with 2D imaging
- Chamber remodelling can be assessed by 2D and M-mode imaging
- Disturbed blood flow can be assessed by colour and spectral Doppler imaging
- Pressure gradients, flow rates and orifice area can be calculated with a combination of spectral Doppler, colour Doppler and 2D imaging.

Methods used to assess valvular stenosis may differ slightly from those used for valvular insufficiency, but a combination of methods is always more reliable than a single method.

Valvular regurgitation

Mitral regurgitation

Valve lesions: 2D echocardiography can provide an enormous amount of information on structural abnormalities of the mitral valve, abnormal motion and secondary effects on chamber remodelling. DCM can also cause severe mitral regurgitation, so it is important to assess mitral valve morphology. In myxomatous mitral valve disease (MMVD) the mitral valve leaflets may prolapse, with thickening and distortion developing as structural changes become more severe. In very severe cases, a flail segment may indicate a previously ruptured chord. In DCM, valve leaflets will not be thickened, and may be 'tethered' rather than prolapsed. A summary of methods used for grading mitral regurgitation is given in Figure 11.14.

Chamber remodelling: LA and LV diameter will be increased with severe mitral regurgitation, although this is unreliable in acute regurgitation.

Disturbed flow: Colour flow Doppler can be used to identify jets of mitral regurgitation. A semi-quantitative estimate of mitral regurgitation severity can be made by relating the *jet area* to the LA area, as mild mitral regurgitation produces a small narrow jet. Large jets filling the LA are likely to indicate severe mitral regurgitation. Care should be taken with eccentric jets, where the jet area will be less than expected for the severity of the mitral regurgitation. It should be noted that *jet area is strongly influenced by colour gain controls.*

With a large regurgitant orifice (i.e. a large opening in the closed mitral valve), a large volume of blood will flow backwards from the LV to the LA. The blood accelerates as it passes through the regurgitant orifice, aliasing if the regurgitant volume is large. This hemispherical line of aliasing is termed the *proximal flow convergence region* (Figure 11.15). The diameter of this hemispherical region of aliasing is used in quantitative assessment of regurgitant flow (using the proximal isovelocity surface area technique or 'PISA').

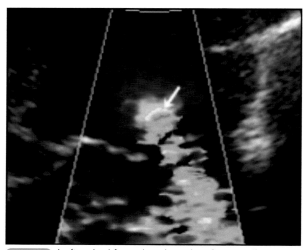

11.15 Left apical four chamber view (zoomed) showing a jet of mitral regurgitation at the closed mitral valve. The colour aliases from blue to yellow at the proximal flow convergence region (white arrow). The 'neck' of the jet (vena contracta, black arrow) corresponds with the regurgitant orifice diameter.

Technique	Feature	Normal	Myxomatous mitral valve disease		
			Mild	*Moderate*	*Severe*
2D	Valve prolapse	None	Just extending beyond annular line	Partial prolapse beyond annular line	Large segments prolapsing with fixed distortion
	Flail leaflets	None	None	None	±
	LA size	Normal	Normal	Normal/mildly dilated	Dilated
Colour Doppler	Jet position	None or trace	Single central	Multiple or eccentric	Filing chamber
	Jet area	None or trace	Narrow or short	Less than half LA area	More than half LA area
	Vena contracta width	N/A	N/A	<2 mm	>2 mm
	Proximal flow convergence	N/A	None	None	Present
Spectral Doppler	Mitral E wave velocity	<1.2 m/s	<1.2 m/s	<1.2 m/s	>1.2 m/s

11.14 Grading of mitral valve severity in MMVD.

The regurgitant flow meets a bottle-neck at the valve's regurgitant orifice, which forms the 'neck' of the regurgitant jet. The width of this 'neck' is called the *vena contracta*, and its width corresponds with the size of the regurgitant orifice. It is difficult to obtain a view of the regurgitant orifice that includes the vena contracta, but this is most easily achieved with left apical views. The vena contracta width is not affected by colour Doppler gain controls or eccentric jets.

Pressure gradients and flow rates: The larger the systolic regurgitant volume, the greater the forward flow of blood across the mitral valve in diastole, so that with severe mitral regurgitation the velocity of early mitral filling (*E wave*) is increased (>1.2 m/s).

Tricuspid regurgitation

Valve lesions: Many of the principles used in mitral regurgitation also apply to tricuspid regurgitation. MMVD can also affect the tricuspid valve, sometimes causing prolapse and flail (see Figure 11.17).

Chamber remodelling: Severe tricuspid regurgitation results in an increase in right atrium (RA) and right ventricle (RV) diameters.

Disturbed flow: The jet of tricuspid regurgitation can be viewed with colour flow Doppler in the same way as mitral regurgitation.

Pressure gradients and flow rates: The main clinical importance of tricuspid regurgitation is in assessing *pulmonary hypertension* (Figure 11.16) (Serres *et al.*, 2007). Although not always present with pulmonary hypertension, tricuspid regurgitation blood flow velocity allows estimation of RV pressure (which is equivalent to pulmonary artery pressure in the absence of pulmonic stenosis).

Aortic regurgitation
Aortic regurgitation is rarely clinically significant in small animals unless infective endocarditis affects the aortic valve, or a ventricular septal defect is present and an aortic valve leaflet prolapses into the defect.

Valve lesions: Causative lesions such as aortic endocarditis can usually be imaged with 2D echocardiography. Sometimes myxomatous valve degeneration also affects the aortic valve, resulting in diffuse thickening and mild aortic regurgitation.

Chamber remodelling: Severe aortic regurgitation may cause an increase in LV volume.

Disturbed flow: One of the best ways to assess the severity of aortic regurgitation is to measure the width of the aortic insufficiency jet at the valve leaflets (vena contracta) relative to the aortic valve diameter.

Pressure gradients and flow rates: The rate of deceleration of the aortic insufficiency jet is related to equilibration of pressures across the aortic valve (i.e. the severity of aortic regurgitation). More rapid deceleration indicates more severe aortic regurgitation.

Pulmonic regurgitation
Pulmonic regurgitation is normal in many dogs and is usually without any haemodynamic significance. Pulmonic regurgitation jet velocity may be useful when assessing severity of pulmonary hypertension, as the pressure gradient across the pulmonic valve gives some indication of mean or diastolic pulmonary artery pressures (see Figure 11.16).

Valvular stenosis

Aortic stenosis
Subvalvular and/or valvular lesions are usually evident on 2D images with moderate to severe aortic stenosis.

Chamber remodelling: LV hypertrophy may be appreciated on 2D or M-mode images.

Disturbed flow: Variance begins at the site of stenosis (e.g. the LV outflow tract with subaortic stenosis, and at the valve with valvular stenosis). Mild aortic regurgitation is often also present.

Pressure gradients and flow rates: Severity of aortic stenosis is generally measured in terms of the magnitude of pressure gradient across the aortic valve, calculated using the simplified Bernoulli equation (see Figure 11.16). It should be noted that pressure gradients are affected by flow as well as the stenotic valve area. This means the *pressure gradient will be underestimated under low-flow states* (i.e. with systolic dysfunction or under anaesthesia).

Condition	Measurements necessary	Formula	Normal values (mmHg)
Pulmonary hypertension	Peak TR velocity	Systolic PA pressure = $(4 \times TR \text{ velocity}^2) + RA$ systolic pressure	<32
	Peak PR velocity	Mean PA pressure = $4 \times PR \text{ velocity}^2$	<20
Aortic stenosis	Peak aortic valve velocity	Aortic valve PG = $4 \times$ aortic valve velocity^2	Mild: <50 Moderate: 50–80 Severe: >80
Pulmonic stenosis	Peak PA velocity	PA PG = $4 \times PA \text{ velocity}^2$	Mild: <50 Moderate: 50–80 Severe: >80

11.16 Calculation of common pressure gradients using Doppler echocardiography. PA = Pulmonary artery; PG = Pressure gradient; PR = Pulmonic regurgitation; TR = Tricuspid regurgitation.

Pulmonic stenosis

The same techniques used for aortic stenosis are applicable to pulmonic stenosis.

Interpretation

The above measurements may be helpful when applying echocardiography to clinical cases, in conjunction with other diagnostic findings. Although a standard approach builds up expertise in the various views, it may be necessary to alter the echocardiography study protocol according to findings. In particular, the different causes of lesions and chamber remodelling should be considered *during* the echocardiography study, which will guide the echocardiographer in selection of the most appropriate measurements. The most common differential diagnoses for cardiac lesions and different patterns of chamber remodelling are given in Figure 11.17.

Abnormality	Image	Differential diagnosis
LA dilatation		Volume overload: • Mitral regurgitation (see image) • Left-to-right patent ductus arteriosus or ventricular septal defect Congenital mitral stenosis LV systolic dysfunction: • Dilated cardiomyopathy LV diastolic dysfunction: • Hypertrophic cardiomyopathy • Restrictive cardiomyopathy • Unclassified cardiomyopathy
LV dilatation		LV volume overload: • Mitral regurgitation • Left-to-right patent ductus arteriosus or ventricular septal defect LV systolic dysfunction: • Dilated cardiomyopathy (see image) • End-stage hypertrophic cardiomyopathy
LV hypertrophy		LV pressure overload: • Aortic stenosis • Systemic hypertension Idiopathic: • Hypertrophic cardiomyopathy (see image)
Mitral valve abnormalities		Myxomatous mitral valve disease (see image) Infective endocarditis Congenital mitral dysplasia

11.17 Differential diagnosis for abnormalities of chamber dimensions and valves. LA = Left atrium; LV = Left ventricle; RA = Right atrium. (continues)

Abnormality	Image	Differential diagnosis
Aortic valve abnormalities	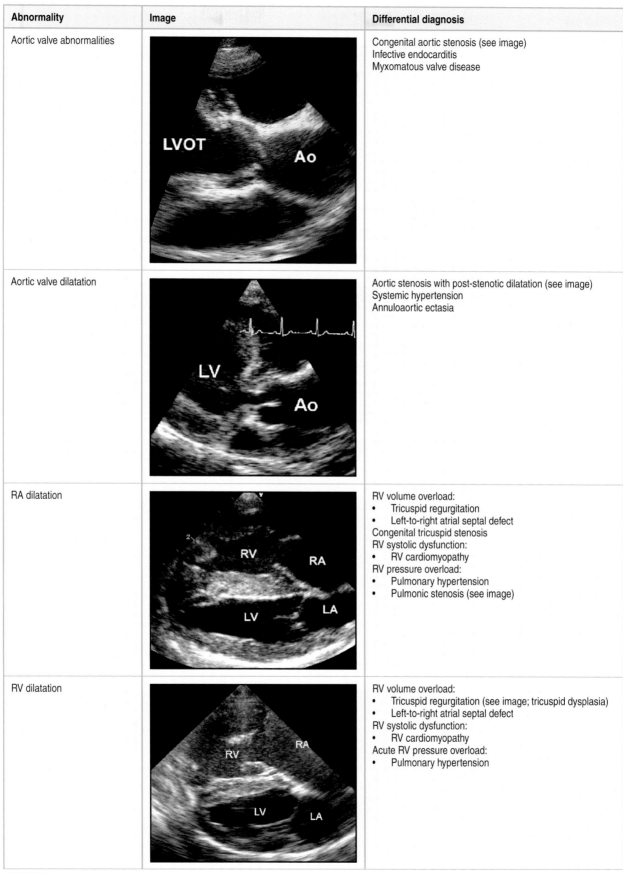	Congenital aortic stenosis (see image) Infective endocarditis Myxomatous valve disease
Aortic valve dilatation		Aortic stenosis with post-stenotic dilatation (see image) Systemic hypertension Annuloaortic ectasia
RA dilatation		RV volume overload: • Tricuspid regurgitation • Left-to-right atrial septal defect Congenital tricuspid stenosis RV systolic dysfunction: • RV cardiomyopathy RV pressure overload: • Pulmonary hypertension • Pulmonic stenosis (see image)
RV dilatation		RV volume overload: • Tricuspid regurgitation (see image; tricuspid dysplasia) • Left-to-right atrial septal defect RV systolic dysfunction: • RV cardiomyopathy Acute RV pressure overload: • Pulmonary hypertension

11.17 (continued) Differential diagnosis for abnormalities of chamber dimensions and valves. Ao = Aorta; LA = Left atrium; LV = Left ventricle; LVOT = Left ventricular outflow tract; RA = Right atrium; RV = Right ventricle. (continues) ▶

Abnormality	Image	Differential diagnosis
RV hypertrophy		RV pressure overload: • Pulmonary hypertension (see image) • Pulmonic stenosis • Double-chambered RV
Tricuspid valve abnormalities		Myxomatous valve disease (see image) Congenital tricuspid dysplasia Distortion of tricuspid valve by RV chamber remodelling
Pulmonic valve abnormalities		Congenital pulmonic stenosis (see image)
Pulmonary artery dilatation		Pulmonic stenosis with post-stenotic dilatation Left-to-right patent ductus arteriosus or ventricular septal defect Pulmonary hypertension (see image)

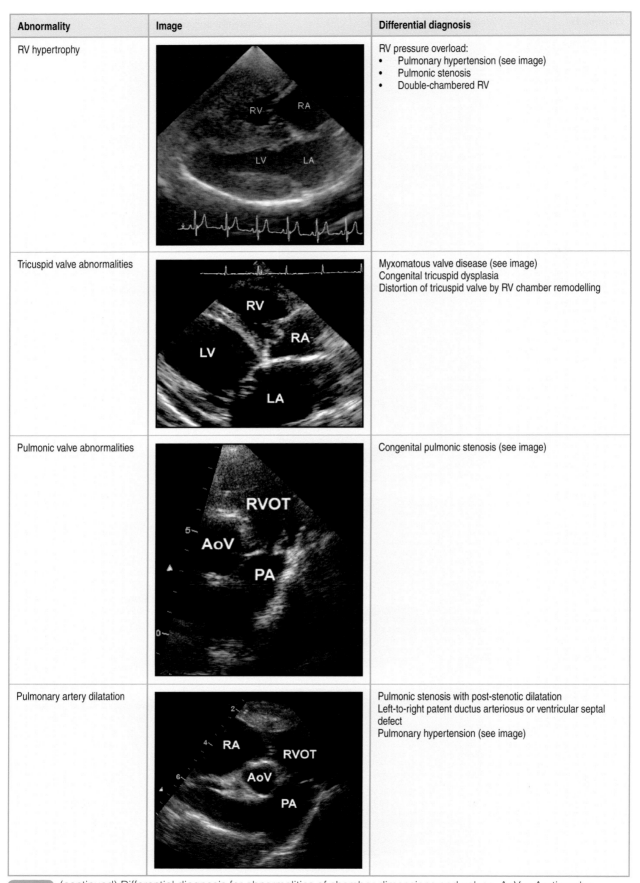

11.17 (continued) Differential diagnosis for abnormalities of chamber dimensions and valves. AoV = Aortic valve; LA = Left atrium; LV = Left ventricle; PA = Pulmonary artery; RA = Right atrium; RV = Right ventricle; RVOT = Right ventricular outflow tract. (continues) ▶

Abnormality	Image	Differential diagnosis
Dilatation of all four chambers		Dilated cardiomyopathy Atrial fibrillation High-grade atrioventricular block (see image) Anaemia Hyperthyroidism

11.17 (continued) Differential diagnosis for abnormalities of chamber dimensions and valves. LA = Left atrium; LV = Left ventricle; RA = Right atrium; RV = Right ventricle.

References and further reading

Boon JA (1998) *Manual of Veterinary Echocardiography.* Williams & Wilkins, Baltimore

Brown DJ, Rush JE, MacGregor J *et al.* (2003) M-mode echocardiographic ratio indices in normal dogs, cats, and horses: a novel quantitative method. *Journal of Veterinary Internal Medicine* **17**, 653–662

Cornell CC, Kittleson MD, Della Torre P *et al.* (2004) Allometric scaling of M-mode cardiac measurements in normal adult dogs. *Journal of Veterinary Internal Medicine* **18**, 311–321

Dukes-McEwan J, Borgarelli M, Tidholm A, Vollmar AC and Haggstrom J (2003) Proposed guidelines for the diagnosis of canine idiopathic dilated cardiomyopathy. *Journal of Veterinary Cardiology* **5**, 7–19

Hansson K, Haggstrom J, Kvart C and Lord P (2002) Left atrial to aortic root indices using two-dimensional and M-mode echocardiography in cavalier King Charles spaniels with and without left atrial enlargement. *Veterinary Radiology & Ultrasound* **43**, 568–575

Schober KE and Baade H (2000) Comparability of left ventricular M-mode echocardiography in dogs performed in long-axis and short-axis. *Veterinary Radiology & Ultrasound* **41**, 543–549

Serres F, Chetboul V, Gouni V *et al.* (2007) Diagnostic value of echo-Doppler and tissue Doppler imaging in dogs with pulmonary arterial hypertension. *Journal of Veterinary Internal Medicine* **21**, 1280–1289

12

Blood gas analysis and pulse oximetry

Amanda Boag

Introduction

Physical examination alone can provide a wealth of information about the presence, nature and severity of cardiorespiratory disease; however, findings are subjective and may on occasion be misleading. Arterial blood gas analysis and pulse oximetry are objective methods used to identify and quantify hypoxaemia and to assess progression over time. Arterial blood gas analysis also provides objective information about ventilation.

Oxygen carriage

Both arterial blood gas analysis and pulse oximetry are methods for evaluating the ability of the lungs to oxygenate arterial blood; however, the information these tests provide is not equivalent. Understanding the difference requires knowledge of the way oxygen is carried in the circulatory system. Oxygen in arterial blood is either bound to haemoglobin or dissolved in plasma. The vast majority of the oxygen is carried in association with haemoglobin in red blood cells, with each molecule of haemoglobin carrying up to four molecules of oxygen. Pulse oximeters measure the percentage of haemoglobin saturated with oxygen (S_aO_2). In contrast, arterial blood gas analysers measure the amount of oxygen dissolved in plasma (partial pressure of oxygen or P_aO_2). The relationship between the P_aO_2 and S_aO_2 is sigmoidal (Figure 12.1). After the first molecule of oxygen binds to haemoglobin, it undergoes a conformational change allowing the subsequent three oxygen molecules to bind more easily. This curve may be shifted left or right by differing physiological conditions, therefore it is not possible to predict accurately the S_aO_2 from the P_aO_2 and *vice versa*.

The total oxygen content of the blood (C_aO_2) can be calculated if the P_aO_2 and S_aO_2 are known. The equation to calculate oxygen content in mlO$_2$/dl is:

$$C_aO_2 = (1.34 \times S_aO_2 \times [Hb]) + (0.003 \times P_aO_2)$$

Where:

- 1.34 is the amount of oxygen (ml) held by each gram of haemoglobin, if the haemoglobin is 100% saturated
- S_aO_2 is the measured haemoglobin saturation
- [Hb] is the concentration of haemoglobin in g/dl
- P_aO_2 is the amount of oxygen dissolved in plasma in mmHg
- 0.003 is the solubility of oxygen in plasma.

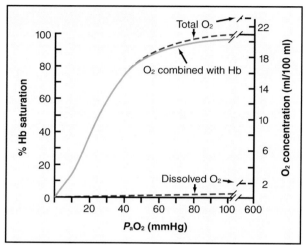

12.1 Oxyhaemoglobin dissociation curve demonstrating the sigmoidal relationship between the P_aO_2 and the S_aO_2.

Thus, oxygen content is dependent on both pulmonary function and the amount of haemoglobin present.

Arterial blood gas analysis

Arterial blood gas analysis is the definitive method of assessing lung function, allowing measurement of the partial pressure (concentration) of both oxygen (P_aO_2) and carbon dioxide (P_aCO_2). Widespread access to 'bench-top' blood gas analysers has increased the use of arterial blood gas analysis as a diagnostic and monitoring tool.

Sample collection and storage

Collection
Arterial samples are most commonly obtained by direct arterial puncture. Any palpable artery can be used; typically the dorsal metatarsal artery is used in dogs and the femoral artery is used in cats and small dogs (<7 kg).

- When using the dorsal metatarsal artery, the patient should be restrained in lateral recumbency.
- The artery on the dependent (lower) leg is easiest to puncture as the dorsal metatarsal

artery runs between metatarsal bones II and III towards the medial aspect of the metatarsus.

- The artery should be palpated and the area clipped and lightly cleaned with antiseptic and alcohol wipes. Vigorous scrubbing of the area will tend to cause the artery to spasm, rendering puncture more difficult.
- One hand should be used to palpate the artery whilst the other hand directs the needle on a pre-heparinized syringe into the arterial lumen. A small-gauge needle should be chosen, typically 25-gauge for a small dog or 22-gauge for a larger patient.
- The needle should be inserted at approximately a 60 degree angle (Figure 12.2). As arterial walls are thicker than venous walls, a purposeful directed motion through the arterial wall is generally needed.
- Once in the artery, a flash of blood will be seen in the hub of the needle and aspiration can begin. Use of proprietary arterial sampling syringes can simplify this part of the procedure. These syringes have a plunger that allows air to be displaced; the syringe is prefilled with air to the volume of blood required, and once the artery is punctured the syringe fills directly under arterial pressure with no need for further manipulation of the plunger (Figure 12.2).
- Once the sample has been obtained, the needle should be withdrawn and firm pressure applied to the site for 2–5 minutes.

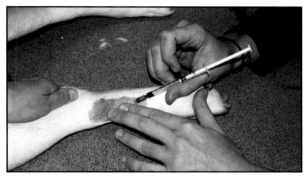

12.2 Taking an arterial sample from the dorsal metatarsal artery. Note the use of a syringe specifically designed for arterial sampling. The syringe is prefilled with air to the volume required and once the artery is punctured it fills under arterial pressure.

Multiple samples: If multiple arterial samples are required for monitoring disease progression, or if the patient would also benefit from measurement of direct arterial blood pressure, an arterial catheter (20–22-gauge) can be placed in the dorsal metatarsal artery. The catheter is placed in an identical manner to venous catheters, although the thicker wall and narrower lumen of the artery makes placement more technically challenging. Once in place, arterial catheters should be carefully secured and flushed frequently (either every 1–2 hours or continuously via a pressure bag and microtubing). When taking samples from an arterial catheter, a small (2–5 ml) pre-sample should be withdrawn first to ensure the diagnostic sample is a true representation of arterial blood.

Storage

Once an arterial sample has been obtained, it must be analysed immediately or stored on ice and analysed within a few hours to ensure that *in vitro* metabolic activity of the cells does not interfere with results. Anaerobic glycolysis by the red blood cells tends to increase the PCO_2 with time, whereas oxygen utilization by the white blood cells reduces the PO_2. The sample must also be handled anaerobically and any air bubbles within the syringe must be removed immediately. If the sample is exposed to room air or even air within bubbles, the PCO_2 tends to decrease and the PO_2 may also change as the gases in the sample equilibrate with the air.

P_aO_2 and hypoxaemia

P_aO_2 represents the concentration of oxygen dissolved in plasma. As a rule of thumb, in an animal with normal lungs, the P_aO_2 should be approximately five times the fractional inspired oxygen (F_iO_2). A normal animal breathing room air (F_iO_2 21%) should have a P_aO_2 of approximately 100 mmHg, and an anaesthetized animal on 100% oxygen should have a P_aO_2 of approximately 500 mmHg. If the F_iO_2 is changed, the P_aO_2 will equilibrate within a few minutes.

The finding of a low P_aO_2 (<80 mmHg on room air) defines hypoxaemia. Typically the S_aO_2 does not drop below 90% until the P_aO_2 is in the region of 60 mmHg (Figure 12.3). Once the P_aO_2 falls below this level, the S_aO_2 drops rapidly and oxygen delivery to the tissues is seriously compromised. Measurement of the P_aO_2 provides a more sensitive and accurate assessment of the severity of hypoxaemia than pulse oximetry.

P_aO_2 (mmHg)	S_aO_2 (%)	Relevance to patient
80–110	95–100	Normal
~60	~90	Moderate hypoxaemia. Risk for rapid deterioration in oxygen delivery to tissues with only small fall in P_aO_2
~40	~75	Life-threatening hypoxaemia

12.3 Relationship between the P_aO_2, the S_aO_2 and the clinical relevance to patient.

Differential diagnoses

The identification of hypoxaemia should lead the clinician to consider the possible causes. Causes of hypoxaemia include:

- Hypoventilation (i.e. reduction in the delivery of oxygen to the alveoli)
- Venous admixture, secondary to:
  - Ventilation–perfusion mismatch
  - Shunting
  - Diffusion impairment.
- Decreased F_iO_2 (e.g. malfunctioning anaesthesia equipment, altitude).

Hypoventilation: This is a relatively common cause of hypoxaemia. The presence of hypoventilation is defined by an increased level of arterial carbon dioxide and is discussed further below.

Venous admixture: This is the term used when venous blood moves from the right side of the circulation to the left side of the circulation without becoming fully oxygenated. A low level of venous admixture is normal as a certain proportion of venous blood (e.g. that in the bronchial or Thebesian veins) does not pass through the pulmonary capillaries. However, numerous pathological processes lead to increased venous admixture and hypoxaemia.

Ventilation–perfusion mismatch: This is the commonest cause of increased venous admixture in veterinary patients and is seen in many patients with parenchymal disease (e.g. pneumonia, congestive heart failure, thromboembolic disease). In healthy animals, the body matches ventilation with perfusion of the alveoli. In disease, local alterations in ventilation and/or perfusion lead to worsening ventilation–perfusion mismatch and hypoxaemia. Patients with ventilation–perfusion mismatch generally remain responsive to oxygen supplementation to some degree.

Shunting: This is the term used when blood completely bypasses functional alveoli. This may occur due to direct venous–arterial shunts (e.g. reverse patent ductus arteriosus) or due to blood flow through unventilated areas of the lungs (e.g. neoplastic masses, completely atelectatic lung lobes). These patients do not tend to respond to oxygen supplementation as an increase in F_iO_2 will not reach unventilated lung regions.

Diffusion impairment: Diffusion impairment secondary to a thickened alveolar capillary membrane is the least common cause of venous admixture as there is a large reserve capacity for oxygen diffusion.

P_aCO_2 and ventilation

Carbon dioxide is the end waste product of aerobic metabolism and is excreted in vast quantities daily through the lungs. Carbon dioxide is a very soluble gas (approximately 20 times more soluble than oxygen) and diffuses easily from the blood into the alveoli. Arterial carbon dioxide levels can be considered to be an accurate indication of alveolar carbon dioxide levels, even in a patient with significant pulmonary parenchymal disease. Arterial carbon dioxide will only change with abnormalities of ventilation, i.e. with changes in fresh gas delivery to the alveoli. Thus, the P_aCO_2 defines whether a patient is hypo- or hyperventilating (Figure 12.4).

P_aCO_2 (mmHg)	State of arterial blood	State of alveolar ventilation
<32	Hypocarbia	Hyperventilation
32–43	Eucarbia	Normal
>43	Hypercarbia	Hypoventilation

12.4 Relationship between the P_aCO_2 and ventilation for the dog. Cats have slightly lower normal P_aCO_2 (26–36 mmHg).

Hypoventilation leads to respiratory acidosis and hypoxaemia. Hypoventilation may be mild and of little clinical consequence. Severe hypoventilation requires intervention, generally with institution of assisted ventilation. A P_aCO_2 of >60 mmHg should prompt consideration of supportive measures. Severe hyperventilation (P_aCO_2 <20 mmHg) is less common, but can lead to respiratory alkalosis and cerebral vasoconstriction that can be life threatening. Differential diagnoses to consider upon identification of ventilatory disturbances are given in Figure 12.5.

Hypoventilation (respiratory acidosis)

Upper airway obstruction (e.g. laryngeal paralysis)
Lower airway obstruction
Central nervous system disease with respiratory centre depression
Spinal cord injury cranial to C4/C5
Drugs (e.g. anaesthetic agents)
Neuromuscular disease (e.g. myasthenia gravis)
Restrictive disease (e.g. pneumothorax, pleural effusion)
Respiratory muscle fatigue (e.g. with prolonged severe parenchymal disease)
Inadequate mechanical ventilation
Compensation for metabolic alkalosis

Hyperventilation (respiratory alkalosis)

Hypoxaemia (severe)
Pulmonary parenchymal disease
Hyperthermia
Pain
Fear/stress
Exercise
Neurological disease
Excessive mechanical ventilation
Compensation for metabolic acidosis

12.5 Differential diagnosis for hypo- and hyperventilation.

Oxygen tension-based indices

A major benefit of arterial blood gas evaluation is the ability to track the progression of disease with time and treatment. As the P_aO_2 is expected to change with both F_iO_2 and alveolar ventilation, a number of equations have been described that allow interpretation of the P_aO_2 in the face of these changes.

P_aO_2/F_iO_2 ratio

The P_aO_2/F_iO_2 ratio is a way of expressing the oxygenating efficiency of the lungs in the face of changing F_iO_2. The measured P_aO_2 is divided by the F_iO_2 expressed as a decimal (i.e. 0.21–1.0).

- An animal with normal lungs will have a P_aO_2/F_iO_2 ratio of >500.
- Values of 300–500 represent a mild decrease in oxygenating efficiency.
- Values of 200–300 represent a moderate decrease in oxygenating efficiency.
- Values <200 are cause for serious concern.

The P_aO_2/F_iO_2 ratio is one of the criteria for defining the presence of acute respiratory distress syndrome (ARDS).

Alveolar–arterial PO_2 gradient

The alveolar–arterial PO_2 gradient (A–a gradient) is an estimation of the difference between the calculated alveolar oxygen level and the measured arterial oxygen level. Theoretically, if lungs were 100% efficient, the A–a gradient would be zero; however, even in healthy animals a small degree of venous admixture occurs and a value <15 is considered acceptable for a normal animal breathing room air. The alveolar oxygen level (P_AO_2) is calculated from the alveolar gas equation:

$$P_AO_2 = F_IO_2 (Pb-P_{H2O}) - P_aCO_2/RQ$$

Where:

- F_IO_2 is the fractional inspired oxygen concentration
- Pb is the barometric pressure
- P_{H2O} is the saturated water vapour pressure at body temperature
- RQ is the respiratory quotient.

At sea level, in room air, and assuming the RQ for the dog to be approximately 0.9 on typical diets, the alveolar gas equation can be simplified as:

$$P_AO_2 = 150 - (P_aCO_2)1.1$$

The A–a gradient is then calculated by subtracting the P_aO_2 from this value.

The principal use of the A–a gradient is to allow an assessment of the oxygenating efficiency of the lungs, whilst removing the variable effect of ventilation on the degree of hypoxaemia (Figure 12.6). The simplified

---

Case example

An arterial blood gas sample is taken from two patients both showing evidence of respiratory distress. Both patients are breathing room air. Which patient has more severe lung dysfunction?

Patient 1:
P_aO_2 70 mmHg
P_aCO_2 65 mmHg

Patient 2:
P_aO_2 75 mmHg
P_aCO_2 23 mmHg

Both patients are hypoxaemic with Patient 1 having slightly worse blood oxygen levels; however, Patient 1 is hypoventilating and Patient 2 is hyperventilating. The A–a gradient should be calculated for both patients:

Patient 1:
$P_AO_2 = 150 - (1.1 \times 65) = 78.5$
A–a gradient = 78.5 – 70 = 8.5

Patient 2:
$P_AO_2 = 150 - (1.1 \times 23) = 125$
A–a gradient = 125 – 75 = 50

Patient 1 has a normal A–a gradient, indicating that the oxygenating efficiency of the lungs themselves is adequate and the hypoxaemia is entirely secondary to hypoventilation. A patient with an upper airway obstruction may present with these arterial blood gas values.

Patient 2 has a greatly elevated A–a gradient, indicating that the lungs have poor oxygenating efficiency. A patient with pneumonia may present with these arterial blood gas values. The A–a gradient can be used to assess improvements or deteriorations in lung function in the face of changing ventilation.

12.6 Use of the A–a gradient for assessing oxygenating efficiency of the lungs in patients.

---

form of the alveolar gas equation cannot be used if the patient is receiving supplemental oxygen.

Pulse oximetry

Pulse oximetry is a non-invasive method used to identify and quantify hypoxaemia. It relies on the differential absorption of light by oxyhaemoglobin and deoxyhaemoglobin. Pulse oximeter probes consist of a light-emitting diode, which emits light of two different wavelengths, and a photodetector. The machine calculates the percentage of arterial oxygen saturation (S_aO_2) by comparing the proportion of the two wavelengths transmitted through the tissues with each arterial pulse. Some machines also display the pulse oximeter waveform.

Patient preparation and probe positioning

To provide an accurate result, pulse oximeter probes must be placed on a tissue bed that is adequately perfused and of a suitable thickness to allow transmission of light. Most probes are designed for use on human ear lobes or fingers. Several sites can be used in the dog and cat, including the lip, pinna, prepuce, vulva, toe webs and skin folds. The tongue is often the most reliable site but can only be used in anaesthetized or heavily sedated patients. Both the transmitting and detecting surfaces of the probe must be in close contact with the skin or mucosa. If needed, hair should be clipped and the skin cleaned with alcohol solution prior to probe placement. The presence of icterus or moderate anaemia does not preclude pulse oximetry as long as the tissue bed is well perfused; however, pulse oximetry is not possible in some darkly pigmented animals (e.g. Chow Chows).

Comparison with arterial blood gas analysis

Pulse oximeters have some advantages over arterial blood gas analysis. They are inexpensive, easy-to-use and can provide a continuous real-time estimation of the S_aO_2. As many machines have a visual and audible output, pulse oximeters can be particularly useful for monitoring patients in which the probe can be maintained in one position for prolonged periods (i.e. anaesthetized patients). They also provide a way of assessing oxygenation in patients in which more invasive monitoring is not possible or unwarranted.

There are several practical and theoretical disadvantages to the use of pulse oximetry. In conscious patients, it can be difficult to maintain the probe in place for long enough to obtain a reliable reading. Motion artefacts are a significant problem inherent to all conventional pulse oximeters, as movement adds another signal to the pulse waveform signal, changing the apparent amounts of light transmitted. Newer generation pulse oximeters have been developed which use an algorithm designed to reduce the artefacts associated with movement and poor perfusion. These have not yet been validated in a clinical veterinary environment but appear to perform well in children. A further practical problem relates to the dependence of pulse oximeters on the detection of variations in light absorption with each pulse. It is essential that the tissue bed used is well perfused; this limits their reliability for assessing oxygenation in patients with concurrent cardiovascular abnormalities. This also accounts for the deterioration in signal with time that occurs when the tissue is 'blanched' by prolonged pressure from the probe. Machines that display the heart rate and pulse oximeter waveform alongside the S_aO_2 are preferred. The operator can then compare the displayed heart rate and the counted heart rate (physical examination or electrocardiogram); if these values are discordant, the displayed S_aO_2 value should be interpreted with great caution. The waveform display also allows the operator to make an assessment of the strength of the signal.

Pulse oximetry is less sensitive than arterial blood gas analysis in detecting mild to moderate hypoxaemia. A pulse oximeter reading of 91% corresponds to a P_aO_2 of approximately 60 mmHg (see Figure 12.1) and should give serious cause for concern. Pulse oximetry is not useful for monitoring oxygenation in patients receiving supplemental oxygen, as a value of close to 100% corresponds to a P_aO_2 of between 100 mmHg and 500 mmHg. The presence of other forms of haemoglobin (e.g. carboxyhaemoglobin with carbon monoxide toxicity) can also lead to misleading results. The absorption spectrum of carboxy-haemoglobin is very similar to that of oxyhaemoglobin, thus the measured S_aO_2 in patients with high levels of carboxyhaemoglobin may be within an acceptable range when a high proportion of the haemoglobin is in a non-functional state. Finally, pulse oximetry does not provide any information on the ventilatory status of the patient.

References and further reading

Haskins SC (2004) Interpretation of blood gas measurements. In: *Textbook of Respiratory Disease in Cats and Dogs*, ed. LG King, pp. 181–192. Saunders, Missouri

Hendricks J (2004) Pulse oximetry. In: *Textbook of Respiratory Disease in Cats and Dogs*, ed. LG King, pp. 193–197. Saunders, St. Louis

Townshend J, Taylor BJ, Galland B and Williams S (2006) Comparison of new generation motion-resistant pulse oximeters *Journal of Paediatrics and Child Health* **42,** 359–365

West JB (2000) *Respiratory Physiology: the Essentials, 6th edn.* Lippincott, Williams and Wilkins, Pennsylvania

13

Blood pressure measurement

Rebecca L. Stepien

Introduction

The increasing recognition of systemic hypertension as a cause of clinical signs and a complication of common medical conditions makes blood pressure measurement an important diagnostic test in clinical veterinary medicine. Reliable measurement techniques, accurate assessment of results and effective therapeutic choices are needed to manage hypertension in dogs and cats successfully.

Direct blood pressure measurement (i.e. intra-arterial needle or catheter) is accurate but technically challenging in dogs and cats. Measurement of blood pressure using non-invasive methods requires less technical skill but results may be inaccurate if careful attention is not paid to technique. The advantages enjoyed by physicians in measuring human blood pressure (i.e. generally cylinder-shaped appendages that easily allow cuff placement at the level of the heart; heart rates usually <150 beats/minute; lack of panting; and patient familiarity with the procedure) are not routinely present in conscious pet dogs and cats. Patient anxiety or excitement due to unfamiliarity with the procedure, rapid heart rates and the requirement that the patient remain motionless in what may be an abnormal position may lead to results that are inconsistent and difficult to interpret. These problems may be lessened, if not completely ameliorated, by excellent and consistent measurement techniques.

Key points

- Indications for blood pressure measurement:
  - Presence of target organ damage (see Figure 13.1)
  - Presence of disease known to be associated with systemic hypertension (see Figure 13.1)
  - Strong clinical suspicion of disease known to be associated with systemic hypertension.
- Commonly available techniques:
  - Invasive (direct) measurement
  - Indirect measurement techniques:
    - Doppler sphygmomanometry
    - Oscillometry
    - High-definition oscillometry.

- Technical aspects:
  - Patient calming prior to measurement
  - Multiple measurements, use average as 'representative value'
  - Repeat measurement on separate occasion if results are ambiguous (e.g. borderline, mismatched to clinical signs).

Indications

Development of hypertension in cats and dogs is almost always associated with the concurrent presence of one or more identifiable underlying diseases. The search for an underlying condition responsible for the development of hypertension is an essential component of the diagnosis of hypertension in cats and dogs.

'Screening' healthy patients

Routine blood pressure measurement in asymptomatic patients that do not have a disease associated with hypertension is controversial. Individual patients may have 'characteristic' blood pressures; theoretically, routine evaluation on every patient would establish a 'normal' blood pressure for each animal. A significant increase in blood pressure from one measurement period to the next would conceivably trigger a more detailed diagnostic work up to search for a cause. The prevalence of hypertension in the healthy population is likely to be quite low, and tests of high sensitivity carry a higher risk of false-positive findings when used in a low-risk population. Therefore, healthy patients with apparently elevated blood pressure should have this finding confirmed on multiple test occasions before proceeding with a diagnostic work up or therapy. In most cases, elevated blood pressure measured in an outwardly healthy patient will be proven to be a false-positive finding.

Patients at risk for hypertension

Patients with clinical signs related to target organ damage (TOD) or a disease that is known to be associated with hypertension should have their blood pressure measured at the time of initial diagnosis. Clinical signs and risk factors for canine and feline hypertension are presented in Figure 13.1.

TOD is most likely to be noted as ocular, neurological, cardiovascular or renal abnormalities. Ocular

Dogs and cats

If clinical signs of target organ damage are present:
• Ocular signs:
   – Acute blindness
   – Hyphaema
   – Retinal haemorrhage or detachment
   – Papilloedema.
• Intracranial neurological signs:
   – Depressed mentation or obtundation
   – Seizures (generalized or focal facial)
   – Nystagmus.
• Auscultable cardiac abnormalities in patients at risk for systemic hypertension based on concurrent disease (e.g. renal disease):
   – Gallop rhythm
   – Left-sided systolic heart murmurs.
• Renal signs:
   – Physical or biochemical evidence of renal insufficiency
   – Proteinuria in the absence of infection.
 	
If causal or related disease is documented or suspected:
• Renal disease, especially if associated with proteinuria
• Diabetes mellitus
• Unexplained left ventricular hypertrophy
• Use of hypertensive medications (e.g. phenylpropanolamine, corticosteroids).

Dogs
Hyperadrenocorticism Acromegaly Phaeochromocytoma Primary hyperaldosteronism
Cats
Hyperthyroidism Suspected hypertrophic cardiomyopathy New heart murmur Age >12 years Primary hyperaldosteronism

13.1 Clinical indications for blood pressure measurement in dogs and cats.

haemorrhage, retinal haemorrhage or detachment (Figure 13.2), neurological signs such as depression, obtundation or seizures, the presence of renal disease or unexplained left ventricular hypertrophy should lead to blood pressure evaluation in both dogs and cats. Hypertension may develop in association with diabetes mellitus, and with the use of some medications.

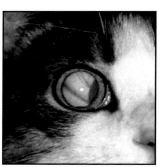

13.2 Feline eye with detached retina visible on basic penlight examination. The cat was presented for acute blindness. (Courtesy of E. Bentley.)

In cats, a diagnosis of hyperthyroidism should include blood pressure evaluation. Screening blood pressure measurements in any cat with left ventricular hypertrophy is required before a diagnosis of idiopathic hypertrophic cardiomyopathy (HCM) can be made with confidence, and blood pressure measurement is a reasonable diagnostic test in any cat >10 years old with a new heart murmur.

In dogs, (in addition to the findings listed above for both species) a diagnosis of hyperadrenocorticism (Cushing's disease), acromegaly, phaeochromocytoma or primary hyperaldosteronism should result in blood pressure evaluation.

In all cases, evidence of ocular damage typical of hypertension or neurological manifestations of hypertension is considered an emergency and treated as such, with a goal of rapid reduction of blood pressure *prior* to pursuit of further diagnostics. Measurement of elevated blood pressure on one occasion is diagnostic for hypertension when clinical signs are present, but should be confirmed with measurement on a second occasion when clinical signs are absent or underlying disease is ambiguous.

Hypotensive patients

Hypotension (as diagnosed by systolic blood pressure <100 mmHg in most species) may occur with dehydration, shock, excessive use of vasodilators or decreased cardiac output due to cardiac dysfunction. Results delivered by indirect methods of blood pressure measurement (Doppler or oscillometric methods, see below) become increasingly unreliable as systolic blood pressure decreases below 100 mmHg. In critical and emergency situations, hypotensive patients will require invasive blood pressure measurement to deliver accurate results and monitor therapy.

Techniques

Invasive measurement

Invasive blood pressure measurement (Figures 13.3 and 13.4) involves arterial puncture (for acute measurement) or arterial cannulation with use of a blood pressure monitor providing pressure tracings for longer-term monitoring. Invasive blood pressure measurement provides a direct reflection of true intra-arterial pressure, but can be cumbersome for clinical use. With rare exceptions, direct blood pressure monitoring is mainly used for anaesthetic or acute critical care monitoring, or in research situations, and is recommended in clinical patients with life-threatening acute hypertension, or significantly ill animals undergoing general anaesthesia.

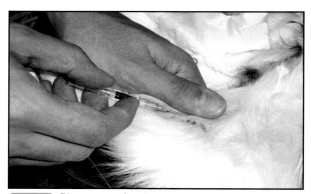

13.3 Placement of an intra-arterial catheter into the femoral artery of a dog. Once in place, the catheter is attached by stiff-walled tubing to a pressure transducer. The 'flash' of blood in the needle hub indicates successful arterial puncture.

Arterial puncture site

Hindlimb:
- Femoral artery at the level of the femoral triangle (most common)
- Dorsal pedal artery (arterial cannulation in dogs).

Patient position

Lateral recumbency with upper hindlimb elevated as needed to expose site of arterial puncture/measurement

Patient preparation

1. Clip hair at intended puncture or cannulation site.
2. Infiltrate skin and subcutaneous tissue with 0.5–1 ml of 2% lidocaine for local anaesthesia (allow approximately 5 minutes prior to arterial puncture).
3. Spray or wipe the site with surgical spirit. Excessive scrubbing/ wiping of the skin should be avoided, as this may result in spasm of the artery.

Technique and measurement

Arterial puncture:
1. Attach a 22-gauge needle to the transducer, and flush the transducer, attached needle and tubing with heparinized saline.
2. Zero the transducer at the level of the sternum in the laterally positioned animal.
3. Palpate femoral artery and advance needle until characteristic pressure trace is noted on the monitor.
4. Print sample of blood pressure trace for offline measurement.
5. Withdraw needle and apply firm pressure to the puncture site for at least 5 minutes.
6. Monitor site closely for haematoma formation after pressure withdrawn.

Arterial cannulation:
1. Flush and zero pressure transducer prior to arterial cannulation.
2. Pre-flush an appropriately sized short over-the-needle catheter.
3. Palpate dorsal pedal artery and advance needle and catheter into artery until intra-arterial position is ascertained ('flash' of blood in needle hub; Figure 13.3).
4. Advance catheter into artery and withdraw needle.
5. Attach catheter to pre-flushed arterial (stiff-walled) tubing previously attached to transducer.
6. Check for characteristic blood pressure trace on monitor, then secure catheter site.
7. Blood pressure tracings are recorded with catheter site level with heart.

13.4 Invasive method for blood pressure measurement.

Indirect measurement

Doppler method
Doppler blood pressure measurement using piezoelectric crystal detection of arterial pulsation and a hand-inflated cuff (sphygmomanometer) is commonly used and at present is the preferred method in cats (Figures 13.5 and 13.6).

Limb used

Right or left forelimb (preferred)
Hindlimb

Patient position

Sternal recumbency with forelimb extended
Sitting with forelimb extended
Lateral recumbency with forelimb or hindlimb extended

13.5 Doppler method for measuring blood pressure. (continues) ▶

Cuff position

Forelimb: radius
Hindlimb: proximal to hock

Patient preparation

1. Clip hair over palmar metacarpal or metatarsal arterial arch (if needed).
2. Allow patient to acclimate and rest comfortably.
3. Measure limb and choose cuff width of approximately 40% of limb circumference at site chosen for cuff placement.

Technique

1. Apply cuff snugly around preferred limb.
2. Attach (short) tubing to sphygmomanometer.
3. Apply acoustic coupling gel to Doppler crystal.
4. Place and hold (or secure with tape) gelled crystal position over clipped area (palmar metacarpal or metatarsal arterial arch).
5. Turn on Doppler sound amplifier.
6. Position crystal until easily audible, clear sounding pulse is heard.

Measurement

1. Turn sphymomanometer dial to close valve for inflation.
2. Inflate cuff gradually to at least 20 mmHg higher than needed to cut off the audible signal.
3. Release sphymomanometer valve a small amount to allow air to escape and the needle to fall gradually (<5 mmHg per second).
4. The pressure at which the Doppler sound is again audible is recorded as the systolic blood pressure value for that inflation.

Replicates

1. Record heart rate after every blood pressure measurement to allow for assessment of patient agitation.
2. Record 6 replicates with approximately 30 seconds between measurements.
3. Discard the first blood pressure/heart rate reading.
4. Discard any clearly false readings.
5. Record the averages of the remaining readings for each category as the representative value for blood pressure and heart rate.

13.5 (continued) Doppler method for measuring blood pressure.

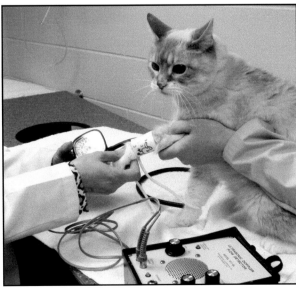

13.6 The cuff is fitted snugly around the cat's forelimb at the level of the radius and is held at the level of the heart for measurement. The Doppler crystal (with gel) is gently held in place over the ventral metacarpal arterial arch. The technician inflates the cuff with a hand-inflated bulb (lower left) while listening for the audible Doppler signal from the amplifier (bottom right).

Accuracy is dependent on user experience and meticulous attention to technique; even with experience diastolic pressures can be difficult to discern in some animals. In dogs, Doppler estimates of systolic blood pressure may underestimate those obtained by arterial cannulation by 5–20 mmHg.

Oscillometric measurement

Oscillometric blood pressure measurement is a common and useful technique that relies on detection of arterial pulsation through the use of an automatically inflating and deflating cuff that is wrapped around a distal limb or tail (Figures 13.7 and 13.8).

Oscillometric techniques have been shown to track trends in blood pressure accurately over time in conscious dogs, but individual measurements obtained oscillometrically may underestimate direct systolic blood pressure measurements by 5–20 mmHg. Oscillometric diastolic pressure results in conscious dogs are poorly correlated with invasively measured diastolic pressure, and are relatively unreliable using present technologies and techniques. So-called high-definition (HD) oscillometry is a more

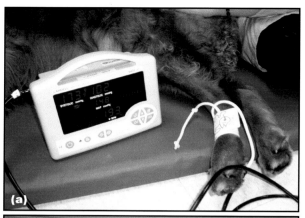

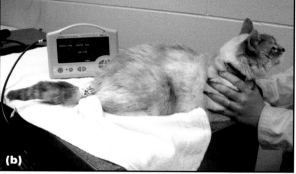

13.8 **(a)** The cuff is fitted at the level of the metatarsus and is level with the dog's sternum during measurement in lateral recumbency. The oscillometric device delivers systolic, diastolic and mean blood pressure with heart rate. **(b)** The cuff is positioned at the base of the tail in a cat. Note that the tailhead is at the level of the heart when the cat is resting comfortably in sternal recumbency.

recent technique that purportedly delivers more accurate results than 'regular' oscillometric techniques but is methodologically similar. At this time, little information has been published on the relative accuracy of HD oscillometry compared with other accepted techniques in conscious pet animals.

Technical aspects of clinical use of indirect methods

Patient preparation

Acclimation of the patient to the surroundings is essential before blood pressure measurement. Indirect measurement should be performed after a short acclimation period in the examination room, but before any other examination, with the owner holding the pet, if possible. The pet should be held in a comfortable position and calmed until relaxed and quiet. Whining or hissing leads to unpredictable elevations in blood pressure.

If blood pressure measurement must be delayed until after initial examinations or other procedures have been performed, blood pressure readings should be separated from blood sampling, radiographic/echocardiographic examinations or temperature-taking by at least 30 minutes. In these situations, special attention to patient acclimation in

Limb used
Hindlimb (preferred)
Right or left forelimb
Tailhead

Patient position
Sternal recumbency with forelimb/hindlimb extended
Sitting with forelimb/hindlimb extended
Lateral recumbency with forelimb or hindlimb extended
Tail cuff can be used in sternal or lateral recumbency. A standing position can be used but is less desirable

Cuff position
Forelimb: radius (either species); humerus in cats if HD oscillometric method is used
Hindlimb: proximal metatarsals or proximal to the hock

Patient preparation
1. Allow patient to acclimate and rest comfortably.
2. Measure limb and choose cuff width of approximately 40% of limb circumference at site chosen for cuff placement.

Technique
1. Apply cuff snugly around preferred limb with bladder of cuff centred over palpable pulse if possible.
2. Attach tubing to oscillometric machine.
3. Clear machine of any previously stored measurements.

Measurement
1. Set machine for correct inflation pressure, cuff size, etc. (variable by manufacturer).
2. Set machine to pause at least 30 seconds between readings.
3. Allow machine to perform consecutive readings.

Replicates
1. Record 6 replicates with approximately 30 seconds between measurements.
2. Discard the first blood pressure/heart rate reading.
3. Discard any clearly false readings.
4. Record the representative blood pressure and heart rate as the averages of the remaining readings.

13.7 Oscillometric or high-definition oscillometric methods for blood pressure measurement.

a quiet room and use of a talented restrainer will increase the accuracy and reliability of blood pressure readings even in anxious patients.

Choice of measurement method

Dogs
In dogs, oscillometric cuffs can be used at the metatarsal (see Figure 13.8a) or radial level of limbs, or at the tailhead. Doppler methods are frequently used in dogs, deliver a measure of systolic pressure reliably and may be the preferred method in dogs that are very anxious and trembling. Both Doppler and oscillometric methods underestimate true blood pressure, and measurements should be repeated multiple times; obvious outliers should be discarded and the results recorded should represent an average of several (at least three) individual readings.

Cats
The most commonly used method in cats is Doppler flow detection using an ultrasound flow detector and a cuff placed at the level of the radius. Cuff placement on the upper forelimb in cats is recommended when using HD oscillometric devices and some clinicians find that a cuff placed at the base of the tailhead is useful (see Figure 13.8b).

Regardless of cuff position, oscillometric methods may have trouble reliably detecting blood pressure in cats when very rapid heart rates or irregular heart rhythms are present. Oscillometric readings correlate less well with invasive measurements of blood pressure in conscious cats than in dogs. Overall, Doppler methods are preferred at this time in cats due to ease of application and the existence of a body of data correlating findings with this method to clinical signs of hypertension.

Cuff size and location
Cuff size is critical to accurate blood pressure measurement. Undersized cuffs will overestimate blood pressure and oversized cuffs will underestimate blood pressure. The circumference of the cuff site is measured prior to placement, and a cuff with a width ~40% of the circumference of the cuff site should be used.

For oscillometric readings, the bladder of the cuff should be positioned over the artery for maximum sensitivity to oscillations. Cuff location (forelimb *versus* hindlimb *versus* tailhead; proximal limb *versus* distal limb) may alter blood pressure measurement results, especially systolic blood pressure, and so the same cuff position should be used and recorded in the medical record each time a given patient's blood pressure is measured.

The cuff should be at the level of the right atrium (RA) during measurements: at the level of the thoracic inlet when the animal is in sternal recumbency; or at the level of the sternum when the animal is in lateral recumbency.

- A cuff positioned *lower* than the RA during readings falsely increases the blood pressure reading.
- A cuff positioned *higher* than the RA during readings falsely lowers the blood pressure reading.

Blood pressure should not be measured with a leg cuff in a standing animal. Sitting patients should be in the 'shake hands' position during readings (see Figure 13.6).

Follow-up
The natural and often unknown variability of blood pressure in veterinary patients plays a role both in diagnosis of hypertension and in management of therapy. Extremely excitable animals may have volatile blood pressure when measured in the clinic that is not reflective of their blood pressure in other settings. A follow-up blood pressure measurement taken when the animal is in a different state of consciousness (awake *versus* sleep) may return false evidence of benefit or lack of benefit of medication. Timing of follow-up blood pressure measurements should take into account the expected onset of action of medications taken prior to measurement. Intra-patient variability can be lessened by having well trained personnel using consistent and repeatable techniques to measure blood pressure.

14

Respiratory pathophysiology

Brendan M. Corcoran

Introduction

The respiratory system is designed to deliver atmospheric oxygen to the body and to remove the waste product of metabolism, carbon dioxide. It achieves this by using a bellows system to draw air into the alveoli and gas exchange mechanisms to transfer oxygen into the pulmonary venous capillaries. Carbon dioxide is then transferred from the pulmonary arterial circulation to the alveoli and expelled into the atmosphere during expiration by the inherent elastic recoil of the lungs.

Respiratory cycle

Inspiration starts from the functional residual capacity (FRC) (Figure 14.1) with active contraction of the diaphragm, which results in expansion of the thoracic wall. At the same time there is contraction of the laryngeal muscles, resulting in a widening of the glottis. Increased thoracic volume leads to a reduction in interpleural pressure, generating a more negative pressure relative to the atmosphere, and resulting in expansion of the lungs. Traction on the intrathoracic airways by the expanding lungs leads to a reduction in airway resistance, and air flows into the respiratory

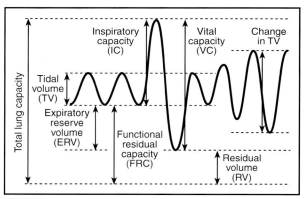

14.1 Lung volume divisions. Tidal volume (TV) is the amount of air that enters the lung with each breath. Inspiratory capacity (IC) is the maximal volume that can be attained from resting lung volume. Expiratory reserve volume (ERV) is the volume that can be exhaled starting at the resting end-expiratory point. The residual volume (RV) is that volume that cannot be exhaled from the lung. The functional residual capacity (FRC) is the combination of the ERV and RV, and is the resting volume during normal tidal breathing.

bronchioles and alveoli with a minimal drop in alveolar pressure. At the end-inspiratory point, tidal volume has been achieved and expiration begins immediately, driven by elastic recoil of the lungs. Once the lungs have returned to their resting volume, the process starts again.

Increasing ventilation

In the event of increased ventilatory demand during exercise, excitement and disease, the respiratory system can increase ventilation by several means. Firstly, an increase in tidal volume can be attempted to satisfy ventilatory demand. The extent to which tidal volume can increase is determined by the inspiratory capacity. Following this, but usually in conjunction with a change in tidal volume, the respiratory rate can be increased. However, at high respiratory rates (hyperpnoea) and large tidal volumes (hyperventilation), the efficiency and balance of gas exchange is compromised, and there is excessive 'blow-off' of carbon dioxide, which is the main stimulus for ventilation. This can result in hypoxaemia with hypocapnia, which depresses respiration. The development of respiratory alkalosis occurs with hypocapnia and this adversely affects cerebrovascular blood flow.

Increased respiratory drive results in recruitment of the internal and external intercostal muscles and the abdominal wall musculature to support respiration, but if sustained, will result in increased metabolic activity and muscular exhaustion. With exhaustion, alveolar hypoventilation can occur, resulting in hypoxaemia and hypercarbia. Hypercarbia then stimulates respiration to prevent the development of respiratory acidosis.

To further improve ventilation, body position can be altered to ease breathing. This is typically seen as open mouth-breathing in a sternal or standing position with the elbows abducted. However, in some dogs it may be appreciated as a reluctance/inability to lie down (orthopnoea), and the dog will remain standing for prolonged periods of time.

The respiratory system has a major capability to increase the volume of air that can be used in gas exchange (minute ventilation) and when demand increases, large areas of under-ventilated lung can be recruited to meet this demand. To match this ventilatory capacity, the pulmonary arterial system can deliver up to six times the amount of venous blood typically used at rest, with only marginal changes in pulmonary arterial pressure and with minimal load on the right ventricle.

Respiratory mechanics

The capacity of the respiratory system is constrained by a variety of mechanical limitations. At resting lung volume, the lung contains the expiratory reserve volume (the volume of air that can be additionally expelled from the end-tidal point) and the residual volume (the volume of air that cannot be expelled). Combined together, the expiratory reserve volume and residual volume are the FRC. The FRC exists because the recoil of the chest wall opposes the elastic recoil of the lung, preventing the lung from collapsing totally after expiration (Figure 14.2). This obviates the need for excessive muscular energy to re-expand the lung during the next inspiratory phase of the cycle. In conjunction with this, the distal airways and alveoli are lined with surfactant, a phospholipid secreted by type II pneumocytes, which reduces surface tension and decreases the pressure needed to re-expand the lung during each inspiration. It can be appreciated that when there is significant lung consolidation or alveolar flooding with exudate or oedema, re-expansion of such lung units can be difficult due in part to loss of surfactant. In the event that the thoracic cage is punctured and the pleural space is opened to the atmosphere, the chest wall can be seen to recoil outwards and the lung to collapse inwards. This illustrates the important role the pleural space has in maintaining the correct mechanical interface between the lung and thoracic cage, and this can be adversely affected by diseases causing pleural effusion and by pneumothorax.

Compliance

The energy required to inflate the lung is related in part to the inherent compliance of the lung. Compliance is a measure of lung distensibility or stiffness, and is a function of volume and pressure (l/kPa). The reciprocal of compliance is elastance, which is the main contributor to the lungs' tendency to recoil. In diseases where the lung parenchyma is stiffer, as with idiopathic pulmonary fibrosis or pneumonia, compliance is reduced and more effort is needed to expand the lungs. This is further complicated by reduced inspiratory capacity because of loss of functional lung. Consequently more energy is expended during inspiration.

With reduced compliance, and conversely increased elastance, there is an increase in lung recoil. This results in a rapid uncontrolled expiration. In some instances expiration is so fast that the lung does not have enough time to empty properly, resulting in inefficient gas exchange. To overcome this problem, the patient may try to slow expiration by use of inspiratory muscles to 'brake' expiration or, more probably, recruit abdominal muscles to force air out of the lung. This latter action is due to activation of stretch receptors by the still inflated lung.

The forced expiration may result in exhaling beyond the normal expiratory point and encroachment into the FRC. If this occurs in normal individuals (as occurs normally in horses), the reverse recoil of the lung reduces the energy required to begin inspiration. However, in a diseased patient this results in increased work to begin the next respiratory cycle. Rapid forced expiration can also result in complete airway collapse, which stimulates coughing (see Chapter 2). When increased expiratory effort occurs in dogs with intrathoracic tracheal or airway collapse, the intrathoracic trachea collapses because of the lack of structural rigidity and not because of compression by a non-complaint lung. However, an increase in lung stiffness may induce airway collapse in a dog that would be otherwise unaffected.

The compliance of the chest wall is also important in ventilation and can be severely compromised by pleural disease, thoracic trauma, a ruptured diaphragm, neuromuscular disease and obesity, typically resulting in hypoventilation.

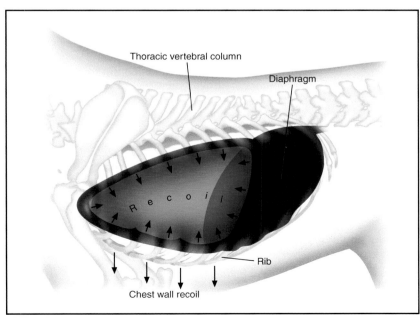

14.2 Recoil forces on the lung and chest wall. The elastic forces of the lung have a tendency to make the lung return to its minimal volume, whilst the chest wall has a tendency to recoil outwards. The balance between the opposing recoil forces of lung and chest wall allows the lung to empty adequately during expiration but prevents lung collapse. In addition, preventing the lung from collapsing facilitates lung re-expansion during inspiration.

Resistance

The main contributor to respiratory resistance is that provided by the airways (Raw). Resistance is a function of pressure and flow (kPa/l/s) and the upper airways make up approximately 50% of Raw. This is particularly important with brachycephalic airway syndrome and laryngeal paralysis, and minor surgical improvement of an upper airway obstruction can have a marked effect on ventilation. Airway resistance is intimately associated with airway diameter and, in terms of flow mechanics, the tracheobronchial tree is considered a non-laminar (turbulent) system. This means that flow is proportional to the pressure gradient between the mouth and alveoli, and to the radius^2 of the conducting airways (radius^4 if the system was laminar).

With a small reduction in diameter of the airway lumen, the pressure must increase markedly to maintain the same level of flow. In ventilatory terms, this means more forceful inspiratory or expiratory effort. However, there is a finite limit to which pressure can be raised, and consequently resistance rises and flow falls with small changes in airway diameter. This effect is best illustrated in dogs with a hypoplastic trachea, where the airway diameter is reduced and fixed, and in feline bronchial disease where the airway diameter is reduced by bronchoconstriction but can vary marginally during the respiratory cycle. For dogs with a hypoplastic trachea, the strategy to maintain adequate ventilation is to reduce activity. Cats that suffer a bronchoconstrictive event may adopt an orthopnoeic posture in order to reduce total airway resistance.

Pulmonary ventilation

Pulmonary ventilation is the total amount of gas available for exchange at the level of the alveoli, and roughly equates to minute ventilation (tidal volume multiplied by the respiratory rate) minus anatomical dead space. For each breath, two-thirds of the tidal volume contributes to ventilation while the remainder occupies anatomical dead space, which consists primarily of the volume of the large conducting airways. Situations where anatomical dead space is increased, as with intubation during anaesthesia, can compromise pulmonary ventilation.

Alveolar ventilation

Alveolar ventilation (VA) is the portion of inspired air that is available for gas exchange. However, not all of the VA will be utilized for gas exchange because there will be areas of under-perfused lung that do not participate in gas exchange, despite adequate ventilation. VA is maximized when increased pulmonary arterial flow opens under-perfused lung units. This region represents physiological dead space, and in normal resting animals can be of equal magnitude to anatomical dead space. Physiological dead space is affected by gravity, posture and position. It can also be increased where there is significant lung disease, but the more likely outcome in that scenario is a mismatch between ventilation (V) and perfusion (Q). This typically results in hypoxaemia due to mixture of blood from under-perfused and normally perfused lung units (venous admixture). V/Q mismatch is often seen with pneumonia, pulmonary oedema and pulmonary thromboembolism. These cases tend to develop hypo- or normocapnia.

Alveolar hypoventilation

Alveolar hypoventilation results in hypercarbia. If this becomes severe, it can cause depression, coma and death. However, since arterial carbon dioxide is the main stimulus for ventilation, hypercarbia will increase respiration, and hypoventilating patients can then be found to be normo- or even hypocapnic. Typical causes of alveolar hypoventilation are diseases resulting in an upper airway obstruction (such as brachycephalic airway syndrome or laryngeal paralysis), but it can also occur with diseases of the lower airway (such as feline bronchial disease with airway trapping), severe pleural effusion and diseases of the thoracic cage (such as rib fractures).

Diffusion impairment

Diffusion impairment can also affect gas exchange, but diseases that reduce diffusion capacity by affecting only the alveolar wall appear to be more common in human patients than in dogs and cats. Alveolar wall diseases in dogs and cats usually extend to include the alveolar space. Conditions that initially affect the alveolar wall (such as interstitial oedema, interstitial pneumonia and idiopathic pulmonary fibrosis) affect diffusion capacity, but by the time the problem is clinically recognizable, V/Q mismatch will be a major contribution to hypoxaemia.

Respiratory failure

Irrespective of the underlying cause of arterial blood gas abnormalities, respiratory failure will eventually occur if disease progression cannot be stopped or reversed.

- Type 1 respiratory failure is defined as hypoxaemia with normo- or hypocapnia. Affected patients tend to respond to supplemental oxygen.
- Type 2 respiratory failure is associated with hypercarbia. Oxygen supplementation has to be administered with caution as this might suppress respiratory drive and worsen hypercarbia.

Type 1 respiratory failure tends to be associated with lung parenchymal diseases. Type 2 respiratory failure tends to be associated with airway obstruction. More detailed discussion of gas exchange and interpretation of blood gas abnormalities can be found in Chapter 12.

Airway and lung protective mechanisms

Since the respiratory system is exposed to the atmosphere, it has to have the capacity to protect itself from inhaled noxious substances and infectious agents. It also has to have the capacity to repair damaged tissue. In the event that damage is extensive, progressive and irreparable, respiratory failure will result irrespective of how well the system performs mechanically.

Large particulate material

The anatomy of the upper respiratory tract is designed to protect the lungs from inhaled particulate material. This includes the conformation of the external nares, nasal passages and oropharynx, and the normal function of the larynx, which all contribute to filter out large particulate matter. This material is trapped in nasal mucus and saliva and can be expectorated or swallowed. Additionally, reflex sneezing and coughing can remove this material or prevent further inhalation.

Small particulate material

Smaller particles that gain entry to the trachea and larger airways tend to collide with the airway walls and stimulate mucus secretion from the submucosal glands and interepithelial goblets cells, leading to trapping of the debris. This material is then moved rostrally using the mucociliary escalator, with activation of the cough receptors, and the material is expectorated and swallowed. This is a very effective and continuously active method of maintaining airway hygiene. Airway mucus is a complex visco-elastic material composed of sol and gel layers that sits on top of the cilia on the airway epithelial surface. The rhythmic beating of the cilia moves this mucus blanket forward in an oral direction. In more distal airways, there are very few ciliated cells, and in the respiratory bronchioles and alveoli there are none; however, mucus from these sites can be moved rostrally through a combination of coughing and capillary action, which is aided by the presence of surfactant. This mechanism of maintaining airway hygiene can be significantly compromised by disease.

Respiratory infections such as *Bordetella bronchiseptica* reduce ciliary activity. With chronic bronchitis, ciliated epithelium can be lost completely, and this is complicated by an associated increase in the quantity and thickness of airway mucus. In these circumstances, coughing is crucial to the removal of airway material and suppression of the coughing may in fact be detrimental.

Small particulate material (typically <5 μm in diameter) that gains entry into the distal airways and alveolar spaces is phagocytosed by alveolar macrophages, transported across the alveolar wall, and drained into the pulmonary lymphatic system for effective removal. In conditions where there is excessive material and/or inflammation, this system may be overwhelmed and rostral removal using the mucociliary escalator and coughing are needed. In such circumstances, clinical disease tends to be evident, with bronchopneumonia being one of the best examples.

Inflammation

Inflammation also results in the recruitment of neutrophils and/or eosinophils and activation of local innate and acquired immune responses. The type of response depends on the type of insult, with neutrophil migration into the airways and lungs being associated with non-specific inflammation and bacterial proliferation, whilst eosinophils are recruited in cases of hypersensitivity and parasitism. If the inflammatory reaction becomes chronic, activation of resident myofibroblasts in the alveolar walls can result in interstitial thickening, fibrosis and the loss of functional lung. When acute inflammation can be readily treated and quickly controlled, there is minimal lung damage, but repeated and sustained lung insult, even at a mild subclinical level, is likely to result eventually in irreparable damage and respiratory failure.

15

Heart failure

Mark A. Oyama

Introduction

Heart failure arises when structural or functional abnormalities prevent the heart from properly filling with or ejecting blood, so that the heart cannot meet the metabolic needs of the peripheral tissue or can do so only in the face of elevated filling pressures. Additional terminology describing failure of the cardiovascular system is based upon the specific organs or tissues involved:

- The term *circulatory failure* encompasses abnormalities of the heart, blood volume or concentration of oxygenated haemoglobin
- The term *myocardial failure* specifically denotes deficiencies of myocardial contraction.

The haemodynamic and circulatory consequences of heart failure involve decreased cardiac output, vasoconstriction, retention of sodium and water, and activation of neurohormonal pathways, including the sympathetic nervous system and the renin–angiotensin–aldosterone axis.

Mechanisms of heart failure

In early disease, the activation of compensatory mechanisms represents an attempt to maintain normal cardiac performance, but heightened neurohormonal activity quickly leads to maladaptive changes that hasten the progression of disease. The mechanisms of heart failure include:

- Alterations in autonomic tone
- Myocardial remodelling and hypertrophy
- Myocyte necrosis and apoptosis
- Abnormal calcium ion cycling and contractility
- Activation of neurohormonal pathways
- Abnormalities in myocardial energy production.

As disease progresses, these mechanisms contribute to the development of clinical signs of heart failure, such as respiratory distress, cough and activity intolerance, as well as to abnormal physical examination findings, such as tachycardia, heart murmur, pulmonary crackles, and ascites. In most cases, the predominant signs of heart failure are manifest as either congestive (i.e. backwards) failure or low output (i.e. forwards) failure. The hallmark of congestive heart failure (CHF) is the presence of effusion or oedema, whereas in patients with low output heart failure, signs of weakness, syncope, hypotension and poor perfusion dominate. Following initial examination, a patient's level of clinical debilitation is often described using a clinical scoring system, such as that recommended by the International Small Animal Cardiac Health Council (ISACHC, 1998). This and other clinical classification systems help standardize disease severity as well as guide treatment decisions.

Alterations in autonomic tone

Heart disease is characterized by activation of the sympathetic nervous system and simultaneous withdrawal of parasympathetic activity. This change occurs early in the course of disease and is one of the clinical hallmarks of heart failure. Decreases in cardiac output and blood pressure are detected by baroreceptors (pressure receptors) and mechanoreceptors (stretch receptors) located in the carotid sinus, aortic arch and atrial walls, leading to a reduction of inhibitory afferent impulses produced by these receptors, which are normally transmitted to the central nervous system (CNS) and vasomotor centres. Withdrawal of these inhibitory signals increases activity of the sympathetic nervous system and suppresses activity of the parasympathetic nervous system, resulting in increased delivery of cardiac noradrenaline (norepinephrine).

As disease progresses, spillover of cardiac noradrenaline into the circulation occurs. In humans with heart disease, the plasma concentration of noradrenaline is a powerful predictor of mortality. Elevated sympathetic nervous system activity results in tachycardia, increased cardiac contractility, vasoconstriction and activation of the renin–angiotensin–aldosterone axis. These effects initially support dwindling cardiac performance by improving cardiac output and maintaining arterial blood pressure; however, these effects are countermanded by the detrimental effects of chronic activation of the sympathetic nervous system. Chronic stimulation ultimately depletes cardiac noradrenaline stores, induces downregulation and uncoupling of myocyte beta adrenergic receptors, as well as causing myocardial cell loss through apoptosis or necrosis. Thus, what begins as a useful compensatory response ultimately desensitizes the heart to adrenergic stimulation and promotes further myocardial cell damage and loss. The seemingly paradoxical response of the heart to chronically heightened adrenergic tone can be viewed in light of the teleological development of the sympathetic nervous system as a means for short-term adaptation (the classic 'fight or flight' response) as opposed to the persistently increased activity seen in cases of heart failure.

Myocardial remodelling

Remodelling of the myocardium, in the form of alterations in mass and geometry, represents one of the primary responses of the heart to increased workload. Remodelling of the ventricle occurs in two classic forms: concentric and eccentric hypertrophy.

Concentric hypertrophy develops in response to pressure overload (i.e. increased afterload), as in the case of systemic hypertension or aortic stenosis. Increased afterload triggers replication of sarcomeres in parallel, resulting in an increase in the relative thickness of the ventricular walls. According to the law of Laplace, ventricular wall stress is elevated by two main factors: increased pressure and an increase in diameter of the ventricular chamber; whereas wall stress is decreased as the ventricular wall thickens. Thus, concentric hypertrophy can be viewed as a means to normalize ventricular wall stress in the face of elevated pressure. Elevated ventricular wall stress increases myocardial oxygen demand, disrupts myocardial collagen and the extracellular matrix, and reduces the intrinsic contractility of individual myocytes.

Eccentric hypertrophy develops in response to volume overload, such as in the case of mitral regurgitation or patent ductus arteriosus. The sarcomeres replicate in series, leading to elongation of the myocytes, dilatation of the ventricular chamber and a small increase in myocardial wall thickness. Thus, in some ways, eccentric hypertrophy is 'less adaptive' than concentric hypertrophy insofar as dramatic increases in ventricular chamber diameter tend to increase ventricular wall stress beyond the point where the mild increases in wall thickness can compensate.

In both forms of hypertrophy, myocardial remodelling is limited by eventual loss of viable myocytes through necrosis or apoptosis, abnormalities in calcium ion cycling, and dysfunction of myocardial energy production.

Myocyte necrosis and apoptosis

The heart has limited ability to regenerate myocytes lost to necrosis or apoptosis. Studies have identified cardiac muscle progenitor cells, but the source, nature, number and robustness of these populations is unknown. In general, loss of large numbers of myocytes is irreversible and exacerbates the stress on the remaining viable cells.

Myocyte necrosis is triggered primarily by ischaemia (as in the case of excessive concentric hypertrophy) or by toxins (such as doxorubicin), and is accompanied by an inflammatory response. Lost cells are replaced by fibrosis, which further impairs systolic and diastolic function.

Apoptosis, which is commonly referred to as programmed cell death, is non-inflammatory and triggered by high catecholamine levels, mitochondrial damage and mechanical stress. The percentage of cells undergoing apoptosis in human cardiac disease ranges widely; most estimates are in the neighbourhood of 0.01%. Although this seems like an extraordinarily low proportion, it must be realized that because the apoptotic process is completed within several hours, a rate of 0.01% over months and years of disease begins to represent a significant number of myocardial cells (Khoynezhad *et al.*, 2007).

Abnormal calcium ion cycling

Contraction of the sarcomere is depressed in heart failure, largely due to abnormalities in intracellular handling of calcium ions. The myocyte's primary calcium store is within the sarcoplasmic reticulum, with much lesser amounts coming from the mitochondria or through the sarcolemmal membrane via specific calcium channels. During cell depolarization, calcium is released from the sarcoplasmic reticulum and binds to the troponin-C apparatus on the actin-myosin filaments, triggering contraction of the sarcomere. Immediately following contraction, the calcium is quickly extruded from the troponin-C molecule and taken back up into the sarcoplasmic reticulum, allowing the sarcomere to relax during cardiac diastole. Calcium release from the sarcoplasmic reticulum is mediated by the ryanodine receptor2, and calcium uptake back into the sarcoplasmic reticulum is mediated by the transporter molecule SERCA2a and its regulatory partner, phospholamban. Figure 15.1 shows the intracellular calcium cycle with respect to its basic regulatory molecules and channels.

In heart failure, sarcoplasmic reticular calcium release and uptake is prolonged, resulting in both systolic and diastolic dysfunction. In addition, in most studies of human and experimental animal heart failure, the expression, protein levels and function of ryanodine receptor2, SERCA2a and phospholamban are decreased (Winslow *et al.*, 1999). Abnormal calcium cycling is exacerbated by tachycardia and the diseased heart experiences a negative force–frequency relationship; that is cardiac contractility worsens as heart rate increases, which is exactly the opposite of healthy heart tissue. This negative force–frequency relationship mitigates much of the positive effect that heart rate normally has on cardiac output.

Activation of neurohormonal pathways

Sympathetic nervous system

The heart is a rich endocrine organ, both as a source and a target. The primary adrenergic receptor on myocardial cells is the beta-1 receptor, which mediates increases in heart rate, contractility and relaxation in response to sympathetic tone. As previously

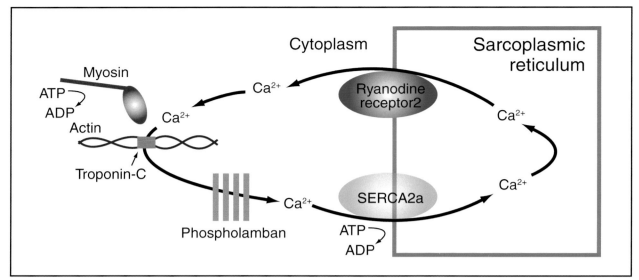

15.1 Calcium cycling in the myocardial cell. The majority of intracellular calcium is stored in the sarcoplasmic reticulum. During cardiac depolarization, calcium is released through the ryanodine receptor2 channel into the cytosol, where it is free to bind to troponin-C. The troponin complex normally inhibits interaction between the myosin head and actin filaments, preventing crossbridging and contraction. Binding of calcium to troponin-C relieves this inhibition and initiates systolic contraction. Once contraction is complete, calcium is released from troponin-C and taken back up into the sarcoplasmic reticulum by the SERCA2a transporter, regulated by phospholamban. The uptake of calcium by SERCA2a as well as crossbridging of myosin and actin utilize a large amount of energy, hence both systole and diastole are energy-dependent events. ADP = Adenosine diphosphate; ATP = Adenosine triphosphate.

mentioned, chronic adrenergic activation leads to downregulation of beta-1 receptor density as well as depletion of cardiac efferent noradrenaline stores. Thus, the failing heart becomes desensitized to sympathetic input even as high noradrenaline levels induce myocardial apoptosis and activation of the renin–angiotensin–aldosterone axis.

Renin–angiotensin–aldosterone axis
The renin–angiotensin–aldosterone axis acts in tandem with the sympathetic nervous system to help maintain arterial blood pressure and adequate organ perfusion. One of the primary triggers for activation is decreased renal blood flow and decreased sodium chloride delivery to the macula densa within the kidneys. Renin from the macula densa converts angiotensinogen to angiotensin I, which is then converted to angiotensin II by angiotensin-converting enzyme (ACE). Angiotensin II is the effector molecule for many of the maladaptive processes that promote heart failure, including vasoconstriction, renal sodium and water retention, elaboration of aldosterone, myocardial hypertrophy, increased thirst and water intake, apoptosis, and potentiation of the sympathetic nervous system.

Elevated activity of the renin–angiotensin–aldosterone axis has been consistently demonstrated in dogs with heart failure (Tidholm *et al.*, 2001; Sisson 2004). The importance of this system in the pathophysiology of heart failure is evidenced by the success of ACE inhibitors in improving longevity in both humans and dogs with heart disease (SOLVD investigators, 1992; Ettinger *et al.*, 1998). In addition to the classic circulating renin–angiotensin–aldosterone axis, a separate tissue-contained renin–angiotensin–aldosterone axis is thought to exist within the myocardial tissue itself. It is likely that this tissue system contributes to myocardial remodelling and hypertrophy, and may be activated much earlier in disease than the circulating system. In addition, ACE-independent pathways that convert angiotensin I to angiotensin II, via an enzyme called chymase, exist within the myocardium in the dog and cat, imparting a certain level of ACE inhibitor 'resistance' to the tissue system.

Angiotensin II induces aldosterone release from the adrenal cortex, which contributes to salt and water retention within the distal segments of the nephron. Importantly, aldosterone is also a potent mitogenic factor, and contributes to vascular and myocardial hypertrophy and fibrosis.

Natriuretic peptides
Two natriuretic peptides, atrial natriuretic peptide (ANP) and B-type natriuretic peptide (BNP), are produced by the heart. The peptides are primarily produced and stored in the atrial muscle and released in response to increased wall stretch. Both natriuretic peptides elicit vasodilatation, natriuresis and diuresis; thus, they serve as counterbalances to the renin–angiotensin–aldosterone axis and sympathetic nervous system. Circulating levels of both ANP and BNP are increased in dogs and cats with heart disease, roughly in proportion to disease severity. However, in advanced cases of disease, the effect of the natriuretic peptides is overwhelmed by the vasoconstrictive and water-retaining activity of the other neurohormonal systems. In addition to physiological effects, ANP and BNP may serve as markers of underlying pathology and aid in the diagnosis, staging and prognostication of various forms of heart disease.

Arginine vasopressin

Arginine vasopressin is elaborated from the pituitary gland in heart failure and increases resorption of free water in the collecting duct of the nephron. Plasma levels of vasopressin tend to mirror circulating levels of noradrenaline. Excess vasopressin leads to expansion of the extracellular fluid volume, contributes to signs of congestion and dilutes total body sodium and chloride levels, leading to hypo-osmolarity. In patients with advanced disease, hyponatraemia and hypochloraemia are often detected on routine blood chemistry, and excessive vasopressin levels are the likely cause. This particular biochemical finding does not indicate deficiencies of either solute, rather that excessive free water retention (dilutional hyponatraemia) is present. This finding is generally thought to represent a poor prognostic sign.

Endothelin-1

Endothelin-1 is a potent vasoconstrictor and is elevated in patients with heart failure. Endothelin-1 is primarily produced by vascular endothelial tissues in response to angiotensin II, shear stress, and various vasoactive cytokines. Endothelin-1 may be particularly important in the pulmonary bed and contribute to pulmonary hypertension in cases of heart failure. Together with angiotensin II, endothelin-1 contributes to increased afterload and increased myocardial workload. Finally, endothelin-1 may be directly toxic to myocardial cells and interfere with normal calcium ion cycling.

Abnormalities in myocardial energy production

The heart can utilize a variety of substrates for energy production, including free fatty acids, glucose and lactate. Interestingly, except in the most severe cases of heart failure or acute ischaemia, the heart appears to maintain adequate perfusion and oxygen and substrate delivery. The adenosine triphosphate (ATP) produced by the heart fuels contraction and relaxation of the sarcomere, operation of the ion pumps and exchangers (especially those involved in calcium cycling), propagation of the action potential, maintenance of the resting cell membrane, and phosphorylation of various enzymes and proteins.

In dogs with myocardial failure, cytochromes and enzymes critical to mitochondrial oxidative phosphorylation are variably absent, and a deficiency of ATP production potentially contributes to the heart failure state (Lopes *et al.*, 2006). Energy stores in the form of creatine phosphate and ATP are depleted in advanced disease and this may also contribute to the development of heart failure. At rest, the heart obtains the majority of its energy from beta-oxidation of free fatty acids. This substrate preference shifts in the face of disease towards greater utilization of glucose and lactate, which despite being less energy dense than fatty acids, are more efficiently converted to ATP per unit of oxygen consumed.

Global cardiac function

The molecular mechanisms previously described form the basis for overall or global function of the heart. It is this global function that the veterinary surgeon is attempting to assess during clinical examination of patients with heart failure. The three primary clinical determinants of global cardiac performance are:

- Preload – the volume of blood or hydrostatic pressure within the ventricles at the end of diastole
- Afterload – the force that opposes ejection of blood into the peripheral arterial system, of which arterial blood pressure is the primary factor
- Contractility – the intrinsic ability of the myocardium to generate force to eject blood.

True contractility is a difficult variable to quantify as its measurement is influenced greatly by both preload and afterload. The clinical cardiac examination evaluates each of these three determinants as follows: preload through assessment of jugular venous distension, effusions, oedema or ascites, and degree of cardiac eccentric hypertrophy using radiography or echocardiography; afterload by measuring systemic arterial blood pressure and chamber dimensions; and contractility by echocardiography and calculating systolic performance indices such as fractional shortening. In patients with heart failure, the molecular mechanisms tend to increase preload and afterload and decrease contractility. The interplay among these variables is elegantly described by a simple physiological relationship, the Frank–Starling mechanism, an understanding of which helps explain the clinical syndrome of heart failure.

Frank–Starling mechanism

In 1914 Ernest Starling, an English physiologist, noted "… the rise of venous pressure [that accompanies increased demands on the heart] must be regarded as one of the mechanical means which are operative in enabling the heart to maintain an output corresponding to the blood it receives from the venous system". This 'discovery' was actually the culmination of research from many previous investigators, including the German physician Otto Frank and perhaps, first of all, Carl Ludwig, another German physician and physiologist who reported in 1856 "… a strong heart that is filled with blood empties itself more or less completely, in other words, [filling of the heart with blood] changes the extent of contractile power".

Regardless of its exact origin, the Frank–Starling Law of the Heart, as it is now widely known, relates cardiac performance to the initial preload condition of the ventricle; in essence, the more volume within the ventricle at the end of diastole, the better the subsequent contraction. This relationship describes both global cardiac performance and the origin of heart failure (congestive and low output), as well as conveying how various types of therapy can be employed to improve cardiac function.

Systolic dysfunction

In health, the Frank–Starling relationship is steep, i.e. small increases in ventricular volume elicit considerable improvement in cardiac function (Figure 15.2a). For example, this relationship describes improved cardiac output during periods of exercise. In the diseased heart, the Frank–Starling curve becomes more flattened as various molecular mechanisms reduce the heart's response to adrenergic drive, decrease the number of viable myocytes, increase afterload and cardiac work, reduce energy production and alter the normal extracellular matrix. In effect, the heart operates in an environment of increased afterload and decreased contractility.

Activation of the renin–angiotensin–aldosterone axis causes sodium and water retention, which (i) maximizes ventricular volume, (ii) shifts the heart's operating point farther to the right along the Frank–Starling curve, and (iii) thereby acts to improve cardiac performance. However, increased preload comes at a

cost in the form of increased ventricular and venous pressure. Once venous pressure rises above approximately 25 mmHg, transudation of fluid occurs across the capillary membrane and effusion or oedema (i.e. CHF) develops (Figure 15.2b). In patients with severely diminished contractility, the Frank–Starling curve may be depressed below a point of adequate cardiac output and clinical signs of low output heart failure (i.e. weakness, shock, organ failure, syncope) predominate (Figure 15.2c). In the very worst of circumstances, both congestive and low output failure may be simultaneously present.

Treatment

Treatment of heart failure aims to reduce preload and afterload and increase contractility. Preload reduction through the use of diuretics and venous vasodilators moves the heart's operating point back to the left, thereby lowering venous pressure and alleviating signs of congestion (Figure 15.2d). Afterload reduction

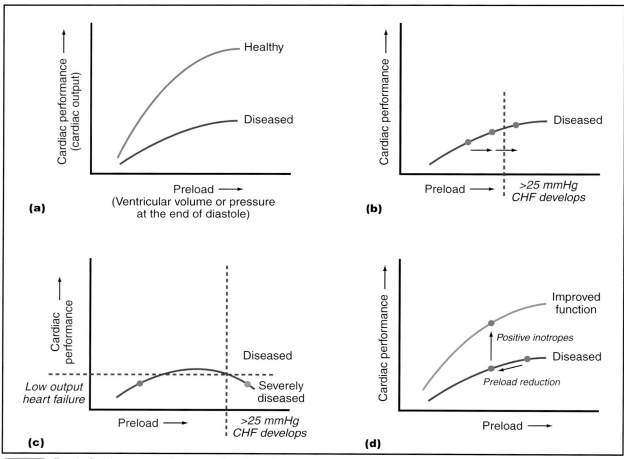

15.2 Frank–Starling curves demonstrating the relationship between preload (ventricular volume or pressure and end-diastole) and cardiac performance (cardiac output). **(a)** In healthy patients, the Frank–Starling relationship is curvilinear and steep, such that small increases in preload effect significant improvements in cardiac output. In diseased patients, the Frank–Starling relationship is depressed and flattened such that cardiac output is decreased for any given level of preload, and the incremental gains in cardiac output for any increase in preload are less than in a healthy patient. **(b)** Development of CHF occurs as the kidneys retain sodium and fluid, and preload increases above approximately 25 mmHg in the pulmonary veins and capillaries. **(c)** Low output heart failure (blue circle) and combined low output and CHF (green circle) in instances of severely depressed myocardial function. **(d)** Treatment of heart failure with preload reducers (i.e. diuretics or venous vasodilators) shifts a patient leftward along the Frank–Starling curve, helping to reduce signs of congestion. Treatment of heart failure with afterload reducers (i.e. arterial vasodilators) or positive inotropes (i.e. dobutamine, pimobendan) shifts the Frank–Starling curve upwards with a steeper slope, helping to restore the normal relationship between preload and cardiac performance.

through the use of arterial vasodilators and positive inotropes increases the slope of the Frank–Starling curve, improving cardiac output for any given level of preload (Figure 15.2d). For many clinicians, understanding the simple relationship described by Frank and Starling helps clarify both the problem and the solution for clinical patients that present with heart failure. However, for all its simplicity and elegance the Frank–Starling mechanism largely ignores an important cause of heart failure: diastolic dysfunction.

Diastolic dysfunction

Many forms of heart disease are primarily due to diastolic dysfunction, as opposed to systolic myocardial failure. The prototypical diastolic heart disease in veterinary medicine is feline hypertrophic cardiomyopathy (HCM). Diastolic heart disease manifest itself as signs of congestive or low output heart failure in the face of normal or near normal systolic function, and can be due to primary impairments of ventricular relaxation, filling or compliance, or secondary to pericardial disease. Diastole comprises three main phases (Figure 15.3a):

- Early ventricular relaxation and filling
- Mid-diastole wherein filling rate slows
- Late-diastole that coincides with atrial contraction and a final surge of ventricular filling.

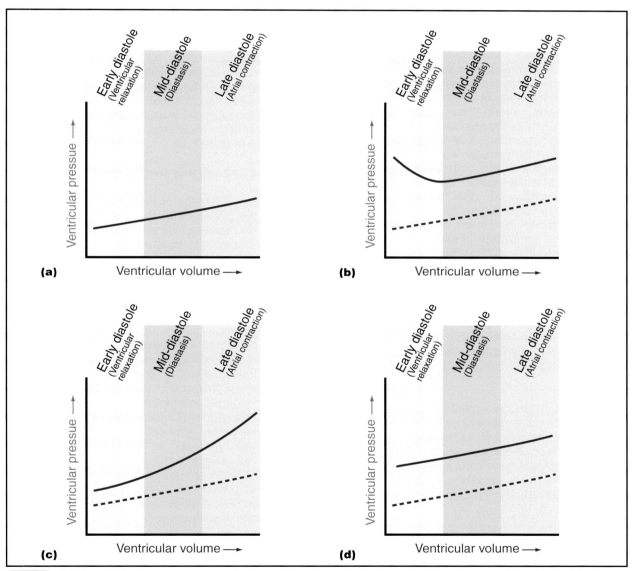

15.3 Relationship between pressure and volume within the ventricle during the three phases of diastole. **(a)** In the healthy patient, increases in ventricular volume are achieved with little change in ventricular pressure because of normal early ventricular relaxation and high ventricular compliance during mid- and late-diastole. **(b)** In patients with impaired ventricular relaxation, early filling is only achieved at the expense of higher ventricular pressures. **(c)** In patients with poor ventricular compliance, mid- and late-diastolic filling is hindered and only achieved at the expense of higher ventricular pressures. **(d)** In patients with pericardial restraint (i.e. pericardial tamponade), the entirety of diastole is affected by external compression of the ventricle, and filling throughout all phases of diastole is accomplished only at higher ventricular pressures.

The early phase of diastole is primarily dependent on relaxation of the ventricular myocardium. This process relies on consumption of energy (i.e. ATP) to move calcium ions back into the sarcoplasmic reticulum and to detach the actin filaments and myosin heads from each other. Thus, in instances of myocardial ischaemia or energy deficit, active relaxation is delayed and early filling of the ventricle is diminished (Figure 15.3b). Subsequent reduction of cardiac output triggers activation of the same neurohormonal and adrenergic responses that are seen in cases of systolic dysfunction, and fluid and sodium retention leads to CHF.

In the normal heart, the ventricle expands readily due to a high degree of compliance (the ability of the ventricle to accommodate blood volume at a low hydrostatic filling pressure). In mid- and late-diastole, ventricular filling is increasingly affected by the compliance properties of the myocardium (Figure 15.3c). The compliance of the ventricle is chiefly a function of wall thickness (concentric hypertrophy decreases compliance), changes in the cytoskeleton and extracellular matrix (fibrosis decreases compliance), and function of the pericardium (pericardial disease or effusion reduces ventricular distensibility). Unlike ventricular relaxation, compliance is generally considered a passive property of the myocardium.

Atrial systole occurs in late-diastole and contributes approximately the final one-fifth of ventricular filling. It is dependent on both the vigour of atrial systolic contraction as well as the compliance of the ventricle. Synchrony of atrial contraction is also important insofar as atrial systolic contribution is lost in patients with atrial fibrillation, complete heart block and ventricular arrhythmias. Finally, the pericardium can adversely affect diastolic function by externally compressing the ventricle, as in cases of pericardial tamponade or constrictive pericarditis. In these cases, diastolic filling is impaired either throughout the entirety of diastole (tamponade) (Figure 15.3d) or only in the mid- and late-phases of diastole (constrictive pericarditis). In both instances, diastolic filling is reduced, cardiac output falls and activation of compensatory responses is triggered.

Treatment

Treatment of diastolic dysfunction is aimed at improving ventricular relaxation, increasing ventricular compliance, maintaining or restoring atrial synchrony, and alleviating any existing pericardial disease. In the absence of obvious pericardial disease, treatment is generally aimed at suppression of arrhythmias and alleviation of congestion through the use of diuretics.

Clinical presentation of heart failure

History and physical examination

When assessing a patient with suspected cardiac disease, an accurate history with regard to the onset and nature of clinical signs, rate of progression, risk factors, previous medical examinations and treatment should be obtained. Importantly, the owner should be specifically questioned regarding the patient's activity tolerance, respiratory effort and rate.

The physical examination should be performed systematically and include:

- Observation of respiratory rate, pattern and effort
- Inspection of the jugular veins
- Palpation of the systemic arterial pulses
- Auscultation of the heart and lungs
- Determination of hydration status
- Detection of pleural or abdominal effusions through percussion, palpation and/or auscultation.

Signs in patients with CHF may range from subtle (e.g. mild tachypnoea, slight abdominal effort, decreased appetite) to overt (e.g. severe respiratory distress, haemoptysis, shock). Signs of disease chronicity may include weight loss, muscle wasting or severe cachexia. Whereas most dogs with heart failure have either an obvious heart murmur or a diastolic gallop, many cats with significant disease have intermittent murmurs or soft gallop sounds that are difficult to detect, particularly in an animal in respiratory distress. Careful attention to history taking and physical examination should allow the practitioner to predict the probability of existing heart disease/failure and to formulate an appropriate plan for further diagnostics or treatment.

Congestive *versus* low output heart failure

The majority of cases of heart failure in companion animals predominantly involve CHF. In these patients, sodium- and water-retaining mechanisms can expand plasma volume by as much as 30 percent. The increased volume is accompanied by increased pressure within the systemic and pulmonary venous system, and once intracapillary pressures rise above plasma colloidal osmotic pressures, fluid is allowed to transude across the capillary membrane and into the interstitial space (Figure 15.4). Typically, pulmonary venous pressures >25 mmHg and systemic venous pressures >20 mmHg are sufficient to produce congestion. Patients with CHF operate on the far right side of the Frank–Starling curve (see Figure 15.2) and resolution of signs is accomplished via preload reduction (i.e. diuretics and venous vasodilators). CHF can manifest as pulmonary oedema, pleural effusion, abdominal effusion (ascites) or occasionally pericardial effusion (especially cats). Peripheral oedema that affects the limbs or subcutaneous tissues is uncommon, and is seen only in the most severe cases of right-sided CHF in small companion animals.

In cases of severe myocardial dysfunction, global cardiac performance may be insufficient to provide adequate cardiac output, and patients present with signs of low output heart failure. This can manifest as depressed mentation, skeletal muscle weakness, oliguria or anuria, hypothermia and cardiac shock. Patients with low output failure operate on the bottom portion of the Frank–Starling curve (see Figure 15.2c) and resolution of signs is accomplished by increasing contractility (i.e. positive inotropes). Judicious arterial vasodilation may also help to improve cardiac output,

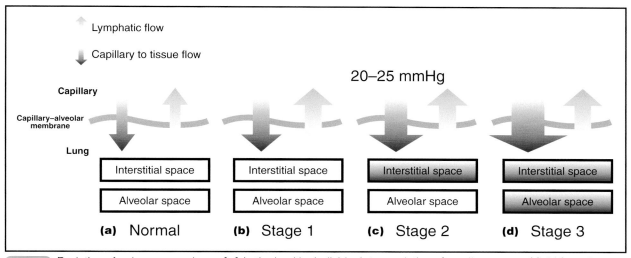

15.4 Evolution of pulmonary oedema. **(a)** In the healthy individual, transudation of small amounts of fluid from the capillary across the capillary–alveolar membrane and into the interstitial space is balanced by removal of the fluid by the lymphatic system. **(b)** In Stage 1 of pulmonary oedema formation, elevated hydrostatic pressure within the capillary system increases the transudation of fluid into the interstitial space; however, no oedema forms due to increased lymphatic removal of fluid from the tissue. **(c)** In Stage 2, the degree of transudation overwhelms the capacity of the lymphatic system to clear fluid, and interstitial oedema results. This occurs when capillary hydrostatic pressures achieve 20–25 mmHg. **(d)** In Stage 3, the degree of transudation is sufficient to accumulate in both the interstitial space as well as in the pulmonary alveoli, and overt clinical signs would be anticipated in these patients.

if it does not compromise arterial blood pressure. In rare instances, patients with low output failure actually benefit from volume (preload) *expansion* to shift their operating point rightward and higher on the Frank–Starling curve. Conversely, overly aggressive diuretic use in a patient with depressed myocardial function could actually precipitate or worsen low output failure.

Left *versus* right heart failure

CHF can manifest as predominantly left- or right-sided failure, or occasionally as biventricular failure. In dogs, acquired mitral valve disease, mitral regurgitation and volume overload affects the left ventricle (LV), left atrium (LA), pulmonary veins and capillaries; thus, heart failure is manifest as left-sided heart failure in the form of pulmonary oedema. In both dogs and cats, pulmonary oedema is exclusively a sign of left-sided heart failure. In dogs, right heart failure is manifest as pleural effusion and/or ascites. In the cat, pleural effusion can occur as a result of either left- or right-sided heart failure, and in most cases is actually due to left-sided heart disease. The explanation for this discrepancy between species is because a portion of the visceral pleural surface actually empties into the pulmonary veins, and this anatomic arrangement appears to be more prominent in cats than in humans and dogs. Ascites as a sign of right heart failure in the cat is relatively uncommon, and most cats with ascites suffer from non-cardiac diseases.

Clinical staging of heart failure

Once the history, physical examination and other confirmatory diagnostic tests are complete, it is useful to classify patients using a scheme based on clinical signs and history of heart failure. Classification allows the practitioner to communicate the severity of disease as well as providing guidance regarding treatment or monitoring decisions. Several classification systems exist, each with their own advantages and disadvantages. One of the most commonly used schemes, the modified New York Heart Association (NYHA) system, describes patients based on tolerance for activity or exercise.

- Patients in NYHA Class I demonstrate no limitations either at rest or during ordinary physical activity.
- Patients in NYHA Class II are comfortable at rest but are fatigued during ordinary physical activity.
- Patients in NYHA Class III remain comfortable at rest but demonstrate marked limitations during ordinary physical activity, and exhibit fatigue or respiratory distress even at lower than normal levels of activity.
- Patients in NYHA Class IV show signs of discomfort and distress even at rest, and all physical activity is severely limited.

Application of the NYHA system to veterinary patients is problematic as many patients do not routinely exert themselves for a myriad of reasons other than cardiac debilitation; this is especially true in naturally sedentary animals such as cats. Thus, detection of early stages of heart failure is often masked, and it is not until animals are overtly affected at rest do owners realize something is wrong. Moreover, whereas the term 'ordinary activity' is well defined in human medicine (i.e. capacity to walk a certain distance or up a certain number of stairs), this term can be widely interpreted in veterinary medicine depending on the breed and lifestyle of any individual dog (i.e. the hunting Labrador Retriever *versus* the handheld Toy Poodle).

In an effort to complement the NYHA system, the American Heart Association (AHA) and American College of Cardiology (ACC) published a system in 2001 that emphasizes the evolution and progression of heart disease. Four stages of disease were described:

- Stage A – patients with no identifiable cardiovascular abnormalities but are at high risk for developing disease (i.e. patients with familial history or with many risk factors such as cigarette smoking or hypertension)
- Stage B – patients with structural heart disease but have yet to develop any clinical signs
- Stage C – patients with structural heart disease and current or prior clinical signs
- Stage D – patients with advanced structural disease and signs at rest despite maximal therapy.

This paradigm, which emphasizes clinical signs rather than capacity for exercise is better adapted to veterinary patients. It should be noted that Stage A is unique in that it identifies patients *before* they have any detectable disease. In veterinary medicine, patients belonging to breeds with a known high incidence of myocardial or valvular disease would be appropriately placed in AHA/ACC Stage A (e.g. Dobermanns, Boxers and Cavalier King Charles Spaniels).

Finally, a veterinary-specific clinical classification system has been proposed by the International Small Animal Cardiac Health Council (ISACHC, 1998) in order to better reflect the signs and evaluation of veterinary patients with heart failure. The ISACHC system contains the following classes:

- Class Ia – animals with structural heart disease, are asymptomatic and possess no radiographic or echocardiographic signs of heart enlargement
- Class Ib – animals as in Class Ia, but with radiographic or echocardiographic signs of heart enlargement
- Class II – animals with mild clinical signs of heart failure at rest or during mild activity
- Class IIIa – animals with overt clinical signs; death or severe debilitation is likely without immediate therapy; homecare is still possible
- Class IIIb – animals as in Class IIIa, but hospitalization is required to effectively treat clinical signs.

Which classification system should practitioners use and why? The author prefers the ISACHC system with the added inclusion of AHA/ACC Stage A. Once a patient's clinical class is established, general guidelines regarding monitoring and therapy can be employed.

- Animals in AHA/ACC Stage A as well as ISACHC Class Ia benefit from client education regarding the incidence and early signs of disease, and from periodic monitoring.
- Animals in Stage Ib should receive closer and more frequent monitoring and may receive treatment as they approach Stage II.
- Animals in Stage II should receive treatment to alleviate clinical signs and undergo routine monitoring.
- Animals in Stage III should receive both urgent care and intensive monitoring.

References and further reading

Ettinger SJ, Benitz AM, Ericsson GF, Cifelli S, Jernigan AD, Longhofer SL, Trimboli W and Hanson PD (1998) Effects of enalapril maleate on survival of dogs with naturally acquired heart failure. The Long-Term Investigation of Veterinary Enalapril (LIVE) Study Group. *Journal of the American Veterinary Medical Association* **213**, 1573–1577

International Small Animal Cardiac Health Council (ISACHC) (1998) Recommendations for the diagnosis of heart disease and the treatment of heart failure in small animals. In: *Manual of Canine and Feline Cardiology, 2nd edn*, ed. MS Miller and LP Tilley, pp. 469–502

Khoynezhad A, Jalali Z and Tortolani AJ (2007) A synopsis of research in cardiac apoptosis and its application to congestive heart failure. *Texas Heart Institute Journal* **34**, 352–359

Lopes R, Solter PF, Sisson DD, Oyama MA and Prosek R (2006) Correlation of mitochondrial protein expression in complexes I to V with natural and induced forms of canine idiopathic dilated cardiomyopathy. *American Journal of Veterinary Research* **67**, 971–977

Sisson DD (2004) Neuroendocrine evaluation of cardiac disease. *Veterinary Clinics of North America: Small Animal Practice* **34**, 1105–1126

SOLVD Investigators (1992) Effect of enalapril on mortality and the development of heart failure in asymptomatic patients with reduced left ventricular ejection fractions. *New England Journal of Medicine* **327**, 685–691

Tidholm A, Haggstrom J and Hansson K (2001) Effects of dilated cardiomyopathy on the renin-angiotensin-aldosterone system, atrial natriuretic peptide activity, and thyroid hormone concentrations in dogs. *American Journal of Veterinary Research* **62**, 961–967

Winslow RL, Rice J, Jafri S, Marban E and O'Rourke B (1999) Mechanisms of altered excitation-contraction coupling in canine tachycardia-induced heart failure – II: model studies. *Circulation Research* **84**, 571–558

16

Arrhythmias

Simon Dennis

Introduction

Electrical impulses control the intracellular movement of calcium ions that regulate contraction and relaxation of cardiac myocytes. Organization of these impulses therefore determines the pattern and timing of contraction and relaxation, which is important to optimize cardiac output. Coordinated electrical activity is vital for this and is achieved by the cardiac conduction system.

Cardiac conduction system

The cardiac conduction system comprises the sinoatrial (SA) node, atrioventricular (AV) node, bundle of His, bundle branches and Purkinje fibre network (see Figure 9.1). Each part of the conduction system can generate an electrical impulse by spontaneous diastolic depolarization.

Cells of the SA node have the fastest rate of diastolic depolarization, making the SA node the dominant *pacemaker* of the heart under normal conditions.

1. An electrical impulse generated by the SA node spreads across the atria in radial fashion, resulting in coordinated atrial contraction and a *P wave* on the surface electrocardiogram (ECG).
2. When the impulse reaches the AV groove it is unable to traverse the electrically inert 'fibrous skeleton' that encircles the AV and semilunar valves. It is therefore channelled via the AV node, which is located on the atrial side of the septum. Some preferential intra-atrial (nodal-to-nodal) conduction occurs via internodal tracts. AV node cells propagate the impulse slowly to the bundle of His. This delay in impulse conduction is important to allow atrial emptying before ventricular activation. It is reflected as a *PR interval* on the surface ECG. The bundle of His penetrates the AV groove before bifurcating into the bundle branches.
3. Finally, the impulse is conducted rapidly to the ventricular myocardium via the bundle branches and Purkinje fibre system. This results in simultaneous depolarization of both ventricles, and contraction in an apical-to-basilar direction. A relatively narrow *QRS complex* on the surface ECG reflects this organized pattern of depolarization, compared with the wide *T wave*

that reflects the less coordinated ventricular repolarization.

Normal heart rhythms result from normal impulse generation (*firing*) within the SA node and normal impulse conduction along the specialized conducting system. An arrhythmia is any cardiac rhythm which is considered to be abnormal for an individual animal. Abnormalities of cardiac electrical activity result in arrhythmias (the terms 'arrhythmia' and 'dysrhythmia' are used synonymously). Arrhythmias occur with abnormalities of impulse generation, abnormalities of impulse conduction, or both.

- *Bradyarrhythmias* are caused by decreased firing from the SA node, or decreased conduction through the atria or AV junction.
- *Tachyarrhythmias* are caused by increased firing from ectopic sites or the phenomenon of re-entry, in which an impulse passes through a region of tissue multiple times by travelling circumferentially.
  - Mechanisms of increased firing are subdivided into automaticity and triggered activity.
  - Re-entry is a disorder of impulse conduction, which requires that the pathway that an impulse traverses divides into two; these two pathways then meet distally, forming a circuit. One of the pathways has slow conduction and the other pathway has unidirectional block. Despite seeming to have complex and implausible criteria, re-entry is the most common mechanism for tachyarrhythmias in cardiac disease.

Normal heart rhythms

Normal sinus rhythm
Normal sinus rhythm results from impulse generation in the SA node at a normal rate (Figure 16.1).

ECG characteristics

- Normal atrial (P) and ventricular (QRS) rate (approximately 70–160 beats/minute in dogs, 140–240 beats/minute in cats).
- Regular atrial (P) rhythm (difference of <0.12 seconds between successive PP intervals for dogs, <0.1 seconds for cats).

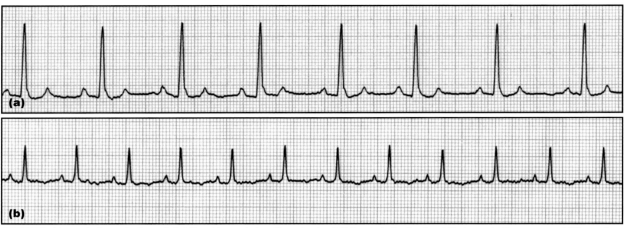

16.1 Normal sinus rhythm. **(a)** Mixed-breed dog (heart rate 125 beats/minute; lead II shown). Paper speed 50 mm/s; gain 1 cm/mV. **(b)** Domestic Shorthaired cat (heart rate 190 beats/minute; lead II shown). Paper speed 50 mm/s; gain 1 cm/mV.

- Regular ventricular (QRS) rhythm (difference of <10% between RR intervals).
- Normal P wave morphology (positive in lead II).
- Normal PR interval and relationship (PR interval duration has slight inverse relationship with heart rate).
- Normal QRS complex morphology (positive in leads II and aVF).
- T wave morphology variable.

Clinical features

- Can be present in healthy animals and those with disease (cardiac or systemic).

Sinus arrhythmia

Sinus arrhythmia results from a variable rate of SA nodal firing. It occurs with phasic acceleration and deceleration of diastolic depolarization of the SA node pacemaker (Figure 16.2). It most frequently occurs with elevated vagal tone. *Respiratory sinus arrhythmia* is characterized by an increase in heart rate with inspiration (due to reflex inhibition of vagal tone) and a decrease with expiration. *Non-respiratory sinus arrhythmia* is characterized by variation in the heart rate unrelated to ventilation.

Causes

- Normal predominance of vagal tone in healthy dogs.
- Abnormally increased vagal tone (cats, some dogs):

  - Severe respiratory disease (particularly upper respiratory obstruction)
  - Intrathoracic mass lesions
  - Severe gastrointestinal disease
  - Central nervous system (CNS) disease
  - Increased intraocular pressure (e.g. ocular surgery).

ECG characteristics

- Irregular PP and RR intervals with a difference of ≥0.12 seconds between successive PP intervals for dogs and ≥0.1 seconds for cats, or a difference of ≥10% between RR intervals (Tilley, 1992ab).
- May or may not be related to phase of respiration.
- P wave morphology may vary if wandering pacemaker present.
- Otherwise criteria for sinus rhythm met.

Clinical features

- Sinus arrhythmia is a common finding in healthy dogs and is a reasonable indicator of the absence of congestive heart failure (CHF) in non-brachycephalic breeds.
- Marked sinus arrhythmia is often present in dogs with respiratory tract disease.
- Sinus arrhythmia in conscious cats is almost invariably abnormal unless the cat is very relaxed or in its home environment. It is often associated with nasopharyngeal or laryngeal disease.

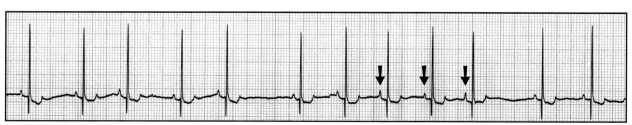

16.2 Sinus arrhythmia in a 10-year-old West Highland White Terrier (lead II shown). Note the variable amplitude P waves, with taller P waves (arrowed) during faster heart rates. This is a wandering pacemaker and indicates a varying site of origin of the sinus impulse. Paper speed 25 mm/s; gain 1 cm/mV.

Wandering pacemaker

The SA node is a large diffuse structure in the dog, and wandering pacemaker occurs when there is beat-to-beat variation in the site of the dominant pacemaker (see Figure 16.2). It most frequently occurs with sinus arrhythmia, in association with elevated vagal tone.

Causes

As for sinus arrhythmias (see above).

ECG characteristics

- Variable P wave morphology (positive, isoelectric, biphasic, negative). P wave is generally positive with intranodal pacemaker sites, but is more variable with perinodal sites.
- PR interval is normal with intranodal pacemaker sites, but may shorten, or occur within the QRS complex with ectopic pacemaker sites in the low right atrium (RA) (near the AV node).
- Otherwise criteria for sinus rhythm/arrhythmia met.
- Note:
  - Pacemaker sites higher in the RA usually have taller, positive P waves in lead II and are typically preceded by shorter RR intervals than sites lower in the RA or at the AV junction
  - It can be difficult to differentiate sinus arrhythmia with a wandering pacemaker from supraventricular premature complexes.

Bradyarrhythmias

A bradyarrhythmia is any arrhythmia causing a heart rate that is inappropriately low for the physiological demands of the body. This results from failure of impulse generation from the SA node, or failure of impulse conduction through the atria or AV junction (AV node and bundle of His).

Sinus bradyarrhythmias

Sinus bradyarrhythmias result from decreased firing of the SA node or decreased conduction of the SA node impulse to the atrial myocardium. Causes can be physiological, pathological or pharmacological. Physiological causes result in an *appropriate* brady-arrhythmia. These result from a normal predominance of vagal tone in certain states (e.g. sinus bradycardia and sinus arrhythmia in a fit dog). Pathological causes are due to disease (cardiac or systemic) and pharmacological causes include anaesthetic or antiarrhythmic drugs. Both result in an *inappropriate* bradyarrhythmia.

Sinus bradyarrhythmias can be caused by:

- Normal (physiological) elevation in vagal tone:
  - Rest/sleep
  - Trained/physically fit dogs
  - Some giant-breed dogs.
- Abnormally increased vagal tone (see Sinus arrhythmia, above)
- Intrinsic SA node disease:
  - Idiopathic degenerative fibrosis
  - Structural heart disease (myocardial disease, atrial dilatation)
  - Inflammatory disease (atrial myocarditis)
  - Infiltration (neoplasia).
- Metabolic abnormalities:
  - Hypothermia
  - Hypoglycaemia
  - Hyperkalaemia
  - Hypothyroidism
  - Severe uraemia.
- Autonomic nervous system disorders
- Drugs (usually in high or toxic doses):
  - Beta-blockers
  - Digitalis glycosides
  - Non-dihydropyridine calcium-channel blockers (diltiazem, verapamil)
  - Sedative and anaesthetic agents (e.g. alpha-2 agonists, phenothiazines, opioids).

Sinus bradycardia

Sinus bradycardia occurs with decreased firing of the SA node (Figure 16.3). It may be present with sinus arrhythmia in animals with elevated vagal tone.

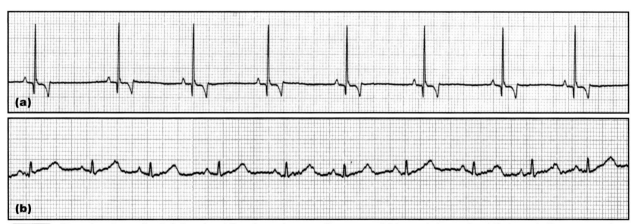

16.3 Sinus bradycardia. **(a)** A trained Greyhound at rest (heart rate 60 beats/minute; lead II shown). Paper speed 25 mm/s; gain 1 cm/mV. **(b)** A 1-year-old Domestic Shorthaired cat with signs of lethargy, anorexia and vomiting, indicating probable gastrointestinal disease (heart rate 130 beats/minute; lead II shown). Paper speed 50 mm/s; gain 1 cm/mV.

ECG characteristics:

- Slow atrial (P) and ventricular (QRS) rate (approximately <70 beats/minute in dogs, <140 beats/minute in cats).
- Otherwise criteria for sinus rhythm/arrhythmia met.

Clinical features:

- A slow regular rhythm is a typical auscultation finding (unless sinus arrhythmia is also present).
- Clinical signs as a result of the bradycardia are uncommon.
- Sinus bradycardia of 60–70 beats/minute may be present in trained/physically fit dogs.
- Cats with low cardiac output can develop sinus bradycardia, particularly if cardiogenic shock is present (results in bradycardia, hypothermia and hypotension).
- Sinus bradycardia in critically ill patients can be a precursor to cardiac arrest.

Sinus arrest

Sinus arrest is a disorder of impulse generation, occurring with temporary cessation of SA nodal firing (Figure 16.4). It most commonly occurs with increased vagal tone or intrinsic SA node disease. It may also occur following tachycardia, which temporarily depresses the pacemaker function of the SA node (overdrive suppression).

ECG characteristics:

- Pause in sinus rhythm of >2 PP intervals that is not a multiple of the underlying PP intervals.
- May have junctional or ventricular escape complexes if pause of sufficient duration occurs.
- Otherwise criteria for sinus rhythm/arrhythmia met.

Clinical features:

- Auscultation reveals pause(s) in the heart rhythm of variable duration.

Sinoatrial block

SA block is a disorder of impulse conduction. Unlike sinus arrest, the SA node continues to fire, but the impulse is not conducted to the atrial myocardium. It is therefore also referred to as *SA exit block*. On the ECG, SA block can be differentiated from sinus arrest based on pause duration. SA block results in a pause that is an exact multiple of the underlying PP interval (2 or more). Sinus arrest results in a pause that is not an exact multiple of the underlying PP interval. However, when SA block is associated with the Wenckebach phenomenon, progressive shortening of the PP intervals may occur prior to the pause. Furthermore, the high frequency of sinus arrhythmia in dogs means that the underlying PP interval duration is rarely regular, so it is usually not possible to accurately differentiate sinus arrest and SA block. Fortunately such differentiation is rarely of clinical relevance.

ECG characteristics:

- Pause in sinus rhythm of multiples of PP intervals (2 or more).
- Progressive shortening of the PP interval may occur prior to pause (Wenckebach phenomenon: usually associated with high vagal tone).
- May have junctional or ventricular escape complexes if pause of sufficient duration occurs.
- Otherwise criteria for sinus rhythm/arrhythmia met.

Clinical features:

- Auscultation reveals pause(s) in the heart rhythm of variable duration.

Sick sinus syndrome

Sick sinus syndrome (SSS, sinus node dysfunction) is a term given to a combination of arrhythmias, of which foremost is decreased SA nodal firing. Inappropriate sinus bradycardia and sinus arrest of long duration (>2–3 seconds in the conscious dog) are typical findings. Commonly associated with this condition is disease of the cardiac conduction system, resulting in failure or delay in firing of latent pacemakers within the

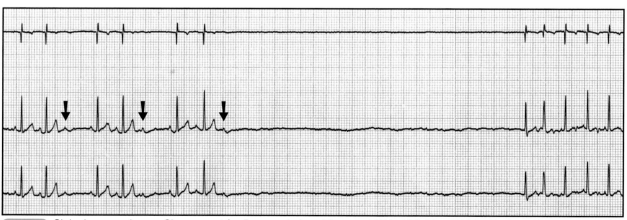

16.4 Sick sinus syndrome. Sinus arrest for 5 seconds in a 12-year-old West Highland White Terrier with syncope and exercise intolerance (leads I–III shown). Note the second-degree AV block with 3:2 conduction prior to the sinus pause (arrows indicate non-conducted P waves). Paper speed 25 mm/s; gain 1 cm/mV.

AV node and His–Purkinje system, and occasionally low-grade AV block (see Figure 16.4). SSS is therefore a disorder of both impulse generation and conduction. Supraventricular tachycardia (SVT) may also occur with SSS. This has been referred to as 'tachycardia–bradycardia syndrome'.

Causes: The cause of SSS is generally unknown. Most cases are idiopathic, with degenerative fibrosis of the SA node, AV node, perinodal tissue and bundle branches as typical histological findings (Miller and Tilley, 1984). Breed predisposition has been reported for West Highland White Terriers, Miniature Schnauzers and Cocker Spaniels (Oyama *et al.*, 2001). Most affected dogs are >6 years of age. Bitches may be over-represented. SSS has not been described in cats.

ECG characteristics: Variable combination of:

- Inappropriate sinus bradycardia (<70 beats/minute)
- Sinus arrest (often with prolonged pauses preceding escape rhythms)
- First- or second-degree AV block (see below)
- SVT.

Clinical features:

- Affected animals may show clinical signs or be asymptomatic.
- Signs of haemodynamic compromise (exercise intolerance, weakness, syncope), resulting from hypoperfusion of the brain and muscles, may occur with sinus arrest or SVT.
- Auscultation may reveal any combination of slow or fast, regular or irregular rhythms, but a slow rhythm with frequent pauses is most common.
- Sudden death is very unusual.

Atrioventricular block

AV block is a disorder of impulse conduction; typically a delay or failure of conduction of a sinus or atrial impulse through the AV node or His bundle (AV junction). The AV node itself is susceptible to 'block' since it conducts very slowly and has a long refractory period. High vagal tone predisposes to AV block as it causes further slowing of AV nodal conduction and prolongation of the refractory period. High adrenergic tone has the opposite effects. Different types of AV block can occur, termed first-degree, second-degree and third-degree.

AV block can be caused by:

- Elevated vagal tone (physiological or abnormal)
- Intrinsic AV node or His–Purkinje disease:
  - Idiopathic degenerative fibrosis
  - Congenital AV block
  - Structural heart disease (myocardial disease)
  - Inflammatory disease (infective endocarditis, Lyme carditis as a result of borreliosis)
  - Infiltration (neoplasia).
- Drugs (usually high or toxic doses):
  - Alpha-2 agonists
  - Beta-blockers
  - Digitalis glycosides
  - Non-dihydropyridine calcium-channel blockers (diltiazem, verapamil)
  - Low-dose atropine (short-term effect).
- Hyperkalaemia
- Autonomic nervous system disorders.

First-degree atrioventricular block

First-degree AV block is characterized by a delay of conduction through the AV junction, resulting in a prolonged PR interval (Figure 16.5). Mild prolongations are commonly seen with elevated vagal tone. Severe prolongations usually occur with structural disease.

ECG characteristics:

- Prolonged PR interval.
- Otherwise criteria for sinus rhythm/arrhythmia met.

Clinical features:

- Clinical abnormalities due to the arrhythmia are rare.

Second-degree atrioventricular block

Second-degree AV block is characterized by intermittent failure of AV conduction, resulting in non-conducted P waves (see Figures 16.4 and 16.5). Single or multiple non-conducted P waves may be present. AV block can be classified according to the width of the conducted QRS complexes.

- *Type A block* has QRS complexes of normal width and is considered to be caused by block above the bifurcation of the His bundle.
- *Type B block* has wide QRS complexes and is considered to be caused by block below the bifurcation of the His bundle.

Different patterns of block can also occur. *Mobitz type I block* is usually caused by elevated vagal tone. *Mobitz type II block* and type B block are generally associated with pathological causes.

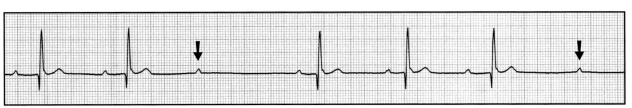

16.5 Second-degree AV block (Mobitz type I) in a 3-year-old Lurcher (lead II shown). Non-conducted P waves are indicated by arrows (second-degree AV block). Prolongation of the PR interval for the conducted sinus complexes is also present (first-degree AV block). Paper speed 50 mm/s; gain 1 cm/mV.

ECG characteristics – Mobitz type I block:

- Intermittent, single, non-conducted P waves.
- PR interval lengthens prior to block (often no pattern to lengthening, but incremental lengthening can occur with Wenckebach phenomenon).
- Conducted QRS complex morphology normal.

ECG characteristics – Mobitz type II block:

- Single or multiple, non-conducted P waves.
- PR interval constant prior to block.
- Often a fixed relationship of P waves to conducted QRS complexes (e.g. 2:1, 3:1, 4:1).
- Conducted QRS complex morphology normal or wide.
- May have junctional or ventricular escape complexes (see below) if pause of sufficient duration occurs.

Clinical features:

- Signs of haemodynamic compromise may be present (exercise intolerance, weakness, syncope) in patients with higher grades of AV block.
- Auscultation reveals pause(s) in the heart rhythm of variable duration.

Third-degree atrioventricular block

Third-degree AV block (complete AV block) is characterized by persistent failure of conduction through the AV junction (Figure 16.6). The ventricles are depolarized by a junctional or ventricular escape rhythm that is independent of the atrial rhythm (P waves). Failure of escape rhythm results in ventricular standstill. Third-degree AV block is almost invariably caused by myocardial damage.

ECG characteristics:

- No conducted P waves.
- Ventricular (QRS) rhythm (i.e. escape rhythm) usually regular and at rate slower than P waves.
- QRS complexes may be of normal morphology if a junctional rhythm is present (block is above the bifurcation of the His bundle), or wide and bizarre if a ventricular rhythm is present (block is below the bifurcation of the His bundle).
- No association between atrial (P) and ventricular (QRS) rhythms (AV dissociation).
- In cats, escape rhythms are usually stable and at a rate of 80–140 beats/minute.

Clinical features:

- Signs of haemodynamic compromise are generally present in dogs (exercise intolerance, weakness, syncope, collapse) with more severe signs in patients with slower escape rhythms.
- CHF may be present, particularly right-sided failure.
- A proportion of cats have third-degree AV block without signs of haemodynamic compromise or CHF; the arrhythmia is detected during routine examination (Kellum and Stepien, 2002).
- There is risk of sudden death due to failure of the escape rhythm. Risk may be greater with very slow escape rhythms (<40 beats/minute), ventricular escape rhythms and unstable escape rhythms.
- Slow heart rate and hyperdynamic pulses are present on examination. Faint atrial (S4) sounds may be audible at the heart base on auscultation.
- Systolic arterial pressure may be elevated in dogs with third-degree AV block, reflecting the increased stroke volume with a longer diastolic filling period rather than systemic hypertension.
- Dilatation of all four heart chambers is a common echocardiographic finding.

Physiological atrioventricular block

Physiological AV block is the mechanism by which the ventricles are protected against rapid stimulation from atrial tachyarrhythmias (e.g. atrial fibrillation). Rapid, repetitive impulses are conducted poorly through the AV node as a result of its long refractory period, which is lengthened further during faster atrial rates. In addition, some atrial impulses are only conducted partially through the AV node, resulting in a further decrease in excitability of nodal tissue. This phenomenon is referred to as *concealed conduction*. Physiological AV block is not in itself a disease, but is rather the normal response of the AV node to rapid stimulation rates.

High-grade atrioventricular block

High-grade AV block has been defined as either third-degree AV block, or second-degree AV block with an AV conduction ratio of 3:1 or higher, in the absence of rapid atrial tachycardia (atrial rate >200 beats/minute) that causes physiological AV block. Dogs with high-grade second-degree AV block have a similar frequency of clinical signs and duration of survival to dogs with third-degree AV block (Schrope and Kelch, 2006).

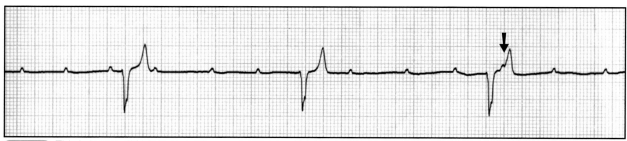

16.6 Third-degree AV block in a 10-year-old Golden Retriever with concurrent signs of right-sided CHF (lead I shown). A ventricular escape rhythm of rate 60 beats/minute is present. A non-conducted P wave is seen to be superimposed on the ST segment of the last escape complex (arrowed). Paper speed 50 mm/s; gain 1 cm/mV.

Atrioventricular dissociation

AV dissociation refers to any situation in which the atria and ventricles are depolarized by separate independent foci: a sinus or atrial focus controls the atria; and an AV junctional or ventricular focus controls the ventricles. Each focus is unable to depolarize the region of the heart controlled by its counterpart. It is important to understand that AV dissociation is *not* an arrhythmia and therefore *not* an electrocardiographic diagnosis. Rather it is a sign of an underlying arrhythmia where the atrial depolarizations are either at a faster or slower rate than the ventricular depolarizations. AV dissociation can result from one or more of the following situations:

- High-grade AV block with escape rhythm
- Rapid junctional rhythm (e.g. junctional tachycardia)
- Ventricular arrhythmia (e.g. accelerated idioventricular rhythm, ventricular tachycardia)
- Severe sinus bradycardia with escape rhythm.

Isorhythmic AV dissociation refers to AV dissociation in which the atrial and ventricular rates are the same or very similar. P waves may cycle back and forth across the QRS complex and are often visible within the Q wave (see Figures 16.11 and 16.18). Baroreceptor feedback control of SA nodal firing has been proposed as a potential mechanism for this phenomenon.

Atrial standstill

Atrial standstill occurs when the SA node fires but the impulse is not conducted to the atrial myocardium. It results in a complete absence of P waves on the surface ECG. In hyperkalaemic atrial standstill, the SA node impulse continues to be conducted to the AV node via the internodal pathways. This results in a slow sinoventricular rhythm. In persistent atrial standstill, a junctional or ventricular escape rhythm results.

Causes

Atrial standstill can be the result of primary myocardial disease (persistent), or secondary to severe hyperkalaemia or digitalis toxicity (temporary). Persistent atrial standstill may be the result of an atrial myopathy (e.g. fascioscapulohumeral muscular dystrophy in English Springer Spaniel) or atrial myocarditis. Terminal atrial standstill may occur with cardiac arrest.

ECG characteristics

- Complete absence of P waves.
- Slow, regular ventricular (QRS) rhythm (usually <70 beats/minute in dogs, <140 beats/minute in cats).
- In hyperkalaemic atrial standstill, QRS complexes may be of normal morphology (Figure 16.7a) or wide and bizarre (Figure 16.7b) with a sinoventricular rhythm.
- In normokalaemic atrial standstill, QRS complexes are of normal morphology with a junctional escape rhythm, or wide and bizarre with a ventricular escape rhythm.

Clinical features

- Affected animals invariably demonstrate clinical signs, as a result of the arrhythmia and/or underlying disease process.
- Clinical signs result from haemodynamic compromise and typically include collapse, exercise intolerance, weakness and syncope.
- Hyperkalaemic atrial standstill is an urgent arrhythmia that requires immediate treatment (see Chapter 20).

Escape rhythms

Escape rhythms occur when the SA node fails to generate an impulse (sinus arrest, sinus bradycardia) or the impulse fails to be conducted (SA block, AV block, persistent atrial standstill). In this circumstance the site with the next most rapid spontaneous

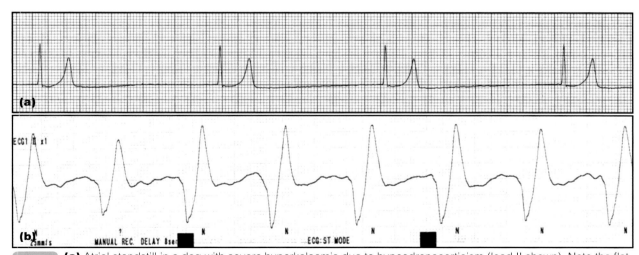

16.7 **(a)** Atrial standstill in a dog with severe hyperkalaemia due to hypoadrenocorticism (lead II shown). Note the flat baseline indicating lack of atrial activity. A sinoventricular rhythm is present at a rate of about 50 beats/minute. Paper speed 50 mm/s; gain 1 cm/mV. **(b)** Atrial standstill in a cat with severe hyperkalaemia due to urinary obstruction (lead II shown). A wide complex, sinoventricular rhythm is present at a rate of 60 beats/minute. This is a very unstable rhythm that requires urgent treatment. Paper speed 25 mm/s; gain 1 cm/mV.

diastolic depolarization takes over as the cardiac pacemaker (i.e. it 'escapes' suppression by the SA node). These are referred to as *latent pacemakers*. Latent pacemakers within the distal AV junction give rise to junctional escape rhythms. Those in the His–Purkinje system result in ventricular escape rhythms. Working atrial and ventricular myocardium does not undergo spontaneous diastolic depolarization in normal conditions. Escape rhythms are not the cause of an arrhythmia; they are an example of normal firing within the myocardium as a consequence of a brady-arrhythmia. Single or multiple consecutive escape complexes may occur. Failure of escape rhythms can result in asystole.

Associated arrhythmias include:

- Sinus arrest/SA block
- Sinus bradycardia
- SSS
- Persistent atrial standstill
- High-grade AV block.

Junctional escape rhythm (idiojunctional rhythm)

ECG characteristics:

- Slow, regular escape rate. Intrinsic rate of AV junction is approximately 50–70 beats/minute in dogs and 100–140 beats/minute in cats.
- Ectopic QRS complex morphology normal.
- Ectopic P waves (P' waves) are usually not seen, either because retrograde conduction of AV impulse to the atria does not occur, or because the P' wave is superimposed on the ectopic QRS–T complex (pacemaker originates from distal AV junction). When visible, P' waves are negative in lead II and have a short P'R interval if preceding an ectopic QRS complex (pacemaker originates from proximal AV junction).
- AV dissociation may be present (e.g. third-degree AV block).

Accelerated idiojunctional rhythm: Accelerated idiojunctional rhythm (or enhanced AV junctional rhythm) is a term used for a faster junctional escape rhythm. It results from increased firing of pacemaker tissue within the AV junction in combination with a low sinus rate. It is typically present in patients with abnormalities of autonomic tone (e.g. systemic

disease or following abdominal surgery). ECG characteristics are as above, but typically at a rate of 70–100 beats/minute in dogs.

Ventricular escape rhythm (idioventricular rhythm)

Ventricular escape rhythms tend to occur when an underlying disease process is also affecting both the SA node and the AV junction.

ECG characteristics:

- Slow, regular escape rate. Intrinsic rate of His–Purkinje system is approximately <50 beats/minute in dogs and <100 beats/minute in cats.
- Ectopic QRS complex morphology abnormal (wide and bizarre).
- Ectopic P waves (P' waves) are either not present as retrograde conduction of AV impulse to the atria does not occur, or not visible when retrograde AV conduction does occur as the P' wave is superimposed on the ectopic QRS–T complex.
- AV dissociation may be present (e.g. third-degree AV block).

Sinus tachycardia

Sinus tachycardia results from increased SA nodal firing. It is most commonly an *appropriate* response to increased sympathetic tone secondary to physiological stresses or systemic disease. However, an *inappropriate* sinus tachycardia may occur with some drugs or toxins. Heart rates approaching 300 beats/minute can be seen in athletic dogs with sinus tachycardia during peak performance (Figure 16.8).

Causes

- Physiological:
  - Exercise
  - Fear/anxiety
  - Pain.
- Systemic:
  - Hypotension
  - Shock
  - High output cardiac states (e.g. pyrexia, anaemia, thyrotoxicosis)
  - Hypokalaemia
  - Heart failure.

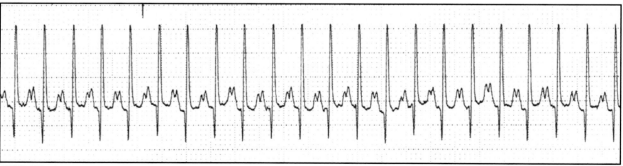

16.8 Sinus tachycardia of 250 beats/minute in a racing Greyhound immediately after finishing a race (lead II shown). The P wave of each sinus complex occurs on the terminal portion of the preceding T wave. Paper speed 25 mm/s; gain 1 cm/mV. (Courtesy of A. Boswood.)

- Drugs:
  - Vasodilators
  - Sympathomimetic agents
  - Parasympatholytic agents (in combination with another cause for elevated heart rate).
- Toxins:
  - Methylxanthines (e.g. caffeine)
  - Theobromine (e.g. chocolate).

ECG characteristics

- Fast atrial and ventricular rate (>160 beats/minute in dogs, >240 beats/minute in cats).
- Otherwise criteria for sinus rhythm met.
- Gradual onset and termination: progressively shorter PP and RR intervals occur at onset ('warm-up'), with progressively longer PP and RR intervals at termination ('cool-down').

Clinical features

Affected animals do not have signs of haemodynamic compromise as a result of the tachycardia, but may have signs of underlying disease/toxicity (if present).

Supraventricular arrhythmias

These are arrhythmias that originate from an ectopic focus or foci involving atrial or junctional tissue (see Figures 16.9 to 16.13).

Atrial tachyarrhythmias

Atrial tachyarrhythmias result from either abnormal firing or re-entry, and are localized to the atrial myocardium only. They may occur in structurally normal hearts, but are more common with atrial dilatation. Single premature ectopy (atrial premature complexes) or multiple consecutive ectopy (atrial tachycardia, flutter and fibrillation) can occur.

Atrial tachyarrhythmias are caused by:

- Atrial dilatation (secondary to cardiac disease) (most common)
- Structural disease of the atria (myocardial disease, infiltration, neoplasia, inflammation, fibrosis)
- Trauma to the atria (e.g. trauma during pericardiocentesis, cardiac catheterization)
- Autonomic imbalance
- Electrolyte imbalances (hypokalaemia)
- Drugs (digitalis glycosides, quinidine, sympathomimetic agents, phosphodiesterase inhibitors, anaesthetic agents).

Atrial premature complexes

Atrial premature complexes (APCs) are single premature atrial ectopy (Figure 16.9). They usually occur as isolated complexes during sinus rhythm and may arise from single or multiple ectopic foci. They can be difficult to differentiate from non-respiratory sinus arrhythmia. They appear to increase in frequency with age.

ECG characteristics:

- Heart rate usually normal but may be increased if there are frequent premature complexes.
- Rhythm irregular due to premature ectopic complexes.
- Ectopic P wave (P' wave) morphology is usually different from the sinus P wave. May be positive, isoelectric, biphasic or negative. May be superimposed on the preceding T wave.
- Ectopic P'R interval usually ≥ sinus PR interval.
- Ectopic QRS complex morphology usually the same as or very similar to sinus QRS complexes.
- APCs usually occur between two sinus-initiated complexes that are separated by a time period of <2 normal RR intervals. The period following the premature complex is referred to as a 'non-compensatory pause' because APCs depolarize the SA node and reset the rhythm. This may not be apparent in patients with sinus arrhythmia.
- Very premature APCs may result in non-conducted P' waves (physiological AV block) because of insufficient time for AV nodal recovery. Partial recovery of the AV node or bundle branches may result in a long P'R interval or a wide and bizarre QRS complex (aberrant conduction, see later), respectively.

Clinical features

- Affected animals typically have extrasystolic beats on auscultation. Pulse deficits may also be present.
- Signs of haemodynamic compromise as a result of the arrhythmia itself are unusual. Frequent APCs may herald the presence of a more severe atrial arrhythmia (e.g. paroxysmal atrial tachycardia), resulting in clinical signs.

Atrial tachycardia

Atrial tachycardia is defined as multiple consecutive APCs, and results from rapidly firing ectopic foci within the atria. Atrial tachycardia can be classified as focal or multifocal.

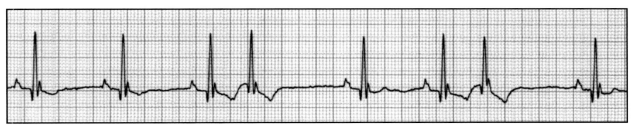

16.9 APCs in a 9-year-old Doberman pinscher with dilated cardiomyopathy (lead II shown). The 4th and 7th complexes are APCs and have similar QRS morphology to sinus complexes. Ectopic P waves (P' waves) are negative and superimposed on the T wave of preceding sinus complexes. Paper speed 50 mm/s; gain 1 cm/mV.

- *Focal atrial tachycardia* occurs when the arrhythmia originates from a single ectopic site. This is the most common form of atrial tachycardia.
- *Multifocal* atrial tachycardia is diagnosed when the tachycardia is caused by ≥3 coexisting ectopic foci. This is less common, but can be present with pulmonary disease or CHF.

Atrial tachycardias are an example of a narrow complex tachycardia. They are usually paroxysmal (spontaneously terminating), may be non-sustained (duration <30 seconds) or sustained (duration >30 seconds), and can be a precursor to atrial fibrillation.

With sustained narrow complex tachycardias, it is difficult to differentiate focal atrial tachycardia from SVT involving the AV node based on ECG findings alone (see Figure 16.13). When AV node conduction is slowed (by a vagal manoeuvre or drugs) then it may become easier to differentiate atrial tachycardia from AV node-dependent SVT, as unconducted P waves may be identified (focal atrial tachycardia) or the rhythm may terminate (SVT involving the AV node).

ECG characteristics:

- Fast atrial (P') and ventricular (QRS) rates (approximately >160 beats/minute in dogs, >240 beats/minute in cats). Maximum ventricular rates often exceed 250–300 beats/minute. Atrial rates may be even more rapid if physiological AV block present.
- Ectopic atrial (P') rhythm usually regular in focal atrial tachycardia and irregular in multifocal atrial tachycardia.
- Ventricular (QRS) rhythm can be regular in focal atrial tachycardia due to the presence of 1:1 AV conduction or fixed physiological AV block (i.e. fixed AV conduction pattern of 2:1, 3:1, 4:1.).
- Ventricular (QRS) rhythm can be irregular if variable physiological AV block is present, or with multifocal atrial tachycardia.
- P' wave morphology all the same in focal atrial tachycardia and usually superimposed on the preceding ST segment or T wave.
- P' wave during focal atrial tachycardia is typically positive in leads II, III and aVF, and negative in lead aVR (Santilli *et al.* 2008a). However, identification of P' waves requires comparison of the ST segment and T waves during the tachycardia and during normal sinus rhythm.
- P' wave morphology highly variable in multifocal atrial tachycardia, with at least three different morphologies identified.
- Constant P'R interval with focal atrial tachycardia, but variable interval with multifocal atrial tachycardia.
- Ectopic QRS complex morphology usually same as or very similar to sinus QRS complexes.
- Gradual onset ('warm-up') and termination ('cool-down') with atrial tachycardia caused by abnormal atrial firing. P'R interval may lengthen during 'cool-down' period. Sudden onset and termination with focal atrial tachycardia caused by re-entry.

Clinical features:

- Signs of haemodynamic compromise (exercise intolerance, weakness, syncope, collapse) may be present, particularly with very rapid rates.
- Sustained tachycardias may cause systolic dysfunction (tachycardia-mediated cardiomyopathy) and result in a dilated cardiomyopathy phenotype.
- Rapid heart rate on auscultation. Apical impulse may be weak.
- Weak arterial pulses may be present.

Atrial flutter

Atrial flutter is a form of atrial tachycardia that results from a large (macro-) re-entrant circuit located entirely within the atria. Atrial flutter is therefore also referred to as macro-re-entrant atrial tachycardia.

- Typical atrial flutter results in flutter waves with a 'saw-tooth' pattern on the surface ECG.
- Atypical forms of atrial flutter also exist, in which flutter waves have a more variable morphology on the surface ECG, sometimes appearing as discrete atrial waves.

Atrial flutter may occur during quinidine therapy for atrial fibrillation. Atrial flutter is rare and often transient in small animals. It may be seen following surgery that requires atrial incision.

ECG characteristics:

- 'Saw-tooth' flutter waves ('F' waves) with no discernible isoelectric baseline are present in typical atrial flutter. F waves are often most evident in leads II and rV$_2$. Atrial waves can be variable in atypical atrial flutter.
- Very fast atrial (F) rate (usually 300–600 beats/minute).
- Ventricular (QRS) rhythm can be *regular* due to the presence of 1:1 AV conduction or fixed physiological AV block (2:1, 3:1, 4:1), and *irregular* if variable physiological AV block is present.
- Ventricular (QRS) rate is highly variable, depending upon the degree of physiological AV block. Usually rapid (>160 beats/minute in dogs, >240 beats/minute in cats), but may be normal or even slow.
- FR interval highly variable and often prolonged. The F wave that precedes the last fully formed F wave immediately before the QRS complex is generally the one that is conducted to the ventricles.
- Normal QRS complex morphology, although superimposed F waves may alter QRS morphology.
- Sudden onset and termination.

Clinical features: As for atrial tachycardia.

Atrial fibrillation

Atrial fibrillation is the most common persistent arrhythmia seen in small animals. It is more common in the dog than in the cat. It is characterized by chaotically irregular depolarizations throughout the atria (Figure 16.10).

Proposed mechanisms are either multiple atrial re-entrant circuits, or a single tachycardic focus that is conducted heterogenously across the atrial myocardium due to the variable conduction and refractory properties of the atria (fibrillatory conduction). Both mechanisms result in multiple wavelets depolarizing the atria randomly and therefore no coordinated atrial contraction. The number of stable wavelets present in the atria is proportional to the size of the atria.

Therefore, atrial fibrillation is more common in larger atria (e.g. large-breed dogs, atrial dilatation) than smaller atria (e.g. cats). It is also influenced by processes that affect conduction velocity and refractory period within the atria, such as autonomic tone and certain drugs. Atrial fibrillation can be paroxysmal, persistent or permanent, depending upon whether atrial fibrillation terminates spontaneously (*paroxysmal*), due to treatment (*persistent*), or not at all (*permanent*).

ECG characteristics:

- Absence of P waves. Presence of fine or coarse, irregular undulations of the baseline (often referred to as 'f' waves). Undulations not always easily discernible in small dogs or cats, and may be indistinguishable from baseline artefact.
- Irregular RR intervals (QRS rhythm).
- Normal QRS complex morphology unless intraventricular conduction defect is present.
- Ventricular (QRS) rate usually rapid (>160 beats/minute in dogs, >240 beats/minute in cats) in patients with atrial fibrillation secondary to structural cardiac disease. Rate may be normal if no underlying cardiac disease or following antiarrhythmic medications.
- Very fast atrial ('f') rate (usually >600 beats/minute).

Clinical features:

- Signs of haemodynamic compromise may be present, due to rapid heart rate and loss of atrial contribution to ventricular filling, which accounts for up to 20% of cardiac output.

- Animals with underlying cardiac disease often have concurrent signs of CHF.
- A chaotically irregular heart rhythm is present on auscultation with variable strength apical impulses.
- Frequent pulse deficits are usually present.
- Less common in cats than dogs, even with severe atrial dilatation.
- In patients with underlying cardiac disease or CHF, the ventricular response rate tends to be rapid due to elevated adrenergic tone and low vagal tone.
- Can be present in large-breed dogs (e.g. Irish Wolfhound) without identifiable structural cardiac disease. Initially the ventricular response rate is usually slower (<120 beats/minute) as vagal tone predominates. Some dogs progress to develop rapid atrial fibrillation and CHF.

Supraventricular tachycardia involving the atrioventricular node

These are arrhythmias that result from increased firing within the AV node, or a re-entrant circuit whose pathway includes the AV node. They may be present in structurally normal hearts, or associated with myocardial disease resulting in systolic dysfunction. Paroxysmal, sustained tachycardias appear more common than single ectopy or runs of short duration.

Junctional tachyarrhythmias

These arrhythmias arise from an ectopic focus within the AV junction. The AV junctional area ranges from the transitional cell zone of atrial-to-nodal tissue, through the compact AV node, to the bifurcation of the His bundle. Distal AV junctional tissue (lower AV node and His bundle) is the site of most rapid spontaneous depolarization outside of the SA node, making it prone to arrhythmias from increased firing.

Junctional tachyarrhythmias can be caused by:

- Metabolic diseases (hypoxaemia, hypokalaemia, hypomagnesaemia, acidosis)
- Structural disease affecting the AV junction (myocardial disease, infiltration, neoplasia, inflammation, ischaemia)
- Catecholamine excess
- Drugs (especially digitalis glycosides).

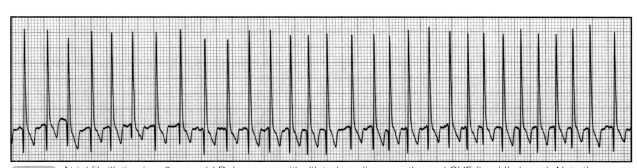

16.10 Atrial fibrillation in a 6-year-old Dobermann with dilated cardiomyopathy and CHF (lead II shown). Note the absence of detectable P waves and irregular RR intervals, which are the hallmarks of atrial fibrillation. Ventricular rate is rapid at 240 beats/minute. Paper speed 50 mm/s; gain 1 cm/mV.

Junctional premature complexes: Junctional premature complexes occur with increased firing within the AV junctional tissue. These usually occur as isolated complexes during sinus rhythm. As with APCs, they can be difficult to differentiate from non-respiratory sinus arrhythmia.

ECG characteristics:

- Heart rate may be increased if frequent premature complexes.
- Rhythm irregular due to premature ectopic complexes.
- Ectopic QRS complex morphology usually normal.
- Ectopic P waves (P' waves) are usually not present, as either retrograde conduction of AV impulse to the atria does not occur, or the P' wave is superimposed on the ectopic QRS–T complex (arrhythmia arises from distal AV junction). When visible, P' waves are negative in lead II and have a short P'R interval if preceding ectopic QRS complex (arrhythmia arises from proximal AV junction).

Clinical features: As for APCs.

Focal junctional tachycardia: Focal junctional tachycardias are caused by increased firing (Figure 16.11). They are the most common junctional tachycardia in small animals, particularly dogs. An association with myocardial failure and an over-representation of Labrador Retrievers has been reported (Santilli *et al.*, 2008b).

ECG characteristics:

- Normal or fast ventricular (QRS) rate. Focal junctional tachycardia is often <250 beats/minute in the dog, with a mean rate of 110–150 beats/minute (Santilli *et al.*, 2008b).

- Rhythm usually regular, but RR intervals can vary slightly.
- Ectopic QRS complex morphology usually normal.
- Ectopic P waves (P' waves) are usually not seen, as either retrograde conduction of AV impulse to the atria does not occur, or the P' wave is superimposed on the ectopic QRS–T complex. When visible, P' waves are negative in lead II and have a short P'R interval if preceding ectopic QRS complex.
- Often have isorhythmic AV dissociation, with normal P waves superimposed on ectopic Q waves (Figure 16.11).

Clinical features: As for atrial tachycardia.

Accessory pathway-mediated arrhythmias
Accessory pathways are anomalous bands of excitable tissue that connect the atrial and ventricular myocardium across the electrically inert fibrous AV skeleton in a site separate from the AV node. Accessory pathways can conduct anterograde (atria to ventricles only), retrograde (ventricles to atria only), or both. Most accessory pathways exhibit rapid conduction, similar to His–Purkinje or working myocardium. These arrhythmias are typically congenital.

Ventricular pre-excitation: Ventricular pre-excitation is the term given to the premature activation of the ventricular myocardium by anterograde conduction of a supraventricular impulse via an accessory pathway. Ventricular pre-excitation results in early activation of only a small portion of the ventricles. The remainder of the ventricular myocardium is depolarized by the normal AV nodal route. This combined activation pattern results in a shortened PR interval and wide QRS complex with a 'slurring' of the upstroke, referred to as a *delta wave* (Figure 16.12). Ventricular pre-excitation can only occur with accessory pathways capable of anterograde conduction.

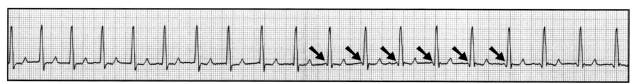

16.11 Focal junctional tachycardia in a 9-year-old Labrador Retriever with myocardial failure and CHF (lead II shown). Note that at the beginning of the trace no P or Q waves are visible, as they are superimposed. Both become visible towards the end of the trace (arrowed) as the ventricular rate slows from 220 to 180 beats/minute. This indicates separate atrial and ventricular rhythms and is termed isorhythmic AV dissociation. Paper speed 50 mm/s; gain 1 cm/mV.

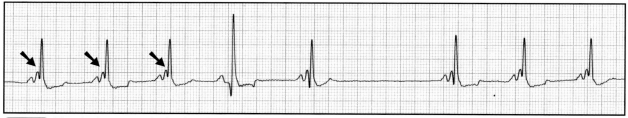

16.12 Ventricular pre-excitation in a 3-year-old Labrador Retriever with SVT (Wolff–Parkinson–White syndrome) (lead II shown). The SVT was treated successfully with diltiazem and this recording was taken during the following 24 hours. The fourth complex is a sinus complex with conduction through the AV node; all other complexes exhibit pre-excitation – short PR interval, delta wave (arrowed) in the upstroke of the R wave, and abnormal QRS complex morphology. This is consistent with an accessory pathway between the atria and ventricles. Paper speed 50 mm/s; gain 1 cm/mV.

These are referred to as *manifest* accessory pathways, due to their detection on the surface ECG during sinus rhythm. Accessory pathways capable of only retrograde conduction are referred to as *concealed*, since they do not affect the surface ECG during sinus rhythm.

ECG characteristics:

- Normal heart rate and rhythm.
- Normal P wave morphology.
- Shortened PR interval.
- Wide QRS complex with slurred upstroke (delta wave).
- Usually sustained, but can be paroxysmal or alternate with sinus rhythm.

AV reciprocating tachycardia: AV reciprocating tachycardia (AVRT) is a re-entrant arrhythmia, with a circuit that includes the atrium, AV node, ventricle and an accessory pathway. It is also referred to as an *accessory pathway-medicated tachycardia*. AVRTs are typically initiated by atrial or ventricular premature complexes. They are further subdivided into *orthodromic* (OAVRT) and *antidromic* (AAVRT) forms. Delta waves are not seen during these tachycardias.

ECG characteristics:

- Fast atrial (P') and ventricular (QRS) rates (approximately >160 beats/minute in dogs, >240 beats/minute in cats). Maximum ventricular rates often exceed 250–300 beats/minute in dogs.
- Very regular rhythm with 1:1 atrial-to-ventricular conduction.
- Sudden onset and termination; usually requires premature atrial or ventricular complex to initiate.

Clinical features: As for atrial tachycardia.

Orthodromic atrioventricular reciprocating tachycardia: During OAVRT, the re-entrant circuit conducts anterograde across the AV node to the ventricles and retrograde across the accessory pathway to the atria. QRS complexes are normal as ventricular conduction occurs entirely via the normal AV nodal route. The majority of dogs (and humans) with AVRT have no evidence of pre-excitation during sinus rhythm (concealed OAVRT). They have a concealed accessory pathway that conducts in a retrograde direction only during the tachycardia.

It should be noted that, with sustained narrow complex tachycardias, it is difficult to differentiate focal atrial tachycardia from SVT involving the AV node based on ECG findings alone (Figure 16.13). Also, when AV node conduction is slowed (by a vagal manoeuvre or drugs) it may become easier to differentiate atrial tachycardia from AV node-dependent SVT, as unconducted P waves may be identified (focal atrial tachycardia) or the rhythm may terminate (SVT involving the AV node).

ECG characteristics: Same as for AVRT, plus:

- Ectopic P waves (P' waves) occur after the QRS complex, but may not be readily visible due to superimposition of the ST segment or T wave
- P' wave during OAVRT is typically negative in leads II, III and aVF, and positive in lead aVR (Santilli *et al.*, 2008a). However, identification of P' waves requires comparison of the ST segment and T wave during the tachycardia and during normal sinus rhythm
- QRS amplitude alternans (difference in R wave height of >1 m/s in at least 1 lead) more likely to be present with OAVRT than with focal atrial tachycardia (Santilli *et al.*, 2008a)
- RP' interval is fixed and usually less than the P'R interval (unless accessory pathways exhibit slow conduction)
- Ectopic QRS complex morphology is generally normal.

Antidromic atrioventricular reciprocating tachycardia: During AAVRT the reverse of OAVRT occurs, with retrograde AV nodal conduction and anterograde accessory pathway conduction. QRS complexes are wide and bizarre as ventricular activation occurs entirely via the accessory pathway. This is very rare in the dog.

ECG characteristics: Same as for AVRT, plus:

- Ectopic P' waves are negative in lead II. They usually precede the QRS complex and may be hidden in the preceding T wave
- RP' interval is fixed and usually more than the P'R interval (unless accessory pathways exhibit slow conduction)
- Ectopic QRS complex is abnormal (wide and bizarre). Morphology will depend upon location of the accessory pathway.

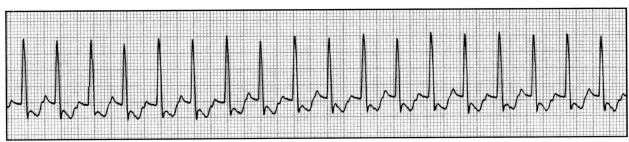

16.13 Narrow complex tachycardia in a 2-year-old Labrador Retriever (lead II shown). Ventricular rate is very rapid at 300 beats/minute. Orthodromic AV reciprocating tachycardia was later confirmed, but focal atrial tachycardia can have a similar ECG appearance. Paper speed 50 mm/s; gain 1 cm/mV.

Wolff–Parkinson–White syndrome: Wolff–Parkinson–White (WPW) syndrome refers to patients with both ventricular pre-excitation and paroxysmal supraventricular arrhythmias. OAVRT is the most common tachycardia in WPW, but other forms of SVT may occur. Patients with WPW are prone to atrial fibrillation and flutter, presumably triggered by the fast tachycardia. These arrhythmias may be particularly dangerous with WPW syndrome, as anterograde accessory pathway conduction can result in very rapid ventricular rates and even ventricular fibrillation. Both WPW syndrome and concealed OAVRT have been reported in Labrador Retrievers, possibly in association with tricuspid dysplasia.

ECG characteristics: As for ventricular pre-excitation, plus SVT (AVRT, atrial or junctional tachycardia).

Ventricular arrhythmias

Ventricular arrhythmias originate from an ectopic focus or foci located entirely within the ventricular myocardium, distal to the bifurcation of the His bundle. They have an abnormal pattern of ventricular activation and do not usually depolarize the atria. Re-entrant arrhythmias are more common with structural heart disease; those caused by abnormal firing are more common with systemic disease. Single premature ectopy (ventricular premature complexes) or multiple consecutive ectopy (ventricular tachycardia, flutter and fibrillation) can occur.

Ventricular arrhythmias can be caused by:

- Structural heart disease:
    - Acquired heart disease (particularly myocardial disease)
    - Congenital heart disease (particularly aortic and pulmonic stenosis)

- Heart failure
- Trauma/inflammation (traumatic or infective myocarditis, infective endocarditis, pericarditis)
- Neoplasia
- Myocardial ischaemia/infarction
- Myocardial fibrosis.
- Systemic disease:
    - Hypoxia (anaemia, hypoxaemia due to respiratory disease)
    - Electrolyte/acid–base imbalances (hypokalaemia, acidosis, hypomagnesaemia)
    - Autonomic imbalance (particularly catecholamine excess)
    - CNS disease (secondary to head trauma or cervical spinal surgery)
    - Systemic inflammation (sepsis, immune-mediated disease, parvovirus)
    - Abdominal organ disease (gastric dilatation–volvulus, splenic disease, pancreatitis).
- Drugs (particularly digitalis glycosides, sympathomimetic agents, anaesthetic agents, anthracycline toxicity)
- Specific causes in canine breeds:
    - Boxer arrhythmogenic right ventricular cardiomyopathy
    - Dilated cardiomyopathy in Dobermanns
    - Inherited ventricular arrhythmias in young (<18 months old) German Shepherd Dogs.

Ventricular premature complexes

Ventricular premature complexes (VPCs) are single premature ventricular ectopy (Figure 16.14). They usually occur as isolated complexes during sinus rhythm, but may occur as two consecutive VPCs, referred to as *couplets*, or as three consecutive VPCs, referred to as *triplets* (Figure 16.15a). A ventricular *run* or *salvo* is a term used to describe

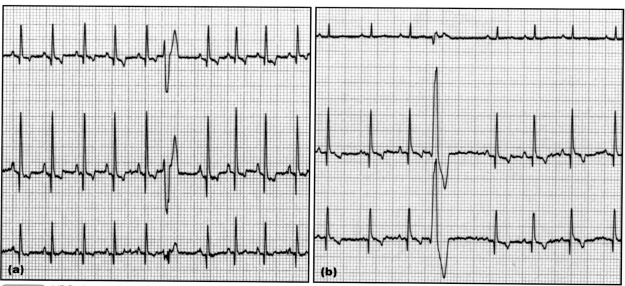

16.14 VPCs in two dogs (leads I–III shown). In **(a)** the sixth complex is a VPC; in **(b)** the fourth complex is a VPC. The morphology of each VPC differs, indicating different sites of origin within the ventricles. However, both are of wide and bizarre conformation compared with their respective sinus complexes. Note the presence of compensatory pauses for both VPCs (VPC is flanked by sinus complexes separated by a period of two RR intervals). Paper speed 25 mm/s; gain 1 cm/mV.

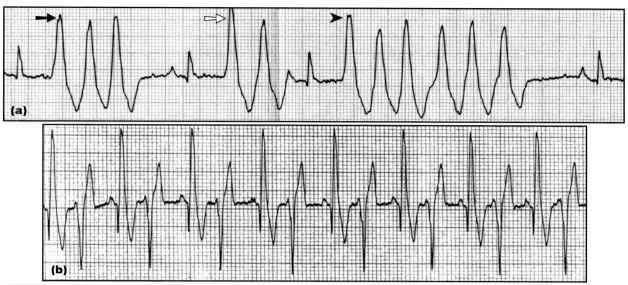

16.15 Complex ventricular ectopy. **(a)** Ventricular arrhythmia in a 4-year-old Dogue de Bordeaux (lead III shown). A triplet (filled arrow), couplet (open arrow) and ventricular run/salvo of six complexes (arrowhead) are seen. Ventricular complexes exhibit R-on-T phenomenon. An idiopathic ventricular arrhythmia was diagnosed as no underlying cardiac or systemic disease was detected. Paper speed 50 mm/s; gain 1 cm/mV. **(b)** Ventricular bigeminy in a Boxer with cardiomyopathy (lead II shown). Sinus complexes alternate with ventricular complexes (bigeminy). Paper speed 25 mm/s; gain 1 cm/mV. (Courtesy of V. Luis Fuentes.)

four to six consecutive VPCs (Figure 16.15a). Pairs of alternating sinus and premature complexes are referred to as *bigeminy* (Figure 16.15b). A single premature complex alternating with two sinus complexes is referred to as *trigeminy*.

VPCs are the most common pathological arrhythmia in small animals. They can occur in animals without identifiable underlying disease and their frequency tends to increase with age.

ECG characteristics

- Heart rate usually normal, but may be increased if frequent premature complexes.
- Ventricular (QRS) rhythm irregular due to premature ectopic complexes.
- P waves are normal in morphology and unrelated to the ectopic QRS complexes.
- Ectopic QRS complexes are premature relative to the sinus rhythm and of abnormal morphology (wide and bizarre). The morphology of an ectopic complex will depend upon the site of origin of the arrhythmia – left ventricular (Figure 16.14a), right ventricular (Figure 16.14b) or septal. Wide QRS complexes are most commonly seen, as the ectopic impulse is conducted slowly through the working myocardium rather than rapidly via the specialized His–Purkinje system. Narrow QRS complexes can occur, the putative explanation being an ectopic focus located in the proximal His–Purkinje system within the septum at a point equidistant between both ventricles.
- Ectopic T waves typically of large amplitude and opposite direction to the ectopic QRS complexes.
- VPCs may have the same morphology or multiple different morphologies. The former are referred to as *monomorphic* or *uniform* VPCs and originate from the same focus. The latter are referred to as

pleomorphic or *multiform* VPCs and originate either from different foci or from the same focus with variable conduction.
- VPCs usually do not disturb the atrial rhythm. These premature complexes are found between two sinus-initiated complexes that are separated by either a single RR interval or exactly two RR intervals. VPCs that occur between a single RR interval are referred to as *interpolated*; those that occur between two RR intervals are said to be followed by a *compensatory pause*. However, due to occasional retrograde AV conduction and the presence of sinus arrhythmia in many patients, this generalization can be unreliable.

Clinical features

- Affected animals typically have extrasystolic beats or post-extrasystolic pauses on auscultation. Pulse deficits are usually present.
- Signs of haemodynamic compromise as a result of the arrhythmia itself are unusual. Frequent VPCs may herald the presence of a more severe ventricular arrhythmia (e.g. paroxysmal ventricular tachycardia) resulting in clinical signs.

Ventricular tachycardia

Ventricular tachycardia is defined as three or more consecutive VPCs, and results from rapidly firing ectopic foci within the ventricles (Figure 16.16). The complexes can be monomorphic, pleomorphic or polymorphic depending on the number of foci and variability of conduction. Monomorphic ventricular tachycardia has a similar QRS morphology from beat to beat within the same episode of ventricular tachycardia. Pleomorphic ventricular tachycardia has >1 QRS morphology from within the same episode. Polymorphic ventricular tachycardia has a continually

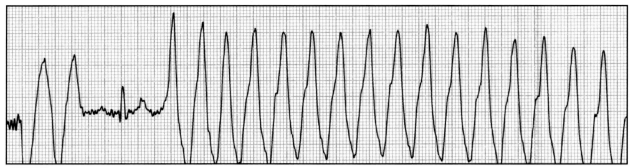

16.16 Rapid ventricular tachycardia (350 beats/minute) in the same dog as in Figure 16.15a (lead II shown). The trace starts with a couplet of different QRS morphology to the tachycardia, followed by a sinus complex, then the tachycardia. Ventricular complexes exhibit R-on-T phenomenon. This is a dangerous arrhythmia that requires immediate treatment. Paper speed 50 mm/s; gain 1 cm/mV.

changing QRS morphology from beat to beat. Ventricular tachycardia is arbitrarily termed *sustained* if lasting for >30 seconds, *non-sustained* if terminating within <30 seconds, and *paroxysmal* if terminating spontaneously. Ventricular tachycardia tends to indicate the presence of more severe cardiac or systemic disease than VPC alone.

ECG characteristics

- Fast ventricular (QRS) rate (>160 beats/minute in dogs, >240 beats/minute in cats).
- Ventricular (QRS) rhythms generally regular, but can have variable RR intervals, particularly with pleomorphic or polymorphic ventricular tachycardia.
- Ectopic QRS complexes of abnormal morphology, typically wide and bizarre, but may be relatively narrow. Morphology may be the same (monomorphic) or vary (pleomorphic/polymorphic).
- P waves often hidden due to superimposition of the tachycardia. P waves that are visible are normal in morphology and unrelated to the ectopic QRS complexes.
- Ectopic T waves typically of large amplitude and opposite direction to the ectopic QRS complexes.
- Gradual or sudden onset and termination may occur. Sudden onset and termination is more likely to be associated with a re-entrant mechanism.
- Fusion and capture complexes may occur (see below).
- R-on-T phenomenon may be present (see below).

Clinical features

- Signs of haemodynamic compromise (e.g. exercise intolerance, weakness, syncope, collapse) may be present, particularly with faster rates and polymorphic tachycardias.
- Animals with underlying heart disease may have concurrent CHF.
- Rapid heart rate on auscultation and weak apical impulse.
- Arterial pulses are typically weak and pulse deficits are common.

- Usually require treatment due to haemodynamic or electrical instability (see Chapter 20).

Fusion and capture complexes

Fusion complexes result from simultaneous activation of the ventricles by both a ventricular and atrial impulse. *Capture complexes* result from normal activation of the ventricles for one complex by a sinus impulse. Both require the sinus impulse to arrive at the AV junction when it has recovered excitability. Fusion complexes require a portion of the ventricular myocardium to have recovered. Capture complexes require the entire ventricular myocardium to have recovered. Fusion complexes are characterized by a QRS complex of intermediate morphology between a normal sinus complex and a ventricular complex, which is preceded by a normal P wave (Figure 16.17). Capture complexes have a P–QRS–T complex resembling the normal sinus complex.

R-on-T phenomenon

This refers to the superimposition of an ectopic R wave on the T wave of a preceding complex (see Figures 16.15a and 16.16). The presence of R-on-T phenomenon is considered to be an increased risk factor for the development of a malignant arrhythmia, such as ventricular fibrillation. This is because the terminal portion of the T wave represents the time of greatest heterogeneity of ventricular repolarization. A depolarization occurring during this time is therefore more likely to result in the development of multiple re-entrant circuits.

Accelerated idioventricular rhythms

Accelerated idioventricular rhythms (AIVRs) are slow ventricular tachycardias that usually occur from a single ventricular focus with abnormally increased firing. Often the firing rates of the ectopic ventricular focus and SA node are similar, resulting in control of the cardiac rhythm alternating between these two competing pacemaker sites (Figure 16.18). AIVR tends to be present in patients with severe systemic illness and typically following major surgery. Autonomic imbalance, hypoxaemia, electrolyte abnormalities and systemic inflammation are common causes. AIVRs can also occur with structural heart disease. They are usually paroxysmal and can be non-sustained or sustained.

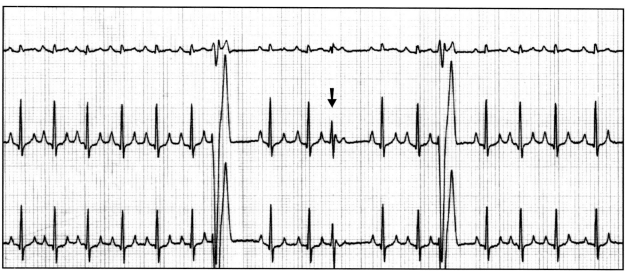

16.17 Fusion complex in a 6-year-old Golden Retriever with monomorphic VPCs (leads I–III shown). The fusion complex (arrowed) is flanked by sinus beats and occurs midway between two VPCs. This timing is suggestive of ventricular parasystole, in which an ectopic ventricular focus fires at a regular rate irrespective of the concurrent sinus rhythm. VPCs or fusion complexes will occur if the ventricular focus fires during diastole (between sinus T wave and QRS complex). If the ventricular focus fires during systole, no ectopic complexes are seen as the ventricle is depolarized by the sinus rhythm. Paper speed 25 mm/s; gain 1 cm/mV.

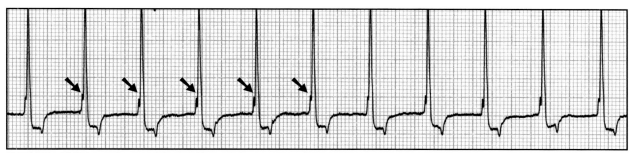

16.18 AIVR in an 8-year-old mixed-breed dog 3 days after abdominal surgery to remove a ruptured splenic haemangiosarcoma (lead II shown). An ectopic ventricular focus and the sinus node are firing at about the same rate of 100 beats/minute, but they are unrelated. Note that P waves (arrowed) are visible, superimposed on the upstroke of the ectopic R waves, and appearing to move in and out of the ectopic ventricular complexes. This is another example of isorhythmic AV dissociation (see Figure 16.11). Paper speed 25 mm/s; gain 1 cm/mV.

ECG characteristics

- Slow to normal ventricular (QRS) rate (50–160 beats/minute in dogs, 100–240 beats/minute in cats).
- Ventricular (QRS) rhythm usually regular.
- Ectopic QRS complexes of abnormal morphology, typically wide and bizarre, but may be relatively narrow.
- P waves usually superimposed on the QRS complexes and may be hidden. Visible P waves normal in morphology and unrelated to the ectopic QRS complexes.
- Ectopic T waves typically of large amplitude and opposite direction to the ectopic QRS complexes.
- Gradual onset and termination usual. Onset occurs when the ectopic rate exceeds the sinus rate. Termination occurs when the reverse occurs. Onset may be precipitated by a VPC.
- Ventricular fusion and capture complexes are common due to the slow ectopic rate. Fusion complexes often occur at the onset and termination of the arrhythmia.

Clinical features

- Clinical signs are usually limited to the underlying disease process.
- Signs of haemodynamic compromise are unusual as the rate is normal.
- Often associated with systemic disease, particularly following abdominal or thoracic surgery.

Torsades de pointes

Torsades de pointes is a rapid, polymorphic ventricular tachycardia that is characterized by: (i) continuously changing amplitude QRS complexes that appears to 'twist' around the isoelectric baseline; and (ii) sinus QT interval prolongation reflecting prolonged ventricular repolarization. The underlying mechanism is not fully understood; both abnormal firing and re-entry may be responsible. Drugs and conditions that prolong the QT interval are commonly implicated in humans, including class Ia and III antiarrhythmic agents, tricyclic antidepressants, some antihistamines, hypokalaemia and hypomagnesaemia. Congenital

Long-QT syndromes are well documented in humans, but have not been reported in small animals. A morphologically similar ventricular tachycardia that occurs in a patient without sinus QT prolongation is *not* torsades de pointes and should be referred to as a polymorphic ventricular tachycardia.

Ventricular flutter

Ventricular flutter is the name given to a ventricular tachycardia that is so rapid that each QRS complex merges with the preceding T wave, resulting in a 'sine wave' appearance. No isoelectric baseline is visible between complexes. The distinction between a very rapid ventricular tachycardia and ventricular flutter can be difficult, but is largely academic as cause, effect and treatment options are the same (see Chapter 20).

Cardiac arrest rhythms

Cardiac arrest rhythms are arrhythmias that are associated with absent cardiac output. Immediate recognition and treatment are essential to prevent irreversible hypoxic damage to the brain. With few exceptions, patients generally require cardiopulmonary–cerebral resuscitation (CPCR). They may occur in animals with severe systemic and/or cardiac disease. Arrest rhythms are:

- Ventricular standstill (asystole)
- Pulseless electrical activity
- Ventricular fibrillation.

Ventricular standstill

Ventricular standstill (asystole) refers to a complete absence of ventricular electrical activity. It may be preceded by ventricular fibrillation, severe sinus bradyarrhythmia, AV block or atrial standstill. Transient ventricular standstill commonly occurs with failure of an escape rhythm, but may become permanent (Figure 16.19).

ECG characteristics

- Complete absence of QRS complexes.
- Normal P waves may be seen with concurrent third-degree AV block.

Clinical features

- Transient ventricular standstill may occur in dogs and cats with third-degree AV block and unstable escape rhythms. This can be a cause of syncope in these patients.
- Patients with prolonged ventricular standstill require immediate CPCR.

Pulseless electrical activity

Pulseless electrical activity (PEA) refers to any coordinated cardiac electrical activity that does not result in discernible cardiac output. The ECG rhythms are usually pulseless bradyarrhythmias (typically atrial standstill with an escape rhythm), but sinus rhythm may also be present with PEA. PEA used to be referred to as electrical-mechanical dissociation. It most commonly occurs with severe acidosis, hypoxaemia or hyperkalaemia.

Ventricular fibrillation

Ventricular fibrillation is characterized by chaotically irregular ventricular depolarizations. It can be caused by multiple foci of re-entry or abnormal firing. There is an absence of coordinated ventricular activity (Figure 16.20). Ventricular fibrillation may develop unpredictably from less severe ventricular arrhythmias.

ECG characteristics

- Distinct P waves and QRS–T complexes absent.
- Baseline oscillations of varying contour and amplitude (fibrillatory waves).
- *Fine* ventricular fibrillation characterized by low amplitude (<0.2 mV) fibrillatory waves (Figure 16.20a). It can be difficult to differentiate from asystole and may be less amenable to electrical defibrillation than coarse ventricular fibrillation.

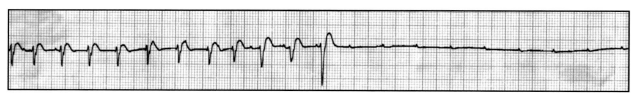

16.19 Ventricular standstill (asystole) in a cat (lead II shown). The first half of the trace shows AV dissociation with an irregular ventricular escape rhythm. Only P waves are present during the second half of the trace as no ventricular electrical activity occurs. Paper speed 25 mm/s; gain 1 cm/mV.

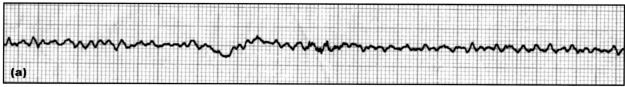

(a)

16.20 Ventricular fibrillation. **(a)** Fine ventricular fibrillation in a dog (lead II shown). Note the absence of coordinated electrical activity and replacement with baseline oscillations of variable contour and amplitude (fibrillatory waves). The amplitude of these oscillations is low, <0.2 mV (fine). Attempts to resuscitate were unsuccessful. Paper speed 25 mm/s; gain 1 cm/mV. (continues) ▶

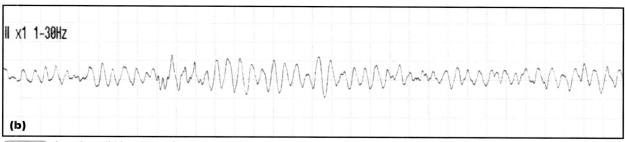

II x1 1-30Hz

(b)

16.20 (continued) Ventricular fibrillation. **(b)** Coarse ventricular fibrillation in a dog with dilated cardiomyopathy (lead II shown). In comparison with (a) the amplitude of these oscillations is high, >0.2 mV (coarse). Paper speed 25 mm/s; gain 1 cm/mV.

- *Coarse* ventricular fibrillation characterized by high amplitude (>0.2 mV) fibrillatory waves (Figure 16.20b).

Intraventricular conduction defects

QRS complexes of supraventricular origin are usually narrow and positive in leads II and aVF due to normal impulse conduction through the ventricles. Some QRS complexes of supraventricular origin can be wide and/or have bizarre morphology. This can occur with any of the following four scenarios:

- Severe right or left ventricular enlargement (see Chapter 9)
- Ventricular pre-excitation (see Accessory pathway-mediated arrhythmias)
- Bundle branch block (BBB)
- Aberrant conduction.

BBB and aberrant conduction are both examples of *intraventricular conduction delay* (IVCD), which refers to slowing of impulse conduction distal to the AV junction.

Bundle branch block

BBB refers to failure or delay of impulse conduction through one or more branches of the His bundle. The His bundle is divided into right and left branches, and the left bundle branch is divided into anterior and posterior fascicles. Block in a bundle branch or fascicle results in delay in depolarization of the region of ventricular myocardium supplied by it, resulting in a QRS complex of abnormal (wide and bizarre) morphology (Figure 16.21).

BBB can be caused by:

- Structural heart disease:
  - Cardiomyopathy (hypertrophic, dilated, restrictive, unclassified)
  - Diseases resulting in ventricular hypertrophy (e.g. aortic or pulmonic stenosis)
  - Other cardiac disease (e.g. ventricular septal defect, neoplasia, ischaemia, endocarditis, myocarditis).
- Hyperkalaemia
- Hypocalcaemia
- May be found in otherwise healthy animals.

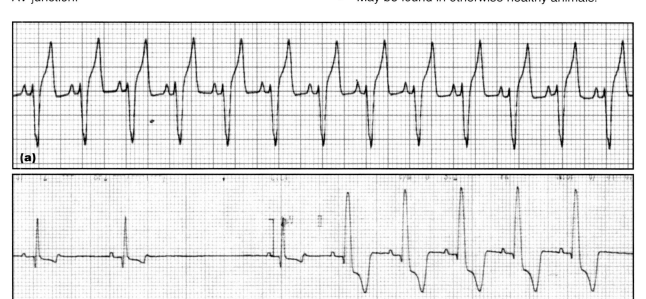

(a)

(b)

16.21 **(a)** RBBB in a dog. QRS complex duration is prolonged (0.08 seconds) with deep S waves and right axis deviation (lead II shown). Paper speed 25 mm/s; gain 1 cm/mV. **(b)** Intermittent LBBB in an 8-year-old Boxer with paraparesis (lead II shown). The first three sinus complexes are conducted normally, the next five with LBBB. The development of aberrant conduction in complexes with a short RR interval following a long RR interval is called Ashman's phenomenon (or long–short aberrancy). Paper speed 25 mm/s; gain 1 cm/mV.

Right bundle branch block

The right bundle branch connects the AV junction to the right ventricle (RV). It is a discrete structure that runs most of its course just beneath the endocardial surface. It is therefore susceptible to damage from disease affecting the RV, such as pulmonic stenosis and pulmonary hypertension causing right bundle branch block (RBBB). RBBB is also commonly seen during right-sided cardiac catheterization.

ECG characteristics:

- Prolonged QRS duration (>0.07 seconds in dogs, >0.06 seconds in cats).
- QRS complex positive in lead aVR and right precordial leads.
- S wave deep (negative) in leads I, II, III, aVF and left precordial leads.
- Right axis deviation (>100 degrees in dogs, >160 degrees in cats).

Left bundle branch block

The left bundle branch is larger than the right, with division into anterior and posterior fascicles. Left bundle branch block (LBBB) can occur at the proximal main branch or at both fascicles (bifascicular block). Because of the large size and extensive nature of the left bundle branch, lesions that result in block are also usually extensive, such as myocardial disease.

ECG characteristics:

- Prolonged QRS duration (>0.07 seconds in dogs, >0.06 seconds in cats).
- QRS complex positive in leads I, II, III, aVF and left precordial leads, and negative in lead aVR and right precordial leads.
- Q wave often absent in leads I and V_2 (leads that record septal electrical activity in right-to-left direction).

Left anterior fascicular block

Left anterior fascicular block (LAFB) is the most common IVCD in cats, particularly in association with hypertrophic cardiomyopathy. The left anterior appears to be more susceptible to fascicle damage as it is longer and thinner than the posterior fascicle. Unlike LBBB, QRS complexes are not particularly wide, but are bizarre.

ECG characteristics:

- Normal QRS complex duration, although usually >0.04 seconds.
- Marked left axis deviation (usually about −60 degrees).
- Q wave small and R wave tall in leads I and aVL.
- S wave deep (negative) in leads II, III and aVF.

Aberrant conduction

Aberrant conduction occurs when a premature impulse originating in the atria reaches a region of the His–Purkinje system that has not fully repolarized and therefore not recovered full excitability. This results in delayed conduction through the non-repolarized region and a BBB pattern. This is referred to as *functional BBB*. Typically RBBB occurs as the right bundle branch has a longer refractory period than the left. Long diastolic (RR) intervals preceding the premature impulse (i.e. slow heart rate) also increase refractory periods, promoting aberrant conduction.

ECG characteristics

- Aberrantly conducted QRS complex has a very short RR interval to the preceding QRS complex (acceleration-dependent aberrancy), or a short RR interval that follows a long RR interval (long–short aberrancy or Ashman's phenomenon) (see Figure 16.21b).
- Aberrant QRS complex wide and of variable morphology.
- T wave of aberrant QRS complex of different morphology or polarity to normally conducted complexes.

Electrical alternans

Electrical alternans refers to a situation in which the P wave, QRS complex or T wave alters in amplitude or morphology in a regular pattern. The most common type of electrical alternans is altering amplitude of every other QRS complex (2:1 QRS alternans). This can occur from either altering anatomical position of the heart within the pericardium, or altering conduction within the myocardium, particularly at fast heart rates. The most common scenarios are therefore large volume pericardial effusion (Figure 16.22a), alternating BBB or SVT (Figure 16.22b).

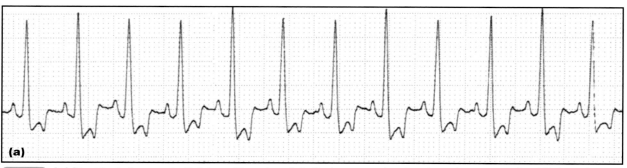

(a)

16.22 **(a)** Electrical alternans in Bulldog with pericardial effusion secondary to a heart base mass (lead II shown). There is one taller R wave alternating with two shorter R waves. This is 3:1 QRS alternans. Paper speed 25 mm/s; gain 1 cm/mV. (continues) ▶

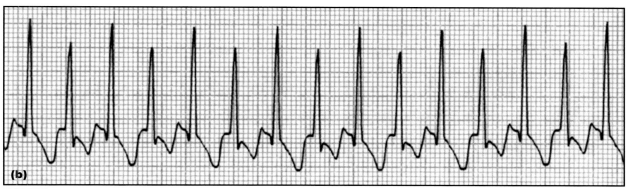

16.22 (continued) **(b)** Electrical alternans (2:1 QRS alternans) in the Labrador Retriever with narrow complex tachycardia shown in Figure 16.13 (lead II shown). Electrical alternans developed when the heart rate exceeded 350 beats/minute. Paper speed 50 mm/s; gain 1 cm/mV.

References and further reading

Fogoros RN (2006) *Electrophysiological Testing, 4th edn*, ed. RN Fogoros. Blakwell Publishing, Oxford

Fox PR, Sisson D and Moïse NS (1999) *Textbook of Canine and Feline Cardiology: Principles and Clinical Practice, 2nd edn*, ed. PR Fox, D Sisson and NS Moïse. WB Saunders, Philadelphia

Kellum HB and Stepien RL (2006) Third-degree atrioventricular block in 21 cats (1997–2004). *Journal of Veterinary Internal Medicine* **20**, 97–103

Miller MS and Tilley LP (1984) ECG of the month. *Journal of the American Veterinary Medical Association* **184**, 423–425

Oyama MA, Sisson DD and Lehmkuhl LB (2001) Practices and outcome of artificial cardiac pacing in 154 dogs. *Journal of Veterinary Internal Medicine* **15**, 229–239

Santilli RA, Perego M, Crosara S, Gardini F, Bellino C, Moretti P and Spadacini G (2008a) Utility of 12-lead electrocardiogram for differentiating paroxysmal supraventricular tachycardias in dogs. *Journal of Veterinary Internal Medicine* **22,** 915–923

Santilli RA, Perego M, Ramera L, Moretti P and Spadacini G (2008b) Focal junctional tachycardia in the dog. In: *Proceedings of the 18th ECVIM-CA Congress, Ghent, Belgium.*

Schrope DP and Kelch WJ (2006) Signalment, clinical signs, and prognostic indicators associated with high-grade second- or third-degree atrioventricular block in dogs: 124 cases (January 1, 1997–December 31, 1997). *Journal of the American Veterinary Medical Association* **228**, 1710–1717

Tilley LP (1992a) Analysis of common canine cardiac arrhythmias. In: *Essentials of Canine and Feline Electrocardiography, 3rd edn*, ed. LP Tilley, pp. 127–207. Lea and Febiger, Philadelphia

Tilley LP (1992b) Analysis of common feline cardiac arrhythmias. In: *Essentials of Canine and Feline Electrocardiography, 3rd edn*, ed. LP Tilley, pp. 208–252. Lea and Febiger, Philadelphia

17

Management of acute respiratory distress

Lindsay M. Kellett-Gregory and Lesley G. King

Introduction

Acute respiratory distress in dogs and cats is a common presenting complaint and can be life-threatening. Early identification of unstable patients and timely therapeutic intervention are essential to limit compromise of tissue oxygenation and deterioration in condition. Oxygen supplementation, appropriate drug therapy, thoracocentesis, thoracostomy tube placement, emergency tracheostomy and positive pressure ventilation (PPV) may be required to relieve respiratory distress. It is important to consider signalment and history, assess posture, observe the pattern of respiration and perform an initial physical examination focused on the cardiorespiratory system (see Chapter 1). Based on these findings, a clinical estimation of the anatomical location of the problem can guide initial therapy.

Acute lung injury and acute respiratory distress syndrome

- Acute lung injury (ALI) is a syndrome of progressive generalized pulmonary inflammation and oedema, resulting in acute respiratory failure.
- Acute respiratory distress syndrome (ARDS) is the most severe form of this pulmonary disease.

Causes

Common inciting causes in dogs include: direct lung injury from aspiration or bacterial pneumonia; pulmonary contusions; smoke inhalation; or any condition associated with a systemic inflammatory response, such as pancreatitis or sepsis. Although specific risk factors in cats have not been identified, severe sepsis has been associated with necropsy findings consistent with ALI/ARDS in this species (Brady *et al.*, 2000).

Aetiology

With ALI, pulmonary inflammation manifests as vascular endothelial injury, interstitial and alveolar permeability oedema, and infiltration with inflammatory cells such as neutrophils and macrophages. With ARDS, this inflammation is further accompanied by proliferation of type-II pneumocytes attempting to restore the damaged epithelium, hyaline membrane formation, and eventually pulmonary fibrosis. Pulmonary arterial hypertension develops secondary to increased pulmonary vascular resistance and due to hypoxaemic pulmonary vasoconstriction. If left untreated, pulmonary hypertension may result in right-sided cardiac dysfunction.

Clinical signs

Clinical findings vary depending on the severity of the syndrome. Respiratory dysfunction may range from subclinical in the mildest form of ALI, to respiratory distress and cyanosis with expectoration of a foamy pink liquid in severe cases of ARDS. Harsh lung sounds progressing to diffuse crackles are usually present on auscultation. The clinical signs of ALI/ARDS may be rapid in onset (hours) or may be delayed by 1–4 days after the inciting event triggers the inflammatory response.

Diagnosis

Diagnosis of ALI and ARDS is based on (Wilkins *et al.*, 2007):

- Acute onset of respiratory distress in the presence of appropriate risk factors
- Bilateral pulmonary infiltrates
- Absence of left atrial hypertension
- Decreased arterial partial pressure of oxygen (P_aO_2): fraction of inspired oxygen (F_IO_2) ratio.

ALI and ARDS can be differentiated by the degree of hypoxaemia as defined by the P_aO_2:F_IO_2 ratio: <300 is diagnostic for ALI; <200 is diagnostic for ARDS. Thoracic radiography and arterial blood gas analysis are therefore helpful indicators of ALI/ARDS. Radiographic evidence of cardiomegaly or enlarged pulmonary vasculature is suggestive of congestive heart failure (CHF) or fluid overload and is not consistent with a diagnosis of ALI/ARDS. In some instances, it may be necessary to perform an echocardiogram to rule out cardiogenic causes of the pulmonary oedema. In some cases, left atrial hypertension can be ruled out by measuring a pulmonary artery occlusion pressure (PAOP) of ≤18 mmHg. Additional diagnostic tests such as haematology or serum biochemistry typically reveal non-specific signs secondary to the underlying cause, although leucopenia and hypoalbuminaemia are common findings in canine ALI/ARDS.

Treatment and prognosis

Animals suffering from ALI have mild to moderate respiratory distress and may respond to oxygen supplementation, fluid restriction, colloid support, low doses of diuretics as needed and treatment of the underlying condition. Despite the fact that ALI is an inflammatory condition, use of corticosteroids in human patients has not been shown to improve survival and they are probably contraindicated due to their immunosuppressive effects. Animals with ARDS have very severe pulmonary dysfunction and poor lung compliance. They usually require PPV to deliver high concentrations of oxygen and prevent respiratory fatigue and subsequent failure. Despite aggressive support, the prognosis is grave with reports of veterinary patients surviving ARDS rare, and mortality rates in humans with ARDS as high as 40–60%.

General principles of therapy

Patients with respiratory distress are often most 'fragile' shortly after presentation to the hospital, owing to the stress of transportation and handling. Additional stress due to handling and diagnostic testing should therefore be minimized to prevent a potentially fatal decompensation in the animal's condition. In many cases, initial stabilization should consist simply of minimal handling and supplemental oxygen therapy.

The aims of initial therapy are to optimize oxygenation and ventilation, thus maximizing oxygen delivery to the tissues and minimizing oxygen consumption. In addition, it is important to limit disease progression and to identify and reverse underlying disease. (For further details on initial stabilization of the animal with respiratory distress, see Chapter 1.) Disease processes are likely to be dynamic, requiring continual reassessment and appropriate adjustments in treatment. Whilst early and aggressive therapy may be needed, consideration should be given to collection of diagnostic samples before treatment reduces the diagnostic potential.

Special considerations for long-term oxygen therapy
In the context of veterinary medicine, 'long-term' is defined as oxygen therapy required for more than 12 hours. Oxygen should routinely be humidified (i.e. saturated with water vapour) to prevent desiccation of the airway mucosa and impairment of normal airway defences. This is especially important if the turbinates are bypassed with nasal or tracheal oxygen catheters. Inspired oxygen is humidified by bubbling through a chamber of sterile distilled water, prior to delivery to the patient. Heating the gas increases the amount of water vapour it contains, and specially designed units that heat and humidify the inspired gas can be placed in anaesthetic or ventilator circuitry.

Long-term therapy with high concentrations of oxygen (F_iO_2 >0.6 for more than 12 hours) causes lung injury due to oxygen toxicity. Both endothelial and epithelial cells are damaged by toxic oxygen metabolites in the form of oxygen free radicals and superoxide molecules. Damage results in increased endothelial permeability, inflammation and cell death. There are no specific clinical signs of oxygen toxicity as changes in the lungs are similar to those of ARDS and difficult to distinguish from worsening parenchymal disease. Other complications reported with prolonged oxygen

therapy include suppression of erythropoiesis, pulmonary vasodilation, systemic arteriolar vasoconstriction and worsening of atelectasis.

To avoid oxygen toxicity, it is important that F_iO_2 is kept to the minimum required to maintain comfort. However, in animals with severe respiratory difficulty, it may not be possible to decrease F_iO_2 without worsening respiratory distress. In such cases, the risk of oxygen toxicity is accepted because use of a lower F_iO_2 can result in hypoxaemia and cell death. Close monitoring of the patient to assess response and the ongoing need for oxygen therapy is essential.

Specific drug therapy

After the patient has been assessed, is receiving oxygen, vascular access has been established, and initial diagnostic tests (if appropriate) have been performed, it may be necessary to administer drugs either to treat a known problem or empirically to treat the most likely disease based on the initial assessment. If the patient is very unstable, it is appropriate to make a list of potential differential diagnoses (see Chapter 1) and empirically treat for all possible treatable disorders. The diagnosis can then be confirmed when the patient becomes more stable.

Diuretics
Diuretics are indicated for the treatment of volume overload and CHF. Furosemide is the most frequently used diuretic in emergency situations as it is readily available and can be administered parenterally. Loop diuretics, such as furosemide, are the most potent and rapidly acting diuretics available.

- Furosemide inhibits the sodium (Na^+)–potassium (K^+)–chloride ($2Cl^-$) co-transporter in the thick ascending limb of the loop of Henle, causing loss of water, hydrogen ions and electrolytes, including sodium, potassium, chloride, calcium and magnesium.
- The dose, route and frequency of furosemide administration is variable, depending on the severity of the pulmonary oedema, but it is typically administered at a dose of 0.5–2 mg/kg i.v., i.m. q4–12h. Response to furosemide administration should be seen within 60–90 minutes of intravenous administration (i.e. urination should occur).
- Furosemide can also be given as an intravenous constant rate infusion (CRI) at a rate of 0.1–1 mg/kg/h. This delivers furosemide continuously, with less variation in serum and renal tubular drug concentrations, and in dogs has been shown to result in more diuresis for an equivalent dose of furosemide given intermittently (Adin *et al.*, 2003). If using a CRI, the infusion should be made up in as small a volume as possible so as to minimize the total volume of fluid administered.
- Cats appear to be more sensitive than other species to the diuretic effects of furosemide, and the authors recommend that a lower dose should be used in these patients.

Emergency use of furosemide is indicated whenever pulmonary oedema is known or suspected to be a cause or contributing factor to respiratory dysfunction. Furosemide is contraindicated in patients with hypovolaemia, severe dehydration or severe depletion of electrolytes. It should also be used with caution in patients with impaired hepatic function or diabetes mellitus. Its use may enhance the effects of concurrent therapy with other diuretics and theophylline. In addition, furosemide-induced hypokalaemia may enhance the chance of digitalis toxicity (Abbott and Kovacic, 2008). Hydration status, renal parameters and electrolytes should be closely monitored when using furosemide. The patient should be encouraged to eat and drink normally during therapy. If there is progressive dehydration or azotaemia during treatment, the drug should be discontinued.

Bronchodilators

Various classes of bronchodilator are available for use in veterinary patients, including:

- Beta adrenoreceptor agonists
- Methylxanthine derivatives
- Anticholinergic drugs.

Beta adrenoreceptor agonists

Terbutaline is a beta-2 adrenoreceptor agonist that causes bronchodilation. In emergency situations, it can be used at a dose of 0.01–0.015 mg/kg i.v., i.m., s.c. q4h in cats and 0.01 mg/kg i.v., i.m., s.c. in dogs. Terbutaline is indicated for emergency management of acute bronchospasm in suspected feline asthma. It may also be used for management of bronchoconstriction in dogs presumed to occur following acute aspiration. Adverse effects potentially include tachycardia and hypotension, and the drug should be used with caution in patients with diabetes mellitus, hyperthyroidism, hypertension, hypertrophic cardiomyopathy (HCM) and seizure disorders. The concurrent use of beta-blockers may antagonize its effects. Salbutamol is a beta-2 adrenoreceptor agonist that can be administered by aerosolization if the patient will tolerate placement of a mask.

Methylxanthine derivatives

Theophylline is a phosphodiesterase inhibitor and alters intracellular calcium levels. In addition to acting as a bronchodilator, it enhances mucociliary clearance, stimulates the respiratory centre and increases the sensitivity to the arterial partial pressure of carbon dioxide (P_aCO_2), increases diaphragmatic contractility, decreases the work of breathing, and has both a mild inotropic effect and diuretic action. Theophylline is administered orally at a dose of 15–19 mg/kg q24h in the evening to cats and 10 mg/kg q12h in dogs. As it is not available for intravenous administration, theophylline is less valuable for emergency management of animals in severe respiratory distress (it is difficult to administer pills to animals in respiratory distress, and there is also the risk of insufficient absorption from the gastrointestinal tract). Side effects are dose-dependent and can include tachycardia and agitation. The concurrent use of theophylline with beta-sympathomimetics is contraindicated as synergism may result in increased adverse effects.

Aminophylline is a stable mixture of theophylline and ethylenediamine that can be given intravenously (5–10 mg/kg q6–8h) if it is diluted and administered slowly. It causes intense pain when injected intramuscularly and should not be given by this route. It is a relatively weak bronchodilator and terbutaline is generally more valuable in an emergency setting.

Etamiphylline is available in the UK in an injectable form that can be administered intramuscularly or subcutaneously in an emergency situation.

Anticholinergic drugs

Anticholinergic drugs, such as atropine and glycopyrrolate, compete with acetylcholine at muscarinic receptor sites. Within the respiratory tract they antagonize vagally mediated bronchoconstriction and decrease secretions, but they have not been studied in the treatment of bronchial disease in animals. Use is restricted to situations when an animal with acute respiratory distress due to bronchial disease is refractory to the treatments listed above, and all other possible differential diagnoses for respiratory distress have been eliminated from consideration.

Anti-inflammatory drugs

Most drugs that induce bronchodilation (see above) may also slightly reduce bronchial inflammation, decreasing mucosal oedema and preventing the release of inflammatory mediators.

Anti-inflammatory drugs used in veterinary practice include corticosteroids and non-steroidal anti-inflammatory drugs (NSAIDs).

Corticosteroids

For a more powerful and global anti-inflammatory effect, corticosteroids are the most commonly used emergency drugs. In addition, they are reported to have 'permissive' effects on beta-2 adrenoreceptors, promoting bronchodilation. Glucocorticoids inhibit the enzyme phospholipase A2, which catalyses the release of arachidonic acid from membrane phospholipids for metabolism into inflammatory mediators. Dexamethasone can be given at a dose of 0.1–0.5 mg/kg i.v., i.m. q12–24h or alternatively, prednisolone can be administered at a dose of 0.2–1.0 mg/kg i.v., i.m., orally q12–24h. Corticosteroids are indicated for acute management of tissue oedema associated with upper airway obstruction and for emergency management of lower airway inflammation due to feline asthma. Treatment with glucocorticoids should be avoided if lymphoma is a possibility, because of interference with the diagnostic quality of samples obtained after administration. Glucocorticoids will also have a negative impact on any infectious process and should be avoided in patients with pneumonia or viral disease.

Non-steroidal anti-inflammatory drugs

NSAIDs do not appear to have clinically significant anti-inflammatory effects in the respiratory tract and, with the exception of use as analgesics, are not indicated for treatment of most types of respiratory distress. They should be avoided until cardiovascular stability has been confirmed and the patient thoroughly evaluated for any underlying renal disease.

Antibiotic therapy

Antibiotic therapy is indicated when bacterial infection is thought to be a primary problem or secondarily contributing to respiratory distress. Ideally, samples should be collected to confirm infection and obtain sensitivity testing prior to antibiotic therapy. Broad-spectrum parenteral treatment can be instituted and later refined on the basis of sensitivity testing results. The choice of antibiotic protocol will depend on the severity of disease, the suspected underlying aetiological agents, and the general health and organ function of the patient. Suggested antibiotic protocols for the treatment of bacterial pneumonia are given in Figure 17.1.

Patient status	Antibiotic protocol
Stable (no hypoxaemia, eating well)	Amoxicillin/clavulanate 14–22 mg/kg orally q12h Enrofloxacin 5–15 mg/kg orally q24h
Unstable (hypoxaemia, anorexia, fever)	Amoxicillin/clavulanate 15 mg/kg i.v. q8h Ticarcillin/clavulanate 50 mg/kg i.v. q6h Cefotaxime 20–50 mg/kg i.v. q6h Amikacin 15 mg/kg i.v. q24h plus ampicillin 22 mg/kg i.v. q8h Enrofloxacin 5–15 mg/kg i.v. q24h plus ampicillin 22 mg/kg i.v. q8h
Bordetella bronchiseptica pneumonia	Azithromycin 5–10 mg/kg i.v., orally q24h

17.1 Antibiotic protocols commonly used in the treatment of bacterial pneumonia.

Mucolytics

N-Acetylcysteine is a mucolytic agent that decreases the viscosity of both purulent and non-purulent airway secretions to facilitate clearance from the respiratory tract (the free sulphydryl group on the drug reduces disulphide bonds in mucoproteins). Although doses are published for nebulization of the drug, that route should be used with caution since it has been associated with bronchospasm (Plumb, 2005). Instead the drug can be administered intravenously or orally at a dose of 70 mg/kg q6h. *N*-Acetylcysteine must be diluted, administered through a filter, and given slowly by the intravenous route to avoid hypotension,

bronchospasm and flushing, which can be seen when given rapidly. *N*-Acetylcysteine is particularly useful when dealing with thick airway secretions that are not readily cleared and risk airway obstruction.

Bromhexine is a mucolytic agent available in the UK. It increases the production of serous mucus within the respiratory tract, thus thinning secretions and facilitating clearance by the cilia. It is available as an intramuscular injection and an oral powder. It is administered to cats at a dose of 1 mg/kg orally q24h and to dogs at a dose of 2 mg/kg orally q12h or 3–15 mg/dog i.m. q12h.

Fluid therapy

It is important to ensure that any patient with respiratory distress has an adequate circulating blood volume in order to maximize oxygen delivery to the tissues and to moisturize airway secretions to facilitate clearance. However, fluid therapy should be provided judiciously so as not to cause pulmonary oedema or pleural effusion to develop. In inflammatory conditions, the pulmonary endothelium may be more permeable than normal, making oedema formation more likely. Fluid therapy must be guided by careful physical examination and frequent monitoring and re-evaluation.

Analgesics and sedatives

When indicated, analgesia is important to minimize oxygen consumption and patient discomfort. When effective analgesia has been achieved, changes in respiration are more likely to be due to respiratory dysfunction than pain. Light sedation can prove useful in facilitating diagnostic procedures and minimizing anxiety associated with respiratory distress.

Pure opioids such as methadone, morphine, fentanyl and pethidine provide effective analgesia that can be titrated to effect and reversed with naloxone if required. Morphine may have an additional centrally mediated effect of decreasing the sensation of 'dyspnoea', and may be useful in the treatment of pulmonary oedema by decreasing preload. Since opioids can have a respiratory depressant effect, doses should be kept to a minimum to achieve the desired response (Figure 17.2). If clinically indicated,

Drug	Dogs	Cats	Comments
Morphine	0.1–0.3 mg/kg i.v., i.m., s.c.	0.1–0.2 mg/kg i.v., i.m., s.c.	
Methadone	0.1–0.3 mg/ kg i.v., i.m., s.c.	0.1–0.2 mg/ kg i.v., i.m., s.c.	
Pethidine	2–5 mg/kg i.m., s.c	2–5 mg/kg i.m., s.c.	Do **not** give intravenously
Fentanyl	CRI: 2–5 µg/kg/h i.v. Bolus: 5 µg /kg	CRI: 2–5 µg/kg/h i.v. Bolus: 2 µg/kg	Titrate to effect from lowest dose
Butorphanol	0.1–0.4 mg/kg i.v., i.m., s.c.	0.1–0.4 mg/kg i.v., i.m., s.c.	For sedation not analgesia
Midazolam	0.2–0.4 mg/kg i.v., i.m.	0.2–0.4 mg/kg i.v., i.m.	
Diazepam	0.2–0.4 mg/kg i.v.	0.2–0.4 mg/kg i.v.	
Acepromazine	0.005–0.02 mg/kg i.v., i.m., s.c.	0.005–0.02 mg/kg i.v., i.m., s.c.	
Naloxone	0.02–0.04 mg/kg i.v.	0.01–0.02 mg/kg i.v.	Reversal of opioids
Flumazenil	0.01–0.02 mg/kg i.v.	0.01–0.02 mg/kg i.v.	Reversal of benzodiazepines

17.2 Suggested doses for analgesia and sedation of patients with respiratory disease.

concurrent use of an analgesic and a sedative may decrease the dose of each drug required, and hence minimize any unwanted depressor activities. In any case, low doses should be used initially and the response closely monitored, as the effect of individual drugs in a critically ill or distressed patient may be greater than that seen in a normal animal.

Ventilation

Indications

A small proportion of animals remain severely hypoxaemic with excessive work of breathing, despite supplemental oxygen therapy and other appropriate medical treatment. In order to manage hypoxaemia effectively and relieve distress, these patients require anaesthesia, intubation and PPV. PPV is indicated for patients in which the P_aO_2 is <50–60 mmHg on supplemental oxygen or those with a P_aCO_2 >50–60 mmHg that cannot be treated in any other way (e.g. reversal of anaesthesia or a tracheostomy) (Vassilev and McMichael, 2004). This is sometimes known as the '50–50 rule'.

PPV is also indicated for animals that are clinically believed to be in danger of impending respiratory arrest due to respiratory fatigue, regardless of blood gas values. In such animals, extreme muscle effort associated with the work of breathing augments energy expenditure, which increases oxygen consumption and may negate the benefits of supplemental oxygen. Further indications for PPV include management of fractious animals that cannot be safely restrained for diagnostic tests or therapy. Finally, PPV may be appropriate in animals that are unstable following cardiopulmonary resuscitation because it permits ongoing control over the airway and decreases the risk of a second cardiorespiratory arrest.

PPV is labour-intensive and patients require constant nursing and monitoring in a critical care unit (CCU) setting. Therefore, it is generally reserved for the patient for which there is no suitable alternative.

The goals of PPV are to stabilize ventilation (P_aCO_2 30–40 mmHg) and oxygenation (P_aO_2 80–100 mmHg) at modest inspired oxygen concentrations, whilst minimizing any deleterious effects. The exact goals also depend on the animal's condition, the acid–base status and whether efforts are being made to wean the animal from ventilatory support.

Induction of anaesthesia

Initial airway access is usually achieved by orotracheal intubation, which requires heavy sedation or light general anaesthesia. Many patients that require PPV have concurrent cardiovascular instability and myocardial irritability secondary to hypoxaemia. Therefore, anaesthetic induction agents that are safe for the cardiovascular system should be chosen. Concerns regarding respiratory depression by induction agents are less important as ventilation will be provided. Rapid control of the airway is required, hence intramuscular drug administration and mask inductions should be avoided due to the time required to obtain airway control.

In the absence of cardiovascular disease, induction with propofol, thiopental, etomidate or ketamine/diazepam combinations would all be suitable. Propofol may cause vasodilation and intrapulmonary arteriovenous shunting, which can temporarily aggravate hypoxaemia. Thiopental does not cause such shunting, but may produce cardiac arrhythmias that can be exacerbated by concurrent myocardial hypoxaemia. In animals with cardiovascular instability, an opioid/benzodiazepine combination is often sufficient for intubation; however, this combination results in a relatively slower induction process and care must be taken to avoid worsened hypoxaemia from the time of drug administration to intubation. Respiratory arrest can result from administration of any drug, in which case the patient must be intubated and ventilated as soon as possible. All patients should be started on an inspired oxygen concentration of 100%, which is then tapered downwards as much as possible.

For ongoing PPV, anaesthesia must be maintained to allow continued intubation. Volatile agents can be used but injectable anaesthetics are preferred, either by repeat injection or ideally by continuous infusion.

Ventilators

Volume-cycled ventilators deliver a specified volume of air–oxygen mixture for every breath. This volume will be delivered regardless of the airway pressure generated, which can be variable depending on the lung disease present. If airway pressure becomes too high (>25–30 cmH$_2$O), alveolar over-distension and lung injury can occur. Therefore, it is essential to monitor airway pressures continually when using this type of ventilator to limit barotrauma.

Pressure-cycled ventilators deliver an air–oxygen mixture until a specified airway pressure is reached, regardless of the volume delivered. Pressure-cycled ventilation is therefore safer for the lung because the risk of barotrauma is lower. However, it is essential that tidal volume is closely monitored when using this ventilator setting. As lung compliance decreases with worsening parenchymal disease, the tidal volume delivered to the patient for a given airway pressure is lower, which can result in hypoventilation, increased P_aCO_2 and respiratory acidosis. The peak pressure needed to achieve adequate ventilation differs among patients and is largely dependent on lung compliance.

Human and animal studies have shown no distinct cardiorespiratory advantage of using volume- or pressure-cycled ventilation. Most ventilators used in veterinary critical care offer both options, and pressure-cycled ventilation is most commonly chosen as a starting point. Alternatively, high-frequency ventilation (HFV) delivers small tidal volumes (1–3 ml/kg) at a high frequency (100–300 breaths/minute). If available, this system of ventilation is useful in the management of hypovolaemic patients because the relatively low peak inspiratory pressure (PIP) does not decrease cardiac output. However, HFV can result in rapid and severe lung injury if there is complete outflow obstruction.

Modes of ventilation

There are two commonly used ventilator modes:

- Assist/control (AC)
- Synchronous intermittent mandatory ventilation (SIMV).

The choice of mode depends on the degree of ventilatory support required by the patient. AC is typically used at the beginning of PPV because it completely controls ventilation, whilst SIMV is useful during weaning (Figure 17.3).

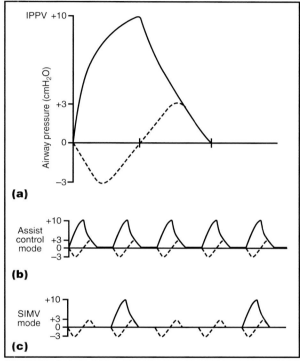

17.3 **(a)** A ventilator breath is compared with a spontaneous patient breath. The spontaneous breath (dotted line) begins as a negative inspiratory effort, followed by a slightly positive airway pressure during exhalation. In contrast, the ventilator breath (solid line) generates exclusively positive airway pressure. **(b)** In *A/C ventilation*, the ventilator delivers a set number of breaths, to a set pressure or tidal volume. The machine delivers these breaths when the patient creates a negative pressure in the airway; if the patient is not breathing, the machine will automatically deliver the set respiration rate. If the patient breathes faster than the set rate, the machine is also triggered, and it will deliver the desired tidal volume for each patient-initiated breath. **(c)** In *SIMV*, the ventilator is set to deliver a desired number of breaths, just as in AC. The breaths are delivered when the machine senses a negative pressure effort by the patient ('synchronous'). Between each breath, if the patient breathes spontaneously, the machine does not 'kick in' with a breath of its own, and the patient-induced breaths only reach the negative pressure and tidal volume determined by the patient. (Reproduced from the *BSAVA Manual of Canine and Feline Emergency and Critical Care, 2nd edition*.)

Assist/control ventilation

In AC ventilation, the machine is set to deliver a minimum number of breaths per minute. The ventilator initiates these breaths when the patient generates a predetermined amount of negative pressure in the airway. However, if a change in pressure is not detected, the machine will deliver a breath as required to achieve the set minimum ventilation rate. If the patient initiates respiratory efforts at a rate higher than the set minimum (i.e. if the patient breathes faster than the set rate), the ventilator is triggered to provide full breaths at this higher rate. In AC mode, the ventilator performs the majority of the work of breathing. However, it can be associated with hyperventilation and dysynchrony if the patient has a rapid and shallow respiratory rate because every patient-initiated breath is supplemented by the ventilator.

Synchronous intermittent mandatory ventilation

In SIMV, the machine is also set to deliver a minimum number of breaths per minute, which occur when the ventilator detects negative airway pressure generated by the patient ('synchronous'). However, in this mode, if the patient-initiated respiratory rate is higher than the set rate, the ventilator does not assist the additional breaths, which only reach the negative pressure and tidal volume determined by the patient. Thus, the animal performs a variable amount of the work of breathing. The amount of work performed by the ventilator can be gradually reduced and that of the patient gradually increased to wean the animal off the ventilator. SIMV is also useful in the management of patients with a rapid and shallow respiratory pattern.

General guidelines for ventilator settings

Normal lungs

Regardless of the type of ventilator used, the general guidelines for initial ventilator settings for patients with normal lungs are:

- Tidal volume of 8–12 ml/kg
- Ventilatory rate of 10–20 breaths/minute
- Minute ventilation of approximately 150–250 ml/kg/minute
- Peak inspiratory pressure of 10–20 cmH$_2$O
- Inspiratory time of approximately 1 second
- End-expiratory pressure of 0–2 cmH$_2$O.

Some patients may require a deep breath (sigh) every 30 minutes to minimize small airway and alveolar collapse, which is given at an airway pressure of 30 cmH$_2$O.

Diseased lungs

Diseased lungs have lower compliance than normal lungs, and the initial ventilator settings for normal lungs are usually inappropriate to adequately ventilate or oxygenate patients with pulmonary parenchymal disease. Diseased lungs are very heterogenous with non-compliant diseased alveoli lying side-by-side with normal alveoli, but both are subject to the same airway pressures. Thus, the healthy compliant alveoli in diseased lungs are significantly at risk of over-distension and barotrauma if 'normal' ventilator settings are used.

When ventilating diseased lungs, tidal volumes should be kept as low as possible (ideally 6–8 ml/kg) and peak airway pressures kept low (<30 cmH$_2$O) to prevent over-distension of the healthier alveoli (The Acute Respiratory Distress Syndrome Network, 2000). It may be necessary to increase the respiratory rate to ensure adequate minute ventilation at low tidal volumes. Care must be taken to ensure that the inspiratory:expiratory (I:E) ratio is <1 to allow full exhalation and avoid air-trapping (so-called 'auto-positive end-expiratory pressure (PEEP)') and the associated volutrauma. The inspired oxygen may need to be as high as 100% for sufficient oxygenation.

Lung protective ventilation strategies (lower tidal volume, low airway pressures) may cause less pulmonary inflammation and improve survival. In addition, the use of PEEP (as described below) can prevent the cycling of alveolar collapse and re-opening, which occurs with each breath and results in inflammation due to stretch and shear injury. *Permissive hypercapnia* relates to the acceptance of higher than normal P_aCO_2 (provided that respiratory acidosis is not too severe), in order to minimize tidal volumes and airway pressures.

Positive end-expiratory pressure

PEEP is commonly used to improve oxygenation in ventilated patients that remain hypoxaemic despite high F_iO_2 values. Small amounts of positive pressure are applied to the airways to prevent complete expiration. This results in increased alveolar size and recruitment, increased functional residual capacity (FRC), and prevention of early closure of the small airways. The application of PEEP should permit the use of a lower inspired oxygen concentration, thus reducing the risk of oxygen toxicity. PEEP is initiated at 5 cmH$_2$O and slowly increased up to a maximum pressure of 20 cmH$_2$O, until the desired P_aO_2 endpoint is obtained. PEEP can decrease cardiac output secondary to decreased cardiac filling, and it is essential to monitor haemodynamic variables closely. PEEP may also increase lung injury due to higher peak airway pressures.

Patient management

Equipment

Every effort should be made to minimize nosocomial infection by means of aseptic technique and use of gloves by operators. The ventilator circuitry must be carefully maintained and securely attached. Traction on the endotracheal tube should be avoided, and the endotracheal tube cuff should be inflated to protect the airway. Ideally, endotracheal tubes with high volume/low pressure cuffs should be used. The cuff should be deflated and the tube moved slightly every 4 hours to prevent pressure necrosis, and any ties securing the tube should be frequently repositioned.

Secretions usually accumulate in the tube over time and can result in obstruction, which can be detected by auscultation or by worsening oxygenation. This is managed by airway suctioning; however, routine suctioning in the absence of obstruction is not advisable because it can result in hypoxaemia for up to 15 minutes following the procedure. In addition, every time the patient is disconnected from the ventilator, PEEP is lost and the alveoli are subject to shear forces when the patient is reconnected to the ventilator. When suction is required, it should be performed in an aseptic manner and care should be taken not to traumatize the airway.

An alternative manual ventilation device should be available at all times in case the power source of the main ventilator fails. In addition, the oxygen supply to the ventilator should be checked frequently. Emergency re-intubation may be required if the endotracheal tube becomes completely obstructed, and the ventilator settings should also be assessed frequently.

Positioning

It is important that the patient is frequently repositioned to avoid pressure necrosis of the extremities and regional oedema secondary to poor lymphatic drainage. The body and all limbs should be well padded and passive range of motion exercises performed frequently.

Head

Artificial tears or lubricating ointment should be applied to both eyes frequently to minimize the risk of corneal ulceration. Both corneas should be stained with fluoroscein daily, and if ulcers are detected antibiotic ointment should be added to the topical therapy. The mouth and pharynx should be lavaged with sterile saline or dilute chlorhexidine and suctioned every 4 hours to limit bacterial colonization. The tongue should be kept clean and moist with glycerine, and care taken to protect against pressure necrosis due to the teeth or pulse oximeter probe.

Nutrition

Animals receiving ventilation also require nutrition, which typically cannot be provided enterally because of the risk of passive regurgitation and aspiration. Ideally, use of a jejunostomy tube (rather than an oesophagostomy or gastrostomy tube) would be the safest way to avoid this problem, but such tubes are not often in place in ventilated patients. Instead, nutrition is usually provided intravenously in the form of total parenteral nutrition (TPN), with careful monitoring of the catheter site for inflammation or infection. Electrolyte levels should also be closely monitored as they may become abnormal as a result of re-feeding syndrome, which can occur with re-introduction of calories to an anorectic patient and results in cardiac, neurological, haematological and muscular abnormalities associated with hypophosphataemia, hypokalaemia and hypomagnesaemia.

Bladder and colon care

Patients on ventilators also require bladder and colon care. A urinary catheter is often placed to facilitate urine quantification, to aid patient monitoring and to minimize soiling and urine scald. The colon should be palpated on a daily basis and warm water enemas administered as necessary to prevent faecal build up.

Patient–ventilator synchrony

Dysynchrony of the patient with the ventilator significantly impairs ventilation and oxygenation, and can be recognized when the patient makes efforts to breathe 'against' the ventilator. When dysynchrony occurs, the clinician must distinguish between one of two possibilities:

- 'Appropriate' patient breathing efforts: the patient is continuing to make efforts to breathe because P_aCO_2 values are too high and ventilator settings are not correct for the patient. In this case, adjusting the settings to ensure adequate ventilation usually resolves the dysynchrony
- 'Inappropriate' patient breathing efforts, which cause desaturation despite ventilator settings known to be correct if the patient was not 'fighting the ventilator'. This most commonly results from too light a level of sedation, but it can indicate the presence of an airway obstruction, pneumothorax or hyperthermia.

When dysynchrony occurs, the first step is to ensure that the patient is sufficiently anaesthetized by checking the palpebral reflex. The next step is to re-assess rectal temperature. To determine whether hypercarbia and/or hypoxaemia is a cause or the effect of the dysynchrony, it may be necessary to use neuromuscular blocking agents, temporarily, to assess respiratory parameters in the absence of patient breathing efforts.

Weaning from ventilatory support

Weaning a patient from ventilatory support can be a slow process. After prolonged periods of ventilatory support, respiratory muscles undergo disuse atrophy and take time to develop strength. In addition, severe diffuse pulmonary disease heals slowly, and withdrawal of support needs to match the gradual improvement in oxygenating capability. Ventilator modes such as SIMV and pressure support allow gradual withdrawal of ventilator support whilst progressively increased work of breathing is assumed by the patient. Continuous positive airway pressure (CPAP) can be another useful adjunct to the weaning process, and spontaneous breathing trials may also be performed. If any of these techniques fail, PPV can be recommenced as necessary, and further weaning efforts resumed later. It can be said that the weaning process begins at the time the patient is put on the ventilator, as settings are continually changed to provide the minimum possible level of support and to challenge the patient as appropriate.

Adverse effects of positive pressure ventilation

Ventilator acquired pneumonia (VAP) is a common consequence of long-term PPV, which occurs due to compromise of the normal airway protective mechanisms and introduction of bacteria into the airways. Intubation and necessary procedures, such as airway suctioning, permit the introduction of bacteria into the respiratory tract. In addition, clearance of airway secretions is impaired by intubation, which results in proliferation of oral and pharyngeal bacteria due to colonization by Gram-negative organisms. These bacteria migrate down the trachea, past the inflated cuff, and gain access to the lower respiratory tract. Finally, atelectasis secondary to recumbency increases the risk of pneumonia.

Mechanical ventilation is not an indication to start antibiotic therapy without a confirmed infection because of the risk of producing resistant organisms. However, the majority of patients will require antibiotic therapy within a week of commencing ventilation. A longer period of time on the ventilator is associated with a higher risk of ventilator-associated complications. Steps to minimize the occurrence of VAP include:

- Regular repositioning of the patient and intermittent 'sighs' to limit atelectasis
- Frequent mouth and pharynx care
- Use of aseptic technique for all airway procedures.

In addition, patients should be closely monitored for evidence of pneumonia, such as development of fever, worsening hypoxaemia or new alveolar infiltrates on thoracic radiographs. Samples should be regularly obtained from the airway using an endotracheal wash technique and submitted for culture and cytology. Appropriate broad-spectrum antibiotics should be commenced in the event of VAP and changed according to sensitivity testing.

The use of high airway pressures (>30 cmH2O) and large tidal volumes in both normal and abnormal lungs can be associated with alveolar septal rupture, pneumothorax, pneumomediastinum, pulmonary haemorrhage, air embolism and pulmonary inflammation. Pneumothorax should be considered in the event of sudden hypoxaemia or ventilator–patient dysynchrony. Tension pneumothorax can develop very quickly in a ventilated patient because positive pressure is being applied to the thorax. In these cases, chest tube placement and continual pleural evacuation is required.

PPV and the use of narcotic sedatives increase the secretion of antidiuretic hormone, thereby decreasing urine output, and PPV also decreases the secretion of atrial natriuretic factor, resulting in fluid retention, which require treatment with a diuretic (Pierce, 1995). As PPV can have adverse cardiovascular effects, perfusion parameters should be closely monitored alongside oxygenation and ventilation parameters. Monitoring of urine output, blood lactate and body temperature should be routine.

Positive pressure ventilation outcomes

PPV can be life-saving in some cases of severe respiratory distress. Outcome, defined as weaning and survival to hospital discharge, varies depending on the reason for mechanical ventilation. In animals with normal lungs ventilated because of neurological dysfunction, reported survival rates vary from 71% (dogs) to 33% (cats) (Beal *et al.*, 2001; Lee *et al.*, 2005). In cases ventilated because of pulmonary parenchymal disease, survival rates are reported to vary from 14–30% (Campbell and King, 2000; Lee *et al.*, 2005).

Ancillary procedures

Emergency techniques can be vital for management of specific patients presenting with acute respiratory distress. These techniques include:

- Thoracocentesis
- Thoracostomy tube placement
- Tracheostomy tube placement
- Nebulization and coupage.

Pre-sterilized packs containing the necessary equipment can save valuable time in an emergency situation.

Thoracocentesis

Thoracocentesis (see Chapter 32) is indicated when pleural space disease is suspected as the cause of respiratory distress. Instances include patients with dull lung sounds either ventrally or dorsally on auscultation, patients with a history of trauma or a fall from a height, and patients being ventilated whose condition acutely deteriorates. When an animal has either pleural effusion or a pneumothorax and is in respiratory distress, supplemental oxygen should be provided and thoracocentesis performed immediately. Radiographic diagnosis is not required and the stress or time associated with obtaining the radiograph may be detrimental to the patient's condition.

Thoracic ultrasonography, if available, may be a rapid means of confirming the presence of fluid but is not a necessary step. Diagnostic imaging following thoracocentesis is more likely to be tolerated by the patient, and allows evaluation of the cardiac silhouette and pulmonary vasculature, as well as identification of the underlying cause, once the pleural fluid has been removed. Thoracic radiographs obtained after thoracocentesis also permit quantification of the remaining fluid, forming a baseline to assess re-accumulation.

Fluid obtained should be placed in an EDTA tube for cytology and cell counts, and a plain tube for further analysis (measurement of total protein, triglycerides). A sample should also be obtained for aerobic and anaerobic cultures if the cytology and gross appearance suggest a septic process.

Thoracostomy tube placement

Thoracostomy tubes (see Chapter 32) should be placed in those animals that require more than two separate thoracocentesis attempts to relieve respiratory difficulty over a short period of time, those in which thoracocentesis fails to yield negative pressure, or in those animals that require repeated drainage for management of the underlying condition (e.g. animals with pyothorax). Tube placement is best performed under general anaesthesia in order to obtain full control of ventilation during tube placement. Alternatively, light sedation and local anaesthesia can be used to good effect in critical patients. If necessary, an assistant may continue to perform thoracocentesis (e.g. tension pneumothorax) to maximize

oxygenation as the patient is prepared and anaesthesia is induced.

Thoracostomy tubes are available in a variety of sizes, ranging from 14–40 Fr, depending on the size of the patient. Smaller tubes may be adequate for removing air, whereas larger tubes may be needed for the drainage of more viscous effusions. Chest tubes are usually made of polyvinyl chloride (PVC) or silicone rubber, although if these are not available, a sterile red rubber feeding tube can be used.

Following placement, orthogonal thoracic radiographs should be obtained and tube placement corrected if necessary. The end of the tube should be located cranial to or adjacent to the heart, but not cranial to the 2nd rib as this could result in obstruction of the tube or irritation of the phrenic nerve. It is important to verify that all the holes within the tube are located within the thoracic cavity. The chest tube should be secured carefully to prevent patient interference, resulting in contamination or disconnection, and if necessary an Elizabethan collar can be used. Patients with chest tubes in place require 24-hour nursing due to the risk of tube disconnection and the development of a potentially fatal pneumothorax.

Indwelling chest tubes cause pain, which can decrease ventilation if not adequately managed. Analgesia should be provided by systemic injection of opioids or NSAIDs, if not clinically contraindicated. In addition, the delivery of local anaesthetic agents (e.g. bupivacaine 1.5 mg/kg q6–8h) through the chest tube can be very useful.

The chest tube should be aspirated as frequently as required by the rate of formation of air or fluid, which is highly variable. When the accumulation of fluid or air is rapid enough to be life-threatening, the tube may need to be connected to a continuous suction device to allow continual emptying of the pleural space. A continuous negative pressure of approximately 10–20 cmH$_2$O is recommended.

Tracheostomy tube placement

There are few indications for a true emergency tracheostomy, as the majority of patients with upper airway obstructive disease can be managed medically or easily intubated. An emergency tracheostomy is indicated only when an airway cannot otherwise be established; for example, if the airway is obstructed by a foreign body or neoplasm, or in cases of severe facial trauma when it may not be appropriate to intubate.

Needle tracheotomy is a simple technique that can be used to bypass an upper airway obstruction and provide oxygen insufflation prior to placement of an emergency tracheostomy tube. Sedation and local anaesthesia are not usually required, but the area is clipped and surgically prepared if time allows. The trachea is stabilized with one hand, and an appropriately sized needle or catheter is advanced on the ventral cervical midline between the tracheal rings at a site distal to the upper airway obstruction. This technique temporarily establishes a small diameter airway for administration of oxygen.

Technique for tracheostomy tube placement

The equipment required for placement of a temporary tracheostomy tube should be gathered prior to anaesthetizing the patient.

1. The patient is placed in dorsal recumbency with the neck extended, and a sand bag or fluid bag positioned under the neck. If time permits, the ventral cervical region is clipped, and aseptic technique should be followed as much as possible.
2. An incision is made on the midline of the ventral cervical region, extending from the caudal edge of the cricoid cartilage of the larynx to approximately the sixth tracheal ring.
3. The paired sternohyoid muscles are separated on the fascial plane and retracted laterally to gain access to the trachea. Additional fascia is dissected away as necessary, staying on the midline to avoid damage to the surrounding structures.
4. The trachea is isolated and a full-thickness stab incision made with a blade through the annular ligament between the third and fourth tracheal rings. The incision is extended laterally to make it large enough to prevent stricture formation upon healing, but no more than 50% of the tracheal circumference.
5. A tracheostomy tube that occupies approximately 50% of the tracheal diameter is placed into the tracheal lumen. Ideally it should have a removable inner cannula to facilitate cleaning. A cuffed tube should be placed if PPV will be required.
6. Stay sutures should be placed around two tracheal rings on either side of the tracheostomy site. The ends of the sutures are tied and left long; sutures are labelled as either cranial or caudal. Placing tension on the sutures will open the tracheostomy site and raise it to the skin surface, exposing the opening in the trachea, in the event that the tube needs to be replaced.
7. The majority of the incision through the skin and subcutaneous tissues is left open, but excess can be closed with sutures. Care should be taken to ensure that enough space remains to allow access for replacement of the tracheostomy tube if needed.
8. The tracheostomy tube is secured using umbilical tape tied around the neck. It should not be sutured to the neck so that it can be easily removed and replaced in an emergency.

Patients with a temporary tracheostomy tube in place require careful 24-hour monitoring. Common complications include obstruction of the tube with mucus and dislodgement of the tube, either of which can lead to severe respiratory distress and death if not detected and rectified immediately. Significant amounts of mucus often accumulate within a short period of time because of inhalation of dehydrated air and because of damage to the mucosa by the physical presence of the tube. Sterile technique should always be maintained when managing the tracheostomy site, tube and suction catheter.

Patients with temporary tracheostomy tubes are at increased risk for pneumonia and should be closely monitored for worsening pulmonary function. If pneumonia is suspected, samples from the airway should be submitted for cytology and culture prior to starting broad-spectrum intravenous antibiotic therapy, which can be subsequently refined based on the results of culture and sensitivity testing. Uncommon short-term complications include:

- Haemorrhage
- Subcutaneous emphysema
- Infection of the site
- Damage to the peritracheal structures, including the recurrent laryngeal nerves, carotid artery, jugular vein, thyroid vessels and oesophagus.

Post-tracheostomy management should include regular nebulization with sterile saline to humidify the airways and encourage clearance of mucus, frequent removal and cleaning of the inner cannula (if present) to decrease the risk of mucus obstructing the tube, and airway suctioning if needed to clear secretions. If airway suction is necessary, the patient should be pre-oxygenated and a small diameter soft catheter should be used. The tracheostomy site should be inspected several times daily for swelling and irritation. After removal of the tracheostomy tube, the wound should be allowed to heal by secondary intention.

Nebulization and coupage

Patients with airway or pulmonary parenchymal disease can benefit from frequent nebulization of the airways with sterile saline, which moistens and encourages clearance of airway secretions. Nebulizers produce tiny droplets (<5 μm in diameter) of saline (as opposed to humidifiers, which saturate the inhaled air with water vapour). The nebulized saline droplets impact the epithelium of the airways and directly moisten the secretions. Patients can be nebulized several times daily or continuously. Nebulization can also be a useful adjunctive method for localized delivery of high concentrations of drugs, although few drugs are specifically formulated for nebulization.

To encourage expectoration of respiratory secretions, coupage can also be performed. The chest wall is percussed with the cupped palms of the hands for approximately 5–10 minutes several times daily, as tolerated by the patient. This should be avoided in patients with rib fractures, a history of thoracic trauma and those with a coagulopathy.

References and further reading

Abbott L and Kovacic J (2008) The pharmacologic spectrum of furosemide. *Journal of Veterinary Emergency and Critical Care* **18(1)**, 26–39
Adin D, Taylor A, Hill R, *et al.* (2003) Intermittent bolus injection *versus* continuous infusion of furosemide in normal adult greyhound dogs. *Journal of Veterinary Internal Medicine* **17(5)**, 632–636
Beal M, Paglia D, Griffin G, *et al.* (2001) Ventilatory failure, ventilator management, and outcome in dogs with cervical spinal disorders: 14 cases (1991–1999). *Journal of the American Veterinary Medical Association* **218(10)**,1598–1602

Brady C, Otto C, Winkle T, *et al.* (2000) Severe sepsis in cats: 29 cases (1986–1998). *Journal of the American Veterinary Medical Association* **217**, 531–535

Campbell V and King L (2000) Pulmonary function, ventilator management, and outcome of dogs with thoracic trauma and pulmonary contusions: 10 cases (1994–1998). *Journal of the American Veterinary Medical Association* **217(10)**, 1505–1509

DeClue AE and Cohn LE (2007) Acute respiratory distress syndrome in dogs and cats: a review of clinical findings and pathophysiology. *Journal of Veterinary Emergency and Critical Care* **17(4)**, 340–347

Hopper K, Haskins S, Kass P, *et al.* (2007) Indications, management, and outcome of long-term positive-pressure ventilation in dogs and cats: 148 cases (1990–2001). *Journal of the American Veterinary Medical Association* **230(1)**, 64–75

Lee J, Drobatz K, Koch M, *et al.* (2005) Indications for and outcome of positive-pressure ventilation in cats: 53 cases (1993–2002). *Journal of the American Veterinary Medical Association* **226(6)**, 924–931

Meuller ER (2001) Suggested strategies for ventilatory management of veterinary patients with acute respiratory distress syndrome. *Journal of Veterinary Emergency and Critical Care* **11(3)**, 191–198

Ogeer-Gyles J, Matthews K and Boerlin P (2006) Nosocomial infections and antimicrobial resistance in critical care medicine. *Journal of Veterinary Emergency and Critical Care* **16(1)**, 1–18

Pierce L (1995) Guide to Mechanical Ventilation and Intensive Respiratory Care. WB Saunders, St Louis

Plumb D (2005) *Veterinary Drug Handbook, 5th edn.* Blackwell Publishing Professional, Iowa

Sauvé V, Drobatz K, Shokek A, *et al.* (2005) Clinical course, diagnostic findings and necropsy diagnosis in dyspnoeic cats with primary pulmonary parenchymal disease: 15 cats (1996–2002). *Journal of Veterinary Emergency and Critical Care* **15(1)**, 38–47

The Acute Respiratory Distress Syndrome Network (2000) Ventilation with lower tidal volumes as compared with traditional tidal volumes for acute lung injury and the acute respiratory distress syndrome. *The New England Journal of Medicine* **342(18)**, 1301–1308

Vassilev E and McMichael M (2004) An overview of positive pressure ventilation. *Journal of Veterinary Emergency and Critical Care* **14(1)**, 15–21

Waddell L and King L (2007) General approach to dyspnoea. In: *BSAVA Manual of Canine and Feline Emergency and Critical Care, 2nd edn*, ed. L King and A Boag, pp. 85–113. BSAVA Publications, Gloucester

Wilkins PA, Otto CM, Baumgardner JE, *et al.* (2007) Acute lung injury and acute respiratory distress syndromes in veterinary medicine: consensus definitions: The Dorothy Russell Havemeyer Working Group on ALI and ARDS in Veterinary Medicine. *Journal of Veterinary Emergency and Critical Care* **17(4)**, 333–339

18

Treatment of congestive heart failure

Virginia Luis Fuentes

Introduction

Although most cardiac diseases have an adverse effect on cardiac output, it is congestive heart failure (CHF) that is usually responsible for clinical signs in dogs and cats. CHF can be defined as abnormal fluid accumulation as a result of heart disease. Increased atrial pressures lead to increased capillary hydro-static pressure, and fluid accumulates in the inter-stitial spaces (pulmonary oedema) or body cavities (pleural effusion or ascites).

Congestive signs are more common than signs of low cardiac output because the main priority of the cardiovascular system is provision of adequate systemic arterial blood pressure, and this is tightly regulated. Arterial blood pressure is maintained in the face of reduced cardiac output via activation of a number of neurohormonal mechanisms. These include increased sympathetic tone, as well as other mechanisms that help to increase cardiac output (such as sodium and water retention) or increase systemic vascular resistance. Importantly, support of arterial blood pressure is often at the expense of increased filling (atrial) pressures, increased risk of pulmonary oedema or effusions, and increased myocardial work.

Treatment according to stage of heart disease

The goals of therapy for heart disease differ markedly according to the stage of disease. In some cases, there are more similarities between treatments for different cardiac diseases at the same stage than for the same disease at different stages. It is therefore essential to stage the heart disease before starting treatment (Figure 18.1), and determining whether an animal has (or has had) CHF is extremely important. Where possible, selection of specific therapies should be based on the evidence of randomized controlled clinical trials carried out in the relevant patient group. Studies evaluating a particular therapy in one stage of heart disease should not necessarily be extrapolated to other stages.

At risk stage
Animals with a genetic predisposition to heart disease are clearly at risk of developing cardiac problems. Early heart disease may be present long before clinical signs are evident and may only be detected by proactive screening.

Management goals
Obviously no treatment is needed for normal animals that are simply at risk of heart disease, but screening may nevertheless be indicated. Breeders of dogs or cats with a genetic predisposition to cardiac disease may wish to screen for heart disease before breeding, and it may also be prudent to screen such animals prior to anaesthesia, aggressive fluid therapy or major surgery. Some cardiac diseases are easier to screen for than others. Careful auscultation may be sufficient for screening for myxomatous mitral valve disease (MMVD) and many congenital diseases. For dilated cardiomyopathy (DCM), echocardiography (with or without 24-hour ambulatory electrocardiogram monitoring) may be more appropriate. Genetic testing for a specific mutation may be recommended to breeders of Maine Coon or Ragdoll cats, but for other cats echocardiography remains the gold standard for detection of cardiomyopathy.

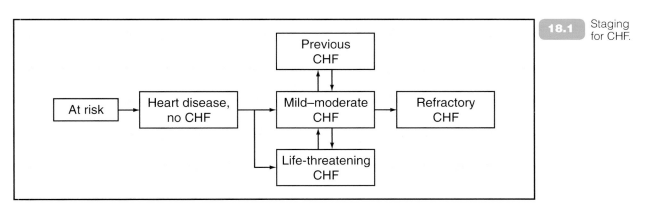

18.1 Staging for CHF.

Heart disease, no congestive heart failure stage

Most animals with heart disease are asymptomatic. In early heart disease, haemodynamic function may be relatively unaffected and there may be little or no neurohormonal activation. There are comparatively few clinical trials available that examine the effects of therapy at this stage in dogs or cats, and there is little consensus on the most appropriate course of action.

Management goals

Therapy at this stage is only worthwhile if it slows or reverses the underlying disease progression, or if the onset of CHF is delayed or prevented. Surgical correction could theoretically achieve this, but is not generally available for most small animal conditions (apart from some congenital defects). It is not known whether neurohormonal blockade alters the disease course in most canine and feline cardiac conditions.

Monitoring

The main goal of monitoring is to detect early signs of heart failure. Owner education is particularly important, as the owner is best placed to identify the earliest signs. A useful way to help the owner to detect early pulmonary oedema is to encourage the owner to record the animal's respiratory rate at home. In MMVD, DCM and feline cardiomyopathy, routine checkups to assess left atrial size can be useful to chart progression of disease and increasing risk of CHF.

Mild to moderate congestive heart failure stage

Animals with mild to moderate CHF will usually show clinical signs, but do not usually require hospitalization for management. It is logical to attempt to counteract the neurohormonal mechanisms leading to sodium and water retention. Most clinical trials in canine heart failure have been carried out with this stage of heart disease and selection of therapy should be evidence-based.

Management goals

Removal of abnormal fluid accumulation (pulmonary oedema, pleural effusion, ascites) is a priority, and the aim is to get the patient 'dry' without causing unacceptable azotaemia or polyuria/polydipsia that compromises quality of life. There is little evidence available from clinical trials for guiding dosages of diuretics in dogs, but the general approach is to titrate a loop diuretic to effect, using the lowest dose that is effective. Neurohormonal blockade may be associated with prolonged survival, and drugs with beneficial haemodynamic effects may also improve outcome.

Monitoring

Goals of monitoring include checking resolution of CHF with thoracic radiographs and respiratory rate at home, and checking for adverse effects of medications by monitoring biochemistry (electrolytes and urea/creatinine). Owners should be questioned about polyuria/polydipsia, as they may not otherwise volunteer information about excessive drinking/urination.

Life-threatening congestive heart failure stage

Many of these cases present acutely, sometimes without any history of prior problems, or sometimes already receiving medical therapy for CHF. With acute deterioration there may be little time for sodium and water retention, and low cardiac output signs may predominate. Therapy must be focused on trying to optimize haemodynamic function. Trying to neutralize neurohormonal activation in this setting may be counterproductive, as the compensatory mechanisms help to support arterial pressures. These cases require rapid aggressive management if they are to survive.

Management goals

The approach is aimed at rapid improvement of oxygenation and haemodynamic function. Critical hypoxaemia must be addressed urgently and cardiac output must be supported in those animals with cardiogenic shock. Hypoxaemia is generally managed by increasing the inspired oxygen concentration and removing pleural effusions or resolving pulmonary oedema. Pleural effusions must be drained and pulmonary oedema is best managed with diuresis, with or without venodilation. Cardiac output can be improved with positive inotropes, but judicious use of arteriodilation can also help. The latter is difficult to judge, as hypotension is one of the most easily measured indicators of low output, and arteriodilators will reduce blood pressure further. Fluid therapy should *not* be used to increase cardiac output, as there is little incremental benefit in stroke volume but considerable potential risk of worsening CHF by elevating atrial pressures.

Monitoring

Monitoring must not compromise patient safety, but the minimum requirement is to monitor respiratory rate/effort to chart resolution of pulmonary oedema and, ideally, blood pressure if low output signs are present. Electrolytes and renal function should also be monitored, as the adverse effects of medications include azotaemia and hypokalaemia (loop diuretics). Heart rate and rhythm (particularly ventricular arrhythmias) should be monitored closely when using catecholamines.

Refractory congestive heart failure stage

This category includes animals that are already receiving 'standard' treatment for heart failure, but heart failure signs persist despite upwards titration of furosemide doses. By this stage there may be surprisingly few signs of diuresis (or polydipsia) as the animal becomes increasingly refractory. Right heart failure signs are common. Addition of other diuretics (without withdrawing the furosemide) will often restore diuresis, but cardiac cachexia becomes a common problem as the disease progresses.

Management goals

The aim is to try to eliminate abnormal fluid accumulation, although by this stage it may not be possible to clear abdominal effusions completely. Some animals will tolerate small abdominal effusions surprisingly well. Sequential nephron blockade is usually necessary, as the combination of multiple diuretics achieves greater diuresis than high doses of a single diuretic. Appetite may be poor by this stage and essential omega-3 fatty acid supplementation can be tried in an attempt to counteract cardiac cachexia.

Monitoring
Both bodyweight and body condition score should be monitored, as they may vary independently with fluid retention and concurrent loss of fat and lean muscle mass (which can lead to dangerously inaccurate drug dosing). Azotaemia and electrolyte disturbances are likely and biochemistry must be monitored more closely than at other stages, particularly with inappetent animals.

At each stage of treatment, the owner should be involved in monitoring if the optimal outcome is to be achieved. Although similar drugs may be given for different conditions, an understanding of the goals of therapy for each stage is essential for optimizing dosages (particularly for diuretics). Many clinicians will involve owners in adjustment of doses according to clinical signs, especially respiratory rate. For treatment of specific diseases, see individual chapters.

Specific treatments

Surgery/catheter interventions
The ideal approach to heart disease is to correct the underlying problem. Some abnormalities can be corrected surgically or via catheter intervention (patent ductus arteriosus (PDA), pulmonic stenosis). Many human valve diseases are considered to be surgical problems and much progress has been made in this field in improving mitral valve repair. Lack of equivalent veterinary facilities and experience is partly responsible for the poor results so far with canine valve surgery, but the small body size of most affected dogs is also a major obstacle to achieving a successful outcome when cardiopulmonary bypass is necessary. Palliative surgical procedures are still indicated for other congenital problems (such as in tetralogy of Fallot), and surgical pacemaker implantation is the optimum treatment for many symptomatic bradyarrhythmias. Nevertheless, in acquired heart disease most management is medical.

Diuretics
Diuretics are indicated in *all* cases with cardiogenic pulmonary oedema. They are also indicated for most causes of CHF, with the exception of CHF due to pericardial effusion (which should be treated by draining the pericardial effusion) and large pleural effusions (which are better managed by thoracocentesis). Diuretics for CHF act by causing sodium excretion (natriuresis), with water following the movement of sodium. *Osmotic diuretics (such as mannitol) are contraindicated in CHF.* Diuretics should be dosed to effect, such that they are titrated both upwards and downwards.

Furosemide
Furosemide is the standard first-line choice for diuresis, whether parenteral or oral. There are very few veterinary clinical trials of furosemide, as it is considered an irreplaceable component of CHF treatment. Nonetheless, there are disadvantages to its use *before* the onset of CHF, including renin–angiotensin system activation.

With observant responsible owners it may be possible to allow an additional dose of furosemide to be given in the event of an increase in respiratory rate and effort. If this becomes necessary, the owner should then seek additional veterinary advice on subsequent maintenance therapy.

Mechanism: Furosemide is a loop diuretic and acts on the sodium–potassium–chloride co-transporter in the ascending loop of Henle, thus leading to loss of potassium and chloride in addition to sodium and water.

Dosage: The dose used is very variable, ranging from 1 to 6 mg/kg q1–24h (i.v., s.c., i.m., orally). It is potent and acts within 20 minutes of parenteral administration. When given intravenously, there are additional venodilating effects (but also a risk of transient deafness when given rapidly). At equivalent doses, the magnitude of natriuresis appears to be greater with constant rate infusions (CRIs) than with intermittent boluses, though it may be easier to judge short-term responses with bolus dosing (Adin *et al.*, 2003). Oral bioavailability is reasonable in dogs and maximum plasma concentrations are achieved within 30 minutes (El-Sayed *et al.*, 1981). The dose is very variable and is judged according to effect. The minimum dose required to eliminate abnormal fluid should be used and the effects (both beneficial and adverse) decrease after chronic dosing. A steady state is usually reached within a couple of weeks, and its effects may be less noticeable after this period. Cats are more sensitive to its effects than dogs.

Adverse effects: Although furosemide can cause prerenal azotaemia, higher doses are actually required to produce an effect in animals with chronic renal disease, though the effects of reducing plasma volume may be particularly poorly tolerated in this group. Adverse effects include excessive polyuria/polydipsia, hypokalaemia, increased urea and activation of the renin–angiotensin system. Hypochloraemia is common.

Spironolactone
Spironolactone has few obvious short-term haemodynamic effects, but is an important part of sequential nephron blockade in chronic CHF therapy, and may have a place earlier in the treatment course in acquired heart disease. Human trials have shown that substantial survival benefits are seen in chronic heart failure when spironolactone is added to standard heart failure therapy (Pitt *et al.*, 1999). Despite promising results in experimental models of hypertrophic cardiomyopathy (HCM), spironolactone did not appear to be helpful in a study of asymptomatic

Maine Coon cats with HCM (MacDonald *et al.*, 2008). Spironolactone is usually used as an 'add-on' therapy in addition to furosemide rather than as a substitute, but can be used in place of potassium supplements for hypokalaemic animals with cardiac disease.

Mechanism: Spironolactone was traditionally viewed as a weak, potassium-sparing diuretic. It is an aldosterone antagonist and, as such, should probably be listed under neurohormonal blockers (see below). The beneficial effects in human heart failure are believed to be associated with blockade of aldosterone-mediated myocardial fibrosis and remodelling.

Dosage: Recommendations for dose rates have been reduced recently to 1–2 mg/kg orally q12–24h, as the original dose rates pre-dated angiotensin-converting enzyme (ACE) inhibitors. The dose used should be sufficiently low to avoid hyperkalaemia.

Adverse effects: Theoretical adverse effects include hyperkalaemia when used with ACE inhibitors, though this appears to be uncommon with standard doses and concurrent furosemide use. Facial skin lesions were reported with use of spironolactone in asymptomatic Maine Coon cats with HCM (MacDonald *et al.*, 2008).

Amiloride
Amiloride is a potassium-sparing diuretic that has no particular other advantages. It is often combined with a thiazide in commercially available diuretics.

Thiazides
Thiazide diuretics act on the sodium–chloride symporter in the distal convoluted tubules of the kidney. They are potent, but not as potent as loop diuretics. They tend to be used in refractory CHF rather than as first-line diuretics and are often used in combination with other diuretics. They should be used with caution, as when added to high-dose furosemide they increase the risk of azotaemia, hypokalaemia and hyponatraemia. As with loop diuretics, they should be used at the minimum dose necessary to achieve a desired effect.

Hydrochlorothiazide is often only available in combination with amiloride. Although bendroflumethiazide is available as a single formulation, there is little published on clinical use of this diuretic in dogs or cats.

Neurohormonal blockers

ACE inhibitors
ACE inhibitors are indicated whenever there is renin–angiotensin–aldosterone system activation, which means they are indicated in most situations where furosemide is prescribed. There may also be beneficial tissue effects before plasma renin activity is increased. The beneficial effects of ACE inhibitors have been well studied in models of systolic dysfunction, systemic hypertension and pressure overload hypertrophy. The effects of blocking angiotensin II have been less obviously beneficial in canine models of volume overload (Perry *et al.*, 2002). ACE inhibitors

have found an established place in management of chronic CHF in cats and dogs. Studies in dogs with naturally occurring CHF have consistently shown clinical improvement or increased survival associated with ACE inhibitor therapy (Ettinger *et al.*, 1998; BENCH Study Group, 1999) and ACE inhibitors are routinely used in conjunction with chronic furosemide therapy in a variety of cardiac conditions.

The evidence in favour of ACE inhibitors is weaker in asymptomatic animals, with a retrospective study suggesting probable benefit for DCM (O'Grady *et al.*, 2009) but two prospective studies in MMVD showing little or no evidence of delay in onset of heart failure or decreased cardiac mortality (Kvart *et al.*, 2002; Atkins *et al.*, 2007). Evidence of benefit in asymptomatic cats is similarly weak. A study of ramipril in asymptomatic Maine Coon cats with HCM showed no reduction in left ventricular mass or diastolic dysfunction after a year of therapy compared with placebo-treated cats (MacDonald *et al.*, 2006).

Mechanism: ACE inhibitors have many effects, including reduction in sodium and water retention, vasodilation, reduction in renal glomerular pressure, and local myocardial tissue effects. They should not be thought of as simply 'vasodilators'. The vasodilatory effects are most prominent when used in animals with activation of the renin–angiotensin–aldosterone system, and so arterial pressures may drop dramatically following their use in animals with low cardiac output signs. In contrast, arterial pressures may barely change with their use in normal or asymptomatic animals.

Dosage: There is little overt benefit of one ACE inhibitor over any other. They mainly differ in their route of excretion, pharmacokinetics and formulation. Enalapril (0.5 mg/kg orally q12–24h) is primarily excreted renally, whereas benazepril (0.5–1.0 mg/kg orally q24h) is excreted partly by the renal and partly by the biliary route. Benazepril is the only ACE inhibitor authorized in cats. Ramipril (0.25 mg/kg orally q24h) and imidapril (0.25 mg/kg orally q24h) are other ACE inhibitors authorized in dogs.

Avoidance of ACE inhibitor-induced coughing is the main indication for angiotensin II antagonists in people. This does not occur in dogs and cats and so there is little reason to choose an angiotensin II antagonist over an ACE inhibitor.

Adverse effects: ACE inhibitors are more likely to cause prerenal azotaemia in hypotensive animals than in normotensive animals, or even those with chronic renal disease (the preferential glomerular efferent arteriolar dilation particularly decreases glomerular filtration rate when renal perfusion pressures are low). Caution is usually warranted with CHF associated with outflow tract obstruction, because of the risk of hypotension. However, this is often more a theoretical than practical concern (Oyama *et al.*, 2003).

Beta adrenergic antagonists
If neurohormonal activation (and sympathetic activation in particular) is harmful, then beta adrenergic

antagonists (beta-blockers) should have a beneficial effect on the myocardium, by preventing progression of myocardial remodelling, apoptosis and fibrosis. The long-term benefits of treatment (after 3 months or more) have been shown in numerous clinical trials in human heart failure (Lechat *et al.*, 1998). Unfortunately the short-term haemodynamic effects of beta-blockers can be disastrous, as they reduce contractility and exacerbate CHF. Although authorized for use in human heart failure, beta-blockers are not recommended in 'uncontrolled heart failure' (i.e. when congestive signs are present) and are started at very low doses and titrated upwards very gradually until a target dose is reached. There have been few published trials of beta-blockade in canine or feline CHF so far and evidence of benefit in clinical patients is still lacking (Oyama *et al.*, 2007).

Inotropes

Positive inotropes increase the strength of myocardial contraction (contractility). This is most commonly achieved by increasing cytosolic calcium concentrations, but may also be associated with increasing the sensitivity of the contractile proteins to calcium. High intracellular calcium concentrations may result in arrhythmias and several long-term human studies evaluating catecholamines or phosphodiesterase III inhibitors have indicated an increased risk of sudden death. This is not true of all positive inotropes, and similar human studies did not find the same risk with low-dose digoxin or calcium sensitizers. Care should also be taken extrapolating the results from human studies of coronary artery disease to canine patients with DCM or MMVD.

Pimobendan

Pimobendan is indicated in canine CHF associated with MMVD and DCM. Beneficial effects on survival have been seen in dogs with DCM and CHF, particularly in Dobermanns (Luis Fuentes *et al.*, 2002; O'Grady *et al.*, 2008). Pimobendan has also performed well in dogs with mitral valve disease and CHF when compared with an ACE inhibitor (Haggstrom *et al.*, 2008). Although few studies have evaluated the combination of furosemide, pimobendan and an ACE inhibitor in dogs with valve disease, this is usually the preferred protocol. Pimobendan has not been studied in cats.

Mechanism: Pimobendan has calcium sensitizing effects and is also an inhibitor of phosphodiesterase (PDE3). Both effects result in increased myocardial contractility, and the PDE3 inhibition also causes vasodilation. The relative inotropic contributions of the two pathways partly depend on the degree of down-regulation of the beta adrenergic signalling system (which produces the cyclic adenosine monophosphate (AMP) that is broken down by PDE3). This beta adrenergic pathway is down-regulated in heart failure and so the calcium sensitization may be a more important mediator of increased contractility in dogs with heart failure compared with normal dogs. The PDE3-mediated vasodilatory effects are *not* down-regulated in heart failure in the same way,

so the vasodilatory effects persist even in heart failure. The vasodilation extends to the venous and arterial system and the systemic and pulmonary circulation. Pimobendan may also have some anti-cytokine effects (Matsumori *et al.*, 2000).

Dosage: The recommended dosage is 0.1–0.3 mg/kg orally q12h. Pimobendan is given orally on an empty stomach, as food interferes with absorption. Peak onset after oral dosing is rapid, with effects evident within an hour. The active metabolites of pimobendan result in a longer duration of action than predicted from its half-life.

Adverse effects: Pimobendan appears to be well tolerated in dogs. There is always concern over proarrhythmia with positive inotropes, but survival studies in dogs with CHF have shown improved survival rather than increased mortality (Luis Fuentes *et al.*, 2002; Haggstrom *et al.*, 2008; O'Grady *et al.*, 2008). Pimobendan is not recommended in asymptomatic MMVD (Chetboul *et al.*, 2007) and should not be used with outflow tract obstruction.

Levosimendan

Levosimendan is another calcium sensitizer which can be administered intravenously or orally (Masutani *et al.*, 2008).

Digoxin

Digoxin has relatively weak positive inotropic effects and is used more for its effects on atrioventricular node conduction in atrial fibrillation than for its positive inotropic effects (see Chapter 20). It is, however, one of the few negative chronotropes that is not a negative inotrope. Few randomized studies have ever been carried out in dogs (Kittleson *et al.*, 1985), but a fairly neutral effect was found in a large placebo-controlled study of digoxin in 5000 human patients (Digitalis Investigation Group, 1997). Further analysis of the data showed that arrhythmic complications were more common at higher serum concentrations and most benefit occurred at lower doses.

Mechanism: Digoxin inhibits the sodium–potassium–adenosine triphosphatase (ATPase) pump and thus results in the increased cytosolic calcium concentrations that lead to its positive inotropic effects.

Dosage: The dosage is unpredictable because of a long half-life (15–55 hours) and the need to dose according to lean bodyweight (important in obese animals or those with large effusions). The dose should also be reduced with renal disease. Currently the ideal serum concentrations are lower than previously recommended (0.6–1.1 ng/ml for trough concentrations at 8–12 hours post-pill) and should be checked 5–7 days after starting treatment. There are few (if any) indications for intravenous digoxin.

Adverse effects: The therapeutic window is very narrow with digoxin and adverse effects are common. These include gastrointestinal effects (inappetence, vomiting, diarrhoea) as well as a wide range of arrhythmias (both bradyarrhythmias and tachyarrhythmias).

Dobutamine

Dobutamine is a catecholamine with potent positive inotropic effects and is indicated in cases with severe low output signs. Although human studies have shown adverse effects on survival (O'Connor *et al.*, 1999), the short-term effects can be life-saving.

Mechanism: Dobutamine has relatively selective beta-1 agonist properties, resulting in an increase in contractility with minimal vascular effects at low doses. Interaction with cardiac beta-1 receptors leads to increased calcium entry and an increase in cytosolic calcium concentrations. This beta adrenergic signalling pathway is down-regulated in chronic heart failure, with a reduction in beta-1 receptors compared with normal animals so that the effects on contractility are weaker in dogs with heart failure.

Dosage: Dobutamine has a very short half-life, so must be given as a CRI. The dose should be started low (≤2.5 μg/kg/minute) and titrated upwards until the desired beneficial effect is reached (improvement in perfusion, blood pressure and attitude) or adverse effects are seen (usually tachycardia or tachyarrhythmias). In dogs with CHF, adverse effects are usually seen at doses >10 μg/kg/minute. The beneficial effects diminish over 48 hours, as down-regulation of the beta-receptors is hastened by the dobutamine. Dobutamine is generally considered to be contraindicated in cats, but it can be helpful in patients with severe low output signs (i.e. with hypotension, hypothermia and bradycardia).

Adverse effects: The main adverse effects are tachycardia or tachyarrhythmias. Nevertheless, dobutamine is not necessarily contraindicated in dogs with poor output signs and fast atrial fibrillation; occasionally heart rate may even decrease with dobutamine if there is sufficient improvement in cardiac output that endogenous sympathetic outflow is reduced. Doses should always be carefully titrated. Other adverse effects include nausea and vomiting, or seizures (particularly in cats).

Vasodilators

Nitroprusside

Nitroprusside is not commonly used, but is a very potent vasodilator. It can be helpful in cases with acute non-responsive alveolar pulmonary oedema, when used in conjunction with furosemide. The potent arteriolar-dilating effects can lower arterial pressures and so direct blood pressure monitoring is ideal. It is often used in conjunction with dobutamine for this reason, to help to maintain blood pressure. It is given as a CRI and the dose should be titrated to effect, starting at low doses (1 μg/kg/minute) and increasing until the desired effect is reached or until systolic blood pressure falls below 90 mmHg. There is cumulative cyanide toxicity with its use and so it is generally only used for about 24 hours. The administration set should be protected from light, as nitroprusside is light-sensitive.

Glyceryl trinitrate

Glyceryl trinitrate is also a nitrate vasodilator, but has mainly venodilatory effects. These effects do not appear to be potent. Glyceryl trinitrate is given as a percutaneous ointment, often on the inside of the pinna or in the groin area. Perfusion, and therefore absorption, may be better from the groin, but the patient should not be allowed to lick the area. There is decreasing responsiveness to glyceryl trinitrate and so it is usually only used for a short period (if at all). Handling the ointment without gloves can lead to headaches.

Amlodipine

Amlodipine is a calcium channel antagonist with predominantly vascular effects. It causes direct arteriodilation, and is the drug of choice for managing systemic hypertension in cats (see Chapter 27). It may also be indicated in MMVD with CHF, although no clinical trials have been carried out with this drug in this patient group.

Hydralazine

Hydralazine is also an arteriodilator that has been used in refractory CHF in dogs with MMVD. It has now been largely superseded by amlodipine.

Diet

Few clinical trials have been carried out to investigate the effect of diet on management of CHF in dogs. Low-salt diets should not be used before the onset of CHF, as low sodium intake can activate the renin–angiotensin–aldosterone system. Low-salt diets tend to be unpalatable and are also difficult to use in advanced CHF, when appetite tend to be poor. Salt loading should be avoided, but modest salt restriction is probably better than aggressive salt restriction.

Other dietary additives include the nutraceuticals (co-enzyme Q10, L-carnitine, taurine). There may be benefit in selected cases (taurine deficiency in cats and American Cocker Spaniels; canine familial L-carnitine deficiency) but in most cases the effect of supplementation appears to be minimal. There is much more justification for omega-3 fatty acid supplementation, which may have an effect in cachexic dogs in particular (Freeman *et al.*, 1998). There may also be some antiarrhythmic benefits (Smith *et al.*, 2007).

Exercise

There are no studies examining the effect of exercise in canine heart failure. Advice for dogs with CHF is generally to restrict exercise as far as possible until signs of CHF resolve. There is less agreement on appropriate advice for animals with a history of previous CHF. In chronic heart failure in humans, regular moderate exercise training improves exercise tolerance (Jonsdottir *et al.*, 2006). Heart failure results in skeletal muscle changes similar to deconditioning, and exercise can reverse this. Both for these reasons and for optimal quality of life, it seems reasonable to recommend continuation of exercise for dogs with stable heart disease. Regular exercise is more likely to be beneficial than intermittent exercise. Conversely, sudden sprinting or extremes of exercise should be avoided in dogs with exertional syncope, or those at high risk of sudden death due to arrhythmias. As always, cats do their own thing.

References and further reading

Adin DB, Taylor AW, Hill RC, Scott KC and Martin FG (2003) Intermittent bolus injection versus continuous infusion of furosemide in normal adult greyhound dogs. *Journal of Veterinary Internal Medicine* **17**, 632–636

Atkins C, Bonagura J, Ettinger S *et al.* (2009) Guidelines for the diagnosis and treatment of canine chronic valvular disease. *Journal of Veterinary Internal Medicine* **23**, 1142–1150

Atkins CE, Keene BW, Brown WA *et al.* (2007) Results of the veterinary enalapril trial to prove reduction in onset of heart failure in dogs chronically treated with enalapril alone for compensated, naturally occurring mitral valve insufficiency. *Journal of the American Veterinary Medical Association* **231**, 1061–1069

BENCH Study Group (1999) The effect of benazepril on survival times and clinical signs of dogs with congestive heart failure: results of a multicenter, prospective, randomized, double-blinded, placebo-controlled, long-term clinical trial. *Journal of Veterinary Cardiology* **1**, 7–18

Chetboul V, Lefebvre HP, Sampedrano CC *et al.* (2007) Comparative adverse cardiac effects of pimobendan and benazepril monotherapy in dogs with mild degenerative mitral valve disease: a prospective, controlled, blinded, and randomized study. *Journal of Veterinary Internal Medicine* **21**, 742–753

Digitalis Investigation Group (1997) The effect of digoxin on mortality and morbidity in patients with heart failure. *New England Journal of Medicine* **336**, 525–533

El-Sayed MG, Atef M, El-Gendi AY and Youssef SA (1981) Disposition kinetics of furosemide in dogs. *Archives Internationale des Pharmacodynamie et de Therapie* **253**, 4–10

Ettinger SJ, Benitz AM, Ericsson GF *et al.* (1998) Effects of enalapril maleate on survival of dogs with naturally acquired heart failure. The Long-Term Investigation of Veterinary Enalapril (LIVE) Study Group. *Journal of the American Veterinary Medical Association* **213**, 1573–1577

Freeman LM, Rush JE, Kehayias JJ *et al.* (1998) Nutritional alterations and the effect of fish oil supplementation in dogs with heart failure. *Journal of Veterinary Internal Medicine* **12**, 440–448

Haggstrom J, Boswood A, O'Grady M *et al.* (2008) Effect of pimobendan or benazepril hydrochloride on survival times in dogs with congestive heart failure caused by naturally occurring myxomatous mitral valve disease: the QUEST study. *Journal of Veterinary Internal Medicine* **22**, 1124–1135

Jonsdottir S, Andersen KK, Sigurosson AF and Sigurosson SB (2006) The effect of physical training in chronic heart failure. *European Journal of Heart Failure* **8**, 97–101

Kittleson MD, Eyster GE, Knowlen GG, Bari Olivier N and Anderson LK (1985) Efficacy of digoxin administration in dogs with idiopathic congestive cardiomyopathy. *Journal of the American Veterinary Medical Association* **186**, 162–165

Kvart C, Haggstrom J, Pedersen HD *et al.* (2002) Efficacy of enalapril for prevention of congestive heart failure in dogs with myxomatous valve disease and asymptomatic mitral regurgitation. *Journal of Veterinary Internal Medicine* **16**, 80–88

Lechat P, Packer M, Chalon S *et al.* (1998) Clinical effects of beta-adrenergic blockade in chronic heart failure: a meta-analysis of double-blind, placebo-controlled, randomized trials. *Circulation* **98**, 1184–1191

Luis Fuentes V, Corcoran B, French A *et al.* (2002) A double-blind, randomized, placebo-controlled study of pimobendan in dogs with dilated cardiomyopathy. *Journal of Veterinary Internal Medicine* **16**, 255–261

MacDonald KA, Kittleson MD, Kass PH and White SD (2008) Effect of spironolactone on diastolic function and left ventricular mass in Maine Coon cats with familial hypertrophic cardiomyopathy. *Journal of Veterinary Internal Medicine* **22**, 335–341

MacDonald KA, Kittleson MD, Larson RF *et al.* (2006) The effect of ramipril on left ventricular mass, myocardial fibrosis, diastolic function, and plasma neurohormones in Maine Coon cats with familial hypertrophic cardiomyopathy without heart failure. *Journal of Veterinary Internal Medicine* **20**, 1093–1105

Masutani S, Cheng HJ, Hyttila-Hopponen M *et al.* (2008) Orally available levosimendan dose-related positive inotropic and lusitropic effect in conscious chronically instrumented normal and heart failure dogs. *Journal of Pharmacology and Experimental Therapeutics* **325**, 236–247

Matsumori A, Nunokawa Y and Sasayama S (2000) Pimobendan inhibits the activation of transcription factor NF-kappaB: a mechanism which explains its inhibition of cytokine production and inducible nitric oxide synthase. *Life Sciences* **67**, 2513–2519

O'Connor CM, Gattis WA, Uretsky BF *et al.* (1999) Continuous intravenous dobutamine is associated with an increased risk of death in patients with advanced heart failure: insights from the Flolan International Randomized Survival Trial (FIRST). *American Heart Journal* **138**, 78–86

O'Grady MR, Minors SL, O'Sullivan ML and Horne R (2008) Effect of pimobendan on case fatality rate in Doberman Pinschers with congestive heart failure caused by dilated cardiomyopathy. *Journal of Veterinary Internal Medicine* **22**, 897–904

O'Grady MR, O'Sullivan ML, Minors SL and Horne R (2009) Efficacy of benazepril hydrochloride to delay the progression of occult dilated cardiomyopathy in Doberman Pinschers. *Journal of Veterinary Internal Medicine* **23**, 977–983

Oyama MA, Gidlewski J and Sisson DD (2003) Effect of ACE-inhibition on dynamic left-ventricular obstruction in cats with hypertrophic obstructive cardiomyopathy. *Journal of Veterinary Internal Medicine* **17**, 400

Oyama MA, Sisson DD, Prosek R *et al.* (2007) Carvedilol in dogs with dilated cardiomyopathy. *Journal of Veterinary Internal Medicine* **21**, 1272–1279

Perry GJ, Wei CC, Hankes GH *et al.* (2002) Angiotensin II receptor blockade does not improve left ventricular function and remodeling in subacute mitral regurgitation in the dog. *Journal of the American College of Cardiology* **39**, 1374–1379

Pitt B, Zannad F, Remme WJ *et al.* (1999) The effect of spironolactone on mobidity and mortality in patients with severe heart failure. *New England Journal of Medicine* **341**, 709–717

Smith CE, Freeman LM, Rush JE, Cunningham SM and Biourge V (2007) Omega-3 fatty acids in boxer dogs with arrhythmogenic right ventricular cardiomyopathy. *Journal of Veterinary Internal Medicine* **21**, 265–273

19

Management of chronic respiratory disease

Lynelle R. Johnson

Introduction

Chronic respiratory disease in the dog or cat is manifest primarily by persistent or recurrent cough, tachypnoea, progressive respiratory effort, and sometimes by loud breathing. The most common diseases that require constant management are asthma in the cat, chronic bronchitis in the dog or cat, bronchiectasis (more common in the dog than the cat), ciliary dyskinesia, eosinophilic lung disease in the dog, and some forms of interstitial lung disease. Appropriate therapy requires a complete diagnostic work up and an individualized approach to treatment. Various options for therapy include corticosteroids (oral or inhaled), bronchodilators (oral or inhaled), antibiotics, antitussives and mucolytic agents. Additional interventions that should be considered include environmental improvements, control of obesity, nebulization and coupage, and home oxygen therapy.

Corticosteroids

Oral therapy

Corticosteroids are indicated for long-term control of feline bronchial disease, canine chronic bronchitis and eosinophilic lung disease. Specific details on the length of therapy required for control of signs are unknown, but most cases require lifelong treatment, either intermittently or continuously. Corticosteroids reduce inflammation through inhibition of phospholipase A2, the enzyme responsible for the initial release of arachidonic acid for metabolism into inflammatory mediators. Corticosteroids also decrease migration of inflammatory cells into the airway and thus the concentration of granulocyte products (major basic protein, eosinophil cationic protein, reactive oxygen species) that lead to airway injury.

Short-acting oral steroids (prednisolone) are preferred for treatment of inflammatory airway disease in the dog or cat to allow an accurate titration of the dose to control clinical signs with minimal side effects. Long-acting glucocorticoids such as dexamethasone, triamcinolone and methylprednisolone acetate do not have a therapeutic advantage over prednisolone, and use of a repositol steroid could result in waxing and waning inflammation between injections. Prednisolone is preferred in the cat, while prednisolone or prednisone can be used in the dog.

The duration and dose of corticosteroid therapy will depend upon the degree and chronicity of respiratory embarrassment, the severity of the pulmonary infiltrate, and the severity of inflammation on cytology. An individualized approach to anti-inflammatory treatment is required for each case.

Cats

In the cat, prednisolone is usually administered orally at 1 mg/kg q12h for 5–10 days. The dosage can be decreased to 1 mg/kg q24h for 10–20 days if a good therapeutic response is seen and then further decreased to 0.5 mg/kg q24h. Although cats are relatively resistant to the side effects of corticosteroids, an attempt should be made to achieve the lowest dose of the drug that will control signs. Approximately one-half to two-thirds of cats will require lifelong medication (Foster *et al.*, 2004ab). Recurrent episodes of coughing or respiratory distress necessitate a return to a higher dosage with a longer taper in the dose. Repeat diagnostic testing may also be indicated.

Dogs

Clinical signs of chronic bronchitis and eosinophilic bronchopneumopathy are also due to airway inflammation, and therapy with glucocorticoids is successful in resolving clinical signs in the majority of dogs. It is important that infectious diseases are ruled out before the initiation of anti-inflammatory treatment, and that coexisting diseases such as severe dental disease or congestive heart failure are controlled before using glucocorticoids.

In dogs with chronic bronchitis, an initial oral dosage of 0.5 mg/kg q12h of prednisolone is usually successful in inducing remission of clinical signs. In dogs with eosinophilic lung disease, a higher dose (0.5–1 mg/kg q12h) is often required. Larger dogs seem to suffer more severe or noticeable side effects with steroids than do smaller dogs, and somewhat lower doses may be appropriate.

The initial dose of corticosteroid is generally employed for 5–10 days, and the dosage should be decreased as clinical signs abate. In dogs with chronic bronchitis, dose reductions can generally be achieved every 10–14 days, but dogs with eosinophilic lung disease often require higher doses of steroid for a longer period of time. As soon as possible, drugs should be tapered to an alternate-day basis to allow normalization of the pituitary–adrenal axis. Long-term therapy (2–3 months for dogs with chronic bronchitis and 4–5 months for dogs with eosinophilic disease) can be anticipated in most cases, but discontinuation of medication may be possible eventually. If disease worsens during lowering of the dose, a return to the higher dose of glucocorticoid that controlled clinical signs is generally required. Alternatively, treatment with inhaled steroids, bronchodilators, or antitussive agents can be added (see below).

Inhaled therapy

Various corticosteroid preparations are available as metered dose inhalers (MDIs) (Figure 19.1).

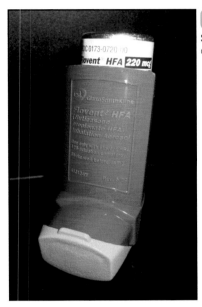

19.1 Standard metered dose inhaler (MDI).

Facemasks and spacers

Because animals will not actively inspire on command, administration of inhaled medication requires attachment of the MDI to a spacer device with facemask. The spacer collects an aerosol cloud from the MDI so that particles will deposit into the lower airways during tidal respirations. In healthy cats, nebulization of a radiolabelled product administered via spacer and facemask resulted in adequate pulmonary deposition (Schulman *et al.*, 2004). Investigation of pulmonary deposition of drug delivery from an MDI attached to a facemask has not been performed and distribution into the airways of dogs or cats with airway disease has not yet been established; however, clinically, this method of drug administration has proved efficacious in controlling clinical signs (Bexfield *et al.*, 2006).

A tightly fitting but comfortable facemask is critical for successful therapy, and it is important to ensure that the dog breathes normally for 8–10 seconds. Another option is to obtain a mask that encloses the nose and lips. Brachycephalic dogs often can be fitted with a facemask built for a cat, or one obtained from a local pharmacy or respiratory supply company as the shape of the face is similar to that in humans. For dolicocephalic breeds, anaesthetic or cone-shaped facemasks are required (Figure 19.2).

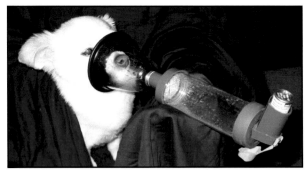

19.2 For deposition of aerosolized particles into the lung, the drug is actuated into a spacing chamber connected to a facemask that conforms tightly to the muzzle or fits over the nose. The animal should take in 8–10 breaths to ensure that the proper dose is inhaled.

Drug dosage and administration

In dogs or cats with moderate to severe clinical manifestations of disease, standard doses of oral steroids are generally recommended during the first several weeks of inhaled therapy because of a delay in the efficacy of inhaled medications. The oral dose can be tapered downwards depending on the clinical response.

The most commonly recommended steroid is fluticasone propionate inhalation powder, which is available in an MDI containing 120 doses. The MDI is usually available in low, medium or high strength, and the medium strength preparation is used most commonly at this time.

The MDI must be well shaken prior to actuation, and must be attached to the spacer before the dose is ejected. Typically, the MDI is actuated once per treatment, and the animal inhales 8–10 breaths (10 seconds) to deposit drug in the airways.

Advantages and disadvantages of inhalants

Some of the side effects noted in human medicine include thinning of skin and perioral dermatitis or infection (particularly with candidiasis). These have not been noted in veterinary patients to date. Clinical adrenal suppression can occur with long-term and high-dose use in human patients; but although suppression of the hypothalamic–pituitary–adrenocortical axis has been reported in cats, systemic side effects are not noted (Reinero *et al.*, 2006) and clinical problems are rarely encountered.

Inhaled medications are more expensive than oral medications, but they may result in improved owner compliance, particularly when animals are difficult to medicate orally and chronic therapy is required. In dogs, this method of therapy is particularly advantageous when side effects of steroids are severe or when concurrent diseases (diabetes, heart disease, pancreatitis, or renal disease) make oral steroid therapy undesirable. Many owners find that animals tolerate inhalation treatment readily, though problems may be encountered. For example, some cats may be frightened by actuation of the MDI, but they can become habituated to the sound with training. In cats suffering an acute asthmatic attack, tolerance of the small facemask is poor and alternative therapy should be considered. An additional concern might be the competence of drug delivery because owners lack ability to deploy the device correctly, or because of a failure of the device to induce deposition of aerosol into constricted or mucus-laden airways. It is unclear whether this is a concern in veterinary patients. Finally, breath holding by the dog or cat can be a reason for treatment failure.

Bronchodilators

The two main classes of bronchodilator used in veterinary medicine are methylxanthine derivatives (theophylline) and beta-adrenergic agonists. While these agents may provide only mild dilation of airway smooth muscle, they are often clinically helpful in reducing signs in dogs or cats with bronchitis, or in allowing a reduction in the dosage of glucocorticoid required to control signs. Both methylxanthine derivatives and beta agonists seem to act synergistically with glucocorticoids in the control of inflammatory lung disease. Theophylline may provide some relief from clinical signs by preventing acute attacks of bronchoconstriction in predisposed cats, by suppressing inflammation, or by reducing the dose of steroid required.

Methylxanthines

Methylxanthine drugs are phosphodiesterase inhibitors that inhibit the breakdown of cyclic adenosine monophosphate (cAMP). However, the dose of theophylline used clinically does not result in accumulation of cAMP sufficient to cause smooth muscle relaxation with resultant bronchodilation. Current research suggests that the clinical effects of methylxanthines likely result from adenosine antagonism or from alterations in cellular sensitivity to calcium. Theophylline may provide other beneficial effects by increasing diaphragmatic muscle strength, improving pulmonary perfusion, reducing respiratory effort and stimulating mucociliary clearance (in dogs, but not in cats). Extended-release theophylline (Inwood Labarotories, 10 mg/kg orally q12h) has been shown to achieve plasma levels in dogs that approximate to the human therapeutic range of 10–20 mg/ml (Bach et al., 2004). In cats, the recommended dosage is 15 mg/kg (tablets) or 19 mg/kg (caplets) q24h in the evening (Guenther-Yenke et al., 2007).

Side effects

Adverse effects of methylxanthines are probably related to adenosine antagonism and include gastrointestinal upset, tachycardia and hyperexcitability. It is essential to individualize drug therapy because there is a wide variation in the dose that causes side effects. Theophylline metabolism is influenced by many factors, including fibre in the diet, smoke in the environment, congestive heart failure and the use of other drugs. In older dogs or dogs with concurrent disease, side effects might be lessened by starting therapy with half the recommended dose (5 mg/kg q12h). If clinical signs improve and the dog tolerates the drug, the dosage may be increased as needed.

Beta agonists

Administration of a beta-2 agonist (terbutaline or salbutamol) results in bronchodilation due to direct relaxation of airway smooth muscle, and intravenous terbutaline has been shown to reduce airway resistance acutely in cats with constricted airways (Dye et al., 1996). Preliminary pharmacokinetic studies have established the safety of the drug, and the recommended dose is 0.01 mg/kg parenterally, or 0.625 mg/cat and 0.625–5.0 mg/dog orally q12h. Active bronchoconstriction does not play a role in canine chronic bronchitis as it does in cats with bronchitis, but salbutamol at 50 µg/kg orally q8h was efficacious in reducing cough in almost half the dogs evaluated in a review of canine chronic bronchitis (Padrid et al., 1990). The bronchodilator also resulted in a reduction in the severity of the pulmonary infiltrate. Theoretically, down-regulation of beta-receptor density could occur with chronic use, resulting in decreased efficacy of the drug, but it is unclear whether this is recognized clinically.

Side effects

As with methylxanthines, beta agonists may result in excitability or tremors during initial therapy, but animals usually become accustomed to the drug. Beta-2 agonists are also widely available for inhaled therapy.

Antibiotics

In general, antibiotic treatment should be utilized for immediate control of infectious lung disease. However, in some situations, chronic antibiotic therapy or intermittent pulse therapy with antibiotics may be required to control clinical signs in dogs with bronchiectasis and animals with ciliary dyskinesia. In these disorders, mucus accumulation with trapping of bacteria in secretions can result in severe pneumonia.

Antibiotic choice should be based on culture and sensitivity results whenever possible and should have a broad spectrum of activity against bacteria commonly found in the lung, such as enteric organisms, anaerobes and *Mycoplasma* spp. (Jameson et al., 1995; Angus et al., 1997; Foster et al., 2004a). The antibiotic chosen should be lipophilic, to facilitate penetration of the airway, and should be relatively free of side effects.

In patients with concurrent bronchiectasis or ciliary dyskinesia that develop signs of pneumonia, intermittent, pulse or chronic antibiotic therapy is often required; broad-spectrum antibiotics or combinations of antibiotics should be chosen because infection may involve various Gram-negative bacteria (especially *Pseudomonas*) and anaerobes.

Chloramphenicol (50 mg/kg orally q8h), trimethoprim/sulphonamide (15 mg/kg orally q12h), metronidazole (10–15 mg/kg orally q12h) or clindamycin (11 mg/kg orally q12h) combined with enrofloxacin (5 mg/kg q24h) can be helpful in resolving disease. Doxycycline (3–5 mg/kg orally q12h) and azithromycin (5–10 mg/kg q24h for 3–5 days and then 2–3 times weekly) are also reasonable alternatives. These drugs have all the desired attributes for treating pulmonary infection, are relatively devoid of side effects, and also have some anti-inflammatory effects. With doxycycline, owners should be instructed to supply water after administering the drug to propel the pill fully into the stomach, thus avoiding the possibility of an oesophageal stricture due to delay in oesophageal transit.

Length of antibiotic treatment depends on whether pneumonia is present or whether bronchial colonization and infection are suspected. True pneumonia generally requires 3–6 weeks of antibiotic therapy, whereas 5–10 days of treatment will usually resolve signs related to bronchial colonization.

If a quinolone is needed in an animal on theophylline, it is important to note that this class of drug inhibits its metabolism, and use of the two drugs together results in toxic plasma levels of theophylline (Intorre *et al.*, 1995). At least a 30% reduction in theophylline dose is recommended when a quinolone is being used concurrently.

Antitussive agents

The cough reflex is of major importance in animals, because it serves the essential function of clearing secretions from the airway. Suppression of this reflex before resolution of inflammation can be deleterious because mucus can become trapped in small airways, and prolonged contact between inflammatory mediators in the mucus and epithelial cells perpetuates airway inflammation. If infection is present, cough suppression may result in more serious pneumonia. When clinical signs suggest that inflammation is resolving yet the cough persists, cough suppression is desirable because chronic coughing can lead to repeated airway injury and syncopal events. Cough suppressants are often required in dogs with resolving chronic bronchitis or airway collapse.

Over-the-counter dextromethorphan-containing compounds are occasionally efficacious in some animals with airway disease. When more potent suppression of a dry cough is required, narcotic agents should be prescribed. Hydrocodone (0.22 mg/kg orally q6–12h) or butorphanol (0.5 mg/kg orally q6–12h) can be used in dogs. These agents must be given at an interval that suppresses coughing without inducing excessive sedation. The drugs are initially given at a higher dose and frequently and then tapered to the lowest dose that controls clinical signs. Long-term therapy may be required in some patients, particularly when airway collapse is also present. Overuse should be avoided since tolerance will develop, necessitating dose escalation.

Mucolytic agents

Marked controversy exists concerning the utility of mucolytic agents in human medicine and there is little information on their use in veterinary patients. Clinical experience suggests that some dogs and cats with excessive production of airway secretions associated with chronic inflammatory disease may benefit from their use. Conditions that might be considered indications for mucolytic agents include chronic bronchitis, bronchiectasis and possibly ciliary dyskinesia. In animals with viscid secretions associated with pneumonia, mucolytics might also be beneficial.

Mucolytic/expectorant agents such as *N*-acetylcysteine, bromhexine, *S*-carboxymethylcysteine, ambroxol and iodinated glycerol can thin the viscosity of mucin-containing secretions. These drugs act by a variety of mechanisms, including breakage of disulphide bonds in airway mucoproteins, stimulation of serous airway secretions, or breakdown of acid mucopolysaccharide fibres in sputum. *N*-Acetylcysteine and *S*-carboxymethylcysteine can be administered orally or by inhalation (although an irritant effect may result in bronchoconstriction) while the remainder of these agents are designed for oral use. *N*-Acetylcysteine also has a variety of antioxidant and endothelial effects that might prove beneficial in respiratory patients. Oral dosing of *N*-acetylcysteine is most convenient, and dosages are generally extrapolated from those used in human patients.

Environmental control

Irritants in the environment, such as smoke, pollens and particulate matter, are known to induce various respiratory diseases in people and in experimental animal models of disease, and it is likely that poor air quality can induce or worsen chronic respiratory diseases in dogs and cats. Therefore, a complete environmental history is essential when developing a list of differential diagnoses for the respiratory patient and when designing a treatment plan. Particular attention should be paid to both indoor and outdoor air quality, with questions directed to exposure to cigarette smoke, the presence of environmental or industrial pollutants, and identification of any unusual agricultural sprays or cooking odours.

Air pollutants or irritants may be much higher indoors than outdoors due to improved insulation during home construction. Indoor air quality can be improved by vigilant upkeep of central-heating boiler filters and air-conditioning vents. If these elements are not maintained, worsened clinical signs may be noted when these units are initially activated at the beginning of the season. Reducing dust or particulate matter in carpets can be beneficial, and installation of an air filter or purification unit may help to control exacerbations of respiratory disease.

Dietary therapy

Obesity is a common finding in the pet population and animals with chronic respiratory disease suffer from worsening of cough and respiratory effort when obesity results in poor lung expansion, reduced thoracic volume and increased work in breathing. Obesity worsens clinical signs in dogs with chronic bronchitis by decreasing thoracic wall compliance and increasing abdominal pressure on the diaphragm.

Improvements in exercise tolerance and arterial oxygenation can be seen with weight loss alone. Owners should be given reasonable goals for the dog's optimal weight and the time in which weight loss can be achieved. The resting energy requirement (RER, in kcal/day) can be used to calculate the daily calories to be provided for an obese dog to start a weight loss programme: RER = 70 × (body weight in kg)$^{0.75}$. A weight loss of 1–2% per week is desirable but highly difficult to achieve (German *et al.*, 2007). Marked energy restriction and rigorous owner compliance are required. Use of a high-fibre, high-protein diet may improve participation in a weight loss programme by enhancing satiety in patients and thus reducing food-seeking behaviour (Weber *et al.*, 2007). When possible, the animal should be encouraged to participate in gradually increasing amounts of exercise. Close monitoring of owner compliance and offering praise for accomplishments in the weight loss programme seem to enhance the overall success.

Nebulization and coupage

Liquefaction and removal of airway secretions from the lower airway can be very beneficial in dogs or cats that suffer from diseases resulting in excessive mucus production or pooling of secretions in the lower airways. An ultrasonic or compressed air nebulizer creates particle sizes that are sufficiently small (1–4 µm) to travel into the small airways and provide added liquid to airway secretions. Sterile water or saline without preservatives can be purchased in single-unit vials. A small aquarium or plastic container can be modified to allow introduction of the nebulized liquid and venting of exhaled carbon dioxide; cats can be easily nebulized in a carrier that is covered with a plastic bag (Figure 19.3). One to four treatments per day can be administered as needed. Gentle exercise or coupage following nebulization will encourage evacuation of airway mucus (Figure 19.4).

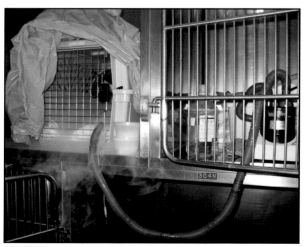

19.3 An ultrasonic nebulizer hose is inserted into a cat carrier covered in plastic wrap to create a nebulization chamber.

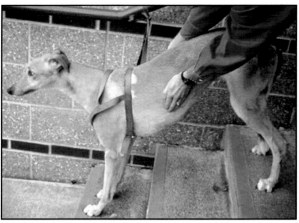

19.4 Using cupped hands, coupage is performed in a ventral to dorsal and caudal to cranial orientation to facilitate expectoration of mucus. Postural drainage can be helpful when performing respiratory therapy.

Home oxygen therapy

Treatment with oxygen at home can be helpful in dogs or cats with severe interstitial lung disease, particularly when the condition is complicated by pulmonary hypertension. This type of therapy requires a very dedicated owner and benefits are not easily quantifiable. However, some owners do indicate that providing supplemental oxygen throughout the night appears to improve the overall wellbeing of their pet. Owners can construct an oxygen chamber from perspex (plexiglass) that contains inlet and outlet valves and provide oxygen through a tank or compressor-driven system. The fraction of inspired oxygen can often be maintained at around 40–50% to provide an oxygen-enriched environment.

References and further reading

Angus JC, Jang SS and Hirsh DC (1997) Microbiologic study of transtracheal aspirates from dogs with suspected lower respiratory tract disease: 264 cases (1989–1995). *Journal of the American Veterinary Medical Association* **210**, 55–58

Bach JE, Kukanich B, Papich MG *et al.* (2004) Evaluation of the bioavailability and pharmacokinetics of two extended-release theophylline formulations in dogs. *Journal of the American Veterinary Medical Association* **224**, 1113–1119

Bexfield NH, Foale RD, Davison LJ *et al.* (2006) Management of 13 cases of canine respiratory disease using inhaled corticosteroids. *Journal of Small Animal Practice* **47**, 377–382

Dye JA, McKiernan BC, Rozanski EA *et al.* (1996) Bronchopulmonary disease in the cat: historical, physical, radiographic, clinicopathologic, and pulmonary functional evaluation of 24 affected and 15 healthy cats. *Journal of Veterinary Internal Medicine* **10**, 385–400

Foster SF, Allan GS, Martin P *et al.* (2004a) Twenty five cases of feline bronchial disease (1995–2000). *Journal of Feline Medicine and Surgery* **6**, 181–188

Foster SF, Martin P, Allan GS *et al.* (2004b) Lower respiratory tract infections in cats: 21 cases (1995–2000). *Journal of Feline Medicine and Surgery* **6**, 167–180

German AJ, Holden SL, Bissot T *et al.* (2007) Dietary energy restriction and successful weight loss in obese client-owned dogs. *Journal of Veterinary Internal Medicine* **21**, 1174–1180

Guenther-Yenke CL, McKiernan BC, Papich MG *et al.* (2007) Pharmacokinetics of an extended-release theophylline product in cats. *Journal of the American Veterinary Medical Association* **231**, 900–906

Intorre L, Mengozzi G, Maccheroni M *et al.* (1995) Enrofloxacin–theophylline interaction: influence of enrofloxacin on theophylline steady-state pharmacokinetics in the Beagle dog. *Journal of Veterinary Pharmacology and Therapeutics* **18**, 352–356

Jameson PH, King LA, Lappin MR and Jones RL (1995) Comparison of clinical signs, diagnostic findings, organisms isolated, and clinical outcome in dogs with bacterial pneumonia: 93 cases (1986–1991). *Journal of the American Veterinary Medical Association* **15**, 206–209

Padrid PA, Hornof W, Kurpershoek C *et al.* (1990) Canine chronic bronchitis: a pathophysiologic evaluation of 18 cases. *Journal of Veterinary Internal Medicine* **4**, 172–181

Reinero CR, Brownlee L, Decile KC *et al.* (2006) Inhaled flunisolide suppresses the hypothalamic–pituitary–adrenocortical axis, but has minimal systemic immune effects in healthy cats. *Journal of Veterinary Internal Medicine* **20**, 57–64

Schulman RL, Crochik SS, Kneller SJ *et al.* (2004) Investigation of pulmonary deposition of a nebulized radiopharmaceutical agent in awake cats. *American Journal of Veterinary Research* **65**, 806–809

Weber M, Bissot T, Servet E *et al.* (2007) A high-protein, high-fiber diet designed for weight loss improves satiety in dogs. *Journal of Veterinary Internal Medicine* **21**, 1203–1208

20

Antiarrhythmic therapies

Simon Dennis

Introduction

Optimal cardiac function is achieved by a coordinated pattern of cardiac contraction and relaxation that is regulated by electrical activity within the heart (see Chapter 16). Severe arrhythmias (or the development of an arrhythmia in a patient with already compromised cardiac function) may result in impaired cardiac output, increased filling pressures and increased myocardial work (haemodynamic instability). Less severe arrhythmias may not cause haemodynamic instability; however, some can be a premonitory sign of a more severe arrhythmia or sudden death (electrical instability).

Haemodynamic or electrical instability may cause one or more adverse clinical sequelae:

- Signs of haemodynamic compromise
- Progression of concurrent cardiac disease
- Sudden cardiac death.

From this, *treatment of arrhythmias appears desirable*.

Antiarrhythmic therapies can come in many forms. The simplest and most effective therapy is treatment of the underlying condition causing the arrhythmia (e.g. gastric dilatation–volvulus, sepsis, heart failure). When this is not possible or effective, specific antiarrhythmic interventions may be necessary. These include antiarrhythmic drugs and electrical therapies (e.g. synchronized DC cardioversion, defibrillation, pacemaker therapy). All antiarrhythmic therapies have limitations, the most important of which is the potential to worsen the arrhythmia or the clinical status of the patient.

Antiarrhythmic drugs are fairly non-selective in action, possessing not only beneficial effects for suppressing arrhythmias in diseased areas of cardiac tissue, but also adverse effects that may potentiate arrhythmias in other areas of the heart (proarrhythmia). Some drugs adversely affect cardiac function or cause adverse non-cardiac effects. External electrical stimulation is inherently painful and therefore limited to patients under general anaesthesia (e.g. transthoracic pacing during pacemaker implantation) or for the treatment of acute, life-threatening arrhythmias (e.g. defibrillation during cardiac resuscitation). Internal pacemaker therapy in small animal cardiology is currently reserved for the treatment of bradyarrhythmias that result in clinical signs and carries a variety of risks, including intra-operative death, lead dislodgement and infection. When used inappropriately any antiarrhythmic therapy has the potential to cause harm, including death. Therefore, *antiarrhythmic therapy should not be considered completely benign*.

This apparent contradiction between the desire to treat an arrhythmia and to 'first do no harm' results in a therapeutic challenge for any clinician faced with managing a patient with an arrhythmia. Critical decision making is the key to appropriate management. Answering a few simple questions can help to determine the most appropriate treatment for any patient with an arrhythmia:

1. Is there a treatable underlying condition?
2. What are the potential adverse effects of the arrhythmia?
3. What are the potential effects (beneficial and adverse) of antiarrhythmic therapy?

Is there a treatable underlying condition?

Conditions that cause arrhythmias do so by altering myocardial structure, intra- or extracellular fluid composition, or neural control and include:

- Structural cardiac disease
- Cardiac trauma
- Autonomic imbalance
- Myocardial hypoxia
- Metabolic abnormalities
- Inflammation
- Drugs/toxins
- Extremes of temperature.

It is extremely important to identify any underlying disease that may cause an arrhythmia, as the most effective antiarrhythmic therapy is to abolish the cause (see Chapter 16). Treatment of the underlying disease alone may be sufficient to resolve the arrhythmia in some cases (e.g. oxygen supplementation in hypoxaemia). In other cases, a concurrent condition may be an important reason for failure of an antiarrhythmic therapy (e.g. hypokalaemia with ventricular tachycardia). It is also important to identify conditions that are not easily treatable and carry a poor prognosis for recovery, such as cardiac neoplasia and end-stage organ failure. Antiarrhythmic therapy may be less effective in these patients.

For patients with arrhythmias secondary to critical systemic disease, it is important to ensure adequate oxygen supplementation and analgesia (if required) and to correct any fluid or electrolyte abnormalities.

What are the potential adverse effects of the arrhythmia?

The potential adverse effects of arrhythmias are the development of signs of haemodynamic compromise, progression of concurrent cardiac disease and sudden cardiac death. These can develop as a consequence of haemodynamic instability, electrical instability, or a combination of both.

Haemodynamic instability
Haemodynamically unstable arrhythmias are those that compromise cardiac function sufficiently to result in poor cardiac output or congestive heart failure (CHF). Poor cardiac output results in clinical signs of hypoperfusion, including:

- Lethargy
- Depressed mentation
- Weakness
- Collapse
- Pallor
- Poor pulse quality
- Cold extremities
- Hypothermia.

Unless concurrent myocardial failure is present, these signs usually only accompany sustained arrhythmias at very rapid rates (e.g. supraventricular tachycardia, ventricular tachycardia) or very slow rates (e.g. third-degree atrioventricular (AV) block). Patients are frequently hypotensive, although some are normotensive with signs of intermittent hypoperfusion. These patients may have no signs of hypoperfusion on examination, but instead have a history of exercise intolerance, episodic weakness or syncope, which develop when there is an increase in metabolic demand (e.g. during exercise) and/or from a transient worsening of the arrhythmia. This can be difficult to identify in animals with a sedentary lifestyle, such as cats and some dog breeds.

If an arrhythmia is suspected to be the cause of episodic collapse, it is important to rule out other conditions that resemble syncope (see Chapter 3). Obtaining a good description of the pattern of signs from the owner is essential. A video recording of collapse episodes may also help to differentiate syncope from seizure or muscular weakness. It is important to make attempts to document the actual cause of collapse in patients with known arrhythmias. Reports of bradyarrhythmia-related syncope in some Dobermanns and Boxers with concurrent ventricular arrhythmias highlight the fact that inappropriate presumptive therapy may be ineffective or even worsen clinical signs (Calvert *et al.*, 1996a; Thomason *et al.*,

2008). To this end, ambulatory (Holter) electrocardiogram (ECG) monitoring, exercise testing with ECG telemetry, or event monitoring with loop recording devices can be useful (see Chapter 9).

CHF tends to occur in patients with sustained tachy- or bradyarrhythmias. When CHF develops in patients without concurrent structural cardiac disease, it is more likely to be right-sided, since oedema develops at lower pressures in the systemic venous system than it does in the pulmonary system (see Chapter 15). Arrhythmias that cause both an abnormal heart rate and absent or asynchronous contractions are particularly likely to cause CHF, since both abnormalities elevate venous pressures independently. Examples include atrial fibrillation (AF) with a rapid ventricular rate, and third-degree AV block. A haemodynamically unstable arrhythmia almost invariably requires treatment. Therefore, a detailed history and thorough physical examination, including evaluation of mentation, inspection of veins, palpation of arterial pulses and assessment for effusions are vital for any animal with an arrhythmia.

Electrical instability
Electrically unstable arrhythmias are those that may result in sudden cardiac death due to the development of a life-threatening arrhythmia, such as pulseless ventricular tachycardia, ventricular fibrillation or asystole (see Chapter 16).

There is no consensus on which criteria are reliable indicators of electrical instability in small animals, and most are based on personal experience or evidence extrapolated from human studies. Most cardiologists agree that rapid, sustained ventricular tachycardia, third-degree or high-grade second-degree AV block (particularly with a ventricular rate <40 beats/minute or periods of ventricular standstill due to an unstable escape rhythm) and hyperkalaemic atrial standstill are potentially unstable arrhythmias, both electrically and haemodynamically. There is also general consensus that infrequent, isolated ventricular ectopy, low-grade AV block and short periods of sinus arrest do not require therapy in a patient without clinical signs, as these arrhythmias rarely result in haemodynamic compromise or electrical instability. Furthermore, supraventricular tachyarrhythmias rarely confer electrical instability and are therefore usually treated based on the presence of haemodynamic compromise or risk of myocardial failure due to tachycardia-mediated cardiomyopathy (see Chronic effects below).

The arrhythmias that present the most difficult therapeutic decisions for the clinician are complex or frequent ventricular arrhythmias that do not result in signs of haemodynamic compromise. Such arrhythmias include non-sustained ventricular tachycardia, ventricular runs, R-on-T phenomenon, polymorphic ventricular premature complexes, couplets, triplets and frequent ventricular premature complexes. It is possible that some or all of these arrhythmias are electrically unstable. From the experiences of human cardiology, couplets, triplets and non-sustained ventricular tachycardia do not confer an increased risk of sudden death in healthy individuals, but do in the presence of myocardial disease, particularly if systolic dysfunction is present (Goldberger *et al.*, 2008). However, it is not known whether the arrhythmias themselves increase risk of sudden death, as their prevention with antiarrhythmic therapy may not necessarily result in improved survival. This has been shown in several studies in humans, in which reduction of arrhythmias and even arrhythmic death was not associated with a reduction in overall mortality (CAST Investigators, 1989). Although there are obvious limitations in direct extrapolation from human studies, this highlights the need to treat the patient rather than simply the arrhythmia. For example, in certain myocardial diseases, even isolated ventricular premature complexes are a marker for more severe, potentially life-threatening arrhythmias. This should always be considered if ventricular arrhythmias are detected in breeds prone to cardiomyopathy with an increased risk of sudden death (such as Boxers and Dobermanns).

Cardiac arrest rhythms
Cardiac arrest rhythms are those that result in no discernable cardiac output. Irrespective of the underlying cause, immediate intervention is essential as death will rapidly ensue. Treatment involves basic cardiac life support (airway, breathing, circulation), followed by advanced cardiac life support (drugs, intravenous fluids, DC cardioversion/defibrillation) as appropriate. For further details, see texts describing cardiopulmonary–cerebral resuscitation (*BSAVA Manual of Canine and Feline Emergency and Critical Care*).

Chronic effects
As well as acute effects, some arrhythmias can have adverse effects in the medium and long term. These are usually seen in patients with sustained tachyarrhythmias or bradyarrhythmias, and treatment should therefore be considered in such cases. *Myocardial failure is an inevitable consequence of a sustained tachyarrhythmia over time* (tachycardia-mediated cardiomyopathy). This typically occurs with supraventricular tachycardias and has been demonstrated in various canine models. For example, rapid ventricular pacing at >240 beats/ minute for 2–3 weeks can cause myocardial failure in a previously healthy canine heart (Wilson *et al.*, 1987). As discussed above, these arrhythmias can also precipitate or potentiate CHF.

Intra-atrial thrombus formation is a potential complication of disease associated with atrial dilatation in cats. Arrhythmias that result in poor or absent atrial contraction are further risk factors for thrombus formation, particularly AF. Low-velocity atrial blood flow predisposes to platelet aggregation.

What are the potential effects of antiarrhythmic therapy?

Pharmacological antiarrhythmic therapies
The most widely used antiarrhythmic therapies in veterinary medicine are drugs. Antiarrhythmic drugs do not act simply to suppress arrhythmias, but instead act by altering the shape of action potentials in cardiac tissue, with the aim of making arrhythmogenesis less likely. Knowledge of the mechanisms behind generation of action potentials in different parts of the heart helps in understanding how different classes of antiarrhythmic agents act, but is not essential for most clinical scenarios.

Cardiac action potentials
The majority of cardiac tissue comprises cardiac myocytes. All myocytes are excitable cells, each with one or more additional functions, such as impulse generation and conduction, cellular contraction and relaxation. Cells with similar functions tend to have similar electrophysiological properties. On this basis, myocytes can be divided into three types of cell: nodal cells; His–Purkinje cells; and working myocardial cells. These three types of cell differ in their ability to generate and conduct an electrical impulse. This is reflected in the shape of their action potential.

An action potential is a graphical representation of the change in potential difference (voltage) across the cell membrane over time. This change in membrane voltage is caused by the movement of ions across the cell membrane, primarily sodium, calcium, potassium and chloride. For the purposes of classification, the action potential is divided into five phases, referred to in chronological order as phases 0–4. For ease of understanding it is better to consider the action potential in three broader phases: threshold depolarization (phase 0); repolarization (phases 1–3); and resting phase (phase 4). Nodal cells, His–Purkinje cells and diseased myocardial cells may also undergo variable degrees of depolarization during phase 4. Figure 20.1 shows typical action potentials in cells of the sinoatrial (SA) node, ventricular myocardium and Purkinje fibres.

The rate of phase 0 depolarization determines the speed at which an electrical impulse traverses a cell. This is referred to as the *conduction velocity*. The rate of phase 4 depolarization is referred to as *automaticity*. The time taken for a cell to recover excitability is referred to as the *refractory period*. This is determined predominantly by the duration of repolarization (phases 1–3).

The differences in ion fluxes, automaticity, conduction velocity and refractory periods in different regions of the heart are important for understanding both the mechanisms of arrhythmogenesis and rationale for antiarrhythmic drug therapies.

Classification of antiarrhythmic drugs
In tachyarrhythmias, the aim of antiarrhythmic drug therapy is to reduce cardiac electrical activity. This is primarily achieved by slowing the rate of depolarization (phases 0 or 4), or prolonging repolarization (phases 1–3) within cells. Antiarrhythmic agents for tachyarrhythmias are broadly classified according to their mechanism of action. The most frequently used classification is the Vaughan Williams system (Vaughan Williams, 1984), which groups drugs into four classes based on their main electrophysiological effects (Figure 20.2). These effects are generally either an action on cardiac ion channels (e.g. sodium, calcium, potassium channels) or receptors (e.g. beta adrenergic receptors).

Cell type	Function	Location	Action potential
Nodal cells	Primary pacemakers	Sinoatrial (SA) node Atrioventricular (AV) node	
His–Purkinje cells	Rapidly conducting tissue	His bundle Bundle branches Purkinje fibre network	
Working myocardial cells	Mechanical work	Atrial myocardium Ventricular myocardium	

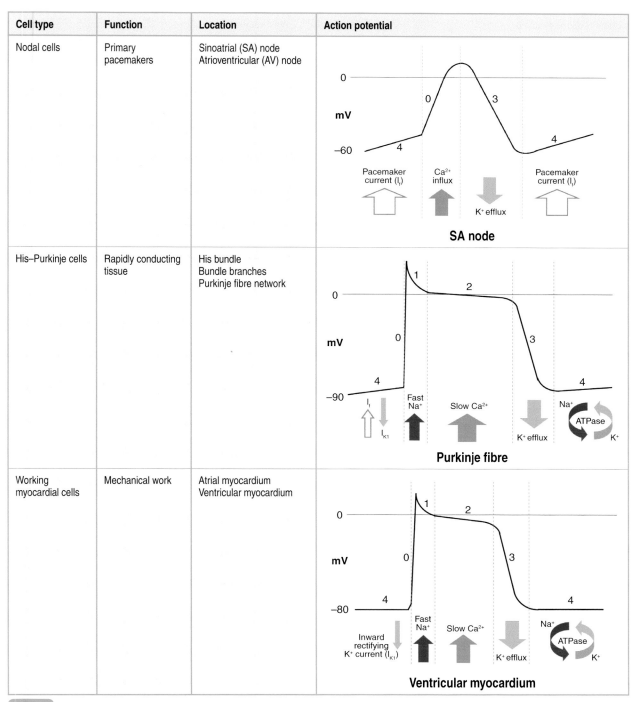

20.1 Cardiac action potentials.

Class	Mode of action	Examples	Main veterinary uses
I	Block sodium channels		
Ia	Depress phase 0 depolarization Prolong repolarization	Quinidine Procainamide Disopyramide	Refractory ventricular arrhythmias Supraventricular arrhythmias (including AVRT and AF conversion)
Ib	Depress phase 0 depolarization in abnormal tissue (little effect on normal tissue) Shorten repolarization	Lidocaine Mexiletine Tocainide Phenytoin	Ventricular arrhythmias May be useful in converting vagally mediated AF and some AVRT

20.2 Vaughan Williams classification of antiarrhythmic drugs. AF = Atrial fibrillation; ARVT = Atrioventricular reciprocating tachycardia (accessory pathway-mediated); AV = Atrioventricular; SVT = Supraventricular tachycardia. (continues)

Class	Mode of action	Examples	Main veterinary uses
Ic	Markedly depress phase 0 depolarization Little effect on repolarization	Flecanide Encainide Propafenone	Little clinical experience in veterinary medicine Experimental efficacy in converting AF
II	Antiadrenergic drugs	Atenolol Propranolol Esmolol Metoprolol Carvedilol	Slow ventricular rate in atrial tachyarrhythmias (especially AF) SVT involving the AV node Ventricular arrhythmias
III	Prolong repolarization	Sotalol Amiodarone Bretylium Ibutilide	Ventricular arrhythmias Supraventricular arrhythmias (including SVT involving the AV node and AF conversion)
IV	Block calcium channels (not dihydropyridines)	Diltiazem Verapamil	Slow ventricular rate in atrial tachyarrhythmias (especially AF) SVT involving the AV node

20.2 (continued) Vaughan Williams classification of antiarrhythmic drugs. AF = Atrial fibrillation; ARVT = Atrioventricular reciprocating tachycardia (accessory pathway-mediated); AV = Atrioventricular; SVT = Supraventricular tachycardia.

- Class I antiarrhythmic agents block sodium channels in working myocardium and His–Purkinje tissue. This inhibits phase 0 depolarization and therefore slows impulse conduction.
- Class II agents are antiadrenergic drugs (mainly beta adrenergic receptor blockers). Catecholamines (via beta adrenergic receptors) cause arrhythmias by increasing myocardial work, activating pacemaker currents and stimulating calcium channels. Class II drugs antagonize these actions.
- Class III agents prolong repolarization in all parts of the heart. This occurs mainly via inhibition of repolarizing potassium currents. For an impulse to propagate from a cell, adjacent cells need to be fully repolarized before they are excitable. Therefore, by delaying repolarization, impulse conduction is slowed or blocked.
- Class IV agents are calcium-channel blockers. They exert their effects via inhibition of slow calcium channels, resulting in a decreased rate of depolarization in nodal cells. Class IV agents therefore slow both the SA nodal pacemaker and AV nodal conduction.

Class I agents are further subdivided according to slight differences in their action.

- Class Ia agents moderately slow conduction in working myocardium and His–Purkinje tissue. They also prolong repolarization (class III action), making them theoretically useful in the more rapid tachycardias.
- Class Ib agents preferentially slow conduction in abnormal (partially depolarized) myocardium. They have little effect on normal myocardium. This may result in a more targeted effect to inhibit depolarization in diseased tissue. They also shorten repolarization in diseased tissue, creating greater homogeneity of refractory periods between different areas of the heart.
- Class Ic agents are the most potent inhibitors of sodium channels. They markedly slow conduction in working myocardium and His–Purkinje tissue, but have minimal effect on repolarization.

There are two major limitations of the Vaughan Williams system. Firstly, it does not account for drugs with multiple classes of action (for example, class Ia agents also have class III actions, sotalol has classes II and III actions, amiodarone has classes I, II, III and IV actions). Secondly, other drugs with important antiarrhythmic actions are not included, such as digitalis glycosides, anticholinergic agents, sympathomimetic agents and magnesium salts. Figure 20.2 shows the main uses in veterinary medicine of antiarrhythmic drugs grouped according to the Vaughan Williams classification. The formulary in the Appendix has a more comprehensive list of antiarrhythmic agents, with suggested doses for dogs and cats.

Adverse effects of antiarrhythmic drugs

Since the actions of all antiarrhythmic drugs are relatively non-selective, they can have a variety of effects on cardiac and non-cardiac tissues, many of which are undesirable. Their effects are rarely targeted only to the area of arrhythmogenic tissue. Consequently, by affecting the electrophysiological properties of normal tissue, antiarrhythmic drugs can promote occurrence of an arrhythmia in one area of the heart, while trying to prevent an arrhythmia in another area (*proarrhythmia*).

Some antiarrhythmic drugs affect cardiac systolic and diastolic function. The negative inotropic effects of beta adrenergic receptor blockers and calcium-channel blockers are typical examples; both have a relative contraindication in patients with overt CHF or myocardial failure. Many antiarrhythmic drugs also have adverse non-cardiac effects. Typical examples of this are central nervous system (CNS) and gastrointestinal effects of many class I drugs. Amiodarone is worthy of specific mention: despite being a drug with classes I, II, III and IV antiarrhythmic effects, and therefore suitable for many ventricular and supraventricular tachyarrhythmias, it is also associated with a variety of adverse non-cardiac effects that limit its use (see below).

Overall, the development of adverse effects in individual patients is variable and unpredictable.

However, precautions to minimize adverse effects (such as administering mexiletine with food) should be followed.

Lidocaine

Lidocaine is a class Ib antiarrhythmic agent. It acts by inhibiting fast sodium channel opening, therefore slowing conduction in His–Purkinje and working myocardial cells. It has a preferential inhibition on cells with a less negative resting membrane potential, which results in a more targeted effect on diseased myocardium, and is effective in arrhythmias caused by all three main mechanisms (automaticity, triggered activity, re-entry). Lidocaine undergoes rapid first-pass hepatic metabolism, so is most effective when administered intravenously. It is mainly protein bound in the plasma.

The rapid onset of action, relative safety and efficacy make lidocaine *the ideal first-choice agent for treatment of ventricular tachyarrhythmias*. In dogs it can be administered at intravenous bolus doses of 2 mg/kg over about 1–2 minutes, up to a maximum of 6–8 mg/kg over 10 minutes. It is advisable to wait for 1–2 minutes between each bolus dose to observe for any resolution of the arrhythmia. Rapid bolus dosing or doses above 6–8 mg/kg should be avoided as they frequently result in neurological signs, ranging from involuntary muscle tremors to generalized seizures. If seizures occur, they can be treated with intravenous diazepam. Hypokalaemia should be corrected, as this is an important reason for a poor response to lidocaine.

The antiarrhythmic effects of lidocaine do not persist beyond 10–15 minutes after bolus therapy. Therefore, if continued therapeutic plasma concentrations are desired, a continuous rate infusion (CRI) at 25–100 µg/kg/minute should be started after bolus doses. The author usually starts at doses of ≥50 µg/kg/minute. Although lidocaine is rapidly metabolized by the liver, tapering may not be required when stopping a prolonged infusion. Active metabolites and distribution of the drug to peripheral tissues (e.g. adipose) lead to an elimination half-life of hours (Kowey *et al.*, 2000).

Although lidocaine has little effect on most supraventricular tachyarrhythmias, it may result in conversion to sinus rhythm in selected cases. These include patients with accessory pathway-mediated supraventricular tachycardia (SVT) (Johnson *et al.*, 2006) and acute-onset vagally mediated AF (Moïse *et al.*, 2005). However, lidocaine is not effective for the vast majority of patients with AF for whom disease of chronic duration is present associated with atrial dilatation and remodelling.

The main adverse effects of lidocaine are neurotoxicity (obtundation, anxiety, tremors, seizures) and gastrotoxicity (anorexia, nausea, vomiting, diarrhoea). There are few cardiac contraindications to the use of lidocaine, as adverse cardiac effects are rarely observed.

Lidocaine can be effective for treating urgent ventricular tachyarrhythmias in cats. However, this species is particularly prone to the adverse neurotoxic effects of the drug. Therefore, it should be administered at a much lower dose in cats (e.g. 0.5 mg/kg bolus, up to 2 mg/kg over 10 minutes).

Mexiletine

Mexiletine is a class Ib antiarrhythmic agent. It therefore has electrophysiological properties, pharmacokinetics and adverse effects similar to those of lidocaine. The main difference is the less rapid hepatic metabolism and longer elimination half-life of mexiletine following oral administration.

Mexiletine is indicated for chronic therapy of ventricular tachyarrhythmias, particularly in patients with arrhythmias that have been successfully treated with lidocaine. Mexiletine can be administered orally at a dose of 4–8 mg/kg q8–12h. *It is important that it is administered with food* or on a full stomach to minimize the most common adverse effects of the drug (i.e. anorexia, nausea, vomiting). Neurological side effects are less common. A combination of mexiletine with a beta adrenergic blocker (e.g. atenolol) may increase efficacy and decrease adverse effects, by allowing administration of both drugs at a lower dose. A combination of mexiletine (5–8 mg/kg q8h) and atenolol (12.5 mg/dog q12h) has been shown to reduce the frequency of ventricular arrhythmias in Boxers with arrhythmogenic right ventricular cardiomyopathy (Meurs *et al.*, 2002). A combination of mexiletine and sotalol has also been used in Boxers with ventricular arrhythmias (Prošek *et al.*, 2006). Mexiletine can also be useful for chronic antiarrhythmic control in cases of accessory pathway-mediated SVT (Johnson *et al.*, 2006).

Class Ib agents can be very neurotoxic in cats. The author has no experience of using mexiletine in this species.

Beta adrenergic blockers

Beta adrenergic blockers (beta-blockers) are class II antiarrhythmic agents and inhibit the binding of potentially arrhythmogenic catecholamines to beta-1 adrenergic receptors on the heart. Catecholamines exert arrhythmogenic effects via increased concentrations of cyclic AMP (cAMP) within the cardiac myocyte. Excess cAMP causes increased cardiac work, increased pacemaker currents and increased calcium-dependent triggered activity. Beta-blockers inhibit all of these effects. There is probably little variation in the antiarrhythmic effect of any beta-blocker in terms of their action on beta-1 adrenergic receptors. Instead beta-blockers vary by their effects on other adrenergic receptors (e.g. atenolol is relatively beta-1 selective, propranolol affects beta-1 and beta-2 receptors), pharmacokinetics (e.g. esmolol has a half-life of minutes, atenolol has a half-life of hours) and additional properties (e.g. sotalol has additional class III effects).

Beta-blockers can be effective for the treatment of supraventricular tachyarrhythmias by inhibiting the initiation of atrial ectopy and slowing conduction via the AV node. The latter action is most useful to decrease the ventricular rate in AF. Beta-blockers are also useful in ventricular tachyarrhythmias, particular those associated with elevated catecholamines. In humans, beta-blockers do not reliably decrease the frequency of ventricular premature complexes, but do decrease clinical signs and mortality as a result of ventricular arrhythmias.

As well as beneficial effects in reducing heart rate and excitability, beta-blockers have short-term adverse effects to reduce contractility and ventricular relaxation. These effects can acutely impair cardiac function in patients with myocardial failure. Consequently they should be used cautiously in patients with systolic dysfunction and generally avoided in patients with poorly controlled CHF. When used in patients with systolic dysfunction, they should be given in very low doses initially, with careful up-titration of the dose and frequency over several weeks to months, depending on the clinical response of the patient. Lethargy, collapse, bradycardia, hypotension and precipitation of signs of CHF are the most common adverse effects. The author usually performs echocardiography and/or radiography in patients with underlying cardiac disease to assess for risk of developing CHF before starting beta-blockers. Respiratory difficulties due to bronchoconstriction may occur with non-selective (beta-1 and beta-2) beta-blockers and high doses of selective (beta-1 specific) beta-blockers.

The most frequently used oral beta-blockers in small animal cardiology are atenolol (beta-1 specific), propranolol (beta-1 and beta-2), metoprolol (beta-1 specific) and carvedilol (beta-1, beta-2 and alpha-1). The author prefers to use atenolol at a dose of 0.2–1.5 mg/kg q12–24h in dogs and 0.5–3 mg/kg q12–24h in cats. Sotalol and amiodarone are considered separately because of their additional actions. Esmolol is an ultrashort-acting beta-1 selective adrenergic blocker that can be given at doses of 50–100 µg/kg intravenously over 5 minutes in both dogs and cats. Esmolol is rapidly converted in the blood to inactive metabolites, resulting in a half-life of minutes. If ongoing beta-blocking actions are required, a CRI (25–100 µg/kg/minute) can be administered after initial bolus therapy.

Sotalol

Sotalol is a class III antiarrhythmic agent with additional class II actions. Commercially available sotalol is a racemic mixture of D- and L-isomers (DL-sotalol), each isomer with differential class II (beta-blocking) and class III (repolarization prolonging) effects. The combined actions result in blockade of beta-1 and beta-2 receptors, and inhibition of repolarizing potassium currents (particularly I_{Kr}) causing prolonged action potentials in all parts of the heart. The beta-blocking effects appear to occur at lower doses than the class III effects. Sotalol is almost entirely unbound in the plasma and therefore has little interaction with other drugs, such as digoxin. It undergoes primarily renal excretion.

Sotalol is effective for both ventricular and supraventricular tachyarrhythmias. In humans, both oral and intravenous sotalol suppresses ventricular ectopy to a similar degree to class I agents, including some prevention of ventricular tachycardia and ventricular fibrillation. It can also be effective in

terminating, slowing, or preventing paroxysmal SVT and AF, with a greater efficacy than beta-blockers. This is probably due to its class III effects that result in an increase in refractory periods in the atria, AV node and accessory pathways. In dogs, sotalol at doses of 1.5–3.5 mg/kg orally q12h appears effective in suppressing ventricular arrhythmias in Boxers, either alone (Meurs *et al.*, 2002), or in combination with mexiletine (Prošek *et al.*, 2006). Intravenous sotalol has anecdotal success in terminating SVT and ventricular tachycardia in dogs and cats; the author has given intravenous bolus doses of 1 mg/kg over 3–5 minutes, repeated as necessary, to either terminate or slow such arrhythmias. This is usually followed by oral sotalol. Doses in dogs can range from 0.5–5 mg/kg orally q12h and in cats from 10–30 mg/cat orally q12h. The author usually starts therapy at the low end of the range in cats.

The main adverse effects of sotalol in small animals are those of all beta-blockers (negative inotropy, negative chronotropy and bronchoconstriction, see above). Negative inotropy can result in exacerbation or precipitation of CHF in patients with advanced heart disease or systolic dysfunction. Administration of sotalol should be avoided in patients with poorly controlled CHF or at risk of developing CHF. Negative chronotropy can result in signs of bradycardia, lethargy and collapse, particularly in patients with concurrent bradyarrhythmias or neurally mediated syncope. QT prolongation is the biggest risk of sotalol use in humans, as this can precipitate sudden death from *torsades de pointes* (see Chapter 16). This complication does not appear to be common in dogs and cats, but consideration of this effect should be given to patients with pre-existing QT prolongation, hypokalaemia, hypomagnesaemia, and with concurrent use of drugs known to prolong the QT interval (e.g. class Ia antiarrhythmics).

Amiodarone

Amiodarone is a drug with classes I, II, III and IV actions according to the Vaughan Williams classification. It therefore has electrophysiological actions on all parts of the heart. Amiodarone is highly lipophilic and very highly protein bound in the plasma. It has poor oral bioavailability, a high volume of distribution to tissues and very long elimination half-life (several weeks) with predominantly hepatic metabolism. These properties result in a slow and variable onset of action after oral dosing, high frequency of non-cardiac effects and continued action for weeks after cessation of dosing. Consequently, most dosing regimens involve loading doses, and the relationship between effects and plasma levels in dogs is poorly defined.

Amiodarone is effective for both ventricular and supraventricular tachyarrhythmias. In humans it has similar efficacy to sotalol for ventricular arrhythmia suppression and treatment of SVT and AF, with a greater efficacy for maintaining sinus rhythm after AF conversion (Singh *et al.*, 2005). In dogs, a number of oral dosing regimens have been described. A loading dose of 10–15 mg/kg q24h for 7–14 days, followed by a maintenance dose of 5–7.5 mg/kg q24h may be effective for chemical cardioversion of AF (Saunders et al., 2006), or to aid maintenance of sinus rhythm with electrical cardioversion (Bright and zumBrunnen, 2008). Similar doses may be effective for ventricular arrhythmias; a loading dose of 10 mg/kg q12h for 1–2 weeks followed by a maintenance dose of 5–10 mg/kg q24h has been described for treatment of ventricular tachycardia in Dobermanns (Calvert and Brown, 2004). Further adjustments may be required on an individual patient basis to achieve the lowest dose for arrhythmia suppression and minimal adverse effects. Given its very long half-life, it is recommended that the effect of any dose adjustment is assessed at least 4 weeks later. Amiodarone has been reported to be variably effective for AF cardioversion when given at doses of 4–8 mg/kg intravenously over 10–15 minutes, albeit with severe adverse effects (Oyama and Prošek, 2006).

Despite its efficacy for treatment of a variety of tachyarrhythmias, amiodarone use is limited by a large number of adverse non-cardiac effects. Toxicity associated with chronic oral administration in dogs includes appetite suppression, gastrointestinal disturbances, keratopathy and a positive Coombs' test (Calvert et al., 2000). Amiodarone also increases serum digoxin concentrations, potentially causing signs of digitalis toxicity. Adverse effects associated with intravenous administration include pain at the injection site, hypotension, hypersalivation and hypersensitivity reactions (erythema, urticaria, swelling, agitation, pruritus); the latter may be a reaction to the carrier solvent (Cober et al., 2009). Amiodarone has fewer negative inotropic effects and a lower risk of torsades de pointes than sotalol. The author prefers amiodarone for treatment of ventricular arrhythmias in dogs with systolic dysfunction and CHF, sometimes in combination with mexiletine. Monitoring of hepatic enzyme activities and thyroid function is recommended.

Diltiazem

Diltiazem is a benzothiazepine calcium-channel blocker or class IV agent according to the Vaughan Williams classification. Its main effects are dose-dependent slowing of the sinus rate and AV node conduction. It also has some arteriodilator actions, although less than dihydropyridine calcium-channel blockers, such as amlodipine. Diltiazem is mainly protein bound in the plasma, has high hepatic metabolism and a relatively short elimination half-life. The latter means that it needs to be administered frequently (q8h) unless sustained-release formulations are used.

Diltiazem is an important agent for treatment of supraventricular tachyarrhythmias. It can be given intravenously for treatment of SVT at a dose of 0.1–0.25 mg/kg over 1–2 minutes, up to a total dose of 0.75 mg/kg over 30 minutes. It can also be given orally for rate-control of AF or atrial tachycardias at a dose of 0.5–2 mg/kg q8h. Diltiazem can be given orally in a loading dose, initially 0.5 mg/kg, followed by 0.25 mg/kg every hour to effect or a 2 mg/kg total dose. Diltiazem is the author's preferred drug for treatment of supraventricular arrhythmias in cats with CHF, given orally at a dose of 7.5–15 mg/cat q8h.

At standard doses, diltiazem has few adverse effects. At toxic doses, signs related to decreased cardiac contractility and vasodilation, such as lethargy, obtundation and hypotension, may occur. Bradyarrhythmias such as sinus bradycardia and AV block are also possible. However, when given to cats at a dose of 60 mg/cat q24h, extended-release diltiazem can cause lethargy, gastrointestinal disturbances and weight loss (Wall et al., 2005). Despite its negative inotropic effects, diltiazem is usually tolerated in patients with CHF or systolic dysfunction, but it should be used cautiously if signs of CHF are not well controlled.

Digoxin

Digoxin is a digitalis glycoside and the oldest antiarrhythmic agent. It has multiple cardiac and non-cardiac effects. The main effects of digoxin are inhibition of the sodium pump (sodium/potassium adenosine triphosphatase (ATPase) pump), improvement in baroreceptor sensitivity, activation of efferent parasympathetic (vagal) tone and inhibition of efferent sympathetic discharge. The neural effects of digoxin account for its antiarrhythmic actions as they result in slowing of the sinus rate and decreased AV nodal conduction. Digoxin inhibits the sodium pump by competing with potassium ions for their binding site. Sodium pump inhibition in the heart results in increased intracellular myocardial calcium concentrations, producing a slight positive inotropic effect, but also an increased risk of tachyarrhythmias, particularly from triggered activity. Sodium pump inhibition at the kidney decreases renin release and exerts a slight natriuretic effect. Digoxin has good oral bioavailability, a very long elimination half-life (1–1.5 days in the dog; 1–3 days in the cat), low protein binding and mainly renal excretion.

Digoxin is mainly used to slow the ventricular rate in persistent atrial tachyarrhythmias. It is the antiarrhythmic agent of choice in dogs with AF and heart failure. Digoxin should be given orally twice daily in dogs and dosed to lean bodyweight, so that the effect of obesity or large volume effusions are accounted for in the dose calculations. The most effective dose of digoxin in terms of clinical response and outcome is unknown in dogs. However, in humans, previous recommendations for dosing to achieve a 'therapeutic concentration' of 1.0–2.0 ng/ml have been superseded by recommendations to achieve a lower concentration of 0.5–1.0 ng/ml. This is based on convincing evidence of decreased mortality and hospitalizations for heart failure in human patients with low (<1.1 ng/ml) versus high (≥1.2 ng/ml) digoxin concentrations (Rathore et al., 2003). Consequently the author uses a dose of 3–5 μg/kg q12h (0.1–0.15 mg/m^2 orally q12h) and aims for a trough (>8h) post-pill serum digoxin concentration of 0.6–1.1 ng/ml. Steady-state serum concentrations are often achieved within 5–7 days. The dose is decreased by 50% for patients with renal failure. There is rarely an indication for 'rapid digitalization', either with intravenous or oral loading doses. The author rarely uses digoxin in cats but, when given, uses a dose of 31.25 μg/cat orally q48h.

Drugs that increase serum digoxin concentrations include quinidine, flecainide, propafenone, amiodarone and verapamil. The effect of diltiazem on digoxin concentrations is usually negligible.

Digoxin has a very narrow therapeutic/toxic window. Most of the non-cardiac signs of digoxin toxicity result from its CNS and parasympathomimetic actions (e.g. depressed mentation, anorexia, vomiting, diarrhoea). Cardiac signs of digoxin toxicity include tacharryhthmias, particularly ventricular bigeminy and trigeminy, and excessively slow sinus rates or slow ventricular rates in AF. Clinical signs of digoxin toxicity can occur at any serum concentration, but are more likely to occur with high doses, hypokalaemia or renal insufficiency. Consequently monitoring of urea, creatinine and electrolytes is recommended in all patients receiving digoxin, particularly those concurrently receiving potassium-losing diuretics (e.g. furosemide, thiazides).

Electrical antiarrhythmic therapies

Electrical cardioversion and defibrillation
The principle behind electrical (DC) cardioversion and defibrillation is the termination of a tachycardia by the delivery of sufficient electrical energy to depolarize all excitable myocardial cells simultaneously. It is hoped that the subsequent uniform repolarization will allow restoration of normal sinus rhythm. Although the principle is the same, both are performed in a similar manner and both use the same equipment, electrical cardioversion and defibrillation are *not* the same.

- *Electrical cardioversion* is the delivery of energy to the myocardium that is *synchronized* to the R wave of the QRS complex.
- *Defibrillation* is the delivery of energy to the myocardium that is *not* synchronized to the underlying rhythm.

Defibrillation should not be performed on a patient with a stable ventricular rhythm, since inadvertent delivery of electrical energy to the myocardium during the T wave can precipitate ventricular fibrillation.

Both electrical cardioversion and defibrillation can be achieved with either monophasic or biphasic energy waveforms.

- *Monophasic* cardiovertor/defibrillators deliver a high-energy pulse across the chest in one direction.

- *Biphasic* cardiovertor/defibrillators alternate the direction of pulses across the chest, allowing a lower energy to be delivered.

Biphasic cardioversion is more effective and safer than monophasic, as it allows the generation of greater transmyocardial current for cardioversion/defibrillation with lower energy levels and therefore less soft tissue and myocardial injury to the patient.

Defibrillation is used during cardiopulmonary–cerebral resuscitation for ventricular fibrillation and asystole. Electrical cardioversion (Figure 20.3) is performed in small animals for the conversion of supraventricular tachyarrhythmias and ventricular tachycardia to sinus rhythm.

Pacemaker therapy
The main indication for pacemaker therapy is a *bradyarrhythmia causing clinical signs of haemodynamic compromise* (see below). Since the vast majority of bradyarrhythmias of this type are permanent, most pacemaker therapy is also permanent. All pacemaker units comprise a pulse generator (battery, pacing circuits, telemetry coil and lead connector) and lead system (internal conducting wire, external insulation and electrodes). For permanent pacemaker implantation the pulse generator is a compact device with a titanium casing and a lithium-anode battery (often lithium–iodine), which has a lifespan of up to 10 years (Figure 20.4). New pulse generators and leads can be purchased from manufacturers. Second-hand equipment may be obtained

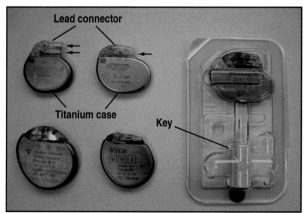

20.4 Pacemaker pulse generators of various sizes, makes and models. The pulse generator at the top left has two lead connectors (arrowed) to allow dual chamber pacing. The pulse generator on the right is in its sterile package, which includes the key to screw the lead into the lead connector.

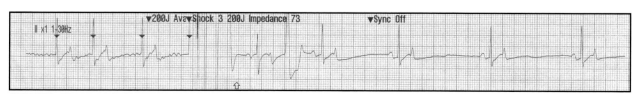

20.3 Electrical (DC) cardioversion in a Labrador Retriever with AF. The first four complexes have arrowheads above the QRS complexes, indicating that the device is correctly identifying the R waves. A shock is delivered synchronous with the R wave of the fourth complex. Sinus rhythm ensues, with a ventricular premature complex interpolated between the first and second sinus complex. Note that synchronous mode automatically turns off after the shock is delivered. Lead II shown. Paper speed 25 mm/s; gain 1 cm/mV. (Courtesy of A. Boswood.)

from human hospitals and should always be gas sterilized prior to use.

All pacing systems require two electrodes (cathode and anode) for an electrical circuit to be maintained and cardiac pacing to occur. The cathode is always located at the tip of the lead. The anode can be located either outside the heart (at the pulse generator) or within the heart (on the lead proximal to the cathode). The former is referred to as *unipolar* pacing and the latter *bipolar* pacing. Most modern pacing systems are bipolar, as there are many disadvantages of unipolar pacing, including: the need for continual contact between the pulse generator and body to maintain a circuit; a susceptibility to interference from normal skeletal muscle activity; and the potential for rhythmic stimulation of skeletal muscles at the site of pulse generator implantation (referred to as 'thumps').

Bipolar leads and pulse generators can be set for either unipolar or bipolar pacing, whereas unipolar systems can only be set for unipolar pacing. Therefore, if bipolar pacing is desired it is always recommended that leads and pulse generators are checked prior to use to ensure that they are compatible. This may require prior programming of the pulse generator. Pulse generator programming is performed by telemetry with a programmer device, which consists of a computer and programming magnet (Figure 20.5). When the magnet is positioned in

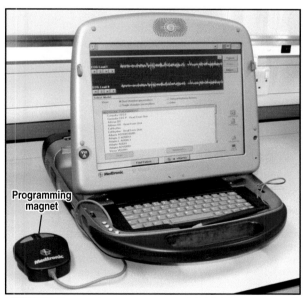

20.5 Pacemaker programmer. A foldable screen and programming magnet are features of all models.

close proximity to a pulse generator, the computer can be used to programme a number of settings depending upon the model and type of generator. These may include polarity, pacing mode, pacing rate, pulse amplitude (voltage), pulse duration, refractory period and sensitivity. Many devices will also provide information on previous use of the pulse generator and an estimation of remaining battery life.

Pacing modes are referred to by a three- to five-letter coding system. Figure 20.6 provides a summary of the more common pacing modes used in veterinary species. For example, a pacemaker may be set to VVI mode at 80 beats/minute, indicating that the pacemaker only fires when the intrinsic heart rate falls below 80 beats/minute. This type of pacing is most useful for patients with clinical signs related to sinus arrest, for whom the heart rate is usually >80 beats/minute at other times. However, in patients with persistently low heart rates (e.g. third-degree AV block) this type of pacing does not account for changes in heart rate that are required in response to physiological needs. Consequently a preferred pacing mode for these patients is VVIR. This mode allows for pacing between a fixed lower and upper rate.

Changes in pacing rate can be based on one of a number of variables. These include movement, right ventricular pressure, or changes in physiological variables within the blood (e.g. oxygen saturation, pH, temperature). Dual chamber pacing can be achieved with an additional lead which is implanted into the right atrium. This provides a more physiological type of pacing in patients with AV block, as both sinus control of the heart rate and AV synchrony are maintained, but increases the potential for complications, particularly lead dislodgement. In an attempt to overcome this, use of a pacing system with a single ventricular lead and attached floating lead in the right atrium has been described in dogs (Bulmer *et al.*, 2006).

Permanent pacemakers can be implanted either transvenously or epicardially.

- Transvenous implantation is the most common route in dogs.
- Epicardial implantation is the most common route in cats.

Transvenous implantation is carried out under fluoroscopic guidance, via a jugular vein, with the lead implanted into the right ventricle and/or atrium, and the pulse generator usually implanted in either the subcutaneous tissues of the neck or in a tissue

First letter	Second letter	Third letter	Fourth letter
Chamber paced	*Chamber sensed*	*Response to sensing*	*Rate modulation/programmable functions*
V = ventricle	V = ventricle	T = triggers pacing	P = programmable (rate and/or output)
A = atrium	A = atrium	I = inhibits pacing	M = multiprogrammable (e.g. rate, output, sensitivity)
D = dual (A+V)	D = dual (A+V)	D = dual (T+I)	C = communicating functions (e.g. telemetry)
O = none	O = none	O = none	R = rate modulation

20.6 Pacing modes.

pocket beneath the omotransversarius muscle. Many cardiologists prefer to implant via the right jugular vein, as this minimizes the risk of inadvertent placement via a persistent left cranial vena cava.

- Endocardial leads maintain contact with the myocardium by either passive or active fixation.
  - Passive fixation leads have tined tips that are designed to hook within the trabeculae of the right ventricle.
  - Active fixation leads have helical tips that screw into the myocardium.
- Epicardial leads require active fixation using a screw-in type of lead. These leads are usually implanted via a transdiaphragmatic approach, with the pulse generator implanted in a pocket within the abdominal muscle wall.

Complications of pacemaker implantation include lead dislodgement, seroma formation, intraoperative mortality, pulse generator or lead failure, and infection. Lead dislodgement is the most frequently encountered major complication, irrespective of the type of lead system used (Oyama *et al.*, 2001; Wess *et al.*, 2006). This usually occurs within the first few days of pacemaker implantation. Complication rates can be quite high, with reported rates ranging from 20% to 60%, and an inverse correlation between complication rate and experience of the operator (Oyama *et al.*, 2001). Therefore, it is preferable that pacemaker implantation is performed by trained and experienced personnel.

Pacemaker implantation requires more than just a skilled operator, pacing equipment and programmer. It also requires a sterile operating room, fluoroscopy unit and a skilled anaesthesia team. Patients requiring pacemakers often develop a more severe bradyarrhythmia or ventricular arrhythmias during induction and maintenance of anaesthesia. These arrhythmias may precipitate cardiac arrest from asystole or ventricular fibrillation. Such arrhythmias may be reduced by the use of temporary pacing, which can be accomplished by either transthoracic or transvenous methods.

Temporary pacing

Temporary transthoracic pacing uses electrode pads attached to clipped areas of skin on either side of the thoracic wall (Figure 20.7). This type of pacing is painful, as it results in skeletal muscle stimulation, and therefore requires anaesthesia to be induced first. Use of skeletal muscle relaxants during anaesthesia reduces the degree of skeletal muscle stimulation and therefore patient movement during subsequent permanent pacemaker implantation. However, this necessitates mechanical ventilation due to relaxation of the intercostal muscles and diaphragm.

Temporary transvenous pacing is usually achieved using a temporary pacing lead implanted into the right ventricle under fluoroscopic guidance via a femoral vein. The pacing lead is passed aseptically via a vascular introducer that is inserted into the vein via a Seldinger technique. This technique can be performed in well restrained patients prior to induction of general anaesthesia, but it is more technically demanding and time-consuming, requires additional radiation exposure and is difficult to perform in poorly cooperative patients without chemical restraint.

Other uses for temporary pacing include general anaesthesia for procedures other than permanent pacemaker implantation in a patient with a less severe bradyarrhythmia, and in patients with unstable bradyarrhythmias associated with a potentially reversible condition (e.g. endocarditis, drug toxicity).

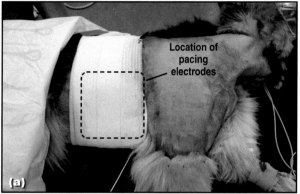

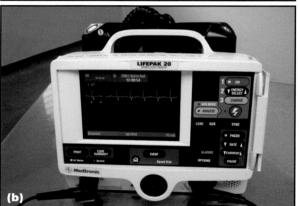

20.7 Temporary transthoracic pacing in a German Shepherd Dog with third-degree AV block, undergoing general anaesthesia for permanent pacemaker implantation. **(a)** Pacing electrodes (adhesive pads) are placed on either side of the thoracic wall, over the heart. Cables attached to the pads run to a cardioverter/defibrillator unit **(b)**.

Management of patients following pacemaker implantation involves minimizing the risk of lead dislodgement in the short term and avoiding damage to the lead and pulse generator in the neck. Exercise restriction is recommended during the first month following implantation, to avoid lead dislodgement. To avoid damage to the lead, blood sampling should not be performed via the jugular vein and the owner should be informed that the dog should never be allowed to wear a collar. Either could result in catastrophic damage to the lead resulting from lead fracture or insulation failure. It is also important to avoid blood sampling from the jugular veins of any dog that may be in imminent need of a pacemaker, since a patent jugular vein is an important prerequisite for pacemaker implantation. In the event of death, the pulse generator should always be removed prior to cremation otherwise the battery will explode!

Therapy for specific arrhythmias

Flowcharts in the following sections show suggested approaches to narrow QRS complex tachycardia (SVT, Figure 20.8), AF (see Figure 20.12), wide QRS complex tachycardia (usually ventricular tachycardia, see Figure 20.13) and bradyarrhythmias (see Figure 20.15).

Supraventricular arrhythmias

Supraventricular arrhythmias usually occur secondary to structural heart disease, most commonly those resulting in atrial dilatation (e.g. AV regurgitation, myocardial disease, patent ductus arteriosus). Some patients will present with concurrent CHF. In this circumstance, treatment of CHF may be effective in reducing the rate, or occasionally result in conversion to sinus rhythm by decreasing circulating catecholamines and reducing atrial pressures. This alone may be sufficient to treat some supraventricular arrhythmias effectively and should therefore be the first therapeutic step. If CHF is not present or therapy is not effective, specific antiarrhythmic therapy should be considered if the arrhythmia is rapid enough to result in haemodynamic compromise in the short term, or is

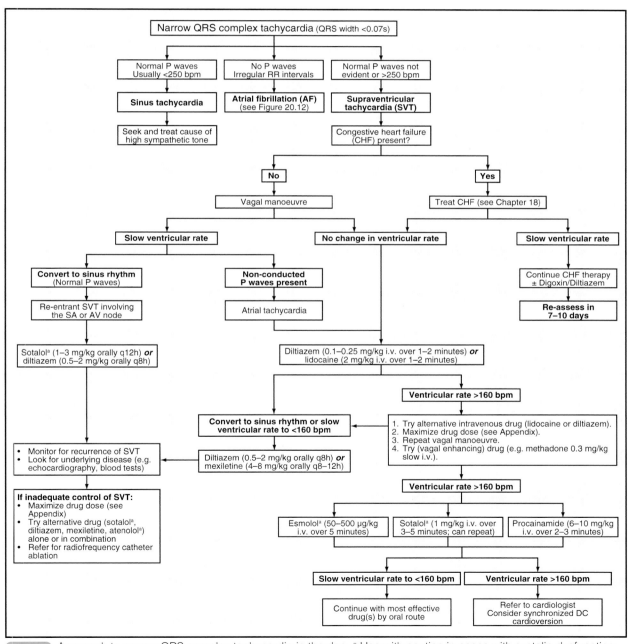

20.8 Approach to narrow QRS complex tachycardia in the dog. [a] Use with caution in cases with systolic dysfunction; avoid use in cases with CHF; do not give together. AV = Atrioventricular; SA = Sinoatrial.

sufficiently rapid and sustained to cause myocardial failure in the long term. Unlike ventricular arrhythmias, supraventricular arrhythmias rarely result in death from electrical instability. However, they can precipitate death in patients with advanced cardiac disease.

Isolated supraventricular premature complexes (atrial or AV junctional) rarely require specific therapy as they do not usually cause measurable haemodynamic effects and do not affect the rate sufficiently to induce myocardial failure. However, they may be a marker for underlying cardiac disease or a precursor for a more sustained arrhythmia (e.g. AF).

A sustained supraventricular arrhythmia usually requires antiarrhythmic drug therapy. *The aim is either conversion to sinus rhythm or to slow the ventricular rate.* Conversion to sinus rhythm is preferable, to optimize cardiac function. However, maintaining adequate rate control may be just as effective clinically. This has been illustrated in several large studies in humans with AF who have not demonstrated a benefit from conversion to sinus rhythm over pharmacological rate control (Wyse *et al.*, 2002).

Supraventricular tachycardia

SVT is usually a narrow QRS complex tachycardia (QRS width <0.07 seconds in dogs). A suggested approach to the management of narrow QRS complex tachycardia is shown in Figure 20.8. Vagal manoeuvres (Figure 20.9) can be useful either to terminate some SVTs involving the AV node, or transiently to slow the ventricular rate in atrial tachycardia (Figure

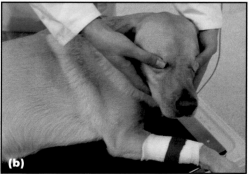
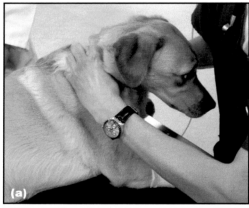

20.9 Vagal manoeuvres. **(a)** Carotid sinus massage is achieved by applying continuous digital pressure to the region of the carotid sinuses, just caudal to the larynx, to stimulate carotid baroreceptors. **(b)** Ocular pressure is achieved by applying firm pressure over both globes for approximately 20 seconds.

20.10). The author finds that carotid massage is usually more effective than ocular pressure. However, in most cases, antiarrhythmic drug therapy (e.g. diltiazem, lidocaine, sotalol) is necessary to terminate the SVT or slow the ventricular rate (Figure 20.11).

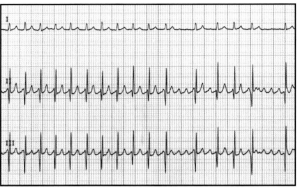

20.10 Vagal manoeuvre in atrial tachycardia/flutter: carotid sinus massage in a 2-year-old Bulldog with SVT. Slowing of the ventricular rate after the ninth QRS complex revealed an atrial rate of about 450 beats/minute. By slowing the ventricular rate independently of the atrial rate, an atrial tachycardia was diagnosed. Leads I–III shown. Paper speed 25 mm/s; gain 1 cm/mV.

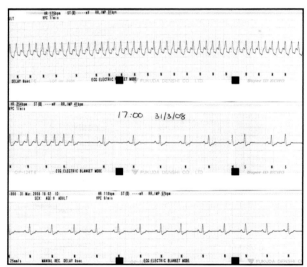

20.11 Pharmacological cardioversion of SVT: conversion of an SVT of >300 beats/minute in a 2-year-old Labrador Retriever following two doses of slow intravenous sotalol, each at a dose of 1 mg/kg given 5 minutes apart. Termination of the SVT and conversion to sinus rhythm occurred shortly after the second dose. Previous attempts at conversion with vagal manoeuvres, intravenous diltiazem, esmolol and lidocaine had been ineffective. The dog was subsequently maintained successfully on oral sotalol. An SVT at 350 beats/minute is seen on the top strip. Conversion to sinus rhythm occurs after the eighth complex in the middle strip. Sinus rhythm at 110 beats/minute is maintained on the lower strip. Lead II shown. Paper speed 25 mm/s; gain 0.5 cm/mV.

Once conversion to sinus rhythm or adequate control of the ventricular rate has been achieved, chronic therapy with the most effective drug(s) should be continued orally. Echocardiography to assess for concurrent structural or functional heart disease and laboratory tests for systemic disease can also be performed. Monitoring for arrhythmia recurrence, ideally with ambulatory (Holter) ECG monitoring, is also important.

Animals with SVT that are refractory to pharmacological therapy may be candidates for electrical (synchronized DC) cardioversion (see above) or intracardiac electrophysiological mapping. The latter is a highly specialized technique that allows identification of a re-entrant pathway or ectopic atrial focus, and radiofrequency catheter ablation of a portion of the re-entrant circuit or arrhythmogenic focus. This technique can result in permanent resolution of AV reciprocating tachycardia or atrial tachycardia in dogs (Wright *et al.*, 2006). A further option in patients with incessant atrial tachycardia is AV node ablation and permanent pacemaker implantation.

Atrial fibrillation

A suggested approach to the management of AF is shown in Figure 20.12. AF is considered separately from other sustained supraventricular arrhythmias as it can differ in its underlying cause, treatment and outcome.

AF is the most common supraventricular arrhythmia. It is more likely to occur in larger atria and under conditions of enhanced autonomic tone; therefore, it is more frequently seen in animals with atrial dilatation secondary to structural heart disease. However, there is also an increased prevalence in giant-breed dogs in the absence of detectable underlying heart disease. The vast majority of cases of AF detected in small animals are persistent or permanent (see Chapter 16). This is in part because AF induces electrophysiological and pathological changes within the atrial myocardium that perpetuate the arrhythmia (Brundel *et al.*, 2005). Consequently *permanent restoration of sinus rhythm is not easily achievable*. The patients with the greatest chance for permanent conversion to sinus rhythm are those with acute-onset AF, particularly if iatrogenic (e.g. following intravenous opioid administration, during general anaesthesia, or

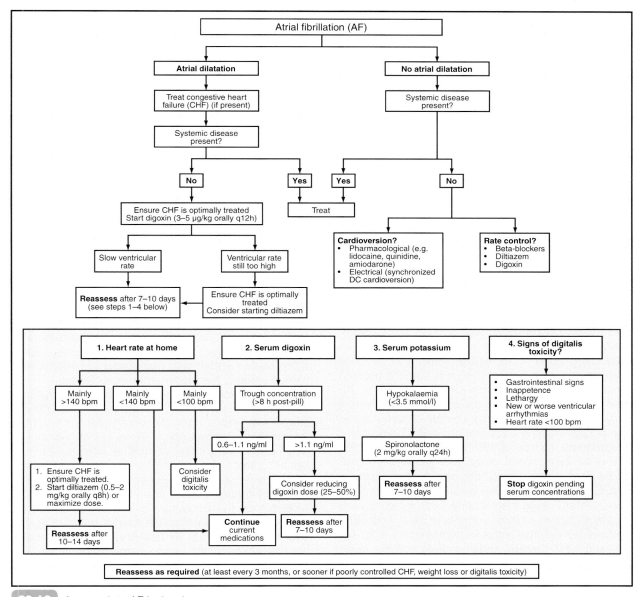

20.12 Approach to AF in the dog.

cardiac catheterization), and in patients without atrial dilatation. Options for cardioversion are either pharmacological (e.g. class I agents, amiodarone) or electrical (synchronized DC cardioversion). Permanent conversion to sinus rhythm is not achievable for most patients with AF. Therefore, the goal for the majority of cases is to control the ventricular rate in order to provide the most effective cardiac output and reduce clinical signs.

The 'ideal' rate is one that maximizes arterial pressure, while minimizing venous pressure and myocardial oxygen demand. Unfortunately the precise 'ideal' rate in the dog and cat is unknown. Furthermore, the rate obtained will vary depending upon temperament, the setting in which the heart rate is taken (in-clinic or at home), the method of heart rate measurement (ECG *versus* auscultation) and the presence or absence of CHF. One study assessing naturally occurring AF in dogs with CHF suggested that an at-home, owner-auscultated heart rate of 130–145 beats/minute (mean 138 beats/ minute) was optimal to allow both effective control of CHF (as measured by respiratory rate) and increased cardiac output (Hamlin, 1995). Since AF is most commonly present in dogs with cardiac disease resulting in CHF, this information is useful. On this basis, the author recommends a target rate of <140 beats/minute at home (owner-auscultated or Holter ECG) as a reasonable aim for most dogs with AF and CHF.

A higher heart rate is often expected in the clinic due to increased production of catecholamines from the stress of a visit. Overestimation of the rate by at least 20 beats/minute for in-hospital ECG *versus* Holter monitoring was found in one study (Gelzer *et al.*, 2009). Therefore, a rate of <160 beats/minute in the hospital/clinic setting may be consistent with good control. Some owners can become adept at counting their animal's heart rate by thoracic palpation or auscultation, but this usually requires some degree of training and practice. As well as being more accurate, 24-hour Holter monitoring provides more information, such as maximum, minimum and mean heart rates, as well as rate response to exercise/excitement, which may be increased in dogs with AF. Some cardiologists advocate more stringent control, such as maintaining rates <120 beats/minute; this is more achievable in dogs without CHF. It is also important to remember that effective rate-control therapy in AF must be one that results in the greatest improvement in clinical signs, particularly control of CHF, rather than purely targeting a specific numerical end-point.

Adequate therapy of CHF is an essential component of AF rate control, since poorly controlled CHF results in elevated sympathetic and decreased vagal tone. Oral digoxin is usually given in addition to CHF therapy. Many dogs also require further rate-control therapy. Diltiazem is most commonly used, and often provides good rate-control in combination with digoxin and CHF therapy. Beta-blockers can be given instead, but should be used with caution as their potent negative inotropic action may impair adequate control of CHF. It is for this reason that diltiazem is preferred by the author.

Non-antiarrhythmic drugs that may be useful in AF include angiotensin-converting enzyme (ACE) inhibitors, aldosterone antagonists (e.g. spironolactone) and omega-3 fatty acids. These drugs may help to reverse some of the structural atrial remodelling and pro-inflammatory cytokines that modulate arrhythmia perpetuation (Brundel *et al.*, 2005).

Supraventricular arrhythmias in cats
Cats with supraventricular arrhythmias almost invariably have underlying cardiac disease. They differ from dogs in that they are less likely to develop sustained supraventricular arrhythmias, presumably due to smaller atrial mass. Additionally, they are more susceptible to the toxic effects of digitalis glycosides. Fortunately, since cats develop cardiac disease with diastolic dysfunction (i.e. hypertrophic and restrictive cardiomyopathy) far more commonly than systolic dysfunction (i.e. dilated cardiomyopathy), the use of drugs with a negative inotropic effect (diltiazem or beta adrenergic blockers) to control ventricular rate is often most appropriate, in addition to optimal control of CHF. As with dogs, the author prefers diltiazem to beta-blockers for rate-control in cats with CHF. If a digitalis glycoside is to be used in a cat, digoxin should be given, but in much smaller doses (e.g. 31.25 µg/cat orally q48h). Digitoxin should not be used in cats due to its extremely long half-life.

Ventricular arrhythmias
Ventricular arrhythmias can result from both cardiac and systemic disease (see Chapter 16) and can range from occasional isolated monomorphic ventricular premature complexes to rapid sustained polymorphic ventricular tachycardia. Holter monitoring studies reveal that isolated ventricular premature complexes may occur infrequently (<24 ventricular premature complexes/day) in otherwise healthy dogs (Meurs *et al.*, 2001). Even when more frequent, ventricular premature complexes do not usually result in haemodynamic compromise. Therefore, isolated ventricular premature complexes by themselves are rarely an indication for antiarrhythmic therapy. However, their presence should prompt further investigation into an underlying disease process and ambulatory (Holter) ECG monitoring to assess for a more severe arrhythmia, particularly in patients with clinical signs of haemodynamic compromise.

The electrical instability of a ventricular arrhythmia is roughly correlated to its frequency and complexity. Dogs with more complex ventricular arrhythmias (ventricular tachycardia, R-on-T phenomenon, polymorphic ventricular premature complexes) may be at greater risk of sudden cardiac death and therefore most likely to benefit from antiarrhythmic therapy, although there is at present no evidence that reduction in the frequency of ventricular ectopy or complexity of arrhythmia results in a reduced risk of sudden cardiac death. More important considerations are the presence of haemodynamic compromise and underlying cardiac disease likely to result in sudden cardiac death, such as cardiomyopathy or CHF. These patients are more likely to benefit from antiarrhythmic therapy.

Those with intermittent signs are managed with oral medications. Drugs that can be effective for the oral treatment of ventricular arrhythmias in dogs include class Ia and Ib agents, beta-blockers, sotalol and amiodarone. Mexiletine (class Ib) is generally now preferred over other class I agents (procainamide, quinidine, tocainide), which have tended to require more frequent dosing and result in greater toxicity (Calvert *et al.*, 1996b). There is also anecdotal evidence of greater efficacy for mexiletine in dogs (Lunney and Ettinger, 1991).

Antiarrhythmic medications may be given alone or in combination. Suitable combinations include a class I drug with either class II or III, or class Ia drug with a class Ib. There is evidence suggesting a benefit for such therapy in Boxers and Dobermanns with ventricular arrhythmias and episodic collapse (Meurs *et al.*, 2002; Calvert and Brown, 2004).

Ventricular tachycardia

Patients with sustained ventricular tachycardia typically present with a wide QRS complex tachycardia (QRS width ≥0.07 seconds). This is an urgent scenario and a suggested approach to wide QRS complex tachycardia is shown in Figure 20.13.

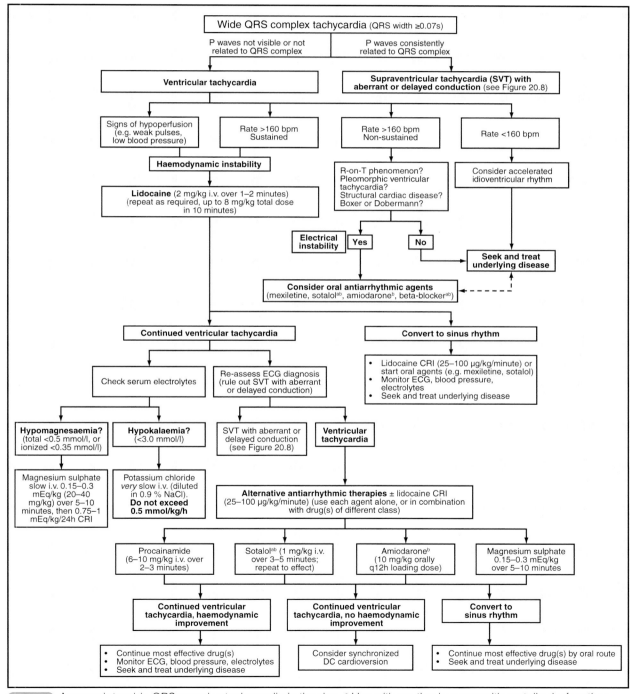

20.13 Approach to wide QRS complex tachycardia in the dog. [a] Use with caution in cases with systolic dysfunction; avoid use in cases with signs of CHF. [b] Do not give together.

Patients with a ventricular rate >160 beats/minute or clinical signs of hypoperfusion should be treated promptly and aggressively with intravenous lidocaine. Boluses of 2 mg/kg should be given to effect, or up to 8 mg/kg total dose in 10 minutes. Failure to convert warrants assessment and correction of electrolyte imbalances, re-evaluation of the ECG or use of an alternative antiarrhythmic agent. Concurrent hypokalaemia is an important reason for failure of lidocaine therapy. Choice of second-line agents is empirical and options include sotalol, procainamide, beta-blockers, magnesium sulphate and amiodarone (oral).

Patients with a ventricular rate <160 beats/minute and no signs of hypoperfusion may have an accelerated idioventricular rhythm (see Chapter 16). These arrhythmias most commonly occur following abdominal surgery and in critically ill patients. Aggressive treatment with antiarrhythmic drugs is not always necessary, as this tends to be a relatively stable rhythm and less likely to result in signs of hypoperfusion. Treatment of the underlying disease process is recommended, including the administration of analgesia, intravenous fluids and oxygen as necessary.

Failure to pharmacologically convert ventricular tachycardia to sinus rhythm confers a poor prognosis, but a reduction in rate and improvement in haemodynamic status following antiarrhythmic therapy are reasonable secondary end-points. In this circumstance, continuation of effective therapy either via CRI or orally is warranted while seeking and treating an underlying cause. Some patients may convert to sinus rhythm after several days if the acute effects of their arrhythmia are adequately managed.

Successful treatment of a ventricular arrhythmia with a parenteral antiarrhythmic usually warrants continued therapy with an oral drug of the same class. Chronic therapy with drugs or combinations that have class II effects is preferred, as this may reduce the likelihood of sudden cardiac death due to ventricular fibrillation. Sotalol, amiodarone, or mexiletine and atenolol are commonly used. The author prefers to use amiodarone for patients with systolic dysfunction or CHF, as these patients may not tolerate more potent beta-blockers.

Ultimately, the goal for any antiarrhythmic therapy is to provide a clinical benefit while minimizing adverse effects. Regular monitoring of patients that have started antiarrhythmic therapy is recommended to assess for continued arrhythmia suppression, any proarrhythmic effect and any other adverse effects. Resolution of both clinical signs and arrhythmia is desired. In those patients for whom a ventricular arrhythmia is present without clinical signs, a reduction in ventricular ectopic frequency of >80–85% on sequential 24-hour ambulatory (Holter) ECG recordings is necessary to provide evidence of an antiarrhythmic benefit. This degree of reduction is required since the day-to-day spontaneous variability in frequency of ventricular ectopy can be up to 80–85% in humans and dogs (Spier and Meurs, 2004).

Ventricular arrhythmias in cats

It is unusual for cats to develop ventricular arrhythmias that require urgent antiarrhythmic therapy. Most cats with ventricular arrhythmias have myocardial disease and, when present, arrhythmias tend to be of low grade.

Treatment options for cats with ventricular tachycardia are limited compared with those for dogs, since cats are far more susceptible to the adverse effects of class I drugs, particularly neurological and gastrointestinal effects. *Hypokalaemia should always be ruled out or treated when present.* Intravenous lidocaine can be given, but in lower doses (0.25–0.75 mg/kg bolus) and slowly (over 2–3 minutes). Beta-blockers are often preferred in cats with concurrent diastolic dysfunction but, as with dogs, they should be avoided in patients with poorly controlled CHF. Sotalol can also be given to cats, both orally and intravenously. In the author's experience this drug appears to be well tolerated in patients without systolic dysfunction or CHF. It can be given in intravenous boluses of 1 mg/kg over 3–5 minutes and repeated to effect. Another option is esmolol, 50–500 µg/kg i.v. over 5 minutes.

For chronic therapy in cats with ventricular arrhythmias, the author prefers atenolol (6.25–12.5 mg/cat orally q12–24h) or sotalol (10–20 mg/cat orally q12h, occasionally up to 30 mg/cat q12h). Procainamide and quinidine have also been used in cats, but recent limited availability, the need for more frequent dosing (three to four times daily) and frequent toxicity limit their clinical utility.

As with dogs, treatment of underlying cardiac or systemic disease is always preferable in cats with ventricular arrhythmias. Consequently, in addition to testing for hypokalaemia, *it is usually worth testing any middle-aged or older cat with a tachyarrhythmia for hyperthyroidism.* Figure 20.14 shows an example of pharmacological cardioversion of ventricular tachycardia in a cat.

Bradyarrhythmias

Bradyarrhythmias are most frequently encountered in small animals as a result of high vagal tone, general anaesthesia or sedation. These rarely require treatment beyond reversal of the underlying condition or drug. Those that require more specific treatment usually result from hyperkalaemia, inadvertent drug toxicity, or cardiac disease affecting the atria, SA or AV nodes.

Bradyarrhythmias can be divided into atrial standstill, sinus bradyarrhythmias (sinus bradycardia, sinus arrest) and AV block. *Sick sinus syndrome* and *sinus node dysfunction* are terms applied to patients with sinus bradyarrhythmias in the absence of disease causing high vagal tone.

Bradyarrhythmias that require treatment are those that are electrically unstable (may result in sudden cardiac death) or result in clinical signs of haemodynamic compromise (hypoperfusion, CHF). Sinus bradycardia, short durations of sinus arrest and low-grade second-degree AV block rarely result in clinical signs; consequently they do not require

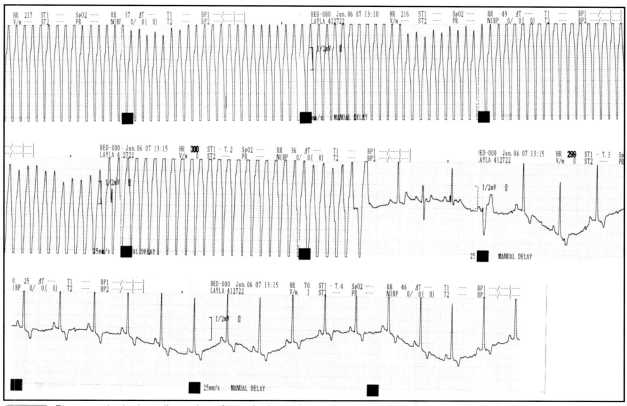

20.14 Pharmacological cardioversion of ventricular tachycardia: conversion of sustained ventricular tachycardia in a 5-year-old Domestic Shorthaired cat following slow intravenous lidocaine at a dose of 0.5 mg/kg. Ventricular tachycardia at 380 beats/minute is seen on the top strip. Conversion to sinus rhythm occurs two-thirds of the way along the middle strip. Sinus rhythm is maintained on the lower strip. Hypertrophic cardiomyopathy with focal ventricular wall thickening was diagnosed on echocardiography. Oral therapy was continued with sotalol. Lead II shown. Paper speed 25 mm/s; gain 1 cm/mV.

treatment. Those that do require treatment include high-grade AV block, sinus node dysfunction and atrial standstill. If an underlying reversible condition is present (e.g. hyperkalaemia), then this should be treated first. Otherwise *the most effective therapy is permanent pacemaker implantation* (see above). Trial therapy with sympathomimetic agents (e.g. terbutaline), phosphodiesterase inhibitors (e.g. theophylline) and/or anticholinergic agents (e.g. propantheline) may be effective in reducing clinical signs in some patients. However, response is variable and adverse effects are common (e.g. gastrointestinal signs with anticholinergic agents, hyperexcitability with phosphodiesterase inhibitors). Figure 20.15 shows an approach to bradyarrhythmias.

Bradyarrhythmias in cats
Cats with sinus bradyarrhythmias (sinus arrhythmia, sinus bradycardia, sinus arrest) usually have concurrent disease causing high vagal tone. Nasopharyngeal obstruction is a common example of this. These patients require treatment of their underlying non-cardiac disease.

Hyperkalaemic atrial standstill is the most common bradyarrhythmia in cats, with urinary obstruction the most common cause. High-grade AV block is the most common idiopathic bradyarrhythmia in cats and can cause signs of hypoperfusion and/or CHF. Third-degree AV block is more common in older cats and is often permanent. However, some cats present with sinus rhythm and syncope associated with transient third-degree AV block. These can be very difficult to distinguish from seizures, but arrhythmic episodes usually have a rapid recovery. Concurrent myocardial disease may be present, but often the disease is idiopathic.

Unlike dogs, cats may have stable and relatively fast escape rhythms (80–140 beats/minute) (Kellum and Stepien, 2006). As a consequence, some cats do not have clinical signs associated with their arrhythmia. Often the only sign is a slow heart rate detected during routine examination. Concurrent systemic disease (e.g. hyperthyroidism) may also be present. Normokalaemic atrial standstill rarely occurs in cats.

If clinical signs are present, permanent pacemaker implantation can be considered for cats with AV block or normokalaemic atrial standstill. This is usually performed via an epicardial approach, due to the technical difficulties of the transvenous route and a higher incidence of thromboembolic complications and obstruction to venous drainage.

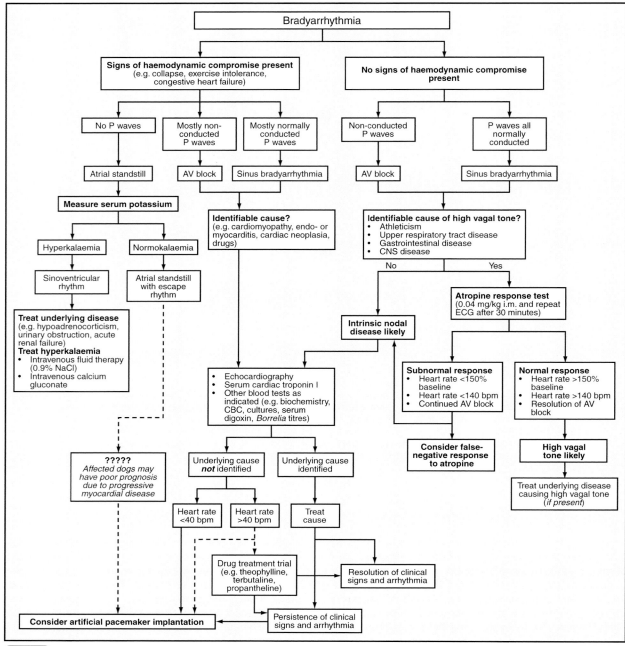

20.15 Approach to bradyarrhythmias in the dog.

References and further reading

Bright JM and zum Brunnen J (2008) Chronicity of atrial fibrillation affects duration of sinus rhythm after transthoracic cardioversion of dogs with naturally occurring atrial fibrillation. *Journal of Veterinary Internal Medicine* **22**, 114–119

Brundel BJJM, Melnyk P, Rivard L and Nattel S (2005) The pathology of atrial fibrillation in dogs. *Journal of Veterinary Cardiology* **7**, 121–129

Bulmer BJ, Sisson D, Oyama MA *et al.* (2006) Physiologic VDD versus non-physiologic VVI pacing in canine third degree atrioventricular block. *Journal of Veterinary Internal Medicine* **20**, 257–271

Calvert CA and Brown J (2004) Influence of anti-arrhythmia therapy on survival times of 19 clinically healthy Doberman Pinschers with dilated cardiomyopathy that experienced syncope, ventricular tachycardia, and sudden death (1985–1998). *Journal of the American Animal Hospital Association* **40**, 24–28

Calvert CA, Jacobs GJ and Pickus CW (1996a) Bradycardia-associated episodic weakness, syncope, and aborted sudden death in cardiomyopathic Doberman Pinschers. *Journal of Veterinary Internal Medicine* **10**, 88–93

Calvert CA, Pickus CW and Jacobs GJ (1996b) Efficacy and toxicity of tocainide for the treatment of ventricular tachyarrhythmias in Doberman Pinschers with occult cardiomyopathy. *Journal of Veterinary Internal Medicine* **10**, 235–240

Calvert CA, Sammarto C and Pickus C (2000) Positive Coombs' test result in two dogs treated with amiodarone. *Journal of the American Veterinary Medical Association* **216 (12)**, 1933–1936

Cardiac Arrhythmia Suppression Trial (CAST) Investigators (1989) The preliminary report: effect of encainide and flecainide on mortality in a randomised trial of arrhythmia suppression after myocardial infarction. *New England Journal of Medicine* **321**, 406–412

Cober RE, Schober KE, Hildebrandt N, Sikorska E and Riesen SC (2009) Adverse effects of intravenous amiodarone in 5 dogs. *Journal of Veterinary Internal Medicine* **23**, 657–661

Gelzer AR, Rishniw M and Kraus MS (2009) In-hospital

electrocardiography overestimates 24-hours ventricular rate in dogs with atrial fibrillation. *Proceedings of the 2009 ACVIM Forum*, Montreal, Canada, pp. 80

Goldberger JJ, Cain ME, Hohnloser SH *et al.* (2008) AHA/ACCF/HRS Scientific Statement on Noninvasive Risk Stratification Techniques for Identifying Patients at Risk for Sudden Cardiac Death. *Circulation* **118**, 1497–1518

Hamlin RL (1995) What is the best heart rate for a dog in atrial fibrillation? *Proceedings of the 1995 ACVIM Forum*, Lake Buena Vista, Florida pp. 325–326

Johnson MS, Martin M and Smith P (2006) Cardioversion of supraventricular tachycardia using lidocaine in five dogs. *Journal of Veterinary Internal Medicine* **20**, 272–276

Kellum HB and Stepien RL (2006) Third-degree atrioventricular block in 21 cats (1997–2004). *Journal of Veterinary Internal Medicine* **20**, 97–103

Kowey PR, Marinchak RA, Rials SJ and Bharucha DB (2000) Classification and pharmacology of anti-arrhythmic drugs. *American Heart Journal* **140**, 12–20

Lunney J and Ettinger SJ (1991) Mexiletine administration for management of ventricular arrhythmia in 22 dogs. *Journal of the American Animal Hospital Association* **27**, 597–600

Meurs KM, Spier AW, Wright NA and Hamlin RL (2001) Use of ambulatory electrocardiography for detection of ventricular premature complexes in healthy dogs. *Journal of the American Veterinary Medical Association* **218**, 1291–1292

Meurs KM, Spier AW, Wright NA *et al.* (2002) Comparison of the effects of four anti-arrhythmic treatments for familial ventricular arrhythmias in Boxers. *Journal of the American Veterinary Medical Association* **221**, 522–527

Moïse NS, Pariaut R, Gelzer ARM, Kraus MS and Jung SW (2005) Cardioversion with lidocaine of vagally associated atrial fibrillation in two dogs. *Journal of Veterinary Cardiology* **7**, 143–148

Oyama MA and Prošek R (2006) Acute conversion of atrial fibrillation in two dogs by intravenous amiodarone administration. *Journal of Veterinary Internal Medicine* **20**, 1224–1227

Oyama MA, Sisson DD and Lehmkuhl LB (2001) Practices and outcome of artificial cardiac pacing in 154 dogs. *Journal of Veterinary Internal Medicine* **15**, 229–239

Prošek R, Estrada AE and Adin DB (2006) Comparison of sotalol and mexiletine versus stand alone sotalol in treatment of boxer dogs with ventricular arrhythmias. *Journal of Veterinary Internal Medicine* **20**, 710–802A

Rathore SS, Curtis JP, Wang Y, Bristow MR and Krumholz HM (2003) Association of serum digoxin concentration and outcomes in patients with heart failure. *Journal of the American Medical Association* **289**, 871–878

Saunders AB, Miller MW, Gordon SG and Van De Wiele CM (2006) Oral amiodarone therapy in dogs with atrial fibrillation. *Journal of Veterinary Internal Medicine* **20**, 921–926

Singh BN, Singh SN, Reda DJ *et al.* (2005) Amiodarone versus sotalol for atrial fibrillation. *New England Journal of Medicine* **352**, 1861–1872

Spier AW and Meurs KM (2004) Evaluation of spontaneous variability in the frequency of ventricular arrhythmias in Boxers with arrhythmogenic right ventricular cardiomyopathy. *Journal of the American Medical Association* **224**, 538–541

Thomason JD, Kraus MS, Surdyk KK, Fallaw T and Calvert CA (2008) Bradycardia-associated syncope in 7 Boxers with ventricular tachycardia (2002–2005). *Journal of Veterinary Internal Medicine* **22**, 931–936

Vaughan Williams EM (1984) A classification of anti-arrhythmic drug actions reassessed after a decade of new drugs. *Journal of Clinical Pharmacology* **24**, 129–147

Wall M, Calvert CA, Sanderson SL *et al.* (2005) Evaluation of extended-release diltiazem once daily for cats with hypertrophic cardiomyopathy. *Journal of the American Animal Hospital Association* **41**, 98–103

Wess G, Thomas WP, Berger DM and Kittleson MD (2006) Applications, complications, and outcomes of transvenous pacemaker implantation in 105 dogs (1997–2002). *Journal of Veterinary Internal Medicine* **20**, 877–884

Wilson JR, Douglas P, Hickey WF *et al.* (1987) Experimental congestive heart failure produced by rapid ventricular pacing in the dog: cardiac effects. *Circulation* **75**(4), 857–867

Wright KN, Knilans TK and Irvin HM (2006) When, why, and how to perform cardiac radiofrequency catheter ablation. *Journal of Veterinary Cardiology* **8**, 95–107

Wyse DG, Waldo AL, DiMarco JP *et al.* (2002) A comparison of rate control and rhythm control in patients with atrial fibrillation. *New England Journal of Medicine* **347**, 1825–1833

21

Myxomatous mitral valve disease

Jens Häggström

Introduction

Myxomatous mitral valve disease (MMVD) of the atrio-ventricular (AV) valves is characterized by the accumulation of glycosaminoglycans (myxomatous proliferation) and fibrosis of the valve leaflets and tendinous chordae (Figure 21.1). The condition has been given many names, including endocardiosis, chronic degenerative valvular disease, chronic valvular disease, chronic valvular fibrosis and acquired mitral or tricuspid regurgitation or insufficiency. The valvular degeneration leads to insufficient coaptation of the valve leaflet, valvular regurgitation and, in some animals, eventually to congestive heart failure (CHF). The condition most commonly involves the mitral valve with or without involvement of the tricuspid valve. Isolated tricuspid myxomatous degeneration occurs but is less common. Likewise, myxomatous changes occur infrequently on the semilunar valves (especially the aortic) but are rarely of clinical importance.

Aetiology

The cause of myxomatous degeneration is currently unknown. The current scientific belief is that the primary factor is a defect in the quality of connective tissue (ground substance) within the valve. Affected individuals are born normal but, because of this inherent weakness of the valve, degenerative changes develop unusually early in life. There is no scientific evidence of any association between the disease and vaccination or haematological spread of bacteria from the oral cavity.

Epidemiology and inheritance

MMVD is the most common cardiac disease in dogs, but the prevalence is highly variable among different breeds. The disease is encountered in all breeds, but is most common in small to medium-sized breeds, such as the Papillon, Poodle, Chihuahua, Dachshund and Cavalier King Charles Spaniel (Egenvall *et al.*, 2006). The condition is uncommon in young individuals but is common in older dogs. Indeed, the prevalence in some affected breeds may be >90% in dogs over 10 years of age, with cardiac mortality exceeding all other causes of death in many affected breeds (Egenvall *et al.*, 2006). The prevalence of MMVD in

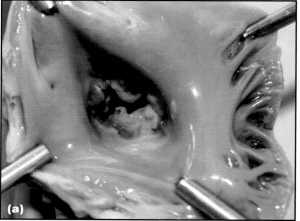

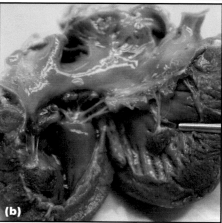

21.1 Post-mortem specimen of a dog with end-stage MMVD. **(a)** The mitral valve leaflets appear thickened and contracted when observed from the atrial side. **(b)** The thickening consists of nodules on the free edges of the leaflets and thickening of the chordae tendineae, and the left ventricle and atrium are dilated. Chordal rupture, particularly of lesser-order chordae, is a common finding but not apparent in this image. Jet lesions are present on the atrial wall, which occur when regurgitant jets of blood from the left ventricle strike the atrial wall.

cats is unknown, but seems to be extremely low and is rarely of clinical importance.

The exact genetic basis for MMVD is unknown. Because of the variable prevalence of the disease in different breeds, a genetic basis has long been suspected. However, it was not until fairly recently that MMVD was shown to be inherited in Cavaliers and

Dachshunds. The mode of inheritance is not simple and the age of disease onset is inherited as a polygenetic trait (Swenson *et al.*, 1996; Olsen *et al.*, 1999), meaning that more than one gene is involved in the disease process. Males have an earlier onset and the disease progresses more rapidly than in females (Häggström *et al.*, 2004; Egenvall *et al.*, 2006). The major role played by genetic factors suggests that other factors (level of exercise, degree of obesity, diet) play only a small role.

Pathophysiology

The progression of the disease in an affected dog involves two pathophysiological events: the progression of valve degeneration and the progression of mitral regurgitation. The latter is dependent on the severity of the former, but mild MMVD may be present without any mitral regurgitation, and mitral regurgitation may be caused by many other underlying types of cardiac disease.

Progression of valve degeneration

- The primary defect leads to abnormal valve motion with prolapse of the leaflets, which in turn increases the shear stress imposed on the leaflets, both directly (abnormal leaflet apposition) and indirectly (increased regurgitant flow).
- Regurgitation and valve stress lead to endothelial damage and subsequent activation of valvular interstitial cells (fibroblasts) in the valve (Black *et al.*, 2005).
- The activation of valvular interstitial cells leads to subendothelial deposition of glycosaminoglycans and fibrosis, resulting in further distortion of valve morphology and regurgitation (Black *et al.*, 2005).
- The abnormal stress on the valve caused by prolapse and the altered ultrastructure of the leaflets predispose to rupture of chordae tendineae, which leads to increased regurgitation.
- The end-stage valve is characterized by thickened, fibrotic and contracted leaflets, usually with evidence of ruptured low-order chordae tendineae (see Figure 21.1).

Progression of mitral regurgitation and congestive heart failure

- With progression, the valvular lesions cause insufficient coaptation of the leaflets, leading to regurgitation into the atrium.
- Severity and progression of mitral regurgitation is dependent on the severity and progression of the valvular lesions (Olsen *et al.*, 1999; Pedersen *et al.*, 1999a).
- Compensatory mechanisms include cardiac dilatation, eccentric hypertrophy, increased force and rate of contraction, increased heart rate, increased pulmonary lymphatic drainage, fluid retention and neurohormonal modulation of cardiovascular function (Häggström and Kvart, 2005).
- Ventricular dilatation further increases the regurgitation by causing secondary valvular regurgitation, so regurgitation begets regurgitation.
- With progression, compensation of the regurgitation is no longer possible, leading to reduced cardiac output and increased venous pressures with subsequent pulmonary oedema (left-sided CHF) or ascites (right-sided CHF).
- Pulmonary hypertension may develop as a consequence of left-sided heart failure.

Clinical signs

The most important clinical manifestation of MMVD is the characteristic *left apical systolic heart murmur* (see Chapter 4). A murmur is a very common incidental finding in middle-aged to old dogs. The progression of MMVD from the development of a soft heart murmur in a dog without clinical signs, to severe heart failure in advanced MMVD often takes years. Some large dogs appear to be less tolerant of the disease, and in these dogs the disease has a more rapid progression.

Coughing in the absence of congestive heart failure

Moderate to severe valvular regurgitation leading to cardiomegaly may cause compression of the mainstem bronchi. Recognition of this situation may be complicated by the fact that MMVD and bronchial collapse or chronic bronchitis frequently coexist.

Valvular regurgitation causing signs of congestive heart failure

This is most commonly left-sided. Any of the following clinical signs may be present in a typical dog with CHF attributable to mitral regurgitation:

- Cough, often worse in the morning or evening
- Tachypnoea, respiratory distress and orthopnoea
- Lethargy
- Anorexia
- Reduced exercise tolerance
- Syncope
- Weight loss (in advanced stages)
- Ascites (right-sided CHF).

Syncope

Syncope may occur via a number of mechanisms with MMVD, most of which are poorly understood (see Chapter 3). Syncope may be vasovagal or associated with supraventricular tachyarrhythmias. Syncope is often triggered by exercise or excitement, as well as by coughing (tussive syncope). Pulmonary hypertension is common in dogs with MMVD and syncope.

Sudden death

Sudden death may occur as a consequence of an acute development of a complication (see below), but is uncommon in the absence of preceding clinical signs of CHF.

Diagnostic approach

The diagnosis of mitral regurgitation caused by MMVD is usually straightforward, because both the characteristic murmur and the echocardiographic changes are easily recognized. Early detection may not be necessary for appropriate management, as the effect of mild mitral regurgitation on the circulation is minimal, and clinical signs usually develop later in the course of the disease. More importantly, it may be a diagnostic challenge to determine whether mitral regurgitation is the true underlying cause for the clinical signs.

Clinical investigation should be tailored to the individual patient and will include tests listed in Figure 21.2.

Physical examination

Dogs without clinical signs of disease

- Systolic click (early stage): high pitched, sharp sound between S1 and S2 heart sounds. This sound is frequently mistaken for a gallop sound.

- Apical systolic heart murmur is present with mitral or tricuspid regurgitation (Figure 21.3).
- A soft, early, late or holosystolic murmur (grades 1–2/6) is consistent with mild regurgitation; a loud murmur (grades 4–6/6) is consistent with moderate to severe regurgitation (Häggström et al., 1994).
- A systolic click and/or a left apical systolic murmur compatible with mitral regurgitation in a middle-aged to old dog of a typical breed is highly suggestive, but not conclusive evidence, of myxomatous valve disease (Häggström et al., 1994; Pedersen et al., 1999b) (Figure 21.3).
- Presence of sinus arrhythmia is usually associated with less severe mitral regurgitation, and is rare with CHF.
- Isolated atrial premature complexes are common in some small dogs and the presence of a few such complexes on the electrocardiogram (ECG) may not necessarily indicate severe disease (see below).

History	Coughing?	See Chapter 2
	Breathlessness?	See Chapter 1
	Syncope?	See Chapter 3
	Signs indicative of concurrent disease?	Additional tests may be necessary
	Previous medication?	Note response and current treatment
Physical examination	Heart rate and rhythm?	Normal heart rate and sinus arrhythmia are less likely to be associated with CHF Tachyarrhythmias indicate more advanced disease
	Murmur?	Left apical holosystolic murmur is typical
	Increased respiratory rate and effort?	May indicate pulmonary oedema
	Pulmonary crackles?	May indicate more severe pulmonary oedema, other causes of airway fluid or pulmonary fibrosis
Thoracic radiography	Left atrial enlargement?	Clinically significant disease is usually associated with left atrial enlargement
	Mainstem bronchus compression?	May be associated with coughing in absence of CHF
	Pulmonary infiltrates?	Consistent with pulmonary oedema (hilar or generalized)
	Signs of non-cardiac disease?	Are alternative causes of coughing/tachypnoea present?
Echocardiography	Thick/prolapsing mitral valve leaflets?	Helps confirm diagnosis of MMVD
	Left atrial enlargement?	Good indicator of prognosis
	Systolic function?	Normal with mild mitral regurgitation, hyperdynamic left ventricle with severe mitral regurgitation in small dogs With reduced systolic function, consider dilated cardiomyopathy
	Mitral regurgitation on colour flow Doppler?	Helps confirm diagnosis of mitral regurgitation, but rule out other causes
Electrocardiography	Tachyarrhythmia?	Atrial premature complexes or atrial fibrillation indicate more advanced disease
Blood tests	Azotaemia?	Pre-renal azotaemia common, may be exacerbated by therapy
	NTproBNP?	Low concentrations suggest mild disease, high concentrations suggest risk of heart failure
Blood pressure	Hypertension?	May exacerbate signs of MMVD
	Hypotension?	May indicate severe output failure or may be associated with vasodilator use or overzealous use of diuretics

21.2 Diagnostic approach to suspected MMVD.

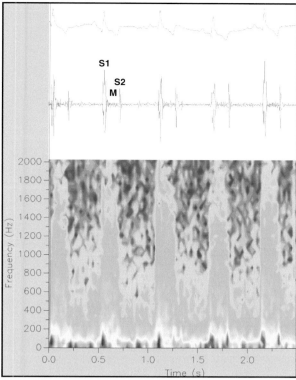

21.3 Phonocardiogram (PCG) from a Cavalier King Charles Spaniel with a moderate intensity murmur due to MMVD. The recording is displayed in two modes: the upper mode shows synchronous PCG and ECG traces; and the lower mode shows a time–frequency graph where different frequencies are displayed according to intensity, with high-intensity frequencies in red and low-intensity frequencies in blue. The two PCG tracings are timed with respect to each other. Note that the murmur is composed of sound with a frequency up to 1400 Hz, but the most intense part of the murmur is composed of low-frequency components (<400 Hz), which gives the murmur a harsh character. M = Murmur; S1 = First heart sound; S2 = Second heart sound.

Dogs with congestive heart failure

- Loud heart murmur (grade 4–6/6) is usually present.
- The first heart sound is loud (Häggström *et al.*, 1994), unless there is significant systolic dysfunction from concurrent myocardial disease, and the second heart sound is decreased in intensity (may often be difficult to hear).
- Tachycardia and loss of respiratory sinus arrhythmia.
- Arrhythmia may be present, most commonly frequent supraventricular premature complexes. Atrial fibrillation or frequent ventricular premature complexes are indicative of severe disease and a poor prognosis.
- Weak femoral pulses and pulse deficits.
- Prolonged capillary refill time and pale mucous membranes.
- Tachypnoea, respiratory distress and orthopnoea.
- Respiratory crackles and wheezes may sometimes be evident with pulmonary oedema.

- Pink froth in the nostrils and oropharynx from acute, severe pulmonary oedema (fulminant CHF).
- Ascites and jugular venous distension if right-sided CHF is present.

Imaging

Echocardiography
Echocardiography is the method of choice to diagnose MMVD and estimate the severity of mitral regurgitation. However, the method cannot accurately diagnose the presence of CHF. Echocardiographic findings include thickening and/or prolapse of the AV valve and identification of a regurgitant jet on spectral or colour flow Doppler (see Chapter 11) (Figure 21.4).

- Determination of the severity of mitral regurgitation includes assessment of the magnitude of left atrial dilatation and left ventricular eccentric hypertrophy (see Chapter 11). Size of the regurgitant jet on colour Doppler is not an exact method to assess severity of regurgitation, but may be used to semi-quantify severity of mitral regurgitation (Kittleson, 1998; Kittleson and Brown, 2003).
- Unlike small-breed dogs, affected large-breed dogs are less likely to present with severe valve prolapse and thickening. Indeed, some of these dogs may present with massive mitral regurgitation but relatively modest valvular changes.

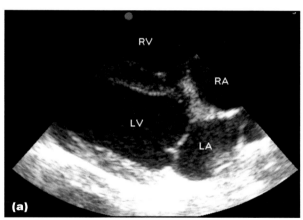

(a)

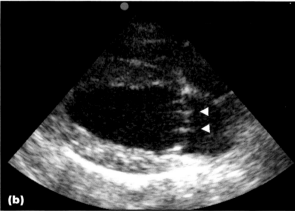

(b)

21.4 Right parasternal long-axis views of the left atrium (LA) and left ventricle (LV) during systole in: **(a)** a normal dog; **(b)** a dog with mild mitral valve prolapse and MMVD. RA = Right atrium; RV = Right ventricle. (continues) ▶

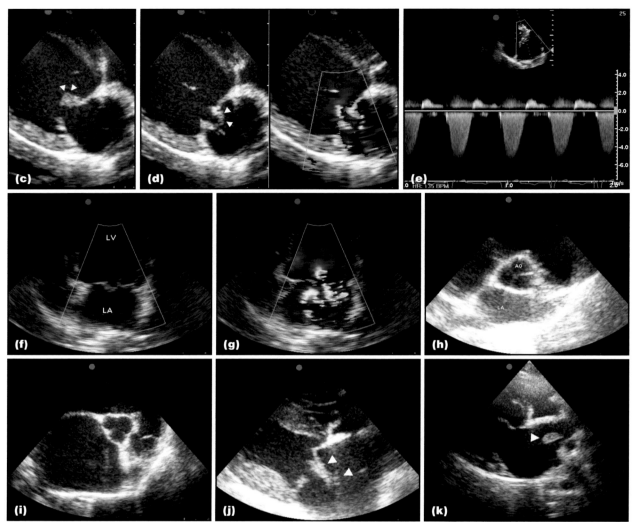

21.4 Right parasternal long-axis views of the left atrium (LA) and left ventricle (LV) during systole in: **(c,d)** a dog with severe mitral valve prolapse and MMVD. In (c) the mitral valve appears thickened in diastole (arrowheads); and prolapse is evident in (b) and (d) as systolic displacement of both leaflets to the atrial side of the mitral annulus (arrowheads). Colour Doppler echocardiography in (d) shows valvular regurgitation during systole. Mitral regurgitation is usually, but not always, best captured in a left apical four-chamber view because of better alignment with the blood flow. **(e,f,g)** Flow velocity of the regurgitant jet (e) is often measured in the same view because of the same reason, and flow velocity in a typical case is often approximately 5.5–6 m/s unless there is significant systolic dysfunction, when the flow velocity is lower, or there is poor alignment. Appearance of the LA in a right parasternal short-axis view at the aortic valve level in: **(h)** a normal dog; and **(i)** a dog with a severely enlarged LA. Complications to the disease include rupture of multiple major chordae tendineae causing: **(j)** a 'flail' mitral valve leaflet (arrowheads); and **(k)** the development of intracardiac blood clots (arrowhead).

Electrocardiography

Electrocardiography does not allow a definitive diagnosis of MMVD, mitral regurgitation or CHF (see Chapter 9). Abnormal duration or amplitude of the PQRS complexes are common findings in severe disease and such findings are usually indicative of secondary changes in cardiac size. Unfortunately, electrocardiography is an insensitive method to detect such abnormalities; echocardiography and radiography are preferred. However, it is the most useful diagnostic test to detect and characterize arrhythmias. Presence of a tachyarrhythmia such as atrial fibrillation or ventricular premature depolarizations on an ECG usually indicates severe disease, presence of a complication (acute chordal rupture or myocardial infarction) or other concurrent

cardiac disease. Atrial premature complexes are the most common arrhythmia in AV regurgitation (see above).

Thoracic radiography

Radiography cannot be used to diagnose MMVD or mitral regurgitation, but it is the method of choice to detect the consequences of MMVD and mitral regurgitation (i.e. to diagnose left-sided cardiomegaly, pulmonary oedema and congestion) (see Chapter 6). Furthermore, thoracic radiography is important for excluding other diseases as a cause for respiratory signs of disease and allows a global estimate of cardiac size. Radiographic findings include left-sided cardiomegaly and left atrial dilatation in dogs with moderate or severe mitral regurgitation (Figure 21.5).

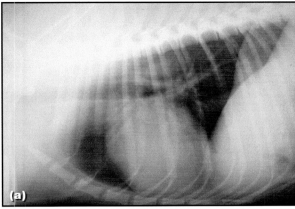

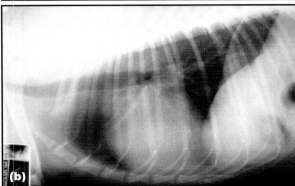

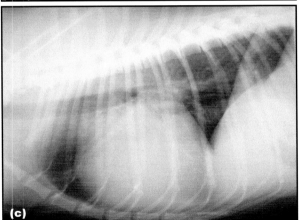

21.5 Left lateral recumbent views of a dog with MMVD and mitral regurgitation. **(a)** The dog was asymptomatic, and the radiograph shows a normal cardiac silhouette and vascular perfusion. **(b)** Radiograph of the same dog 2 years later. The dog was still asymptomatic, but the intensity of the murmur had increased. Left atrial and left ventricular enlargement are evident, with elevation and slight compression of the left mainstem bronchus, but the vascular markings are within normal limits. **(c)** 1 year later the dog had developed respiratory distress and had suffered episodes of syncope. In addition to the findings in (b), there is more obvious cardiomegaly, compression of the left mainstem bronchus and evidence of pulmonary congestion and interstitial oedema. (Courtesy of K. Hansson.)

- A vertebral heart size of >10.5 is suggestive of cardiac enlargement, but some breed variation has been reported (Buchanan and Bücheler, 1995; Lamb *et al.*, 2001).
- Recognition of left atrial dilatation is very important.

- Left-sided CHF is characterized by perihilar to caudodorsal pulmonary infiltrates (interstitial, mixed or alveolar pattern) and pulmonary venous distension.
- Compression of the left mainstem bronchus is seen by widening of the left bronchial angle at the body of the left atrium on dorsoventral (DV)/ventrodorsal (VD) views, and splitting apart of the bronchi on the lateral view.

Blood pressure
Blood pressure should be measured to identify dogs with systemic hypertension (see Chapter 26). Mitral regurgitation is greatly worsened by increased afterload. Hypotension with low output signs may also occur with arrhythmias, secondary systolic dysfunction, excessive vasodilator therapy or overzealous diuresis.

Haematology

Routine blood tests
Haematology and serum biochemistry are useful to detect concurrent disease or secondary consequences of mitral valve disease (e.g. pre-renal azotaemia, electrolyte imbalances, anaemia) and for guiding therapeutic decisions (see Chapter 8). Haematology and biochemistry panels are usually unremarkable in mild cases.

Biomarkers
New blood-based tests are available and may be very valuable for evaluating disease severity (natriuretic peptides) and for identifying active myocardial damage (troponins) (see Chapter 8). Plasma concentrations of natriuretic peptides (NTproANP and NTproBNP) may be useful as a point-of-care test to differentiate dogs with respiratory distress due to CHF from other causes (DeFrancesco, 2007; Prosek *et al.*, 2007), and for staging of disease. Values are often unremarkable in less severe cases (normal reference range varies with particular method). Moderate to severe disease is always associated with increased levels (Häggström *et al.*, 2000). Serum troponin I (cTnl) levels are normal (normal reference range varies between different methods) in mild cases, and mild to moderately increased with moderate to severe disease. Severe elevations are rare, and when present usually indicate myocardial ischaemia, myocarditis, or infarction (Oyama and Sisson, 2004; Prosek *et al.*, 2007).

Differential diagnoses
The differential diagnoses for mitral regurgitation include:

- Mitral regurgitation secondary to a primary cardiomyopathy
- Mitral dysplasia
- Mitral regurgitation secondary to congenital heart disease, resulting in left ventricle dilatation (e.g. patent ductus arteriosus)
- Infective endocarditis of the mitral valve
- Systemic hypertension.

Treatment

The ideal therapy for MMVD would halt the progression of the valvular degeneration, or improve valvular function (e.g. by surgical repair or valve replacement). However, no therapy is currently known to inhibit or prevent the valvular degeneration, and surgery is not technically or economically practical in most veterinary patients. The management of MMVD and mitral regurgitation is therefore palliative, by ameliorating the clinical signs and improving survival. This usually means that therapy is tailored to the individual patient, owner and practitioner, and often involves concurrent treatment with two or more drugs once signs of heart failure are evident (Figure 21.6).

Preclinical dogs

Medical treatment is not indicated in the absence of clinical signs of disease (Atkins *et al.*, 2009). No treatment has convincingly been shown to slow or halt disease progression in preclinical disease (Kvart *et al.*, 2002; Häggström *et al.*, 2004; Atkins *et al.*, 2007).

Dogs with coughing but no evidence of congestive heart failure

For appropriate work up and therapy of dogs with primary airway disease, see Chapter 29.

- Obese dogs should be fed a calorie-restricted diet, as obesity may promote inactivity and exacerbate bronchial compression and tracheal instability (if present).
- Arterial vasodilators such as amlodipine have been used by the author to reduce afterload, reduce regurgitant fraction, and possibly reduce left atrial size. They should not be used in hypotensive patients.
- Cough suppressants can be helpful when primary cardiorespiratory disease has been ruled out:

- Codeine (0.5–2 mg/kg orally q12h)
- Butorphanol (0.5–1 mg/kg orally q6–12h)
- Hydrocodone bitartrate (1–5 mg/dog orally q6–12h).

Dogs with congestive heart failure

The therapeutic goal is to alleviate clinical signs and improve quality of life, as well as life expectancy (see Chapter 18). Treatment involves eliminating pulmonary oedema and/or ascites, improving haemodynamic flow, controlling heart rate in patients with arrhythmias, reducing afterload in an attempt to reduce the severity of mitral regurgitation, providing inotropic support, and protecting the heart from detrimental exposure to neurohormones.

Acute/life-threatening heart failure

Treatment for patients with severe acute pulmonary oedema includes:

- Diuresis with parenteral furosemide: dose depends on the severity of CHF (the author uses 4–8 mg/kg q2–6h, preferably i.v., i.m. or s.c.)
- Oxygen supplementation and cage rest (see Chapter 17)
- Additional treatment options:
  - Glyceryl trinitrate ointment topically
  - Nitroprusside 1–5 µg/kg/minute continuous rate infusion (CRI) (do not use in hypotensive animals)
  - Pimobendan 0.1–0.3 mg/kg orally q12h.

Therapeutic success is preferably monitored by measuring the respiratory rate and assessing the degree of respiratory distress.

Chronic heart failure

Choice of drug and drug combinations depends on the disease severity and clinical signs (see Chapter 18 and Figure 21.6).

Disease stage	Standard treatment	Optional use	Diet/exercise
Heart disease, no CHF	No treatment	No drug has been shown effective at this stage. Suggested drugs include: ACE inhibitors, beta adrenergic receptor blockers, spironolactone	Normal diet and exercise (decrease calorie intake if obese)
Mild to moderate CHF	Furosemide Pimobendan ACE inhibitor	Spironolactone Digoxin	Avoid salt load Restrict exercise until CHF resolved, then avoid extreme exertion
Severe/ life-threatening CHF	Intravenous furosemide Oxygen Pimobendan	Glyceryl trinitrate Sedation (e.g. butorphanol) if distressed Thoracocentesis if large pleural effusions Dobutamine if hypotensive Intravenous nitroprusside plus dobutamine if non-responsive pulmonary oedema Continue with ACE inhibitors/spironolactone if already receiving	Encourage eating Cage rest
Refractory CHF	Furosemide (increase dose until no further effect or 5 mg/kg q8h) Pimobendan ACE inhibitor Spironolactone	Thiazides Parenteral furosemide Abdominocentesis if refractory ascites Amlodipine or hydralazine Sildenafil if severe pulmonary hypertension Digoxin if atrial fibrillation	Avoid salt load Avoid undue exertion

21.6 Therapy for MMVD.

Mild to moderate CHF:

- Oral furosemide: dose to effect (1–3 mg/kg q12–24h).
- Pimobendan: reduced mortality compared with an angiotensin-converting enzyme (ACE) inhibitor in dogs with CHF and MMVD (Häggström *et al.*, 2008).
- ACE inhibitor: indicated in conjunction with furosemide and pimobendan.

Chronic refractory CHF: Increased furosemide doses are necessary to control CHF signs, and additional drugs are added if insufficient (furosemide is continued and *not* replaced by other drugs):

- Oral furosemide: increase dose until no further effect or 5 mg/kg q8h
- Pimobendan
- ACE inhibitor
- Spironolactone.

  Additional therapy includes:

- Thiazide diuretics
- Amlodipine
- Digoxin
- Abdominocentesis may be necessary with severe refractory ascites
- If atrial fibrillation develops, heart rate must be controlled (usually with digoxin).

Monitoring and follow up

Client education is vital for successful management of the dog at home. Owners of preclinical dogs should be taught how to recognize the common clinical signs of CHF and what to do if such signs develop. In moderate to severe cases, it is often useful to instruct an owner to administer an additional dose of furosemide if the dog develops signs of respiratory difficulty. Owners of dogs diagnosed with CHF should be educated on how to measure the respiratory rate when the dog is at rest, the importance of regular administration of drugs and how to adjust the dose of furosemide within a fixed range, based on persistent or dramatic increases in resting respiratory rate.

Frequency of follow up examinations depends on the severity of mitral regurgitation, clinical signs and owner compliance with medications and monitoring.

- Preclinical dogs with slight to moderate regurgitation can be rechecked every 6–12 months and those with moderate to severe regurgitation are rechecked by the author every 3 months.
- Following control of acute heart failure and discharge from the hospital, a follow up examination should be scheduled for 1–2 weeks later to check for resolution of clinical signs, level of dehydration, electrolytes, renal function, radiographic evidence of CHF and the presence of complications. If the dog is stable, follow up examinations are scheduled every 3–6 months thereafter, with more severe cases requiring more frequent monitoring.

Complications

Dogs should be monitored for the following complications:

- The development of CHF in previously preclinical dogs
- Recurrence of CHF in dogs previously stabilized by medical therapy
- Reduced systolic function, as indicated by an increase in end-systolic left ventricular dimension and a reduction of the fractional shortening on serial echocardiographic measurements
- Progression of left-sided CHF to biventricular CHF with ascites (Johnson *et al.*, 1999)
- Development of cardiac cachexia (very common)
- Onset of arrhythmias such as atrial fibrillation, which may worsen CHF
- Rupture of chordae tendineae, which may cause life-threatening pulmonary oedema or sudden death
- Pericardial effusion and cardiac tamponade, which may develop following a left atrial tear (an acquired atrial septal defect may also arise this way)
- Formation of an intracardiac thrombus and/or large myocardial infarction (rare).

Small infarcts caused by arteriosclerotic changes are common, but their clinical significance is currently unknown (Häggström and Kvart, 2005).

Prognosis

Prognosis and outcome are highly variable. Dogs may remain free from clinical signs of CHF for several years.

- Risk factors for progression from mild to severe disease include the severity of valvular lesions, increased age and male gender (increased risk in some breeds; Olsen *et al.*, 1999; Pedersen *et al.*, 1999a).
- Risk factors for the onset of CHF include regurgitation severity, left atrial size and elevations of natriuretic peptides (Häggström *et al.*, 2000).

The prognosis for dogs with CHF (acute or stabilized) is dependent on age, breed, severity of mitral regurgitation (as indicated by left atrial size) and CHF (as indicated by pulmonary oedema and clinical signs), type of CHF therapy, left ventricular systolic function, presence of cardiac cachexia, and the presence of other diseases (e.g. renal failure) (Borgarelli *et al.*, 2008; Häggström *et al.*, 2008). Development of complications such as atrial fibrillation or rupture of major chordae tendineae or thromboembolism and myocardial infarction are associated with a poor prognosis.

Clinical trials have shown a mean survival time after onset of CHF of 6–10 months (Ettinger *et al.*, 1998; BENCH Study Group, 1999; Häggström *et al.*, 2008), but survival time may vary from days to years in different dogs.

References and further reading

Atkins CE, Keene BW, Brown WA *et al.* (2007) Results of the veterinary enalapril trial to prove reduction in onset of heart failure in dogs chronically treated with enalapril alone for compensated, naturally occurring mitral valve insufficiency. *Journal of the American Veterinary Medical Association* **231**, 1061–1069

Atkins CE, Bonagura J, Ettinger P *et al.* (2009) Guidelines for the diagnosis and treatment of canine chronic valvular heart disease. *Journal of Veterinary Internal Medicine* **23**, 1142–1150

BENCH Study Group (1999) The effect of benazepril on survival times and clinical signs of dogs with congestive heart failure: results of a multicenter, prospective, randomized, double-blinded, placebo-controlled, long-term clinical trial. *Journal of Veterinary Cardiology* **1**, 7–18

Black A, French A, Dukes-McEwan J *et al.* (2005) Ultrastructural morphologic evaluation of the phenotype of valvular interstitial cells in dogs with myxomatous degeneration of the mitral valve. *American Journal of Veterinary Research* **66**, 1408–1414

Borgarelli M, Savarino P, Crosara S *et al.* (2008) Survival characteristics and prognostic variables of dogs with mitral regurgitation attributable to myxomatous valve disease. *Journal of Veterinary Internal Medicine* **22**, 120–128

Buchanan JW and Bücheler J (1995) Vertebral scale system to measure canine heart size in radiographs. *Journal of the American Veterinary Medical Association* **206**, 194–199

DeFrancesco, TC (2007) Utility of an ELISA B-type natriuretic peptide assay in the diagnosis of congestive heart failure in dogs presenting with cough or dyspnea. *Journal of Veterinary Internal Medicine* **21**, 243–250

Egenvall A, Bonnett B and Häggström J (2006) Heart disease as a cause of death in insured Swedish dogs less than 10 years of age. *Journal of Veterinary Internal Medicine* **20**, 894–903

Ettinger SJ, Benitz AM, Ericsson GF *et al.* (1998) Effects of enalapril maleate on survival of dogs with naturally acquired heart failure. The Long-Term Investigation of Veterinary Enalapril (LIVE) Study Group. *Journal of the American Veterinary Medical Association* **213**, 1573–1577

Häggström J, Boswood A, O'Grady M *et al.* (2008) Effect of pimobendan versus benazepril hydrochloride on survival times in dogs with congestive heart failure due to naturally occurring myxomatous mitral valve disease: results of the QUEST study. *Journal of Veterinary Internal Medicine* **22**, 1124–1135

Häggström J, Hansson K and Kvart C (1994) Heart sounds and murmurs: changes related to severity of mitral regurgitation in Cavalier King Charles spaniels. *Journal of Veterinary Internal Medicine* **9**, 75–85

Häggström J, Hansson K, Kvart C *et al.* (2000) Secretion patterns of the natriuretic peptides in naturally acquired mitral regurgitation attributable to chronic valvular disease in dogs. *Journal of Veterinary Cardiology* **2**, 7–16

Häggström J and Kvart C (2005) Acquired valvular heart disease. In: *Textbook of Veterinary Internal Medicine. Diseases of Dogs and Cats, 6th edn*, ed. SJ Ettinger and EC Feldman, pp. 1022–1040. WB Saunders, Philadelphia

Häggström J, Pedersen HD and Kvart C (2004) New insights into degenerative mitral valve disease in dogs. *Veterinary Clinics of North America: Small Animal Practice* **34**, 1209–1226

Johnson L, Boon J and Orton, EC (1999) Clinical characteristics of 53 dogs with Doppler-derived evidence of pulmonary hypertension: 1992–1996. *Journal of Veterinary Internal Medicine* **13**, 440–447

Kittleson M (1998) Myxomatous atrioventricular valvular degeneration. In: *Small Animal Cardiovascular Medicine*, ed. MD Kittleson and R Kienle, pp. 297–318. Mosby Inc, St. Louis, Missouri

Kittleson M and Brown W (2003) Regurgitant faction measured by using the proximal isovelocity surface area in dogs with chronic myxomatous mitral valve disease. *Journal of Veterinary Internal Medicine* **17**, 84–88

Kvart C, Haggstrom J, Pedersen HD *et al.* (2002) Efficacy of enalapril for prevention of congestive heart failure in dogs with myxomatous valve disease and asymptomatic mitral regurgitation. *Journal of Veterinary Internal Medicine* **16**, 80–88

Lamb CR, Wikeley H, Boswood A and Pfeiffer DU (2001) Use of breed-specific ranges for the vertebral heart scale as an aid to the radiographic diagnosis of cardiac disease in dogs. *Veterinary Record* **148**, 707–711

Olsen L, Fredholm M and Pedersen HD (1999) Epidemiology and inheritance of mitral valve prolapse in Dachshunds. *Journal of Veterinary Internal Medicine* **13**, 448–456

Oyama M and Sisson D (2004) Cardiac troponin-I concentration in dogs with cardiac disease. *Journal of Veterinary Internal Medicine* **18**, 831–839

Parameswaran N, Hamlin RL, Nakayama T *et al.* (1999) Increased splenic capacity in response to transdermal application of nitroglycerine in the dog. *Journal of Veterinary Internal Medicine* **13**, 44–46

Pedersen HD, Häggström J, Falk T *et al.* (1999b) Auscultation in mild mitral regurgitation in dogs: observer variation, effects of physical maneuvers, and agreement with color doppler echocardiography and phonocardiography. *Journal of Veterinary Internal Medicine* **13**, 56–64

Pedersen HD, Lorentzen K and Kristensen BO (1999a) Echocardiographic mitral valve prolapse in cavalier King Charles spaniels: epidemiology and prognostic significance for regurgitation. *Veterinary Record* **144**, 315–326

Prosek R, Sisson DD, Oyama MA and Solter PF (2007) Distinguishing cardiac and noncardiac dyspnea in 48 dogs using plasma atrial natriuretic factor, B-type natriuretic factor, endothelin, and cardiac troponin-I. *Journal of Veterinary Internal Medicine* **21**, 238–242

Swenson L, Häggström J, Kvart C *et al.* (1996) Relationship between parental cardiac status in Cavalier King Charles spaniels and prevalence and severity of chronic valvular disease in offspring. *Journal of the American Veterinary Medical Association* **208**, 2009–2012

22

Infective endocarditis

Jens Häggström

Introduction

Infective endocarditis (IE) is caused by invasion of the valvular endothelium by microbes, resulting in proliferative or erosive lesions and consequently valvular insufficiency (Figure 22.1). The mitral and aortic valves are almost exclusively infected in small animals (Miller *et al.*, 2004). Vegetative lesions may result in embolism or metastatic infection involving multiple body organs, producing a large variety of clinical signs. Endocarditis has a low incidence (0.04–0.13% of all dogs referred to one veterinary medical teaching hospital) (MacDonald *et al.*, 2004). The incidence in cats is considerably lower.

Aetiology

Transient or persistent bacteraemia is a prerequisite for the development of IE. Common routes of infection include discospondylitis, prostatitis, pneumonia, urinary tract infections, pyoderma, periodontal disease and long-term indwelling central venous catheters. A proportion of cases with IE have no clinically detectable source of infection (Sisson and Thomas, 1984). The condition has been associated with sub-aortic stenosis and high-velocity shunting diseases (e.g. patent ductus arteriosus, ventricular septal defect) (Sisson and Thomas, 1984). There is a possible increased risk associated with corticosteroid use (Calvert, 1982). IE has not been found to have any association with myxomatous mitral valve disease (MMVD) in dogs. Furthermore, the risk of IE seems to be very small following conditions or procedures that cause bacteraemia (e.g. dental cleaning, endoscopy) unless another predisposing factor coexists.

The most common bacteria isolated from diseased patients are:

- *Staphylococcus* spp. (*aureus, intermedius,* coagulase positive and coagulase negative)
- *Streptococcus* spp. (*canis, bovis* and beta-haemolytic)
- *Escherichia coli*.

Less commonly isolated bacteria include:

- *Pseudomonas* spp.
- *Erysipelothrix rhusiopathiae*
- *Enterobacter* spp.
- *Pasteurella* spp.

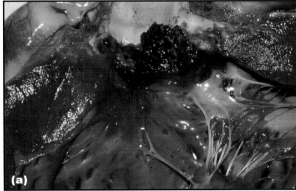

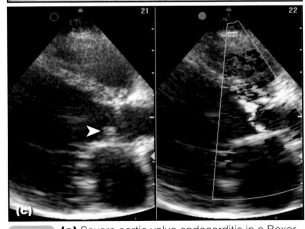

22.1 **(a)** Severe aortic valve endocarditis in a Boxer. (Courtesy of V. Luis Fuentes.) **(b)** Histopathological examination of the aortic valve in a Kelpie showing infiltrates of inflammatory cells within the cusps. (Courtesy of G. Hestvik.) **(c)** Echocardiogram performed during the clinical work up of the dog in (b) showing thickened and immobile aortic valve cusps and significant aortic regurgitation (arrowhead).

- *Corynebacterium* spp.
- *Proteus* spp.

The majority of cases (60–70%) are culture negative, presumably because many dogs are already receiving antibiotic therapy prior to blood culture (Sisson and Thomas, 1984; MacDonald *et al.*, 2004). In addition, *Bartonella* spp. (*B. vinsonii berkhoffii*, *B. henselae*, *B. clarridgeiae*, *B. clarridgeiae*-like, *B. washoensis*) are intracellular bacteria that have recently emerged as an important cause of endocarditis in dogs. *Bartonella* spp. were reported to be the causative agent of endocarditis in 28% (5 out of 18) of dogs with IE in a recent North American study, representing 45% (5 out of 11) of dogs with negative blood cultures (MacDonald *et al.*, 2004). Another study from the same institution found that 19% (6 out of 31) of dogs with negative blood cultures tested positive for *Bartonella* spp. (Sykes *et al.*, 2006). Both studies reported that *Bartonella* spp. infection was always associated with IE of the aortic valve. Recent European reports have demonstrated that infection with *B. henselae* appears to be particularly common in cats in Europe (Barnes *et al.*, 2000), but no association with IE has been made.

Pathophysiology

Non-bacterial thrombotic endocarditis
Endothelial damage and a hypercoagulable state predispose to the development of platelet-fibrin deposition on damaged valve tissue. Disruption of endothelial surfaces may occur secondary to inflammation (e.g. vasculitis) or mechanical damage (e.g. from high-velocity flow secondary to subaortic stenosis). The resulting cellular deposits are referred to as *non-bacterial thrombotic endocarditis* (*NBTE*). During bacteraemia, microorganisms adhere to these sites via exposed fibronectin, converting NBTE to IE.

Colonization of the valve
The inciting event is bacterial adherence to valve structures. This may occur through either a direct adherence of the bacteria with the surface endothelium via the bloodstream, or adherence of bacteria to capillaries within the valve. The coagulum of fibrinogen, fibrin, platelet proteins and fibronectin forms and avidly binds bacteria, protecting them from host defence and antibiotics. Bacterial pathogenicity is also an important factor in both adherence to endothelial surfaces and subsequent valve damage.

Valve tissue destruction
The destruction of valvular tissue can be caused by the action of bacteria or the cellular response of the immune system. Immune complexes form, which primarily consist of immunoglobulins, complement factors and bacterial antigens. These are deposited in the basement membrane and cause further complement activation and tissue destruction. In addition, immune-mediated glomerulonephritis, polyarthritis and skin diseases are common sequelae of immune complex deposition.

Embolization
Septic or aseptic emboli frequently lodge in the kidneys, spleen, heart, brain, systemic arteries and other organs. These emboli do not always cause clinical signs, but evidence of systemic embolization is common at post-mortem examination in dogs with IE.

Effects on heart function
The haemodynamic effects of IE depend on the severity and rate of development of structural changes to valve morphology. Severe mitral or aortic insufficiency leads to elevated left ventricular end-diastolic pressure, left atrial pressure and pulmonary capillary pressure, with subsequent left-sided congestive heart failure (CHF). With severe acute valvular disruption, pulmonary oedema may develop early in the clinical course. With less disruptive lesions, progressive left ventricular remodelling may develop before the onset of CHF.

Clinical signs

IE can easily be overlooked as the history and clinical signs are non-specific and predisposing factors are not always present. Medium to large breeds and middle-aged to older male dogs are more commonly affected with IE. The most common clinical signs include:

- Lameness
- Lethargy
- Anorexia
- Respiratory abnormalities
- Weakness and collapse
- Neurological signs
- Haematuria.

Diagnostic approach

Since the clinical signs of IE are generally associated with septic embolization of other organs rather than the heart, the diagnosis is easily overlooked. The likelihood of a correct ante-mortem diagnosis of IE is increased if it is based on a set of major and minor criteria (Figure 22.2).

Physical examination
Cardiovascular abnormalities are commonly found. A murmur is present in most (89–96%) dogs (Calvert, 1982; MacDonald *et al.*, 2004): a left apical holosystolic murmur occurs with mitral regurgitation; whereas a left basilar diastolic murmur with bounding femoral arterial pulses is highly suggestive of aortic valve involvement. Many dogs (40–70%) have arrhythmias, including ventricular arrhythmias, supraventricular tachycardia, atrioventricular block and atrial fibrillation (Calvert, 1982; Sisson and Thomas, 1984; MacDonald *et al.*, 2004). Respiratory distress, cough, or crackles on lung auscultation may be present in animals with CHF. Fever is present in 70% of dogs and joint effusion and lameness are also common (Calvert, 1982; Sisson and Thomas, 1984; MacDonald *et al.*, 2004).

Major criteria of IE	Minor criteria of IE
Positive echocardiographic findings (vegetative, erosive lesion or abscess) Newly developed moderate to severe aortic insufficiency in the absence of congenital disease, aortic disease or severe systemic hypertension Positive blood culture for typical microorganism (≥2 positive blood cultures)	Fever Medium to large dog (>15 kg) Subaortic stenosis Thromboembolic disease Immune-mediated disease Immunocompromised (such as chronic systemic corticosteroid therapy) Polyarthritis/glomerulonephritis Single positive blood culture or atypical organism

Definitive diagnosis of IE	Possible diagnosis of IE	No diagnosis of IE
Histopathology of valve 2 major criteria 1 major and 2 minor criteria	1 major and 1 minor criterion	Other cardiac disease diagnosed Resolution of regurgitation or valvular abnormality within 4 days of treatment No pathological evidence of IE on post-mortem examination

22.2 Criteria for diagnosis of IE. Modified from the Modified Duke criteria used in human medicine for the diagnosis of endocarditis (Baddour *et al.*, 2005).

Imaging

Echocardiography
Valvular vegetations may be detected using two-dimensional (2D) echocardiography, but small or less advanced lesions may be difficult to distinguish from myxomatous disease (see Figures 22.1c and 22.3). Mitral vegetations do not normally result in valve prolapse. 2D and M-mode echocardiography can also be used to measure secondary changes in cardiac size.

- Echocardiographic identification of a hyperechoic oscillating vegetative lesion on the valve is the principal method of diagnosing endocarditis.
- Erosive lesions may be more difficult to identify.
- The presence and severity of valvular insufficiency is assessed in the same way as valvular insufficiency due to other causes (see Chapter 11).
- Left atrial enlargement may be present with

chronic endocarditis of the mitral valve, but left atrial size may be normal in acute disease.
- Left ventricular eccentric hypertrophy (i.e. increased left ventricular end-diastolic diameter) occurs in response to chronic aortic and mitral endocarditis that causes valvular insufficiency.
- Left ventricular end-systolic diameter and E-point to septal separation may be increased and fractional shortening decreased in animals with systolic failure secondary to chronic aortic (and/or mitral) insufficiency.

Thoracic radiography
Thoracic radiographs are obtained to exclude the presence of coexisting thoracic disease, to assess global cardiac size and to evaluate for CHF, which is reported in approximately 50% of dogs with IE (MacDonald *et al.*, 2004). Perihilar to caudodorsal interstitial to alveolar pulmonary infiltrates and pulmonary venous distension are characteristic of left-sided CHF. Increased global cardiac or left atrial size may be absent in acute disease.

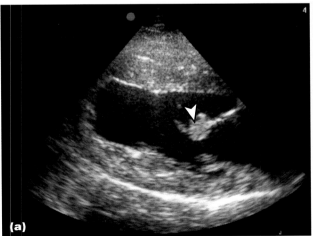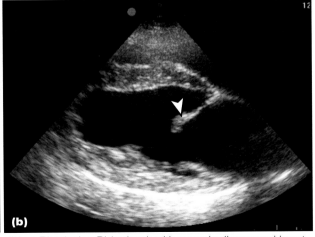

22.3 **(a)** Valvular vegetation of the mitral valve (arrowhead) in a Rhodesian Ridgeback with a newly discovered heart murmur. Multi-drug resistant *Staphylococcus intermedius* was isolated from the blood culture. The dog was treated aggressively with antibiotics according to the resistance pattern for 3 months. **(b)** After 3 months the vegetation had decreased in size considerably (arrowhead), but had not resolved completely.

Blood culture

Positive blood cultures help to confirm the disease. Contrary to previous opinion, it is more likely that the bacteraemia associated with IE is a continuous rather than intermittent event.

- The referral laboratory should be contacted concerning the preferred type of pre-prepared vials before obtaining a sample.
- Paediatric vials are useful because less blood is required, but larger volumes (>20 ml) increase the likelihood of growth.
- To avoid contamination, strict aseptic sampling should be observed, which includes thorough clipping and disinfection of the sampling site and use of sterile gloves.
- Sampling through indwelling catheters should be avoided.
- The bottles should be pre-warmed to 37°C and, after sampling, incubated at the same temperature.
- Three to four blood samples should be aseptically collected from different venous sites, 30–60 minutes apart, and submitted for aerobic and anaerobic bacterial culture.
- Lysis centrifugation tubes may increase the yield of bacteria.

Bartonella species

Serum may be submitted for measurement of antibody titres to *Bartonella* spp. A titre ≥1:1024 is strongly suggestive of bartonellosis. There is strong cross-reactivity between species. Culture is not recommended; *Bartonella* spp. are rarely cultured from dogs despite long-term incubation in an enriched medium. Because of these methodological problems, PCR-based detection of *Bartonella* spp. DNA from blood is also recommended (Duncan *et al.*, 2008).

Other laboratory tests

Other helpful diagnostic tests include haematology, serum biochemistry, urinalysis, urine protein:creatinine ratio (if there is proteinuria) and urine culture.

- Most animals (78%) with IE have leucocytosis with mature neutrophilia and monocytosis (MacDonald *et al.*, 2004).
- A mild non-regenerative anaemia and thrombocytopenia are also common.
- Serum biochemistry often reveals azotaemia (prerenal or renal), metabolic acidosis, hypoalbuminaemia and elevated liver enzyme activities.
- Haemoglobinuria, haematuria, cystitis and proteinuria may also be present.
- Serum troponin-I concentration is often increased

Differential diagnoses

- Mitral regurgitation from MMVD or mitral dysplasia.
- Aortic insufficiency secondary to aortic valve degeneration or a large ventricular septal defect.
- Aortic insufficiency and stenosis due to congenital aortic stenosis.

- Lameness from immune-mediated polyarthritis, septic arthritis, tick-borne diseases or degenerative arthritis.
- Fever from other systemic diseases such as sepsis, pneumonia, neoplasia, or immune-mediated diseases.

Treatment

The goal of therapy is to eradicate the infective microorganism and to treat all secondary complications. A successful outcome of therapy is based on early diagnosis and immediate and aggressive treatment. Long-term bactericidal antibiotic treatment is generally necessary. The ideal duration of therapy is unknown, but at least 4–6 weeks is recommended, and therapy may be required for 3–4 months.

- Selection of the appropriate antibiotic is based on culture and sensitivity testing (minimum inhibitory concentration of the antibiotic), whenever possible.
- Euthanasia should be considered if the isolated bacterium is multi-resistant to antibiotics due to the risk of spread of the microorganism to other dogs and humans, and because of the poor long-term prognosis.
- While the culture results are pending, or if the microbial cause is not known, empirical treatment with broad-spectrum antibiotics is recommended (such as aminoglycosides and beta-lactam antibiotics, fluoroquinolones and beta-lactam antibiotics).
- Initially, intravenous antibiotics are administered for 1–2 weeks, followed by oral antibiotics.
- Intravenous fluids are necessary for animals treated with aminoglycosides; concurrent administration of furosemide should be avoided as it worsens aminoglycoside nephrotoxicity. Aminoglycosides are contraindicated in animals with CHF for these reasons.

Specific antibiotic combinations include the following (including for *Bartonella* spp.):

- Acute endocarditis: amikacin 20 mg/kg i.v. q24h and timentin 50 mg/kg i.v. q6h *or* imipenem 10 mg/kg i.v. q8h for 1–2 weeks
- Chronic endocarditis: amoxicillin/clavulanate 20 mg/kg orally q8h and/or enrofloxacin 5–10 mg/kg orally q12h for 8 weeks, *or* imipenem 10 mg/kg s.c. q8h. In case of bartonellosis, consider doxycycline 5 mg/kg orally q24h for 6–8 weeks, *or* azithromycin 5 mg/kg orally q24h for 7 days then q48h for 6–8 weeks (Rolain *et al.*, 2004).

Congestive heart failure

Treatment of CHF involves the following:

- Furosemide:
  - Stable mild to moderate CHF: 1–4 mg/kg orally q8–12h
  - Acute fulminant CHF: 4–8 mg/kg i.v. q2–4h initially, then reduce.

- ACE inhibitors
- Positive inotropes: digoxin and pimobendan
- Afterload reducers for severe aortic (or mitral) insufficiency: hydralazine, nitroprusside, or amlodipine.

Monitoring and management

- Client education is important. The owners should be informed of prognosis, treatment strategy, possible complications and possible zoonotic risk with multi-resistant infections. In animals with positive blood or urine cultures, the culture should be repeated 1–2 weeks after starting antibiotics and 2 weeks after termination of the antibiotics.
- An echocardiogram may be repeated 1–2 weeks after starting therapy, at 4 weeks, and then 2 weeks after stopping therapy to assess vegetative size, chamber sizes, severity of valvular insufficiency and ventricular function.
- In cases of CHF, this complication may be monitored as in patients with MMVD (i.e. clinical signs and thoracic radiography; see Chapter 21).
- Repeat blood tests and urinalysis should be considered if there is evidence of septic embolization.
- Repeat measurement of antibody titres for *Bartonella* spp. is done after 1 month of treatment. If there is no decrease in the titre, consideration should be given to changing the antibiotic (though titres may sometimes persist even with successful therapy).

Prognosis

Prognosis depends on the infective agent, the aggressiveness and severity of valve colonization, the immunological status of the animal and how promptly therapy has been initiated. The prognosis is grave to guarded, with an overall median survival of 54 days in one study (Sykes *et al.*, 2006). The prognosis was worse for aortic endocarditis (median survival of 3 days *versus* 476 days for mitral IE) in another study that included mostly bartonellosis (MacDonald *et al.*, 2004). Euthanasia, CHF or sudden death are the most common short-term causes of death.

References and further reading

Baddour LM, Wilson WR, Bayer AS *et al.* (2005) Infective endocarditis: diagnosis, antimicrobial therapy, and management complications. *Circulation* **111**, 394–434

Barnes A, Bell SC, Isherwood DR, Bennett M and Carter SD (2000) Evidence of *Bartonella henselae* infection in cats and dogs in the United Kingdom. *Veterinary Record* **147**, 673–677

Calvert CA (1982) Valvular bacterial endocarditis in the dog. *Journal of the American Veterinary Medical Association* **180**, 1080–1084

Duncan AW, Marr HS, Birkenheuer AJ *et al.* (2008) *Bartonella* DNA in the blood and lymph nodes of Golden Retrievers with lymphoma and in healthy controls. *Journal of Veterinary Internal Medicine* **22**, 89–95

MacDonald KA, Chomel BB, Kittleson MD *et al.* (2004) A prospective study of canine infective endocarditis in northern California (1999–2001): emergence of *Bartonella* as a prevalent etiologic agent. *Journal of Veterinary Internal Medicine* **18**, 56–64

Miller MW, Fox PR and Saunders AB (2004) Pathologic and clinical features of infectious endocarditis. *Veterinary Cardiology* **6**, 35–43

Rolain JM, Brouqui P, Koehler JE *et al.* (2004) Recommendations for treatment of human infections caused by *Bartonella* species. *Lancet* **48**, 1921–1933

Sisson D and Thomas WP (1984) Endocarditis of the aortic valve in the dog. *American Veterinary Medical Association* **184**, 570–577

Sykes JE, Kittleson MD, Pesavento PA *et al.* (2006) Evaluation of the relationship between causative organisms and clinical characteristics of infective endocarditis in dogs: 71 cases (1992–2005). *Journal of the American Veterinary Medical Association* **228**, 1723–1734

23

Canine dilated cardiomyopathy

Joanna Dukes-McEwan

Introduction

Dilated cardiomyopathy (DCM) is a primary myocardial disease characterized by ventricular dilatation and systolic dysfunction with eccentric hypertrophy (increased left ventricular mass, but relatively thin walls). Remodelling leads to a round rather than elliptical left ventricle (LV) (increased sphericity). It is important to note that DCM is a diagnosis of exclusion; other congenital and acquired cardiac diseases and systemic conditions that may lead to these changes should be actively excluded prior to making this diagnosis.

Aetiology and inheritance

In humans a variety of insults can lead to a DCM phenotype, including viral and other forms of myocarditis, alcohol abuse, chemotherapeutic agents (e.g. doxorubicin), tachycardia-mediated cardiomyopathy and skeletal myopathies (Maron *et al.*, 2006). However, it is now recognized that at least 30% of human cases have a familial basis, usually inherited as an autosomal dominant trait, with age-dependent, incomplete penetrance.

In dogs, although doxorubicin toxicity and tachycardia-mediated cardiomyopathies occur, the clear breed predispositions and the familial distributions within breeds suggest that genetically determined disease is the most common. As in humans, an autosomal dominant mode of transmission with incomplete, age-dependent penetrance has been reported. In most breeds, the genetic mutations resulting in the DCM phenotype have not been elucidated, although DCM is recognized as part of X-linked Duchenne's muscular dystrophy (dystrophin absence) in the Golden Retriever. In a juvenile form of DCM in the Portuguese Water Dog, transmitted as an autosomal recessive trait, linkage analysis has mapped the critical region to canine chromosome 8, but the causal gene has yet to be identified (Werner *et al.*, 2008). In other breeds, linkage analysis and candidate gene-screening strategies have not so far identified a chromosome locus or the gene defect (Wiersma *et al.*, 2008). In humans, a number of different chromosome loci and genetic mutations have been associated with the familial disease. In most cases, the known mutations encode proteins of the cytoskeleton.

Breeds with a high prevalence of DCM are shown in Figure 23.1. They are predominantly large and giant breeds, but spaniel breeds are also included. In most breeds there is no sex predisposition, but males are more likely to present with signs of congestive heart failure (CHF) at an earlier age, so they appear to be over-represented. Age of onset is typically middle-aged (e.g. 4–8 years), but there is a wide age range and very young dogs have been reported (weeks to months old).

Pathology and histopathology

The left-sided or four-chamber dilatation is apparent on removing the heart at post-mortem examination. The characteristic findings of CHF may also be evident. The ventricular myocardium is often pale and flabby once opened (Figure 23.2). Two distinct histopathological features have been reported in DCM. In most dog breeds with DCM, particularly the giant breeds, attenuated wavy fibres are present with minimal evidence of inflammatory infiltrate or fibrosis. In the Dobermann, there is a striking amount of fibrosis; and in Boxers, adipocyte infiltration with fibrosis can be seen, which has been described as the fibrofatty infiltrative change (Tidholm and Jonsson, 2005). In

Giant breeds	Large breeds	Spaniel breeds	Other
Irish Wolfhound Deerhound Great Dane Newfoundland St Bernard Leonberger	Dobermann Boxer Weimaraner Dogue de Bordeaux Golden Retriever Labrador Retriever Old English Sheepdog German Shepherd Dog	English Cocker Spaniel English Springer Spaniel American Cocker Spaniel	Portuguese Water Dog

23.1 Breeds with high prevalence of DCM.

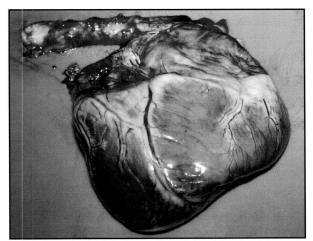

23.2 Post-mortem specimen from a 10-year-old Newfoundland that had been treated for 4 years for CHF associated with DCM with AF. The patient was eventually euthanased due to refractory congestive failure. Note that all four chambers are markedly dilated and the ventricular myocardium is flabby.

this latter form, ventricular arrhythmias are commonly reported, which can result in clinical signs such as syncope or sudden cardiac death. The histopathological changes in Boxers are similar to arrhythmogenic right ventricular cardiomyopathy (ARVC) described in humans and cats (Basso *et al.*, 2004).

Pathophysiology

The final DCM phenotype is similar irrespective of the inciting cause. An initial stage of ventricular remodelling occurs with changes in myocyte structure and function (see Chapter 15) as well as in the extracellular matrix. Individual cardiomyocytes become elongated and attenuated, and cell-to-cell slippage may also occur, ultimately leading to chamber dilatation and compounding systolic dysfunction. Neurohormonal activation results in sodium and water retention, which, together with the abnormal systolic and diastolic LV function, leads to CHF (see Chapter 15).

Applying the Laplace relationship to the LV, wall stress is directly proportional to the radius of the chamber and end-diastolic pressure, and inversely proportional to the wall thickness (see Chapter 15). Therefore, in DCM, there is high ventricular wall stress associated with the dilated chamber, relatively thin walls and elevated filling pressures. This may compromise coronary perfusion, particularly in patients with tachycardia (lack of time for diastolic coronary flow). Both of these factors can lead to ventricular arrhythmias, as well as histopathological alterations (e.g. myocardial fibrosis), forming a substrate for pathological arrhythmias.

A murmur may result from atrioventricular (AV) regurgitation, secondary to stretch of the mitral annulus and altered geometry of the mitral valve apparatus as the LV becomes rounded.

Clinical signs

There are a number of breed-specific variations in the clinical features of DCM. The most common variations are described in Figure 23.3.

Breed	Clinical presentation	Thoracic radiography	Echocardiography	Electrocardiography /Holter	Prognosis
Dobermann DCM	Ventricular arrhythmias; no clinical signs or syncope	Normal	Normal	>50 VPCs/24 hours, ± couplets, triplets, ventricular tachycardia	Risk of sudden death
	Systolic dysfunction; no clinical signs	Mild cardiomegaly	Dilated, hypocontractile LV; LA may be normal	± VPCs	Risk of CHF within 2 years
	Systolic dysfunction and CHF/ low output signs	Severe left-sided enlargement; pulmonary infiltrates if CHF	Dilated, hypocontractile LV, LA dilatation	± VPCs; AF common	Rapidly progressive disease
Boxer ARVC	Ventricular arrhythmias; no clinical signs	Normal	Normal	>50 VPCs/24 hours; usually single VPCs or couplets	May progress or remain preclinical
	Ventricular arrhythmias; syncope	Normal	Normal	Usually >500 VPCs/24 hours ± couplets, triplets, ventricular tachycardia	High risk of sudden death; risk of CHF is low
	'Classic' DCM and biventricular CHF	Left-sided or generalized cardiomegaly; pulmonary infiltrates/ pleural effusion if CHF	Dilated, hypocontractile LV; LA dilatation	± VPCs AF/SVT common	Rapidly progressive disease with refractory CHF

23.3 Breed-specific variations in clinical features of DCM. AF = Atrial fibrillation; LA = Left atrium; LV = Left ventricle; MR = Mitral regurgitation; SVT = Supraventricular tachycardia; VPC = Ventricular premature complex. (continues) ▶

Breed	Clinical presentation	Thoracic radiography	Echocardiography	Electrocardiography /Holter	Prognosis
Irish Wolfhound DCM	AF often with 'slow' ventricular response, so relatively normal heart rate; asymptomatic	Normal	Normal or sometimes mild left or bi-atrial enlargement	AF with slow ventricular rate; intraventricular conduction disturbances may also be documented	May progress or remain preclinical; may progress over 3–4 years to develop CHF
	'Classic' DCM and biventricular CHF; ascites may be present	Left-sided or generalized cardiomegaly; pulmonary infiltrates/ pleural effusion if CHF	Dilated, hypocontractile LV; often severe MR present resulting in low-normal indices of systolic function; severe LA dilatation	AF at a fast rate May have VPCs	Stabilization of CHF and rate control can result in good quality of life for months
Other giant-breed DCM	Preclinical (identified with echocardiographic screening); arrhythmias possible (AF most common)	Normal	Initially impaired systolic function, then rounded LV with increased LV dimensions or volumes; initially no left atrial enlargement	Often shows normal sinus rhythm; less likely than Irish Wolfhound to show 'lone' AF; occasional ectopy	May progress or remain preclinical
	'Classic' DCM and left-sided or biventricular CHF	Left-sided or generalized cardiomegaly; pulmonary infiltrates/ pleural effusion if CHF	Dilated, hypocontractile LV; LA dilatation	AF common; ± VPCs	Stabilization of CHF and rate control can result in good quality of life for months

23.3 (continued) Breed-specific variations in clinical features of DCM. AF = Atrial fibrillation; LA = Left atrium; LV = Left ventricle; MR = Mitral regurgitation; SVT = Supraventricular tachycardia; VPC = Ventricular premature complex.

Arrhythmias/murmur/systolic dysfunction without clinical signs

Abnormalities such as tachyarrhythmias, a murmur or systolic dysfunction on echocardiography may be detected as a result of health screening.

Congestive heart failure

CHF can be either left-sided or biventricular. Left-sided CHF signs dominate and include:

- Breathlessness/severe respiratory distress
- Coughing.

Right-sided CHF signs include:

- Ascites
- Respiratory distress associated with pleural effusion (biventricular failure).

If right-sided CHF signs dominate and there is no evidence of left-sided failure, it is important to exclude pericardial effusion and other pericardial diseases resulting in cardiac tamponade.

Forward failure

Low-output (forward) heart failure is less common than CHF, but when it occurs it often accompanies CHF. Dogs with sustained ventricular tachycardia may have low-output signs without CHF. Affected dogs are usually weak and hypothermic.

Syncope

Dogs with ventricular arrhythmias may present with syncope prior to the onset of CHF, or may have syncopal episodes after CHF has developed. Syncope is usually associated with excitement or exertion, and may indicate an increased risk of sudden death.

Sudden death

Dogs with ventricular arrhythmias and DCM are at high risk of sudden death.

Diagnostic approach

The diagnosis of DCM cannot be made on physical examination alone as the clinical presentation may vary. A diagnostic approach to suspected DCM is summarized in Figure 23.4.

Physical examination

Dogs without clinical signs

- A systolic heart murmur of mitral or tricuspid regurgitation may be detectable, but tends to be low-grade (<grade 3/6).
- A diastolic gallop sound (S3) may be the *only* abnormality in some patients.
- ± Tachyarrhythmias.
- Physical examination may be unremarkable.

Dogs with congestive heart failure

- A systolic murmur may be present: left apical with mitral regurgitation or right-sided with tricuspid regurgitation.

History	Coughing?	See Chapter 2
	Breathlessness?	See Chapter 1
	Syncope?	See Chapter 3
	Weakness? Exercise intolerance?	May indicate heart failure or tachyarrhythmia
	Signs indicative of concurrent disease?	Additional tests may be necessary
	Previous medication?	Previous administration of anthracycline chemotherapy? Response to any cardiac therapy?
	Diet?	Evidence of low taurine diet?
Physical examination	Heart rate and rhythm?	Normal heart rate and sinus arrhythmia are less likely to be associated with CHF Tachyarrhythmias (particularly AF and ventricular arrhythmias) are common, even in the absence of CHF
	Murmur?	Low-grade left apical systolic murmur may be present
	Gallop?	Presence of gallop in a large-breed dog is suggestive of DCM
	Increased respiratory rate and effort?	May indicate pulmonary oedema
	Pulmonary crackles?	May indicate more severe pulmonary oedema, other causes of airway fluid, or pulmonary fibrosis
	Weak pulses? Cold extremities?	May indicate low output failure
	Jugular distension? Ascites?	May indicate right-sided CHF
Thoracic radiography	Generalized cardiomegaly?	Clinically significant disease is usually associated with cardiomegaly, particularly if left-sided Rule out pericardial effusion
	Left atrial enlargement?	LA enlargement is a consistent finding in DCM with CHF Rule out pericardial effusion
	Pulmonary infiltrates?	Consistent with pulmonary oedema (hilar or generalized)?
	Signs of non-cardiac disease?	Are alternative causes of coughing/tachypnoea present?
	Pleural effusion? Ascites?	Indicates right-sided CHF (need to rule out pericardial effusion as a cause)
Echocardiography	Dilated LV?	Diastolic and systolic LV dimensions usually well above breed-specific reference ranges
	Rounded LV?	Indicates ventricular remodelling (eccentric hypertrophy)
	Systolic dysfunction?	Can be difficult to measure and interpret, particularly in the presence of concurrent MR In disease resulting in heart failure, systolic dysfunction is usually obvious
	Dilated LA?	Usually present in patients with left-sided CHF
	MR on colour flow Doppler?	Helps confirm diagnosis of MR as cause of heart murmur
	Presence of concurrent cardiac disease?	Need to rule out degenerative MVD, PDA, or other cause for LV volume overload
	Normal?	May be no echocardiographic abnormalities in Boxers or Dobermanns with ventricular arrhythmias
Electrocardiography	AF?	AF with rapid ventricular rate indicates more advanced disease and heart failure AF with slow ventricular rate may be present prior to evident systolic dysfunction in some breeds (e.g. Irish Wolfhound)
	Ventricular arrhythmias?	Boxers and Dobermanns prone to frequent, severe ventricular arrhythmias, even in the absence of systolic dysfunction May be present in dogs with advanced disease, particularly acute, life-threatening CHF
	Sinus rhythm/SVT?	Some affected dogs may remain in sinus rhythm or have intermittent SVT

23.4 Diagnostic approach to suspected DCM. AF = Atrial fibrillation; LA = Left atrium; LV = Left ventricle; MR = Mitral regurgitation; MVD = Mitral valve disease; PDA = Patent ductus arteriosus; SVT = Supraventricular tachycardia. (continues) ▶

Blood tests	Azotaemia?	Prerenal azotaemia common, may be exacerbated by diuretic therapy
	Electrolyte abnormalities?	Hypokalaemia may be present with loop diuretic therapy Hyponatraemia may indicate increased free water retention from vasopressin release and confers a poor prognosis
	NTproBNP?	Low concentrations suggest mild disease, high concentrations suggest risk of heart failure
Blood pressure	Hypotension?	Commonly present, particularly in low output failure or associated with vasodilator therapy

23.4 (continued) Diagnostic approach to suspected DCM. AF = Atrial fibrillation; LA = Left atrium; LV = Left ventricle; MR = Mitral regurgitation; MVD = Mitral valve disease; PDA = Patent ductus arteriosus; SVT = Supraventricular tachycardia.

- A diastolic gallop sound (S3) is often present with CHF but can be difficult to detect in the presence of tachyarrhythmias.
- Dogs in sinus rhythm may have a metronomically regular heart rhythm, without sinus arrhythmia.
- Pulmonary oedema results in an increase in respiratory rate, with inspiratory crackles if alveolar oedema is present.
- Pleural effusion leads to the absence of respiratory sounds ventrally, and reduced resonance on percussion ventrally.
- With right-sided failure, the jugular veins may be distended or hepatojugular reflux may be evident.
- Ascites and hepatomegaly occur with right-sided failure.
- ± Tachyarrhythmias.

Forward failure
Findings on physical examination may include:

- Hypothermia
- Weak peripheral pulses
- Pale mucous membranes, with slow capillary refill time
- Cold extremities
- 'Quiet' or 'distant' heart sounds on auscultation
- ± Tachyarrhythmias
- ± CHF signs.

Arrhythmias
Tachyarrhythmias are common at all stages of presentation, so the physical findings below may be found in any affected dog. Atrial fibrillation (AF) is particularly common, but ventricular arrhythmias are also frequently seen in Dobermanns, Boxers and some other breeds. Pulse deficits generally accompany tachyarrhythmias, and any systolic heart murmur may vary in intensity. An electrocardiogram (ECG) is essential for correct identification of the arrhythmia (see Chapter 16).

- AF typically sounds completely chaotic with marked pulse deficits.
- Ventricular premature complexes (VPCs) may be audible as 'early' beats, or the post-ectopic pause may be easier to detect.
- Ventricular tachycardia may sound regular, but the relative intensity of S1 and S2 may vary.
- Supraventricular tachycardia and atrial premature complexes may also be heard.

Imaging

Radiography
Thoracic radiographs (Figure 23.5) are indicated to document the presence of CHF (see Chapter 6). Typical features of DCM and left-sided CHF include:

- Generalized cardiomegaly with increased vertebral heart size
- Left atrial and left ventricular enlargement
- Pulmonary veins may be distended
- An interstitial, mixed or alveolar pulmonary infiltrate may be apparent, consistent with pulmonary oedema.

If there is concurrent right-sided congestive failure, one or more of the following may be documented:

- Right atrial and right ventricular enlargement
- Wide caudal vena cava
- Hepatomegaly
- Ascites
- Pleural effusion.

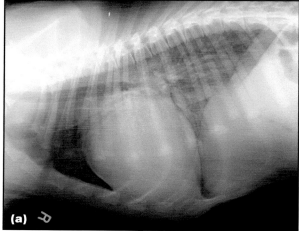

(a)

23.5 Radiographs from a 6-month-old Great Dane with DCM following initial treatment for pulmonary oedema. **(a)** Right lateral recumbent view showing generalized cardiomegaly (vertebral heart size 12.1), particularly due to left atrial and ventricular enlargement. The outline of the cardiac silhouette is very sharp, due to loss of normal systolic–diastolic movement blur. There is a generalized increase in interstitial pulmonary pattern, which is predominantly perihilar, consistent with residual pulmonary oedema. Loss of serosal detail in the abdomen is associated with very poor body condition. (continues) ▶

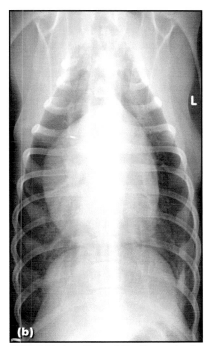

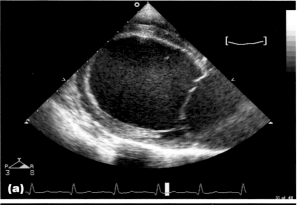

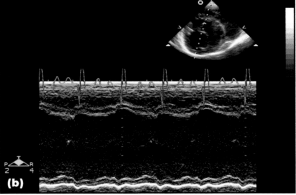

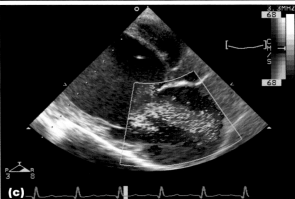

23.5 (continued) Radiographs from a 6-month-old Great Dane with DCM following initial treatment for pulmonary oedema. **(b)** Dorsoventral view confirming four-chamber enlargement of the cardiac silhouette, pulmonary venous distension and a generalized increase in interstitial markings.

Radiographs are also important in monitoring efficacy of CHF therapy. Auscultation alone is not sensitive at detecting residual pulmonary oedema.

Echocardiography

Echocardiography confirms the diagnosis of DCM and also excludes other acquired or congenital heart diseases which could result in four-chamber or left-sided dilatation and impaired systolic function (Figure 23.6ab).

Echocardiographic findings of DCM include:

- Dilated LV:
  - Dimensions are above normal confidence intervals for breed, or for weight where breed-specific data are not available (Figure 23.6b).
- Impaired systolic function:
  - Various methods of assessing contractility using echocardiography are available (see Chapter 11). All of the ejection phase indices are influenced by loading conditions. Severe mitral regurgitation (Figure 23.6c) may affect load to such an extent that systolic dysfunction is underestimated using these conventional measures.
- Rounded LV.

Diastolic function can be assessed; a restrictive filling pattern is associated with a poor prognosis (Borgarelli *et al.*, 2006). It should be noted that echocardiography may be unremarkable in Boxers with ventricular arrhythmias associated with ARVC. Those Boxers with CHF signs usually show the typical echocardiographic features of DCM.

23.6 Echocardiographic images from a 20-week-old Great Dane with DCM and CHF in sinus rhythm. **(a)** Right parasternal long-axis four-chamber view, showing a dilated, relatively thin-walled, rounded left ventricle (LV) in systole. **(b)** Left ventricular M-mode at the level of chordae tendinae, obtained from a short-axis view. The dilated LV chamber, with proportionately thin-walled interventricular septum and left ventricular free wall, and marked hypokinesis can be appreciated. In this case, the mean left ventricular diameter during diastole (LVDd) was 74.5 mm and during systole (LVDs) was 65.9 mm, with a fractional shortening of 11.6%. **(c)** Colour flow Doppler image of the mitral valve/left atrium on a right parasternal long-axis four-chamber view during systole, showing mitral regurgitation as a consequence of altered LV geometry.

Electrocardiography

An ECG is mandatory to make a precise diagnosis of any arrhythmia (see Chapter 16). In patients with sinus rhythm, evidence of chamber enlargement or intraventricular conduction disturbances may be apparent (though this is more easily determined with echocardiography). Common arrhythmias include AF and ventricular arrhythmias.

Atrial fibrillation
Hallmarks of AF are irregularly irregular RR intervals with a normal supraventricular QRS complex and absence of P waves (Figure 23.7). Rate is normally fast, but some giant breeds (e.g. Irish Wolfhound) do not show an accelerated ventricular response with preclinical disease (Figure 23.8).

Ventricular arrhythmias
Ventricular arrhythmias can range from isolated single VPCs to more complex arrhythmias such as couplets, triplets, paroxysms or sustained runs of ventricular tachycardia. They can be multiform (pleomorphic). In general, if the QRS complex is predominantly negative in lead II, it is likely to be of left ventricular origin. If positive, it is likely to be of right ventricular origin (Figure 23.9). The latter is common in Boxer ARVC.

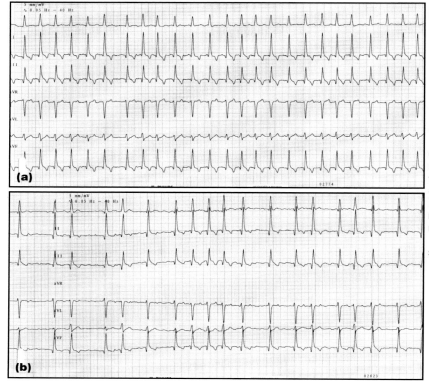

23.7 **(a)** Six-lead ECG from a German Shepherd Dog with AF. Note the normal appearance of the QRS complexes, completely irregular RR interval and the absence of P waves. The ventricular rate in this case is over 260 beats/minute. A cursory glance at the ECG fails to appreciate the very irregular RR intervals at very fast heart rates; human ears are better at detecting the chaotic rhythm. Paper speed 50 mm/s; gain 0.5 cm/mV. **(b)** Six-lead ECG from the same dog following 10 days of treatment with both digoxin and diltiazem. The ventricular rate is now better controlled at about 180 beats/minute. Note that this rate control is still not optimal if the rate persists at 180 beats/minute over 24 hours. Paper speed 50 mm/s; gain 0.5 cm/mV.

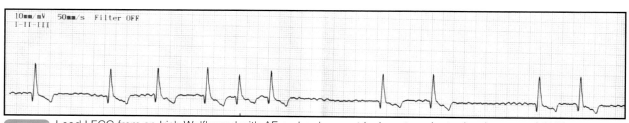

23.8 Lead I ECG from an Irish Wolfhound with AF and a slow ventricular rate, prior to development of CHF or any clinical signs evident to the owner. Ventricular rate is about 120 beats/minute. Note that fibrillation waves are evident affecting the base line, but their presence is not required to make the diagnosis of AF in dogs. Paper speed 50 mm/s; gain 1 cm/mV.

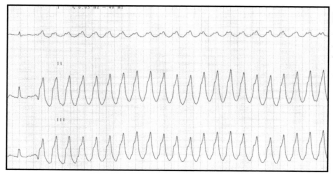

23.9 Leads I, II and III from a Boxer with ARVC. One sinus complex precedes sustained ventricular tachycardia. The left bundle branch-block morphology of the ventricular ectopics suggests right ventricular origin. The rate of the ventricular tachycardia is 340 beats/minute. Paper speed 50 mm/s; gain 0.5 cm/mV.

Holter monitoring

In both Boxers and Dobermanns, ventricular arrhythmias can be evident prior to typical echocardiographic evidence of DCM or development of clinical signs of CHF. Abnormalities on Holter monitoring (24-hour ambulatory ECG recording) can be a sensitive marker of affected dogs, with proposed criteria of the number of ventricular ectopics per 24 hours: >50 VPCs per 24 hours is suggestive of the disease in Dobermanns; and >100 VPCs per 24 hours is consistent with disease in Boxers in the absence of other predisposing causes (Meurs *et al.*, 1999; Calvert *et al.*, 2000; Meurs, 2004).

Although the number of ventricular ectopics over a 24-hour period can be used as a diagnostic criterion in Boxers and Dobermanns, it should be noted that there is considerable day-to-day variation in absolute number of ectopics (>80%) in Boxers with ARVC (Spier and Meurs, 2004). Ambulatory ECG (Holter) monitoring may identify arrhythmias not present during a routine 1–2-minute standard ECG (Figure 23.10); it also has other advantages over a standard ECG (see Chapter 9).

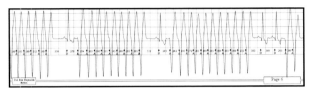

23.10 Channel from an ambulatory ECG recording (Holter monitor) from a Dobermann diagnosed with DCM showing paroxysms of ventricular tachycardia, with only occasional sinus complexes in this section. The initial ECG showed sinus rhythm with occasional VPCs. Paper speed 25 mm/s.

Blood tests

Haematology and biochemistry

Haematology is normally unremarkable in DCM. Pallor of mucous membranes is associated with reduced peripheral perfusion, and a packed cell volume (PCV) or full haematology is indicated to exclude anaemia. Biochemistry may be normal or show findings consistent with CHF (see Chapter 8). In addition, haematology and biochemistry may be useful to exclude significant concurrent disease. Of particular concern in a patient with CHF is coexisting renal disease associated with azotaemia; such patients often fail to tolerate the high doses of diuretics required to alleviate congestive signs. Other conditions that warrant exclusion include hypothyroidism, particularly as many breeds (e.g. Dobermann, Newfoundland) are predisposed to both DCM and hypothyroidism. Specific endocrine testing is therefore indicated in patients with compatible clinical findings.

Cardiac biomarkers

Measuring concentrations of plasma biomarkers may be helpful in staging of DCM (see Chapter 8).

- Elevated serum cardiac troponin-I (cTnI) concentrations may indicate the presence of cardiac disease, but are not specific for DCM, nor for the presence of CHF. Serum cTnI concentrations may be elevated as a consequence of haemodynamically significant arrhythmias, regardless of cause.
- Natriuretic peptide concentrations may be more useful. Although elevated plasma concentrations of NTproANP and NTproBNP are not specific for the diagnosis of DCM, they may be elevated in preclinical disease, and even more elevated in the presence of CHF.

These assays can be useful to indicate whether a patient presenting with clinical signs potentially referable to cardiac disease (e.g. cough) has cardiac disease or another cause for presentation. They may prove useful in screening for and staging DCM.

Blood pressure

Systemic hypertension should be ruled out prior to making the diagnosis of DCM. In addition, blood pressure monitoring gives useful information about the severity of systolic dysfunction, and the response to treatment. Systolic blood pressure can be indirectly assessed by the Doppler technique, and systolic/diastolic and mean arterial pressure can be evaluated by the oscillometric method (see Chapter 13). Systolic pressure is sometimes low in DCM, associated with poor systolic function. Mean arterial pressure is normally preserved as this is a homeostatic priority.

Screening

Clinical DCM is merely the 'tip of the iceberg'. There is a prolonged preclinical phase with progressive systolic impairment and chamber dilatation. The evolution of DCM, therefore, is a continuum from initially phenotypically normal dogs, which become clinically affected over a prolonged period (years). This makes the diagnosis of preclinical DCM difficult. Prospective serial echocardiographic evaluations may identify and confirm progression, but single studies may be equivocal or ambiguous. Mild left ventricular dilatation or mild systolic impairment is not sufficient to confirm a diagnosis in a dog with no clinical signs.

In breeds where dogs are being screened for preclinical DCM prior to breeding, a scoring system has been proposed by the European Society of Veterinary Cardiology (ESVC) DCM taskforce (Dukes-McEwan *et al.*, 2003) (Figure 23.11). For a robust diagnosis of DCM, the score should progress during serial evaluations.

Treatment

It is important to recognize the various stages of DCM, as treatment is markedly different for each phase. Various classifications of the severity of CHF can be used, such as the modified New York Heart Association (NYHA) and International Small Animal Cardiac Health Council (ISACHC) functional classifications, or the American College of Cardiology/American Heart Association (Hunt, 2005) stages of heart disease. However, for simplicity, the stages can be subdivided as:

Criteria		Score
Major criteria		*3 for each*
Left ventricle (LV) dilatation	Systolic or diastolic LV diameter >95% confidence intervals from breed-specific reference range, or weight of dog	3
Increased LV sphericity	LV diastolic length:diameter ratio <1.65	3
Reduced fractional shortening Or Reduced ejection fraction	<20–25% depending on breed-specific M-mode reference values <50% based on 2D volume calculations	3
Minor criteria		*1 for each*
Arrhythmias strongly associated with breed (e.g. ventricular ectopy in Boxer, Dobermann)		1
Atrial fibrillation		1
Increased mitral E point to septal separation (M-mode)		1
LV fractional shortening in equivocal range for breed		1
Left or bi-atrial enlargement		1
Pre-ejection period:ejection time ratio exceeding 95% confidence intervals (>0.4)		1
Interpretation		
Diagnosis consistent with DCM		Total score ≥6
Recommend serial re-evaluation (e.g. annually)		Total score ≤5

23.11 Proposed scoring system to be used when echocardiographically screening dogs for the presence of DCM (European Society for Veterinary Cardiology).

- Breeds at risk of DCM
- Preclinical DCM (heart disease but no CHF)
- Mild to moderate CHF
- Acute, life-threatening heart failure
- Refractory CHF.

It is important to appreciate that treatment of DCM is merely palliative. The goals are: (a) to reduce clinical signs; (b) to improve quality of life; and (c) to increase survival times. Treatment strategies include:

- Treatment based on the stage of CHF
- Management of haemodynamically significant or life-threatening arrhythmias.

Therapy of CHF is discussed in Chapter 18 and details of antiarrhythmic treatment can be found in Chapter 20. Management of DCM at different stages is summarized in Figure 23.12.

In breeds commonly affected with ventricular ectopy (Dobermann, Boxer), Holter monitoring (see

Disease stage	Standard treatment	Optional use	Diet/exercise
Heart disease, no CHF	No treatment	Angiotensin-converting enzyme (ACE) inhibitor Beta-blocker (with care) Taurine/L-carnitine	Normal
Mild to moderate CHF	Furosemide Pimobendan ACE inhibitor	Spironolactone Taurine/L-carnitine	Avoid salt load Restrict exercise until CHF resolved, then avoid extreme exertion
Acute, life-threatening CHF	Intravenous furosemide Oxygen Glyceryl trinitrate Pimobendan	Sedation (e.g. butorphanol) if distressed Thoracocentesis if large volume pleural effusions Dobutamine if hypotensive Intravenous nitroprusside plus dobutamine if non-responsive pulmonary oedema Continue with ACE inhibitors/spironolactone if already receiving	Encourage eating Cage rest
Refractory CHF	Furosemide (increase dose until no further effect or 5 mg/kg q8h) Pimobendan ACE inhibitor Spironolactone	Thiazides Parenteral furosemide Abdominocentesis if refractory ascites Omega-3 fatty acid supplementation if cachexic Taurine/L-carnitine? Digoxin if atrial fibrillation ± diltiazem if persistently elevated heart rate Mexiletine or amiodarone if ventricular arrhythmias	Encourage eating Avoid salt load Avoid undue exertion

23.12 Management of DCM according to stage of heart disease.

above) is a helpful screening tool. Its value has been shown in Dobermanns, where ventricular ectopy can precede echocardiographic evidence of DCM by months (Calvert *et al.*, 2000). Holter monitoring is the main method of screening for ARVC in Boxers, and this condition is defined by the number and complexity of ventricular arrhythmias on Holter recordings in the absence of other predisposing causes (Meurs, 2004).

The role of cardiac biomarkers has yet to be confirmed in screening for preclinical disease. BNP may have most value (Oyama *et al.*, 2007b) but cTnI appears to be more useful in Boxers with ARVC (Baumwart *et al.*, 2007). Screening by biomarkers is certainly more cost and time effective than echocardiographic examinations and would mean that patients needing further investigations are more effectively identified, as has been reported in humans (McDonagh, 2000).

In the future, it is hoped that genetic markers or a genetic test may be available for DCM in certain breeds. This means that breeders can identify puppies at risk of future development of DCM by a blood test or cheek swab. Breeding from genetically susceptible animals can be avoided and at-risk dogs can be monitored.

Preclinical dilated cardiomyopathy

Some dogs may have significant arrhythmias, which may require specific treatment (see Chapter 20).

Treatment of preclinical patients with systolic dysfunction (often identified during echocardiography) is controversial. The aim of treatment is to slow progression into CHF and, ideally, to limit ventricular remodelling. Data to indicate that this is achievable in dogs are sparse. In humans, a large study has shown that in patients with asymptomatic left ventricular dysfunction, angiotensin-converting enzyme (ACE) inhibitors delay the onset of CHF and slow progression of left ventricular dilatation (SOLVD Investigators, 1992; Konstam *et al.*, 1993). Data for Dobermanns showed similar findings (O'Grady *et al.*, 1997). Where there are no cost constraints, the author currently recommends that dogs identified with preclinical DCM are treated with an ACE inhibitor.

Congestive heart failure

Mild to moderate
The goal of treatment in these patients is to improve quality of life by controlling clinical signs of CHF, antagonizing the deleterious effects of neurohormones on the heart and circulatory system, providing inotropic support, and controlling haemodynamically significant or life-threatening arrhythmias. This is best achieved by the use of the following:

- Furosemide (1–2 mg/kg orally q12h) – for diuresis. Titrate dose to effect; once congestive failure signs have resolved, maintain on lowest effective dose.

- ACE inhibitor (see Appendix for specific oral drug doses) – to counteract activation of the renin–angiotensin–aldosterone system associated with both cardiac disease and furosemide use. Shown to improve quality of life and survival times in dogs with DCM and heart failure (COVE Study Group, 1995; BENCH Study Group, 1999).
- Pimobendan (0.1–0.3 mg/kg orally q12h) – for inotropic support and vasodilation. Use in dogs with CHF from DCM has resulted in improvement in survival times when used in addition to ACE inhibitors and standard therapy (Luis Fuentes *et al.*, 2002; O'Grady *et al.*, 2008).
- ± Spironolactone (0.5–1 mg/kg orally q12–24h) – an aldosterone antagonist that acts as a weak potassium-sparing diuretic and may prevent some aldosterone-mediated myocardial fibrosis and remodelling. Should be used in hypokalaemic patients.

Heart rate and rhythm control is also indicated where abnormal rhythms further perturb myocardial function or are judged to be life-threatening (see below).

Acute, life-threatening
Dogs with severe, life-threatening CHF are a genuine emergency. The typical presentation is respiratory distress. Often, this can result in orthopnoea; the dog is unable to lie down or rest, and appears to be exhausted. These patients are susceptible to stress and are very anxious. The two major problems that need to be addressed are acute severe pulmonary oedema and cardiogenic shock.

Acute severe pulmonary oedema: Pulmonary oedema is a major life-threatening presentation.

- Oxygen should be provided without stress (see Chapter 17).
- Intravenous furosemide: the author uses 1–2 mg/kg i.v. q1–2h until respiratory rate reduces to near-normal (e.g. 40 breaths/minute), and then the interval between dosing is increased.
- Furosemide can also be used as a constant rate infusion.

Furosemide is titrated to effect and treatment should not be limited by a theoretical maximal daily dose, but electrolytes and renal function should be monitored. Additional treatment options include:

- Topical glyceryl trinitrate ointment
- Drainage of significant pleural effusions by thoracocentesis
- Anxiolytic drugs (e.g. methadone).

Cardiogenic shock and hypotension: Dogs with CHF and signs of cardiogenic shock are gravely ill. Despite maximal vasoconstriction because of the neuroendocrine activation of CHF, these patients are still hypotensive.

- Positive inotropic support:
  - Dobutamine continuous rate infusion (if continuous ECG available)
  - Oral pimobendan.
- Despite hypotension, fluid therapy should be avoided.
- ACE inhibitors are not commenced until the patient is stable.

If haemodynamically significant or electrically unstable arrhythmias are present, they should be addressed at the same time as treating the signs of heart failure (see below and Chapter 20).

Refractory

Initially, left-sided CHF is treated with diuretics, ACE inhibitors and pimobendan. As the disease progresses and when there is concurrent evidence of right-sided CHF (ascites, with or without pleural effusion), control of the signs of CHF may become more difficult. Pleural effusions should be drained if they compromise respiration, and the dose of furosemide should be increased. Ascites is particularly difficult to manage since it can lead to hypoproteinaemia, which contributes to cardiac cachexia. Bowel oedema may lead to compromised absorption of nutrients and drugs. Pharmacological management of ascites is preferred to mechanical drainage, due to protein loss associated with repeated abdominocentesis. Drainage should be considered a palliative procedure, and undertaken when the weak patient's mobility is compromised by the mass of fluid or respiratory function is impaired.

With refractory CHF signs:

- Furosemide dose should be increased
- ACE inhibitor dose should be optimized
- Spironolactone should be administered at a diuretic dose (1–2 mg/kg orally q12–24h)
- Hydrochlorothiazide/amiloride combination should be considered when the furosemide dose has been maximized
- Digoxin can be considered even in dogs with sinus rhythm, aiming for a trough (>8 hour post-pill) serum level of about 0.6–1.1 ng/ml
- Electrolytes and renal function should be carefully monitored.

Arrhythmias

Patients with no clinical signs may have significant arrhythmias. For example, some giant breeds of dog (particularly Irish Wolfhounds) develop AF. Although this is often at a relatively normal heart rate (e.g. 90–120 beats/minute), it must be distinguished (preferably by an ECG) from sinus arrhythmia (see Chapter 16). Holter monitoring is required to determine whether rate control is necessary; for example, if the ventricular response is excessively fast during excitement or exercise. Uncontrolled ventricular rate in AF can result in worsening of myocardial function (tachycardia-mediated cardiomyopathy).

In breeds at high risk of ventricular arrhythmias with preclinical DCM (especially Dobermanns,

Boxers), evidence may be missed during routine auscultation or a standard ECG. Ambulatory ECG recording (Holter monitoring) (see Figure 23.10) is therefore indicated to assess the severity of arrhythmias and determine whether antiarrhythmic medication should be considered.

Atrial fibrillation

When AF occurs in the presence of DCM, it indicates the presence of atrial myocardial disease and/or significant atrial stretch. Since AF depends on atrial mass, it is more likely in large or giant breeds of dog, and in some breeds it may precede the development of CHF (see Figure 23.8). In other patients, onset of AF may result in CHF in a previously preclinical dog, or recurrence of CHF in a previously stable dog.

Once AF has developed, conversion to a sustained sinus rhythm is difficult to achieve and maintain. The aim, therefore, is to control ventricular response to AF by using agents that slow conduction through the AV node (see Figure 23.7b). These include digoxin, calcium-channel antagonists such as diltiazem, or beta-blockers such as atenolol. It should be noted that beta-blockers are contraindicated in the face of uncontrolled CHF, and most dogs with clinical DCM fail to tolerate a beta-blocker.

- Digoxin is normally the drug of first choice, as it is (uniquely among drugs showing AV conduction) not negatively inotropic. Serum digoxin level should be measured after 5–7 days, aiming for a trough level of about 0.6–1.1 ng/ml (it should be noted that this reference range is much lower than that cited by most laboratories, which give a range of about 1.0–2.5 ng/ml).
- Diltiazem may be added if further rate control is required (see Chapter 20).

Ventricular arrhythmias

VPCs are common in dogs with DCM, with Dobermanns and Boxers most at risk of haemodynamically significant ventricular arrhythmias. Syncopal episodes are common in dogs with complex ventricular arrhythmias.

Ventricular tachycardia, emergency presentation: This requires immediate antiarrhythmic medication.

- Intravenous lidocaine is the first-choice drug for emergency therapy. If successful, lidocaine can be continued as a constant rate infusion (see Chapter 20). If unsuccessful, serum electrolytes (potassium, magnesium) should be checked and corrected if required.
- If lidocaine is unsuccessful, intravenous procainamide, intravenous or oral sotalol or oral amiodarone can be considered (see Chapter 20).

Intermittent ventricular tachycardia, Boxer ARVC:

- Oral sotalol (classes II and III actions)
- Oral mexiletine (class Ib actions) and atenolol (class II actions).

Intermittent ventricular tachycardia, DCM and CHF: Patients with CHF tolerate negative inotropes (such as sotalol or atenolol) poorly. Oral amiodarone (classes I, II, III and IV actions) may be more suitable. This has been used with some success in controlling ventricular arrhythmias in Dobermanns (Calvert and Brown, 2004).

The addition of mexiletine to either sotalol or amiodarone may be necessary to control refractory ventricular arrhythmias in some dogs. It should be noted that all antiarrhythmic drugs are potentially proarrhythmic. Therefore, efficacy should be assessed by Holter monitoring over a 24-hour period after 1–2 weeks.

Potential role of beta-blockers: Humans with DCM show improved systolic function when they are treated with, and manage to tolerate, a beta-blocker. However, this improvement is only evident after 3–6 months and slow up-titration is required. The apparent paradox of improving systolic function with a negative inotrope is probably founded on myocardial protection from the toxic effects of catecholamines. Additionally, certain beta-blockers (particularly metoprolol and carvedilol) are associated with improved survival times in human patients. Beta-blockers may also have a role in canine DCM, but early reports are not encouraging (Oyama *et al.*, 2007a). Most patients with clinical signs of CHF fail to tolerate beta-blockers at all, and owners often report that the dog is markedly lethargic and depressed during beta-blockade. Beta-blockers may well have a role in the preclinical patient, but this requires investigation.

Nutraceuticals: These are substances with both nutritional and possible pharmaceutical effects. The best known of these supplements is taurine: taurine deficiency in cats was a historically important cause of feline DCM, reversible with supplementation. There does not appear to be the same cause/effect relationship in canine DCM. However, certain Boxers with classic DCM have been documented to have myocardial L-carnitine deficiency, and systolic function can be improved in some of these patients with supplementation (though there is no effect on the ventricular arrhythmias) (Keene, 1991). Certain breeds of dog may be taurine deficient and have low whole blood taurine levels, possibly associated with protein source or total protein intake. These include American Cocker Spaniels, Golden Retrievers and Newfoundlands (Kittleson *et al.*, 1997; Backus *et al.*, 2003; Willis *et al.*, 2003; Belanger *et al.*, 2005).

Patients with severe cardiac cachexia are problematic. Studies have shown that these patients have significantly increased cytokine levels, such as tumour necrosis factor-α (TNF-α) and interleukins. Studies indicate that fish-oil (with high omega-3 levels) supplementation, can reduce these cytokine levels and improve patient status and appetite (Freeman *et al.*, 1998). In addition, fish-oil supplementation can reduce ventricular arrhythmias in Boxers with ARVC (Smith *et al.*, 2007).

References and further reading

Backus RC, Cohen G, Pion PD *et al.* (2003) Taurine deficiency in Newfoundlands fed commercially available complete and balanced diets. *Journal of the American Veterinary Medical Association* **223**, 1130–1136
Basso C, Fox PR, Meurs KM *et al.* (2004) Arrhythmogenic right ventricular cardiomyopathy causing sudden cardiac death in boxer dogs: a new animal model of human disease. *Circulation* **109**, 1180–1185
Baumwart RD, Orvalho J and Meurs KM (2007) Evaluation of serum cardiac troponin I concentration in Boxers with arrhythmogenic right ventricular cardiomyopathy. *American Journal of Veterinary Research* **68**, 524–528
Belanger MC, Ouellet M, Queney G and Moreau M (2005) Taurine-deficient dilated cardiomyopathy in a family of golden retrievers. *Journal of the American Animal Hospital Association* **41**, 284–291
BENCH Study Group (1999) The effect of benazepril on survival times and clinical signs of dogs with congestive heart failure: results of a multicentre, prospective, randomised, double-blinded, placebo-controlled, long-term clinical trial. *Journal of Veterinary Cardiology* **1**, 7–18
Borgarelli M, Santilli RA, Chiavegato D *et al.* (2006) Prognostic indicators for dogs with dilated cardiomyopathy. *Journal of Veterinary Internal Medicine* **20**, 104–110
Calvert CA and Brown J (2004) Influence of antiarrhythmia therapy on survival times of 19 clinically healthy Doberman pinschers with dilated cardiomyopathy that experienced syncope, ventricular tachycardia, and sudden death (1985–1998). *Journal of the American Animal Hospital Association* **40**, 24–28
Calvert CA, Jacobs GJ, Smith DD, Rathbun SL and Pickus CW (2000) Association between results of ambulatory electrocardiography and development of cardiomyopathy during long-term follow-up of Doberman pinschers. *Journal of the American Veterinary Medical Association* **216**, 34–39
COVE Study Group (1995) Controlled clinical evaluation of enalapril in dogs with heart failure: results of the Cooperative Veterinary Enalapril Study Group. The COVE Study Group. *Journal of Veterinary Internal Medicine* **9**, 243–252
Dukes-McEwan J, Borgarelli M, Tidholm A, Vollmar AC and Häggström J (2003) Guidelines for the diagnosis of canine idiopathic dilated cardiomyopathy. The ESVC Taskforce for canine dilated cardiomyopathy. *Journal of Veterinary Cardiology* **5**, 7–19
Freeman LM, Rush JE, Kehayias JJ *et al.* (1998) Nutritional alterations and the effect of fish oil supplementation in dogs with heart failure. *Journal of Veterinary Internal Medicine* **12**, 440–448
Harpster NK (1983) Boxer cardiomyopathy. In: *Current Veterinary Therapy. Small Animal Practice. VIII*, ed. RW Kirk, pp. 329–337. WB Saunders, Philadelphia
Hunt SA (2005) ACC/AHA 2005 guideline update for the diagnosis and management of chronic heart failure in the adult: a report of the American College of Cardiology/American Heart Association Task Force on Practice Guidelines (Writing Committee to Update the 2001 Guidelines for the Evaluation and Management of Heart Failure). *Journal of the American College of Cardiology* **46**, e1–82
Keene BW (1991) L-carnitine supplementation in the therapy of canine dilated cardiomyopathy. *Veterinary Clinics of North America. Small Animal Practice* **21**, 1005–1009
Kittleson MD, Keene B, Pion PD and Loyer CG (1997) Results of the multicenter spaniel trial (MUST): taurine- and carnitine-responsive dilated cardiomyopathy in American cocker spaniels with decreased plasma taurine concentration. *Journal of Veterinary Internal Medicine* **11**, 204–211
Konstam MA, Kronenberg MW, Rousseau MF *et al.* (1993) Effects of the angiotensin converting enzyme inhibitor enalapril on the long-term progression of left ventricular dilatation in patients with asymptomatic systolic dysfunction. SOLVD (Studies of Left Ventricular Dysfunction) Investigators. *Circulation* **88**, 2277–2283
Luis Fuentes V, Corcoran B, French A *et al.* (2002) A double-blind, randomized, placebo-controlled study of pimobendan in dogs with dilated cardiomyopathy. *Journal of Veterinary Internal Medicine* **16**, 255–261
Maron BJ, Towbin JA, Thiene G *et al.* (2006) Contemporary definitions and classification of the cardiomyopathies: an American Heart Association Scientific Statement from the Council on Clinical Cardiology, Heart Failure and Transplantation Committee; Quality of Care and Outcomes Research and Functional Genomics and Translational Biology Interdisciplinary Working Groups; and Council on Epidemiology and Prevention. *Circulation* **113**, 1807–1816
McDonagh TA (2000) Asymptomatic left ventricular dysfunction in the community. *Current Cardiology Reports* **2**, 470–474
Meurs KM (2004) Boxer dog cardiomyopathy: an update. *Veterinary Clinics of North America. Small Animal Practice* **34**, 1235–1244, viii
Meurs KM, Spier AW, Miller MW, Lehmkuhl L and Towbin JA (1999) Familial ventricular arrhythmias in boxers. *Journal of Veterinary Internal Medicine* **13**, 437–439
O'Grady M, Horne R and Gordon SG (1997) Does angiotensin

converting enzyme inhibitor therapy delay the onset of congestive heart failure or sudden death in Doberman pinschers with occult dilated cardiomyopathy? *In: Proceedings of the 15th Annual ACVIM Forum. Lake Buena Vista*, p. 685

O'Grady MR, Minors SL, O'Sullivan LM and Horne R (2008) Effect of pimobendan on case fatality rate in Doberman Pinschers with congestive heart failure caused by dilated cardiomyopathy. *Journal of Veterinary Internal Medicine* **22**, 897–904

Oyama MA, Sisson DD, Prosek R *et al.* (2007a) Carvedilol in dogs with dilated cardiomyopathy. *Journal of Veterinary Internal Medicine* **21**, 1272–1279

Oyama MA, Sisson DD and Solter PF (2007b) Prospective screening for occult cardiomyopathy in dogs by measurement of plasma atrial natriuretic peptide, B-type natriuretic peptide, and cardiac troponin-I concentrations. *American Journal of Veterinary Research* **68**, 42–47

Smith CE, Freeman LM, Rush JE, Cunningham SM and Biourge V (2007) Omega-3 fatty acids in Boxer dogs with arrhythmogenic right ventricular cardiomyopathy. *Journal of Veterinary Internal Medicine* **21**, 265–273

SOLVD Investigators (1992) Effect of enalapril on mortality and development of heart failure in asymptomatic patients with reduced left ventricular ejection fractions. *The New England Journal of Medicine* **327**, 685–691

Spier AW and Meurs KM (2004) Evaluation of spontaneous variability in the frequency of ventricular arrhythmias in Boxers with arrhythmogenic right ventricular cardiomyopathy. *Journal of the American Veterinary Medical Association* **224**, 538–541

Tidholm A and Jonsson L (2005) Histologic characterization of canine dilated cardiomyopathy. *Veterinary Pathology* **42**, 1–8

Werner P, Raducha MG, Prociuk U *et al.* (2008) A novel locus for dilated cardiomyopathy maps to canine chromosome 8. *Genomics* **91**, 517–521

Wiersma AC, Stabej P, Leegwater PA *et al.* (2008) Evaluation of 15 candidate genes for dilated cardiomyopathy in the Newfoundland dog. *Journal of Heredity* **99**, 73–80

Willis R, Dukes-McEwan J, Biourge V, Desprez G and Mellor D (2003) The role of taurine in dilated cardiomyopathy in Newfoundland dogs. In: *Proceedings of the 21st ACVIM Forum. Charlotte, North Carolina*, p. 1008

24

Pericardial disease

Anne French

Introduction

Pericardial disease is common, with reports in referral institutions of 8% of cardiac cases in dogs and 6% of feline cases (Tobias, 2005). Congenital, acquired primary and acquired secondary forms have been described. The most common pericardial diseases result in accumulation of pericardial fluid. In dogs, primary acquired disease is most common, where local (often inflammatory or neoplastic) processes are responsible. In cats, secondary acquired disease such as congestive heart failure (CHF) predominates. Pericardial disease can often be mistaken for other cardiac or non-cardiac disorders and diagnosis can be challenging.

Normal pericardium

The pericardium is divided into fibrous and serous pericardia. The fibrous part is the outer covering, which is composed of collagen and elastin. The serous pericardium is composed of a single layer of mesothelial cells. It lines the inner surface of the fibrous pericardium, where it is referred to as the parietal layer of the serous pericardium, and also overlies the heart, where it is called the epicardium or visceral layer of the serous pericardium. The pericardial cavity is the area between the visceral and parietal layers and usually contains a small quantity of fluid; 0.25 (±0.15) ml/kg bodyweight. The main roles of the pericardium are to fix the position of the heart, to maintain optimal cardiac shape and to protect the heart.

Pathophysiology

Pericardial effusion

The rate of fluid accumulation within the pericardium determines the haemodynamic effects. Slow accumulation of fluid results in expansion and hypertrophy of the pericardium, which is tolerated initially but eventually leads to increased intrapericardial pressure with resulting compression of the right atrium and ventricle, known as *tamponade*. Rapid fluid accumulation results in acute tamponade. Cardiac tamponade leads to decreased cardiac output, arterial hypotension and right-sided CHF.

Constrictive pericardial disease

Pericardial constriction occurs when the parietal and visceral pericardial layers become thickened and rigid, adversely affecting diastolic function. In affected cases, even a small quantity of pericardial effusion may result in marked increases in intrapericardiac pressure with resulting tamponade (effusive–constrictive disease). Diagnosis can be very challenging.

Intrapericardial mass lesions

Intrapericardial mass lesions usually cause effusion, but some lesions cause compression of the great vessels or of the outflow tracts, resulting in signs typical of poor cardiac output.

Causes

Congenital

Pericardial defects, complete absence of the pericardium and congenital pericardial cysts have been reported in small animals, but the most commonly reported congenital pericardial disease is peritoneal–pericardial–diaphragmatic hernia (PPDH). PPDH typically presents with gastrointestinal or respiratory signs in young animals and rarely presents with signs of CHF or poor cardiac output. Pericardial cysts may result in pericardial effusion and cardiac tamponade.

Acquired

Pericardial effusion

Pericardial effusion is the main manifestation of acquired pericardial disease. Primary pericardial effusions may be idiopathic, neoplastic, infectious, traumatic, toxic or due to left atrial rupture from chronic mitral regurgitation. Secondary pericardial effusions may occur due to hypoalbuminaemia or CHF. Effusions may be transudates, modified transudates, exudates, haemorrhagic or neoplastic, and characterization of the effusion may aid in diagnosis. Primary effusions often result in tamponade, whilst secondary effusions rarely result in tamponade.

Neoplasia: The most common cause of pericardial effusion in dogs is neoplasia affecting either the heart, heart base or pericardium. Haemangiosarcoma of the right atrium is frequently reported in German Shepherd Dogs (Figure 24.1a). Heart base tumours such as chemoreceptor cell tumours are most often seen in older Boxers (Figure 24.1b). Mesotheliomas appear to have a higher prevalence in small or medium sized dogs. Metastasis of tumours to the heart or pericardium from other sites can also occur.

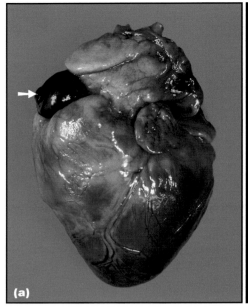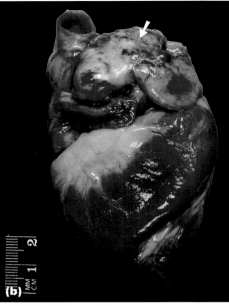

24.1
(a) Gross pathological specimen from a dog with a confirmed right atrial haemangiosarcoma (arrowed). **(b)** Gross pathological specimen from a dog with a confirmed heart base chemodectoma (arrowed). (Courtesy of R. Else.)

In cats, lymphoma, heart base tumours and a variety of metastatic tumours have been reported as causes of pericardial effusion.

Idiopathic: This is the second most common cause of pericardial effusion in the dog but appears to be rare in cats. It has been referred to as chronic proliferative pericarditis, idiopathic haemorrhagic pericardial effusion or idiopathic pericardial haemorrhage. Effusions are haemorrhagic and are commonly found in middle-aged, male, large- and giant-breed dogs, with Great Danes, Newfoundlands, St Bernards, Golden Retrievers and Labrador Retrievers overrepresented. The cause is unknown and recent studies have shown no evidence of a viral or immune-mediated aetiology (Martin *et al.*, 2006; Zini *et al.*, 2007). Interestingly, one case series in Golden Retrievers has shown apparent progression of idiopathic pericardial effusion to mesothelioma over a prolonged time course (Machida *et al.*, 2004).

Other: Bacterial pericardial effusions have been reported associated with migrating foreign bodies, penetrating wounds and concurrent pulmonary infections. Aetiological agents include *Actinomyces*, *Bacteroides*, *Pasteurella*, *Pseudomonas*, *Staphylococcus* and *Streptococcus* species. Fungal pericardial infection with *Coccidioides immitis* has been reported, as have infections due to leishmaniasis and aberrant dirofilariasis. In cats, feline infectious peritonitis is known to cause pericardial effusions. In dogs with myxomatous mitral valve disease, left atrial rupture is a recognized cause of haemorrhagic pericardial effusion; and coagulopathies due to rodenticides such as warfarin may also result in a haemorrhagic pericardial effusion.

Secondary: CHF and hypoproteinaemia may result in pericardial effusions in dogs and cats. The most common cause of pericardial effusion in cats is CHF secondary to myocardial disease (Davidson *et al.*, 2008).

Constrictive
Constrictive pericardial disease has been reported associated with pericardial infections, traumatic pericardial haemorrhage, intrapericardial neoplasia and recurrent idiopathic pericardial haemorrhagic effusion. It has been reported in dogs and cats. At the time of diagnosis the original cause of the disease may not always be apparent.

Clinical signs

Animals are often presented with vague signs of inappetence, lethargy, exercise intolerance, weakness, collapse, respiratory difficulties, weight loss, polydipsia or abdominal enlargement. In some dogs cardiomegaly results in airway compression leading to coughing, and chronic right-sided CHF may cause diarrhoea (Stepien *et al.*, 2000; Stafford Johnson *et al.*, 2004). As signs can be very non-specific, it is important to rule out pericardial disease in any animal presenting with ascites but also in cases of collapse and exercise intolerance. Some animals with small volume effusions can present with no clinical signs.

Diagnostic approach

Physical examination
Poorly audible or muffled heart sounds are often present due to pericardial effusion. With subacute or more chronic cardiac tamponade, right-sided CHF may occur with jugular venous distension, jugular venous pulsation, ascites and pleural effusion. The pleural effusion may result in respiratory distress and may also contribute to the muffled heart sounds. The pulse quality is usually weak due to poor cardiac output, and the quality may vary excessively with respiration (pulsus paradoxus). Sinus tachycardia is frequently present secondary to decreased cardiac output.

In constrictive pericardial disease the physical findings are similar, but the heart may be more clearly audible as there is little or no pericardial effusion. In human medicine a characteristic pericardial 'knock' is described with constrictive pericardial disease; this is rarely reported in dogs.

Electrocardiography

Low-voltage QRS complexes (R wave <1 mV) are common in dogs with pericardial effusion, but this finding is not specific and other conditions such as hypothyroidism, pleural effusion, wide chest conformation and obesity may also cause low-voltage complexes. Low-voltage QRS complexes are normal in cats. Electrical alternans (a variation in the height of the QRS complexes with alternate beats) is relatively common with large pericardial effusions and is due to the swinging motion of the heart within the pericardial fluid (Figure 24.2).

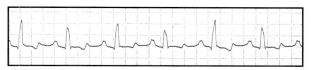

24.2 ECG trace (lead II shown) from a dog with pericardial effusion showing low-voltage QRS complexes and electrical alternans. Paper speed 50 mm/s; gain 10 mm/mV.

Imaging

Radiography

The presence of a primary pericardial effusion results in a more spherical cardiac shape (Figure 24.3). Cardiac size will depend on the quantity of the effusion. The normal chamber contours are usually lost, except in the case of left atrial rupture where left atrial enlargement may still be identifiable. In some cases there will be pleural effusion, which may obscure the cardiac silhouette. The caudal vena cava is distended and there will be evidence of hepatomegaly and ascites if right-sided CHF is present. A mass lesion may be visible at the heart base or on the right atrial wall, and secondary metastasis may be present in the thoracic lymph nodes or lung. Secondary pericardial effusions are often smaller in quantity and result in an enlarged cardiac silhouette, but normal cardiac contours may still be recognizable. In the case of congenital PPDH, abdominal contents may be visible within the cardiac silhouette (Figure 24.3). Fluoroscopy, pneumopericardiography and direct and indirect angiography have all been used in the investigation of pericardial disease in the past, but in recent years these have been largely replaced by echocardiography.

Echocardiography

Echocardiography is the best diagnostic test for pericardial disease (Figure 24.4). Pericardial effusion is visible as a hypoechoic area surrounding the heart. It is important to differentiate pericardial from pleural effusion. Pleural effusions are more diffuse and frequently have fibrin tags, whilst pericardial effusions

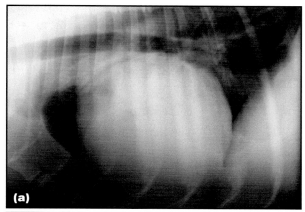

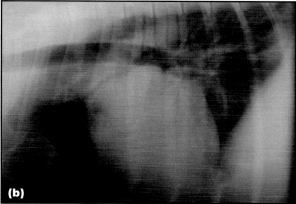

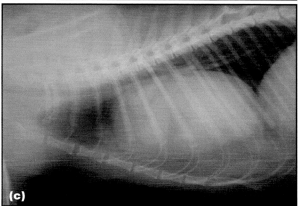

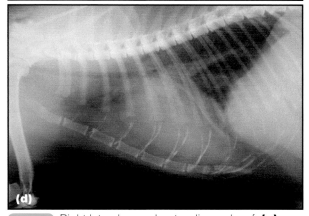

24.3 Right lateral recumbent radiographs of: **(a)** a dog with idiopathic pericardial effusion before pericardiocentesis; **(b)** the same dog following pericardiocentesis; **(c)** a cat with PPDH; and **(d)** a cat with a moderate amount of pericardial effusion due to intrapericardial lymphoma.

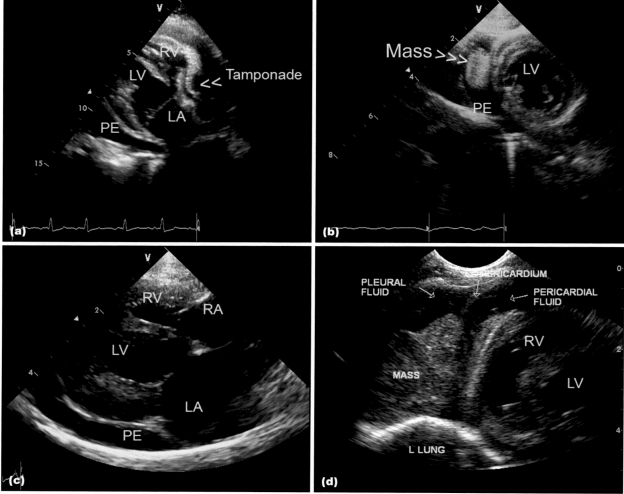

24.4 **(a)** Right parasternal long-axis view of a dog with idiopathic pericardial effusion and cardiac tamponade. The arrowheads demonstrate the collapse of the right atrial wall. **(b)** Right parasternal short-axis view at the level of the papillary muscles of the heart of a cat with pericardial effusion due to intrapericardial lymphoma. The arrowheads mark the tumour. **(c)** Right parasternal long-axis view of a cat with hypertrophic cardiomyopathy and secondary pericardial effusion. **(d)** Right thoracic ultrasonogram in a dog with a thoracic mass causing a pleural and pericardial effusion. LA = Left atrium; LV = Left ventricle; PE = Pericardial effusion; RA = Right atrium; RV = Right ventricle.

may outline cardiac chambers (such as auricular appendages) and rarely have fibrin tags. Fluid accumulation is greater around the cardiac apex than at the base. If both pleural and pericardial effusion are present then the pericardium can be clearly visualized (Figure 24.4d).

Mass lesions are invariably easier to visualize if some pericardial effusion is present (Figure 24.4b). They can be large and very easy to distinguish, or small and difficult to see. Haemangiosarcomas can frequently be seen infiltrating the right atrial wall, whilst heart base tumours are typically found surrounding the aorta and pulmonary artery. Mesotheliomas and small/early cardiac tumours may not always be visible, resulting in a false diagnosis of idiopathic effusion.

Cardiac tamponade is characterized by either diastolic or systolic collapse of the right atrial wall and is best observed in the right parasternal long-axis view (Figure 24.4a). Severe tamponade can lead to a reduction in left ventricular chamber filling and to an apparent increase in left ventricular wall thickness,

referred to as pseudohypertrophy. In the case of constrictive pericardial disease, the pericardial wall is often very thickened with little or no pericardial effusion present. Secondary pericardial effusions are usually of small volume and rarely cause tamponade (Figure 24.4c).

Laboratory tests

Mild hypoproteinaemia (hypoalbuminaemia and hypoglobulinaemia) has been reported in dogs with pericardial effusion and is presumed secondary to right-sided CHF (unless it is the underlying cause). A non-regenerative or poorly regenerative anaemia has also been reported in some cases, presumed to be anaemia of chronic disease. Dogs with haemangiosarcoma may have evidence of schistocytes, acanthocytes and thrombocytopenia. Liver enzymes may be elevated if hepatic congestion is present, and a mild prerenal azotaemia may be present due to poor cardiac output.

Troponin I has demonstrated variable utility, as some studies have shown increased serum troponin I in dogs with pericardial disease compared with normal controls, or higher serum troponin I levels in dogs with haemangiosarcoma compared with dogs with idiopathic effusions (Shaw *et al.*, 2004; Spratt *et al.*, 2005; Linde *et al.*, 2006).

Pericardiocentesis

Pericardiocentesis may be used as a diagnostic test and as a treatment for pericardial effusion. It is the only effective treatment for tamponade. Removal of even a small quantity of pericardial effusion can result in a marked decrease in intrapericardial pressure. Analysis of the pericardial effusion may aid diagnosis.

Secondary pericardial effusions rarely cause tamponade and usually resolve with treatment of the primary disease problem, but on occasion pericardiocentesis may be indicated as an aid to diagnosis if the aetiology is uncertain.

Diuretics should not be given prior to pericardiocentesis, as not only will they be ineffective at relieving signs of CHF but also, by reducing circulating fluid volume and therefore intracardiac pressures, exacerbation of tamponade may occur.

Technique
The animal is placed in left lateral recumbency. Light sedation may be necessary: a combination of pethidine (2–3 mg/kg) and low-dose acepromazine (0.01 mg/kg) intramuscularly usually works very well.

- A large area is clipped on the right thorax. This side is chosen in order to avoid the large coronary artery on the left and also to avoid the lungs by using the cardiac notch.
- The exact location for pericardiocentesis can be identified using ultrasonography, or the procedure can be undertaken without echocardiography. The usual location is the fifth or sixth intercostal space at the costochondral junction.
- Once the site is located, local anaesthetic is injected into the skin, subcutaneous tissues and intercostal muscles. The site is then prepared aseptically. Sterile drapes are used.
- Different techniques have been described with over-the-needle catheters (Nelson and Ware, 2008), through-the-needle jugular catheters and pericardiocentesis catheters placed into the pericardium using the Seldinger technique.

The technique for pericardiocentesis using a veterinary pericardiocentesis catheter kit (Figure 24.5a) is as follows:

1. Make a small stab incision aseptically in the skin.
2. Pass a large needle with a 2 ml syringe attached through the skin and intercostal muscles into the pleural space.
3. Advance the needle carefully until the pericardium can be felt, and then slowly advance further into the pericardium.
4. Remove the syringe and pass a guidewire through the needle into the pericardium.

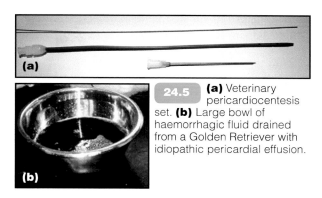

24.5 **(a)** Veterinary pericardiocentesis set. **(b)** Large bowl of haemorrhagic fluid drained from a Golden Retriever with idiopathic pericardial effusion.

5. Withdraw and remove the needle, and advance the catheter over the guidewire into the pericardium.
6. Withdraw the guidewire.
7. Attach a three-way tap and extension set to the catheter and drain the pericardium using either a 20 ml or 50 ml syringe. There are several large holes at the distal tip of the catheter to facilitate drainage.
8. Retain a sample in a plain tube to confirm fluid is pericardial and does not clot: intracardiac blood will usually clot within 5 minutes.

Electrocardiographic monitoring should be used throughout the procedure, as any contact with the myocardium will result in tachyarrhythmias (usually ventricular arrhythmias). If this occurs the catheter should be repositioned. The effusion is frequently very haemorrhagic regardless of the underlying disease and resembles venous blood; however, it does not clot and can thus be differentiated from right ventricular blood (Figure 24.5b).

The volume of pericardial effusion differs considerably and can range from 10 ml up to 2 litres, depending on the size of the patient and the underlying cause. In cases of cardiac tamponade, once the pericardial effusion is removed the preload increases dramatically, and the sudden increase in size of the right atrium may lead to transient atrial fibrillation, which usually resolves without treatment within 24–72 hours. Any ascites will usually resolve in 24–48 hours and diuretics are not necessary, but they will result in more rapid resolution of the right-sided CHF. It is common for some of the pericardial effusion to leak into the pleural cavity during drainage and again this will resolve within 24–48 hours.

Complications
Pericardiocentesis carries a risk of haemorrhage, tumour laceration, coronary laceration, infection, cardiac puncture and arrhythmias, and should always be undertaken with care.

- Ventricular arrhythmias are rarely life-threatening and usually stop once the catheter is repositioned.
- Cardiac puncture and removal of a large quantity of right ventricular blood can lead to hypovolaemic shock and can be avoided by checking that the haemorrhagic fluid is pericardial in origin.

- Aseptic technique should decrease the risk of infection, and use of the right side for pericardiocentesis will decrease the risk of coronary laceration.

Pericardial fluid analysis

Pericardial fluid may be an exudate, transudate, modified transudate, haemorrhagic or neoplastic (Figure 24.6). It can be very difficult to differentiate the type of effusion based on clinical appearance and further analysis should always be undertaken, including total and differential white blood cell count, packed cell volume, cytology, bacterial culture and sensitivity.

Type of effusion	Aetiology
Haemorrhagic	Idiopathic pericardial haemorrhage Neoplasia: haemangiosarcoma, heart base mass, lymphoma, mesothelioma Trauma Coagulopathy Ruptured left atrium
Transudate	Hypoproteinaemia
Modified transudate	Right-sided CHF Neoplasia PPDH
Exudate	Feline infectious peritonitis Infection: bacterial, fungal Foreign body

24.6 Types of pericardial effusion and aetiology.

Haemangiosarcomas rarely exfoliate, which can make diagnosis difficult. Neoplastic mesothelial cells may exfoliate and aid in reaching a definitive diagnosis, but care must be taken as reactive mesothelial cells can mimic neoplastic cells (Figure 24.7) and sometimes a definitive diagnosis can only be made based on histopathology and immunohistochemistry of the pericardium. Lymphoma cells are sometimes found in the effusion. Although other tests (such as effusion pH) have been used in an attempt to differentiate the aetiology, conflicting findings in the literature suggest that this is not helpful (Edwards 1996, Fine *et al.*, 2003, Laforcade *et al.*, 2005, Mellanby and Herrtage 2005).

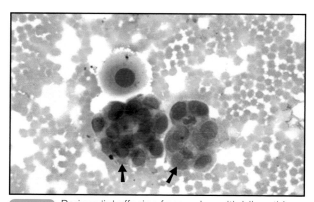

24.7 Pericardial effusion from a dog with idiopathic pericardial effusion. Reactive mesothelial cells are present (arrowed), which can mimic neoplastic cells. May–Grünwald–Giemsa stain; original magnification X40. (Courtesy of E. Milne.)

Long-term treatment and prognosis

Surgery

The most common surgical treatment is a subtotal pericardiectomy using either a lateral or midline approach; a thoracoscopic approach has also been described.

A percutaneous balloon pericardiotomy is an alternative palliative therapy for dogs with neoplastic effusions. Under general anaesthesia a balloon dilation catheter is passed percutaneously through a catheter sheath and positioned across the pericardium. Multiple dilations result in the formation of a small window that allows fluid to drain into the pleural space. At present there is little information in the literature comparing outcome using this technique with that for pericardiectomy.

Idiopathic pericardial effusion

Prognosis is very much dependent on the underlying cause, thus every effort should be made to reach a definitive diagnosis. In the case of idiopathic effusions in dogs, about one-third may not recur following single pericardiocentesis (Stafford Johnson *et al.*, 2004; Mellanby and Herrtage, 2005). Owners should be alerted to the possibility of recurrence, which can be from weeks to years later.

If the effusion recurs, surgical pericardiectomy is recommended as repeat drainage may lead to constrictive pericardial disease. Surgical pericardiectomy carries all the risks of a major thoracotomy, but it is usually curative and dogs with idiopathic pericardial effusions that have had pericardiectomy have a better survival rate than dogs that have not. Thoracoscopic partial pericardiectomy is an alternative option.

Neoplastic pericardial effusion

In the case of neoplastic effusions, the prognosis differs considerably depending on the tumour type. As mentioned previously, confirmation of tumour type is not always easy; however, a combination of echocardiographic location of the tumour within the heart, presence and location of metastatic disease, and pericardial fluid analysis may aid in reaching a definitive diagnosis.

Haemangiosarcomas are very malignant and commonly metastasize. Pericardiocentesis is palliative and recurrence within days is common. Even with palliative tumour resection and chemotherapy, the maximum reported survival time is 7–8 months (Weisse *et al.*, 2005).

Heart base tumours are usually slow growing and survival times are longer. Surgical removal may be an option, but clean margins are difficult to achieve and recurrence is common. Pericardiocentesis is indicated if an effusion is present and palliative pericardiectomy has been shown to significantly prolong survival times, with times of up to 3 years recorded in some cases (Vicari *et al.*, 2001).

Mesothelioma typically results in rapid recurrence of pericardial effusion post-pericardiocentesis. Pericardiectomy, if undertaken, may result in dissemination of the tumour into the pleural space, leading to chronic pleural effusion. Chemotherapy has been shown to decrease postoperative pleural effusion. Survival times of up to 10 months have been reported. Interestingly, in cases where it has been difficult to differentiate mesothelioma from idiopathic pericardial effusion, even with histopathology and immunohistochemistry, the recurrence of significant amounts of pleural effusion within 120 days of pericardiectomy has been shown to be an indicator of mesothelioma (Stepien et al., 2000).

In the case of lymphoma in cats resulting in pericardial effusion, palliative pericardiectomy and chemotherapy are indicated.

Other pericardial effusions and diseases

Pericardial effusion due to a bacterial infection can be managed conservatively using appropriate antibiotic therapy, but there is a high risk of constrictive pericardial disease and pericardiectomy is recommended once the animal is stabilized.

Pericardial effusion due to left atrial rupture may resolve without treatment, but pericardiocentesis may be required and there are reports of surgical repair of the ruptured left atrium. Congenital PPDH and cysts should be treated surgically.

References and further reading

Davidson BJ, Paling AC, Lahmers SL and Nelson OL (2008) Disease association and clinical assessment of feline pericardial effusion. *Journal of the American Animal Hospital Association* **44**, 5–9

Edwards NJ (1996) The diagnostic value of pericardial fluid pH determination. *Journal of the American Animal Hospital Association* **32**, 63–67

Fine DM, Tobias AH and Jacob KA (2003) Use of pericardial fluid pH to distinguish between idiopathic and neoplastic effusions. *Journal of Veterinary Internal Medicine* **17**, 525–529

Laforcade AM, Freeman LM, Rozanski EA and Rush JE (2005) Biochemical analysis of pericardial fluid and whole blood in dogs with pericardial effusion. *Journal of Veterinary Internal Medicine* **19**, 833–836

Linde A, Summerfield NJ, Sleeper MM et al. (2006) Pilot study on cardiac troponin I levels in dogs with pericardial effusion. *Journal of Veterinary Cardiology* **8**, 19–23

MacGregor JM, Faria MLE, Moore AS et al. (2005) Cardiac lymphoma and pericardial effusion in dogs: 12 cases (1994–2004). *Journal of the American Veterinary Medical Association* **227**, 1449–1453

Machida N, Tanaka R, Takemura N et al. (2004) Development of pericardial mesothelioma in Golden Retrievers with a long-term history of idiopathic haemorrhagic pericardial effusion. *Journal of Comparative Pathology* **131**, 166–175

Martin MW, Green MJ, Stafford Johnson MJ and Day MJ (2006) Idiopathic pericarditis in dogs: no evidence for an immune-mediated aetiology. *Journal of Small Animal Practice* **47**, 387–391

Mellanby RJ and Herrtage ME (2005) Long-term survival of 23 dogs with pericardial effusions. *Veterinary Record* **156**, 568–571

Nelson OL and Ware WA (2008) Pericardial Effusion. In: *Kirk's Current Veterinary Therapy, XIV: Small Animal Practice*, ed. JD Bonagura and DC Twedt, pp. 825–831. WB Saunders, Philadelphia

Shaw SP, Rozanski EA and Rush JE (2004) Cardiac troponins I and T in dogs with pericardial effusion. *Journal of Veterinary Internal Medicine* **18**, 322–324

Spratt DP, Mellanby RJ, Drury N and Archer J (2005) Cardiac troponin I: evaluation of a biomarker for the diagnosis of heart disease in the dog. *Journal of Small Animal Practice* **46**, 139–145

Stafford Johnson M, Martin M, Binns S et al. (2004) A retrospective study of clinical findings, treatment and outcome in 143 dogs with pericardial effusion. *Journal of Small Animal Practice* **45**, 546–552

Stepien RL, Whitley NT and Dubielzig RR (2000) Idiopathic or mesothelioma-related pericardial effusion: clinical findings and survival in 17 dogs studied retrospectively. *Journal of Small Animal Practice* **41**, 342–347

Tobias AH (2005) Pericardial Disorders. In: Textbook of Veterinary Internal Medicine, ed. SJ Ettinger and EC Feldman, pp. 1104–1118. Elsevier, St. Louis

Vicari ED, Brown DC, Holt DE and Brockman DJ (2001) Survival times of and prognostic indicators for dogs with heart base masses: 25 cases (1986–1999). *Journal of the American Veterinary Medical Association* **219**, 485–487

Weisse C, Soares N, Beal,MW et al. (2005) Survival times in dogs with right atrial hemangiosarcoma treated by means of surgical resection with or without adjuvant chemotherapy: 23 cases (1986–2000). *Journal of the American Veterinary Medical Association* **226**, 575–579

Zini E, Glaus TM, Bussadori C et al. (2009) Evaluation of the presence of selected viral and bacterial nucleic acids in pericardial samples from dogs with or without idiopathic pericardial effusion. *Veterinary Journal* **179(2)**, 225–229

25

Feline cardiomyopathies

John D. Bonagura

Introduction

Genetic and idiopathic myocardial diseases are often termed primary cardiomyopathies. These include hypertrophic (HCM), dilated (DCM), restrictive (RCM), arrhythmogenic right ventricular (ARVC) and unclassified (UCM) cardiomyopathies, as well as myocarditis (or endomyocarditis) (Figure 25.1). Myocardial infarction is a poorly characterized disorder in cats, which causes regional or global ventricular dysfunction. Of these conditions, HCM is most common.

Secondary myocardial diseases develop from defined disorders such as systemic hypertension, hyperthyroidism, taurine deficiency and growth hormone excess (acromegaly). Echocardiographic findings overlap between primary and secondary myocardial disorders, but these conditions should be distinguished as patient management and long-term prognoses can differ.

Primary (idiopathic/genetic)
Hypertrophic cardiomyopathy (HCM): obstructive *versus* non-obstructive; diffuse *versus* regional *versus* focal Dilated cardiomyopathy (DCM) Restrictive cardiomyopathy (RCM) Arrhythmogenic right ventricular cardiomyopathy (ARVC) Unclassified cardiomyopathies (UCM) Myocarditis/endomyocarditis

Secondary (identifiable cause)
Left ventricular hypertrophy: hyperthyroid heart disease; hypertensive heart disease DCM: taurine deficiency; myocarditis (diffuse); tachycardia-induced High output myocardial disease: anaemia; thyrotoxicosis (chronic) Infiltrative cardiomyopathy: neoplastic infiltration; myocarditis Myocardial infarction Heart disease related to acromegaly

25.1 Clinical classification of feline cardiomyopathies.

Other causes of heart disease must be considered in the differential diagnosis of feline cardiomyopathies. Congenital malformations of the heart and great vessels are observed regularly in cats. Mitral valve malformation, ventricular septal defects (VSDs) and atrial septal defects (ASDs) are encountered most often (see Chapter 26). Although congenital cardiac malformations are usually considered problems of kittens and young cats, these defects may go unrecognized until maturity.

Moderate to severe anaemia is an under-recognized reason for cardiac enlargement. Cats with diabetes mellitus may exhibit myocardial disease, in some cases related to growth hormone excess. Additionally, severe respiratory disease in cats can induce pulmonary hypertension and cor pulmonale (see Chapter 28), sometimes resulting in marked enlargement of the right heart. In contrast to other species, both degenerative valvular disease and infective endocarditis are very rare in cats. Pericardial effusions in cats are generally caused by congestive heart failure (CHF) and often resolve with effective treatment of the underlying condition.

Cardiac rhythm disturbances requiring treatment seem less common in cats when compared with dogs. However, atrial and ventricular ectopic rhythms do develop in association with cardiomyopathies, cardiomegaly, myocardial fibrosis, myocarditis, ischaemia, infarction, increased sympathetic activity, electrolyte disturbances, hyperthyroidism and cardiac or systemic neoplasia (see Chapter 16). Some persistent rhythm disturbances, including atrial fibrillation, can be idiopathic in cats. Atrioventricular blocks are observed most often in older cats.

In terms of vascular disorders, idiopathic aortic dilatation, systemic hypertension and arterial thromboembolism (ATE) are common diseases of mature cats. Idiopathic aortic dilatation (aortoannular ectasia) is a seemingly benign disorder often observed in middle-aged and older cats. Whether or not aortic stiffness is altered in this disease, or whether this vascular change contributes to systolic hypertension, has not been studied. This lesion is frequently associated with subaortic septal hypertrophy and a systolic murmur, clinical findings that can create confusion about the underlying cardiac diagnosis. Systemic hypertension is a common cause of LV hypertrophy as well as cardiac murmurs in cats; it rarely advances to CHF or aortic rupture. When blood pressure is severely elevated, retinal detachment and haemorrhage, renal injury, CNS depression and haemorrhagic stroke are more common outcomes.

Risk factors

There are clearly breed risks for development of HCM (see later). Cats of any age can be affected, including those in their first year. This means that HCM as well as congenital heart defects should be considered in the differential diagnosis of structural heart disease in young cats. Myocarditis can affect feline patients of any age, especially immature cats. Older cats are more likely to manifest a form of RCM or type of UCM. This is also true of the secondary cardiomyopathies, considering that the older population is prone to hyperthyroidism, systemic hypertension and diabetes mellitus.

Stress, fever, moderate to severe anaemia, thyrotoxicosis, anaesthesia, surgical procedures, trauma and fluid therapy may precipitate CHF or ATE in a previously stable cat with cardiomyopathy. Prior therapy with long-acting corticosteroids is considered another risk factor for development of CHF; however, the underlying mechanisms for this association are unresolved.

History

The history of most cats with HCM reveals no signs of heart disease. Conversely, heart failure and ATE are common initial signs associated with a diagnosis of RCM, UCM and DCM. Depression or reduced activity is observed in some cats with cardiovascular disease. Diet is not believed to play an important role, with the exception of now rare cases of taurine-deficiency DCM. This situation is most often observed in home-restricted cats fed non-commercial or custom diets.

Cats with secondary cardiomyopathies are often more affected by the underlying disorder than by any cardiovascular complications. For example, cats with moderate to severe systemic hypertension often demonstrate clinical signs related to target organ injury and to metabolic derangements of renal failure (see Chapter 27). Systemic signs may also be evident when heart disease is caused by hyperthyroidism or anaemia.

With the onset of CHF, respiratory signs consequent to pulmonary oedema or pleural effusion can become evident. Some cats with heart disease have a cough, but this is much less common than in dogs. Chronic coughing in a cat with cardiomegaly is more likely to represent bronchopulmonary disease with cor pulmonale (or dirofilariasis in endemic regions) rather than left-sided CHF.

Emergency presentation to the veterinary hospital is likely following an episode of ATE, owing to the acute onset of pain and paresis in the affected limbs. Syncope is another distressing sign that may prompt an emergency visit. In cats, syncope is commonly mistaken for a seizure disorder. Syncope and sudden cardiac death can occur with cardiomyopathy, myocarditis or primary heart rhythm disturbances. The differential diagnosis of syncope in cats includes: ventricular tachycardia; intermittent complete atrioventricular block with asystole; severe left ventricular outflow tract (LVOT) obstruction related to HCM or mitral dysplasia; and rhythm disturbance due to myocardial infarction. Sudden cardiac death can occur as a consequence of one of these rhythm disturbances. Some cats are reported to have died 'suddenly' when the actual cause was hypoxaemia or shock from unappreciated CHF. Cerebrovascular complications of ATE or systemic hypertension are

probably under-recognized and include altered mental status, syncope, postural changes, seizures and stroke (see Figure 25.3b).

Physical examination

Examination findings in feline cardiomyopathies vary widely (Figure 25.2). Many affected cats are seemingly healthy. Cardiac, vascular and respiratory problems are most often identified in cats with clinical cardiomyopathies, but clinical findings referable to other organ systems may also be evident (Figure 25.3). Often heart disease is discovered

Clinical signs	Possible features
Cardiac auscultation abnormalities	Cardiac murmur Gallop sound Rhythm disturbance: arrhythmia, pauses, bradycardia, or tachycardia Muffled or soft heart sounds
Pulse abnormalities	Hypokinetic, hyperkinetic, variable, or alternating arterial pulse Prominent jugular venous pulse Jugular venous distension
Arterial thromboembolism [a]	Sudden onset of paresis or lameness (rear limbs or forelimb) Signs of limb ischaemia (pulseless, cold, pale limb) Diminished or absent pulse or Doppler flow signals Skeletal muscle firmness or contraction with muscle pain Lower motor neuron neuropathy
Respiratory signs	Tachypnoea Respiratory distress Coughing (less common) Pulmonary adventious sounds Altered bronchial sounds Pulmonary crackles Pleural fluid line
Sudden (cardiac) death	With or without premonitory signs
Central nervous system signs	Depression Syncope Signs of haemorrhagic or thrombotic stroke (altered consciousness, seizures, altered posture associated with brain injury)
Ocular signs	Central retinal degeneration (taurine deficiency) Retinal haemorrhage, detachment, vascular tortuosity, blindness (related to hypertension)
Other potential signs [b]	History of inactivity Pallor or cyanosis of mucous membranes Thyroid enlargement Abnormal renal size or contour Weight loss Hypothermia Abnormal facial appearance (acromegaly)

25.2 Clinical findings associated with primary or secondary feline cardiomyopathies. [a] See Figure 25.5 for a more detailed listing. [b] Some of these signs are related to underlying disorders.

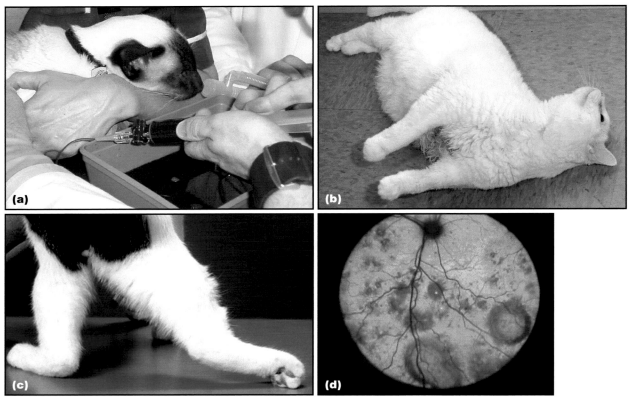

25.3 Clinical signs in feline cardiomyopathy. **(a)** Cat presented with respiratory distress due to congestive heart failure undergoing emergency thoracocentesis. The patient is receiving oxygen and has been sedated. A small butterfly catheter was used to provide partial relief of the effusion. (Courtesy of S. Dennis.) **(b)** Cat with decerebrate type posture following a suspected haemorrhagic stroke. The cat had severe systemic hypertension. Neurological signs improved significantly in this cat with just control of arterial blood pressure. **(c)** Caudal image of a cat during the recovering phase from aortoiliac thromboembolism. The cat is ambulatory but there is extensor weakness in the left limb and proprioceptive deficits in the right limb. **(d)** Ocular fundus of a cat with systemic hypertension. There is mild tortuosity noted in the retinal vessels and numerous focal active retinal detachments evident.

serendipitously following cardiac auscultation or thoracic radiography. Identification of a murmur, gallop sound, arrhythmia, or cardiomegaly usually prompts further investigation. The clinician must be mindful that secondary cardiomyopathies develop and that other organ systems may be affected. Thus, a thorough physical examination and an open mind are critical to accurate and efficient diagnosis.

Auscultation

Gallop sounds
Auscultation of cats with cardiomyopathy often reveals an extra diastolic sound or gallop. Gallops are indicators of abnormal ventricular filling.

* The atrial (S4) gallop is generally a sign of mild to moderate diastolic dysfunction, representing a transient increase in atrial pressure associated with impaired ventricular relaxation. Some older cats develop atrial gallops unassociated with cardiomyopathy, but perhaps indicating an 'ageing' ventricle.
* The ventricular (S3) or summation (S3 + S4) gallop is more ominous and generally indicates advanced diastolic heart failure with a noncompliant ventricle and elevated atrial pressures.

It is very difficult to distinguish atrial from ventricular gallops in cats, because of their rapid heart rate. Sometimes gentle pressure on the nasal planum for about 5 seconds will induce a transient slowing of the heart, and this vagal manoeuvre may help an astute examiner to better determine the timing of the extra sound.

Murmurs
It is also very difficult to distinguish functional (innocent) murmurs from murmurs due to cardiac disease. Both are very common in cats and can sound very similar at the typically high feline heart rate. The genesis of heart murmurs can be difficult to determine, even when a consistent examination approach is undertaken (Figure 25.4; see also Chapter 4).

Heightened sympathetic tone, along with peripheral vasodilatation or altered blood viscosity, are important reasons for physiological murmurs. These situations can develop in thyrotoxicosis, anaemia, fever, volume depletion, following sedatives (ketamine), and with the stress of a veterinary hospital visit. Dynamic right ventricular outflow tract (RVOT) obstruction is a common source of functional murmurs where hyperdynamic contraction of the right ventricle (RV) leads to obstruction to flow in the proximal RVOT.

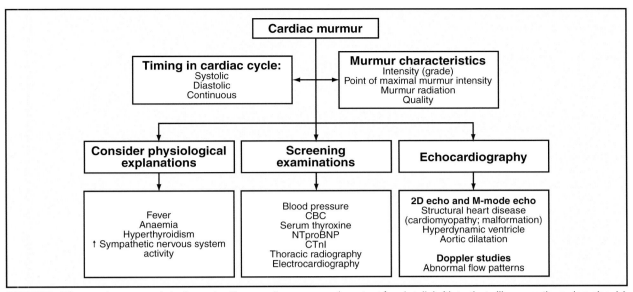

25.4 Diagnostic approach to the cat with a cardiac murmur (see text for details). Note that: (i) serum thyroxine should be measured in cats >7 years of age; and (ii) abnormal NTproBNP, cTnI, thoracic radiographs (cardiomegaly) or ECG (cardiomegaly pattern, axis shift, rhythm disturbance) are indications for obtaining an echocardiographic study. Not all screening examinations are indicated in every case.

Importantly, murmurs due to structural disease are usually related to a form of cardiomyopathy or a congenital heart malformation, as opposed to degenerative valve disease. Another potential source of a systolic murmur is ejection of blood into a dilated aorta – a common finding in older cats. Systolic murmurs in cats often involve dynamic obstruction in the mid-ventricle from hypertrophied muscle, or in the LVOT stemming from mitral–septal contact (dynamic LVOT obstruction caused by systolic anterior motion of the mitral valve). Hyperdynamic contraction due to heightened sympathetic tone can create turbulence in the LV or RV, and can develop in a structurally normal or a hypertrophied chamber. Thus, murmurs that increase in intensity with sympathetic stimulation (as indicated by a higher heart rate) can be functional or organic (secondary to structural cardiac disease).

Almost every murmur in a cat is systolic in timing. Diastolic murmurs are rare, generally resulting from aortic regurgitation due to severe aortic root dilation or infective endocarditis. Continuous (or 'long-systolic') murmurs may be identified cranially in cats with patent ductus arteriosus (PDA). In the author's experience, it is not helpful to designate valve areas for auscultation in cats. Instead, most systolic murmurs are characterized by their location relative to the sternum and palpable cardiac impulse.

- As a gross generality, murmurs loudest at the apex (caudal heart border) are more likely to be caused by mitral regurgitation (MR) from cardiomyopathy or valve malformation.
- In contrast, murmurs more intense at the cranial right sternal edge are suggestive of a VSD, functional murmur, or turbulent flow into the ascending aorta.
- Murmurs stemming from LV obstruction tend to be loud at either location.
- When murmurs are loud, the vibrations can radiate widely, adding ambiguity to the diagnosis.

An emerging, but not unanimous, literature suggests that N-terminal B-type natriuretic peptide (NTproBNP) concentrations may be a cost-effective screening blood test for excluding important structural heart disease in many cats with heart murmurs (see Chapter 8). While some studies support the use of serum cardiac troponin-I (cTnI) as a screening test for cardiomyopathy, in the author's experience too many results fall into a 'grey zone' for this to be consistently helpful in the differential diagnosis of heart murmurs. If all screening examinations shown in Figure 25.4 are conducted, the likelihood of identifying structural heart disease is high; however, the attendant veterinary costs are similarly great. For this reason, many veterinary surgeons simply advocate obtaining an echocardiogram (with Doppler study) when assessing asymptomatic cats with a heart murmur. As a more practical alternative, the NTproBNP test may gain prominence for separating 'normal' from abnormal murmurs.

Respiratory system

Auscultation of the heart should be coupled with examination of the respiratory system. Tachypnoea or respiratory distress in a cat should prompt keen observation of the pattern of ventilation. Significant findings include:

- Presence of loud airway noises (suggesting large airway obstruction)
- Wheezes or rhonchi (suggesting bronchial disease)
- Crackles (suggesting oedema or parenchymal disease)
- Pleural fluid line.

Distressed cats may require oxygen and sedation, along with urgent therapy for upper airway obstruction (intubation), asthma (inhaled or parenteral bronchodilators), pulmonary oedema (diuretics), or pleural effusion (thoracocentesis), before proceeding to radiography or other evaluations.

Pulse abnormalities

Pulse abnormalities may point to a cardiovascular disorder.

- The jugular venous pulse may be prominent or the veins grossly distended in cats with CHF, cardiac tamponade, cor pulmonale, or circulatory volume overload. The latter situation is commonly observed when substantial volumes of intravenous fluids are administered to a cat with anaemia, renal failure or hyperthyroidism.
- Hyperdynamic arterial pulses are typical of bradycardia (heart block), hyperthyroidism and anaemia.
- Irregular pulses should be considered abnormal in cats and prompt an electrocardiogram (ECG) to identify premature complexes or periods of atrioventricular block.

Arterial thromboembolism

Loss of a peripheral arterial pulse in a cat is highly supportive of ATE. Vascular signs of ATE typically stem from an underlying cardiomyopathy (or myocarditis), although thrombi can also develop with multisystemic disorders including pulmonary malignancies. A thromboembolism usually originates in the left atrium (LA) and travels to the terminal aorta. Smaller thrombi may cause myocardial infarction, thrombotic stroke, forelimb monoparesis, renal infarcts or, rarely, mesenteric ischaemia with severe colic. Diffuse intra-abdominal ischaemia also can be caused by a massive aortic thrombosis.

Signs related to embolism to a forelimb can be relatively brief in duration (hours). Terminal aortic embolism is generally more severe, and signs may persist for hours to weeks, though many cats recover limb function if given sufficient time and care (see later). The physical diagnosis of terminal aortic embolism is straightforward and characterized by vascular, musculoskeletal and neurological deficits, and associated laboratory abnormalities (Figure 25.5). Limb oedema is not an early sign of ATE, though it may be observed days after the event as a consequence of severe muscle injury (and predicts a poorer chance for full recovery).

Other physical findings

- Examination of the ocular fundus should be undertaken in cats with cardiac signs, to screen for hypertensive retinopathy in particular, and for retinal degeneration when a diagnosis of DCM has been made.
- The general examination should consider:
  - The cervical region (for thyroid masses)
  - The kidneys (as a risk factor for hypertension or as targets for hypertensive injury or thromboembolic events)
  - The mucous membranes (for signs of anaemia, hypoperfusion, or cyanosis).
- Hypothermia is often observed in cats with ATE and, when profound, is a poor prognostic factor.

Vascular [a]
Cold limbs Pallor or peripheral cyanosis of the skin or toes Diminished or absent arterial pulse Absent Doppler flow signals within the arterial system Identification of aortic embolus using Duplex Doppler ultrasonography Signs of shock, including hypothermia, pallor, metabolic acidosis Signs of progressive reperfusion [b]
Musculoskeletal
Ischaemic muscle contracture Rhabdomyolysis Moderate to severe pain [c] Release into the blood of creatine kinase (CK), aspartate aminotransferase (AST) and alanine aminotransferase (ALT) from damaged muscles [d] Reperfusion hyperkalaemia Flaccid, possibly oedematous muscles (subacute to chronic stage) [e] Tissue necrosis involving muscle, subcutaneous tissues and overlying skin – most common in the toes and distal limb (chronic) Limb contracture (chronic) [f]
Neurological
Pain (likely related to muscle ischaemia and infarction) Sudden onset of paresis (rear limbs or forelimb) Loss of tail function (aortic thromboembolism) Peripheral neuropathy (worse distally) Sensory line (hypalgesia distal; normal to hyperalgesia proximal) Asymmetry of motor loss (common in ATE) Progressive return of limb function (hours to weeks) Permanent neurological deficits (chronic)

25.5 Clinical signs of ATE. [a] Most of these are acute signs of ATE; shock can develop in the most severe cases; [b] Reperfusion can begin within minutes of the ATE event, but typically starts within 24–72 h. [c] Initial pain associated with ATE of the aorta can be very severe and requires aggressive analgesic therapy; pain is generally much diminished by 24–48 h; mesenteric pain related to suprarenal thrombus is relatively uncommon, but can be particularly severe. [d] In typical ATE the CK elevations are very high, often requiring dilution of the sample to quantify; AST is higher (typically 2–3x greater than) ALT, which is derived from striated muscle. [e] Limb oedema typically occurs in cases of severe rhabdomyolysis after 72–96 h, and may be delayed for 1–2 weeks. [f] Contracture can be reduced by physical therapy starting 48–72 h after the injury and, if necessary, bandaging the limb in a functional position to prevent extension. Chronic = signs may not be evident for weeks following the event.

The triad of reduced body temperature, heart rate and blood pressure is highly suggestive of cardiogenic shock, a condition that demands aggressive inotropic therapy (see below).

- Weight loss is compatible with systemic disease of any origin, but is especially common in hyperthyroidism and chronic kidney disease and in some cats with chronic CHF.
- Abdominal distension related to hepatomegaly and ascites can develop in cats with cardiomyopathy, but is relatively uncommon except in cats with atrial standstill, severe right-sided heart disease, or atrial fibrillation.

Diagnostic studies

A number of diagnostic tests can be useful in the evaluation of the cat with signs of cardiovascular disease or cardiomyopathy. These include indirect arterial blood pressure (BP) measurement, the ECG, thoracic radiography, clinical laboratory tests, and echocardiography with Doppler studies.

Blood pressure

Systemic arterial BP is usually normal in cats with cardiomyopathy unless the cause of myocardial disease is systemic hypertension. The cat with profound CHF or ATE may be hypotensive, with hypothermia and reduced peripheral perfusion. Cardiogenic shock is not specific for any particular form of feline cardiomyopathy, but often suggests that an acute event such as a regional wall infarction or a thromboembolic event has supervened. Technical details of indirect BP recording are important and are discussed in Chapter 13.

Electrocardiography

Electrocardiography is insensitive as a screening test for cardiomyopathy and probably has a greater positive than negative predictive value for feline heart disease. In other words, a normal ECG does not exclude a diagnosis of heart disease. Criteria used to identify cardiomegaly patterns in cats are similar to those in dogs qualitatively, but differ in terms of absolute voltages (see Chapter 9). No specific ECG findings can discriminate the various forms of cardiomyopathy in cats. Diagnostic criteria used by the author are noted below.

- Widened (≥0.04 s) or tall (≥0.25 mV) P waves predict the finding of atrial enlargement on echocardiography.
- In the author's experience, R waves or S waves >0.7 in any frontal plane lead or a left axis deviation with voltages of >0.7 mV in leads I or aVL are suggestive of LV hypertrophy or left anterior fascicular block (Figure 25.6).
- When any ventricular waveform is ≥ 1 mV, cardiomegaly is likely.
- Right axis deviation or hypertrophy patterns (S waves in leads I, II, III) and intraventricular conduction disturbances are more common with RCM, ARVC and UCM.
- Congenital heart defects are also a cause of high voltage or altered electrical axis in cats.

Identification of a possible heart rhythm disturbance is the principal indication for an ECG in a cat with suspected cardiomyopathy. Since sinus arrhythmia is uncommon in a cat undergoing veterinary examination, an irregular rhythm as well as a heart rate <160 beats/minute, or a heart rate >240 beats/minute should prompt an ECG. Persistent or recurrent arrhythmias are relatively uncommon in cats, but seem more common with RCM, myocarditis and ARVC. Sometimes an arrhythmia will pre-date the eventual appearance of a structural cardiomyopathy. Hyperthyroidism can lead to premature atrial and

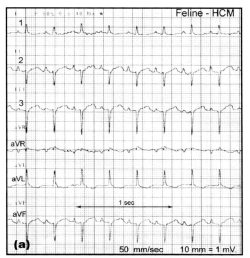

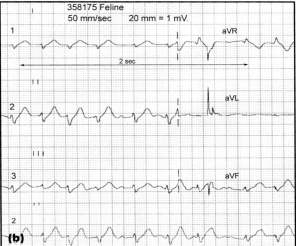

25.6 ECGs in feline cardiomyopathy. **(a)** Sinus rhythm with left axis deviation and increased QRS voltages in a cat with HCM. The frontal axis is left-cranial, with prominent positive voltages in leads aVL and I. There are progressively deeper S waves in leads II, aVF and III. Overall QRS voltages in lead III exceed 1 mV. (Paper speed 50 mm/s and standard calibration) **(b)** Atrial fibrillation and probable right bundle branch block in a cat with cardiomyopathy. The overall rhythm is irregular and there are no consistent P waves evident. The QRS complex is widened, with terminal activation of the ventricle oriented to the right and cranially. Secondary T wave changes are evident.

ventricular complexes that may improve following antithyroid therapy. Complete atrioventricular block can be missed on physical examination since the typical escape rhythm is relatively fast, often in the 120–130 beats/minute range. This rhythm is most common in older cats, probably from degeneration of conduction tissues and perhaps exacerbated by myocardial diseases causing LV concentric hypertrophy.

Thoracic radiography

Thoracic radiography plays a pivotal role in the differential diagnosis of cough, tachypnoea, or respiratory distress. Common diagnostic considerations in feline patients with increased lung density or abnormal thoracic auscultation include pulmonary oedema, bronchial disease/asthma, bronchopneumonia, atypical pneumonia, pulmonary neoplasia and, in some regions, respiratory parasites. Pleural effusions can stem from CHF, thoracic neoplasia, idiopathic chylothorax, pyothorax, feline infectious peritonitis and trauma.

Results of thoracic radiography can be normal in mild disease, but cardiac elongation, apex shifting and atrial enlargement are observed frequently in advanced cardiomyopathies. Typically the apex is shifted towards the midline with enlargement of the LA and LV, but this is variable (Figure 25.7). As with an ECG, there are no specific radiographic findings distinguishing the various forms of myocardial disease. With development of CHF, the cardiac silhouette may be further enlarged by a small to moderate pericardial effusion related to untreated CHF.

The radiographic features of CHF include cardiomegaly with evidence of fluid accumulation in the lung and/or pleural space. Typical cases demonstrate bulging of the LA on the dorsoventral (DV) view, along with elongation or widening of the entire silhouette. A prominent pulmonary vascular pattern (involving both lobar veins and arteries) is anticipated. Pulmonary oedema may manifest as an interstitial, bronchial, alveolar or mixed pattern, and may be focal, patchy or diffuse (Benigni *et al.*, 2009). In cats with a regional rather than generalized lung pattern there is a tendency towards a more caudoventral distribution of cardiogenic oedema, as seen on lateral views. Pleural effusions are common in both acute and chronic cases of CHF and at times can be very large, obscuring the cardiac silhouette.

Laboratory tests

A serum biochemistry profile may demonstrate abnormalities related to heart failure, ATE, recent therapy or an underlying systemic disease. Biomarkers, in particular NTproBNP and cardiac troponin-I (cTnI), may be released from diseased ventricles. Some of the major points are summarized below (see also Chapter 8).

- Renal function is often impaired in cats treated for CHF with diuretics and angiotensin-converting enzyme (ACE) inhibitors. Serum levels of creatinine and urea should be followed whenever dosages are adjusted. Severe uraemia can occur in the setting of suprarenal ATE. Cats with hypertensive heart disease related to chronic kidney disease will often demonstrate uraemia and hypokalaemia, along with an abnormal urinalysis.
- Serum creatine kinase, AST and ALT (of apparent skeletal muscle origin) are often elevated dramatically in ATE. The AST will be significantly higher than ALT when the elevations are related to striated muscle damage. These enzymes may also be helpful in recognizing ATE in a cat with severe but rapidly improving paresis of a forelimb.

Other blood tests can be relevant to the cat with cardiomyopathy:

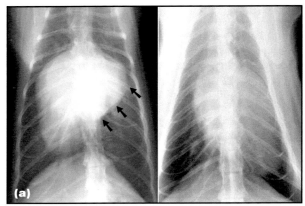
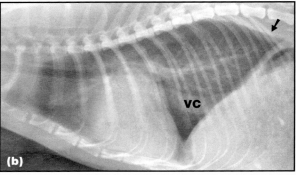
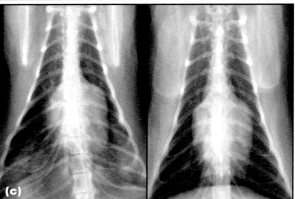

25.7 Radiography in feline cardiomyopathy. **(a)** VD radiographs of two cats with HCM. The cardiac silhouette is significantly enlarged in each cat. The left panel shows marked LA dilatation (arrowed) with the apex shifting to the right. The right panel shows severe elongation of the heart compatible with LV enlargement. **(b)** Lateral radiograph of a cat with RCM. The heart is moderately to severely enlarged. The caudal vena cava (VC) is dilated. The caudal lung lobes demonstrate a prominent pulmonary vascular pattern with interstitial lung densities. There is also a small pleural effusion (arrowed), which was shown to be chylothorax based on chemical analysis. **(c)** VD radiographs of a cat with HCM before (left) and after (right) hospital therapy for CHF. The bilateral pulmonary interstitial and alveolar infiltrates are resolved in the follow-up film; however, the heart is still elongated with slight prominence of the LA.

- Serum thyroxine should be measured in older cats (>7 years of age) showing any cardiac signs, to exclude hyperthyroidism as a potential cause.
- Routine haematology may reveal anaemia or evidence of inflammation, conditions that may result in a functional heart murmur by increasing cardiac output.

- Heartworm antibody and antigen tests are relevant when a cat lives in, has travelled to, or has relocated from a heartworm-endemic area (not the UK).
- In cats with DCM, a whole-blood taurine concentration may indicate whether the aetiology is a dietary deficiency in this amino acid.

A cytological and biochemical evaluation can be instructive in the differential diagnosis of pleural effusion. Analysis generally reveals a modified transudate in CHF, often with a predominant population of small lymphocytes and mesothelial cells.

Chylothorax is another common finding in severe CHF in cats and can be confirmed by measuring serum *versus* fluid triglyceride concentration (the latter is higher). Cats with chylothorax can develop a prominent neutrophilic reaction mixed into a mononuclear cell population, which can be confused with pleuritis.

Biomarkers

NTproBNP concentrations appear in most studies to provide the best balance between specificity and sensitivity in the recognition of cardiomyopathies. As discussed more fully in Chapter 8, the proper handling and shipping of the blood sample is critical for obtaining the best results. Specific optimal 'cut-offs' for distinguishing healthy cats without cardiomyopathy from those with cardiomyopathy are approximately 50 pmol/l (Connolly *et al.*, 2008), but the laboratory should be consulted for specific details as methodologies and reference values may differ. A higher cut-off value (approximately 250 pmol/l) has successfully distinguished cats with respiratory signs caused by CHF from those related to primary respiratory disease (Connolly *et al.*, 2009; Fox *et al.*, 2009). As with any laboratory test, there will be exceptions and ambiguous results, so the clinician must exercise appropriate judgement and integrate all clinical data when interpreting the results of NTproBNP.

Echocardiography

Definitive diagnosis of cardiomyopathy relies on cardiac ultrasonography. Two-dimensional (2D) imaging is most important, supported by M mode and a variety of Doppler studies. The 2D study provides information about lesions and cardiac motion, as well as wall thicknesses, chamber sizes and ventricular systolic function. Details of the echocardiographic examination are provided in Chapter 11. Some points pertinent to all feline myocardial diseases are summarized here and illustrated in Figure 25.8. Specific distinguishing features of the important cardiomyopathies are noted later in the chapter.

Wall thickness

LV diastolic wall thickness in most cats is <5.5 mm, and most cardiologists consider 6 mm or more to indicate LV hypertrophy. The 'HCM phenotype' is most often related to idiopathic/genetic HCM; however, hyperthyroid heart disease and hypertensive heart disease can also lead to papillary muscle thickening and increased wall thickness. A false-positive diagnosis may occur in the setting of diminished LV

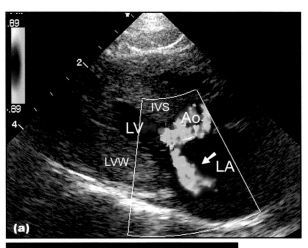

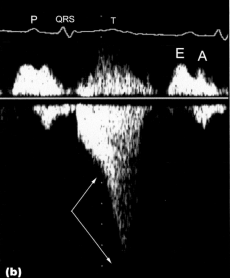

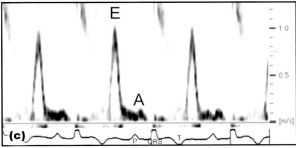

25.8 Echocardiography in feline cardiomyopathy. **(a)** 2D colour Doppler echocardiogram from a cat with HCM of the LV, demonstrating: hypertrophy of the septum (IVS) and LV wall (LVW); LA dilatation; turbulence in the ascending aorta (Ao); and an eccentric jet of mitral regurgitation (arrowed) stemming from systolic anterior motion (SAM) of the mitral valve. **(b)** Continuous wave (CW) Doppler study from a cat with HCM and dynamic LVOT obstruction. The cursor is aligned along a systolic signal that abruptly increases in velocity (arrows) at the time of SAM of the mitral valve. Diastolic flow waves (E and A) are also recorded since the CW cursor crosses the inflow signal of LV filling (these should not be analysed in this plane). **(c)** Pulsed-wave Doppler recording of mitral valve filling from a cat with cardiomyopathy receiving atenolol. The filling pattern has become 'restrictive', characterized by a large E wave and attenuated A wave. These findings are suggestive of elevated pulmonary venous and mean LA pressures.

lumen size caused by diuresis or dehydration, or when an inexperienced examiner measures the papillary muscles instead of the free wall. Wall thinning can be generalized in cats with DCM, or segmental as often observed in regions of infarction. Fibrosis occasionally is evident as a hyperechoic or speckled appearance to the myocardium.

Chamber sizes

Diastolic LV diameter measured by 2D or M mode across the minor axis is generally <18–19 mm in mature cats, but some healthy larger-breed cats (Maine Coon) may exceed this value by 2–3 mm. Left heart or generalized cardiac dilatation is most often observed in DCM or in congenital lesions resulting in left-sided volume overload, such as mitral dysplasia, VSD or PDA. However, states predisposing to volume expansion (moderate to severe anaemia, advanced thyrotoxicosis, chronic bradycardia) can also dilate cardiac chambers. Often one of these underlying conditions is complicated by fluid therapy elevating venous pressures, creating four-chamber dilatation. Isolated right heart enlargement is most often observed with (arrhythmogenic) RV cardiomyopathy, ASD, pulmonic stenosis or cor pulmonale.

Ventricular systolic function

Global LV systolic function is generally in the normal range, with shortening fraction typically 35–50%, in cats with most forms of cardiomyopathy, but there are notable exceptions. Hyperdynamic LV systolic function is common in HCM and in hyperthyroidism. Reduced global function is a requisite for diagnosis of DCM, and most affected cats have a shortening fraction of <25%. Cats with RCM, UCM and 'burned out' HCM often have reduced systolic function, either globally or regionally. Segmental LV systolic dysfunction is common, especially involving the free wall, and may represent ischaemic damage to that part of the myocardium.

Left atrial dilatation

In cats with cardiomyopathy of any type, the size of the LA is a strong indicator of disease severity and the risk for ATE or CHF. In the author's practice, LA dilatation is a factor in considering therapies for otherwise asymptomatic cats (see below). Dilatation (measured across the centre of the chamber by 2D long-axis imaging) is present when the atrial diameter is ≥16 mm. Moderate and severe LA dilatation can be defined arbitrarily as ≥20 mm and ≥25 mm, respectively. Equally important are imaging studies of the atrium that define presence or absence of intramural thrombi or echogenic intra-atrial contrast or 'smoke'. Doppler studies of atrial filling and emptying rates may help to identify cats at higher risk for thromboembolism, with lower values (especially <20 cm/s) indicating a higher chance for blood stagnation and thrombogenesis.

Doppler studies

The various patterns and values of ventricular filling, tissue movement and pulmonary venous flow can be combined to estimate diastolic heart function and ventricular filling pressures. The latter are predictive of CHF in many cats. Mild diastolic dysfunction is characterized by abnormal myocardial relaxation associated with enhanced atrial contraction. Doppler examination is characterized by diminished and delayed early ventricular filling (E waves) and tissue movements (Ea waves) with prominent atrial contraction waves (E/A reversal). As the ventricle becomes less compliant and mean atrial pressure increases, these abnormalities 'pseudo'-normalize. Progressive ventricular disease is associated with decreased compliance and elevated filling pressures, creating high-velocity abbreviated E waves followed by tiny A waves (see Figure 25.8c). Cardiologists frequently use these Doppler methods to identify the various stages of ventricular diastolic dysfunction and to predict impending CHF.

Specific feline cardiomyopathies

Examples of pathological features of feline cardiomyopathies are illustrated in Figure 25.9.

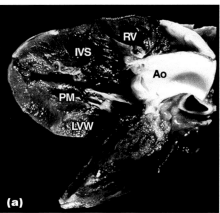

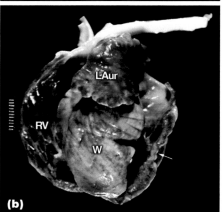

25.9 Pathological features of feline cardiomyopathies. **(a)** Opened LV from a cat with concentric hypertrophy due to HCM. The interventricular septum (IVS), papillary muscles (PM) and ventricular wall (LVW) are all thickened. There is some increase in fibrous tissue along the inner edge of the septum. Ao = Ascending aorta. **(b)** RCM in a cat. The LV wall (W) is discoloured owing to diffuse infiltration with fibrous connective tissue. A segmental infarct is evident in the cut free wall (arrowed). The left auricular appendage (LAur) is moderately dilated. The RV is relatively spared. (continues) ▶

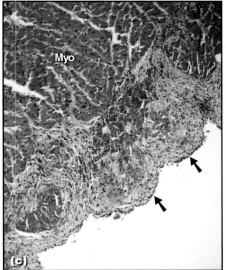

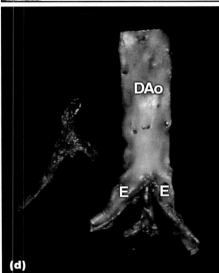

| 25.9 | (continued) Pathological features of feline cardiomyopathies. **(c)** Histological section from a cat with endomyocarditis. Myocardium (Myo) is evident in this low-power photomicrograph. The zones beneath the endocardium (arrowed) are characterized by myocardial fibrosis and infiltration with inflammatory cells. Trichrome stain. **(d)** Segment of descending aorta (DAo) cut near the origin of the internal and external (E) iliac arteries. |

Hypertrophic cardiomyopathy

Feline HCM is characterized by thickening of the LV walls and papillary muscles (see Figure 25.9a) unexplained by congenital disease, hypertension or endocrinopathy. Considering the prominence of HCM in the feline population and prevalence in certain breeds, it is not surprising that genetic mutations have been identified in some affected cats (including mutations of myosin-binding protein C in Maine Coons and Ragdolls). Some limited genetic testing is available currently, but this is mainly of value to breeders. Male cats are predisposed to HCM in some studies; however, there is no reported evidence of a sex-linked mode of inheritance. Specific breeds at risk for HCM include the Maine Coon, Persian, Ragdoll, Bengal, American and British Shorthairs and Norwegian Forest cat.

Lesions and clinical pathophysiology

Pattern of ventricular hypertrophy: The variable pattern of ventricular hypertrophy in this disease, ranging from concentric to focal (segmental) thickening, can be demonstrated at necropsy or by 2D echocardiography (Fox *et al.*, 1995). The pattern can influence prognosis. For example, asymmetrical free-wall hypertrophy is often associated with significant LV dysfunction and progressive LA dilatation. Focal subaortic, focal mid-septal or isolated papillary muscle hypertrophy are often well tolerated; but these lesions will progress in some cats and thus warrant follow up. A specific variant of HCM in older cats is a subaortic septal thickening sometimes associated with a dilated aorta. Whether this is a genetic HCM, or a degenerative aortic dilatation (aortoannular ectasia) in which altered flow stimulates focal hypertrophy is undetermined. In most cases, this form is benign.

Histology: The key histological findings of HCM are hypertrophy of cardiomyocytes with fibre disarray and interstitial fibrosis. Intramural coronary arteries are narrowed, with foci of myocardial infarctions or replacement fibrosis. Some cats with HCM progress to a form of RCM or a type of DCM termed 'burned-out' or 'end-stage' HCM. In each of these conditions, extensive myocardial fibrosis is evident histologically.

Systolic ventricular function: Systolic ventricular function in most cats with HCM is normal to hyperdynamic, but there can be regional or focal reductions that may require advanced echo studies to identify. When HCM evolves to a 'burned-out' form, the entire ventricle may be dilated and hypokinetic. An RCM type phenotype with severe biatrial dilatation can also evolve as a late phase of HCM. Should atrial fibrillation develop, ventricular function is further impaired and this can precipitate severe CHF or ATE.

Pressure gradients: Dynamic and labile pressure gradients between the LV and aorta are found frequently. These gradients stem from the combinations of septal and papillary muscle hypertrophy and systolic anterior motion (SAM) of the mitral valve. The latter is likely related to abnormalities of the papillary muscles or the valve itself. The major differential diagnosis is a primary mitral valve malformation. Intraventricular or midcavitary obstructions often develop between the ventricular septum and papillary muscles and can be identified by Doppler studies.

Diastolic LV dysfunction: The presumptive cause of CHF in feline HCM is diastolic LV dysfunction, which means that elevated LA and venous pressures are required to fill the ventricle. These abnormalities (discussed above) can be documented by advanced Doppler studies and generally evolve gradually, often over years. However, sudden sympathetic stress or abrupt impairment of myocardial perfusion can lead to rapidly developing or 'flash' pulmonary oedema in cats with HCM, with a need for urgent treatment. In some cases, diastolic function seems to improve with elimination of the stress, allowing a reduction in therapy over time.

Clinical findings

Most cats with HCM are asymptomatic and are recognized when a heart murmur or gallop sound is discovered during a routine examination. Some asymptomatic cats have no abnormalities on auscultation. As described previously, there are no unique clinical findings of HCM, and cats can present with any combination of signs listed in Figure 25.2.

Electrocardiography, clinical laboratory and ancillary studies do not sufficiently distinguish HCM from other forms of cardiomyopathy. Thus, a careful clinical work up, including high-quality cardiac ultrasonography, is required for definitive diagnosis. Confirmation of LV hypertrophy, including papillary muscle thickening, is necessary for diagnosis. The presence of significant SAM is invariably associated with an eccentric jet of mitral regurgitation, and may represent an indication for beta adrenergic blockade.

Mild diastolic dysfunction is heralded by an atrial (S4) gallop. Progressive disease leads to decreased LV compliance, high venous pressures, a loud ventricular (S3) or summation gallop and CHF. Progressive atrial dilatation and dysfunction go hand in hand with progressive loss of ventricular function. Thus, atrial size as observed by echocardiography or thoracic radiography remains one of the best indicators of disease severity and short-term prognosis.

The natural history of feline HCM can be benign or lethal, brief or protracted, and some cats remain asymptomatic for many years before succumbing (if ever) to the disease. As in human patients with HCM, *the vast majority of affected cats do not develop overt clinical signs*. Even severely affected cats may be asymptomatic when diagnosed. However, cats with diffuse or regionally severe disease are at high risk for complications, and some cats with mild disease will experience bouts of thromboembolism. When clinical signs do develop, these are explained by left-sided CHF, complications of ATE, outflow tract obstruction, or arrhythmias. The latter can cause syncope or sudden cardiac death.

Management

Management of the cat with clinical signs of CHF, ATE, or arrhythmia related to HCM is discussed toward the end of the chapter (see Figure 25.10).

Treatment of *asymptomatic* HCM is controversial. No data indicate a pivotal benefit of beta-blockers, diltiazem, ACE inhibitors, spironolactone, aspirin or clopidogrel in asymptomatic cats with mild HCM and normal LA size. Neither ACE inhibition (with ramipril) nor inhibition of aldosterone (with spironolactone) altered hypertrophy or estimated volume of fibrosis in controlled studies (MacDonald *et al.*, 2006, 2008). Clients should be advised of this information prior to prescriptions being written for long-term treatment.

LVOT obstruction: While dynamic LVOT obstruction is a risk factor for sudden death in people with HCM, it is unknown whether this is the situation in cats. However, the author does recommend empirical therapy with atenolol for cats with moderate to severe

HCM accompanied by LVOT obstruction. Atenolol appears superior to diltiazem for slowing heart rate, reducing dynamic outflow obstruction and decreasing intensity of murmurs. Beta-blockade also diminishes demand ischaemia, prolongs ventricular and coronary filling times, and carries a lower side-effect profile (when compared with diltiazem). Dosing is adjusted based on heart rate, and many cats take 'split doses'; for example: 12.5 mg in the morning and 6.25 mg in the afternoon. The ultimate daily dosage (6.25–12.5 mg orally q12h) is determined by the examination room heart rate obtained during stable chronic therapy, with a target of 120–160 beats/minute. Beta-blockers are contraindicated in hypotension, bradycardia, thromboembolism and CHF. Beta-blockers can also depress LA contractile function, which may be a problem in cases of severe LA disease or dysfunction.

LA dilatation: When HCM is characterized by significant LV hypertrophy and moderate LA dilatation (diameter ≥20 mm on 2D imaging), the author suggests an ACE inhibitor. In the setting of LV outflow obstruction, atenolol is added; otherwise the calcium-channel blocker diltiazem may be considered. Unfortunately, there is a higher adverse effect profile for diltiazem (including anorexia, weight loss and skin lesions) than for atenolol. Dosing is also problematic for lack of a simple clinical target (since heart rate response is inconsistent). For this reason, the author uses this drug infrequently, while accepting that other cardiologists prescribe it regularly. There are simply no major end-point studies (of survival, CHF, or ATE) on which to base an objective treatment decision. Combining atenolol and diltiazem can cause bradycardia and hypotension and is not recommended. Antiplatelet therapy (see later) is also recommended in this group.

Restrictive cardiomyopathy

Feline RCM represents a heterogenous disorder, and some latitude is used in the classification of cats within this group as opposed to the 'unclassified' category discussed below. The key pathological feature of RCM is myocardial fibrosis (see Figure 25.9b) of uncertain pathogenesis. Antecedent myocarditis may be a cause, but in some cats RCM clearly represents a late stage of HCM. Burmese cats may have a predisposition to RCM.

- Post-mortem lesions in cats with clinical features of RCM are dominated by fibrosis that may be patchy, multifocal, or diffuse.
- The LV cavity is generally normal to reduced in size, with variable but generally unimpressive hypertrophy, sometimes interspersed with regions of thinning or overt infarction. The latter changes are most evident in the LV free wall or apex.
- Prominent endocardial or papillary muscle fibrosis may be evident, with extreme endocardial fibrotic scarring in some cases.
- Large moderator bands may be observed (and are classified by some as a congenital malformation or a separate form of cardiomyopathy – the

endomyocardial form of RCM, with a probable predisposition in Siamese cats).

- A consistent feature of RCM is striking LA or biatrial dilatation.
- Histological lesions include endocardial thickening, endomyocardial fibrosis, myocardial interstitial fibrosis, myocyte hypertrophy, focal myocytolysis and necrosis, and arteriosclerosis.
- Systemic thromboemboli are common, and LA and ventricular mural thrombi may be observed.

Clinical pathophysiology and findings

The clinical pathophysiology of RCM is compatible with a combined diastolic and systolic dysfunction syndrome. Increases of venous and atrial pressures, combined with ventricular dysfunction, atrial stiffness and renal sodium retention, lead to CHF.

Most cats with RCM are presented with overt clinical signs caused by CHF or ATE. Murmurs may not be evident, but loud gallop sounds are the rule, often punctuated by heart rhythm disturbances. The ECG is typically abnormal, with wide P waves, ventricular conduction disturbances and ectopic complexes common. Echocardiography and Doppler studies generally demonstrate the following:

- Mild systolic dysfunction
- Regional LV wall dysfunction
- Mild mitral or tricuspid valvular insufficiency
- Elevated LA pressures
- Impaired LV distensibility with a 'restrictive' filling pattern.

Pulmonary oedema, pleural effusion, jugular venous distension and hepatic congestion are commonly identified through physical examination and diagnostic imaging. The ECG is often abnormal, and atrial and ventricular rhythm disturbances may be observed. Stasis of blood in a dilated LA places affected cats at high risk for atrial thrombi and ATE.

Management

Management of RCM is based on control of CHF and prevention or treatment of ATE (see later). In cats with atrial fibrillation, diltiazem may provide the best control of ventricular heart rate. In the odd case that is diagnosed prior to onset of CHF, empirical use of an ACE inhibitor and an antiplatelet drug seems warranted.

Dilated cardiomyopathy

DCM is now uncommon. Taurine deficiency can cause DCM in cats (Pion et al., 1987) and this is still observed in cats eating off-brand or some 'natural' diets, but most cases are idiopathic or related to diffuse myocarditis. The main post-mortem lesions of DCM are left-sided or four-chamber dilatation, generally with necropsy findings of CHF and with no demonstrable congenital, coronary or valvular heart disease. Histological findings include myocyte loss, prominent interstitial fibrosis, and variable degrees of hypertrophy and myocytolysis or apoptosis. Some cases are characterized by diffuse myocarditis.

The clinical features of DCM in cats can be indistinguishable from those of other cardiomyopathies.

Heart sounds may be soft, owing to impaired contractility or pleural effusion. The principal functional disturbance, as shown by echocardiography, is marked reduction of LV ejection and shortening fractions, often with mitral and tricuspid regurgitation caused by ventricular dilatation and dysfunction. While some cats are detected in the asymptomatic phase, cardiogenic shock, left-sided CHF or biventricular CHF are the most common presentations. These may be complicated by ATE.

Prognosis is poor unless the condition is related to taurine deficiency. Oral taurine supplementation should be administered while awaiting results of a blood taurine test or at a minimum for 2–3 months following diagnosis. Management of DCM is discussed later in the chapter.

Right ventricular cardiomyopathy

This condition, sometimes referred to as arrhythmogenic right ventricular cardiomyopathy, has been observed in cats, and necropsy features have been described (Fox et al., 2000). The RV is replaced by fat and fibrous tissue, with the consequences of right-sided myocardial failure and right-sided dilatation with tricuspid regurgitation. Atrial standstill or atrial fibrillation may be apparent on the ECG. Ventricular ectopic rhythms are also common.

Affected cats are generally presented with pleural effusion, sometimes with concurrent ascites, associated with right-sided CHF. Sudden death can occur. Early cases may demonstrate only atrial or ventricular arrhythmias. Diagnosis hinges on echocardiography and exclusion of other predominantly right-sided diseases such as ASD and cor pulmonale.

Treatment involves control of CHF and possibly antiarrhythmic therapy (see below).

Other acquired myocardial diseases

Unclassified cardiomyopathy

The term unclassified cardiomyopathy describes a myocardial disease of unknown aetiology that does not readily fit into one of the above categorizations. Findings of RCM and UCM are often very similar and what one cardiologist might call RCM is classified as UCM by another. Myocardial infarctions and primary atrial diseases may also lead to a diagnosis of UCM. Assessment and management of the patient with UCM can be 'simplified' by describing completely the clinical, imaging, ECG and biochemical findings evident in the patient and then directing treatments towards managing these abnormalities. Practically, most cases of UCM present with CHF or ATE and are treated for these problems, as discussed below.

Non-suppurative myocarditis

Non-suppurative myocarditis occurs sporadically in cats. The cause is unknown and definitive diagnosis requires microscopic examination of the tissues. There is a tendency for cats with myocarditis to be young. Some are presented for ventricular arrhythmias, while others develop fulminant heart failure, ATE or RCM. Death during anaesthesia is another common scenario.

The clinical diagnosis is based on suspicion and exclusion of other diseases. Blood cTnI is generally elevated, but this is not a specific finding for myocarditis, and there is no 'gold standard' short of myocardial histology to confirm the diagnosis. Myocarditis can also be associated with infectious diseases including toxoplasmosis, so this should be a consideration before anti-inflammatory therapies are considered. No therapies have been shown to be effective in treating myocarditis, and patient management is generally supportive, related to identifiable clinical problems.

Hyperthyroid heart disease

Thyrotoxicosis causes cardiac hypertrophy related to a hypermetabolic state, peripheral vasodilatation and increased demands for cardiac output. Increased sympathetic nervous system activity and elevated thyroid hormone levels may stimulate myocardial hypertrophy. In chronic cases of hyperthyroidism, the LV usually becomes thickened, and concurrent systemic hypertension probably contributes to this in some cases. Echocardiography typically shows LV hypertrophy, often indistinguishable from that in idiopathic HCM. In advanced cases associated with fluid retention, there may be biatrial dilatation with normal or even reduced LV ejection fraction. These cats are at risk for CHF, which is often precipitated by administration of intravenous fluids.

Management: Hyperthyroid heart disease management is centred on controlling the endocrine disorder. In cats with compensated heart disease (as judged by radiography or echocardiography), no specific cardiac treatment is required. For severe sinus tachycardia (>280 beats/minute) or for ectopic atrial or ventricular rhythms, atenolol (6.25 mg orally q12h) can be administered, but this may not be needed if antithyroid medications are given. In cats that cannot receive radioactive iodine treatment and cannot tolerate antithyroid medications (due to hepatic or renal complications), long-term therapy with atenolol is recommended to mitigate the sympathomimetic effects of hyperthyroidism on the cardiovascular system. When volume overload or CHF have developed, beta-blockers should be avoided and management with antithyroid medication, low-dose furosemide (1–2 mg/kg orally q12–24h) and an ACE inhibitor, with or without additional antihypertensive therapy (amlodipine), is suggested.

BP control is important in hypertensive hyperthyroid cases. Hypertension in these cats can be multifactorial: from high cardiac output, aortic stiffness in cats related to aortoannular ectasia, or concurrent renal disease. Atenolol monotherapy is generally insufficient to control hypertension in cats with hyperthyroidism. Furthermore, it should not be assumed that hypertension will resolve following successful treatment of the endocrine disorder with drugs such as methimazole. In some cases BP may even increase following successful therapy (see Chapter 27). When moderate to severe hypertension is evident, treatment with amlodipine (0.625–1.25 mg orally q12–24h) is suggested. Atenolol is a reasonable adjunctive therapy in these cats if more control is needed. An ACE inhibitor may also represent appropriate co-therapy if there is concurrent renal disease. Ventricular changes may improve with effective long-term control of the hyperthyroid state.

Hypertensive heart disease

The heart, along with the brain, eyes, kidneys and small arterioles, are the target organs for elevated systemic arterial BP. Most healthy cats have systolic BP measurements of <150–160 mmHg in the hospital setting, unless they are stressed. Persistent elevation of BP, particularly values >160–170 mmHg in the presence of target organ injury (see Chapter 27), is highly suggestive of hypertensive disease. While systemic hypertension does stimulate LV hypertrophy, neither CHF nor ATE is a common complication. More often, clinical signs of hypertension are referable to the eyes (retinal haemorrhages, detachments), brain (depression, stroke), or kidneys (progressive uraemia). Dissection of the aorta is a rare complication.

The cardiac condition most often resembles mild HCM, with a gallop or murmur detected during examination. Mild cardiac enlargement is often evident by radiography, and LV wall hypertrophy may be demonstrated by echocardiography.

Management is based on treatment of underlying disorders and amlodipine, and is discussed in Chapter 27.

Treating complications of feline cardiomyopathies

Most treatments for feline myocardial diseases have evolved empirically. There are no published trial data regarding optimal management of cats with asymptomatic HCM, CHF, ATE or arrhythmias. The author's empirical choices and recommendations are described below and summarized in Figure 25.10.

Disease stage	Standard treatment	Optional use
Heart disease, no CHF	No treatment	ACE inhibitor if moderate to severe LA enlargement Atenolol if dynamic LVOT obstruction
Mild to moderate CHF	Furosemide (minimum dose to maintain free of CHF) ACE inhibitor	Pimobendan (Not in HCM) Diltiazem if atrial fibrillation Oral taurine initially prior to obtaining serum taurine in DCM

25.10 Treatment of feline cardiomyopathy and CHF (see text for details and dosage information). (continues) ▶

Disease stage	Standard treatment	Optional use
Severe and/or life-threatening CHF	Gentle handling Intravenous furosemide Oxygen Glyceryl trinitrate	Sedation (e.g. butorphanol) if distressed Thoracocentesis if pleural effusion Intravenous dobutamine or pimobendan if hypotensive, hypothermic, bradycardic. If already receiving atenolol or diltiazem, decrease dose by 50%
Refractory CHF	Furosemide (increase dose until no further effect or 5 mg/kg q12h) ACE inhibitor Spironolactone (watch for facial lesions)	Pimobendan if no dynamic outflow tract obstruction Subcutaneous furosemide 1–3 times a week Famotidine if inappetent Rutin if chylothorax

25.10 (continued) Treatment of feline cardiomyopathy and CHF (see text for details and dosage information).

Acute CHF

Management of the cat with acute or severe CHF begins with gentle handling. Thoracocentesis is the treatment of choice for moderate to large pleural effusions. This is most safely done using a small butterfly catheter or needle, with the cat in sternal recumbency and receiving supplemental oxygen by facemask, after sedation. For bilateral pleural effusions it is safest to tap on the right side to avoid puncturing a bulging LA.

Pulmonary oedema

Cats with pulmonary oedema from CHF are managed using the 'FONS' regimen:

- Furosemide is administered (2–4 mg/kg i.v. or i.m.; repeated in 2–4 hours if necessary). Once diuresis occurs and clinical signs improve, the dose is reduced to 1–2 mg/kg i.v., i.m. or s.c., q8–12h. For life-threatening, poorly responsive pulmonary oedema, initial boluses can be followed by a constant intravenous infusion of furosemide of 4–6 mg/kg given over 24 hours
- Oxygen (40–50%) is delivered by cage oxygenator in most cases
- Glyceryl trinitrate (2%) ointment is administered for venodilation (¼ inch (6 mm) cutaneously, q12h) for 24 hours, with the hope of reducing ventricular preload
- Sedation is considered (butorphanol 0.25 mg/kg i.m.; this can be mixed with acepromazine 0.01–0.05 mg/kg, providing rectal temperature is >37.8°C and BP >100 mmHg).

Cardiogenic shock

The cat with cardiogenic shock (hypothermia, often with bradycardia, systolic BP <70 mmHg) is treated with passive warming and intravenous dobutamine infusion for 24–48 hours (regardless of type of cardiomyopathy). Dosing is initiated at 2.5 µg/kg/min and increased to a range of 5–10 µg/kg/min. The final infusion rate targets a rectal temperature of >37.8°C, heart rate >180 beats/minute and systolic BP >90 mmHg. The dose is reduced by 50% every 2–3 hours before discontinuing the drug.

Pimobendan can be considered as an alternative in this setting, and is dosed at 0.625–1.25 mg/cat orally q12h. Furosemide or thoracocentesis are used to treat CHF as appropriate. An ACE inhibitor is started once BP exceeds 90 mmHg.

Cardiogenic shock carries a very guarded prognosis, but survival exceeding 1 year occurs in some cats following this aggressive treatment plan along with diligent homecare. Other cats succumb from unresponsive CHF.

Chronic CHF

The home therapy of chronic CHF provided by cat owners centres on administration of furosemide (usual dosage 1–2 mg/kg orally q12–24h), combined with an ACE inhibitor such as enalapril or benazepril (usual dosage 0.25–0.5 mg/kg orally q12–24h). Occasionally furosemide is given subcutaneously on a regular schedule (1 mg/kg s.c. once to three times weekly in place of an oral dose) for poorly responsive pulmonary oedema or pleural effusion. Spironolactone (6.25–12.5 mg q24h) can be given for possible cardioprotective and potassium-sparing effects (*beware*: anorexia, skin lesions). Neither atenolol nor diltiazem should be administered to cats with recent-onset CHF; such therapy was not beneficial in an unpublished multicentre study reported by P. Fox.

When CHF develops in a cat with HCM receiving chronic atenolol or diltiazem therapy, the daily dosage is reduced by ~50%, but is not stopped unless the cat exhibits cardiogenic shock. In cats with well defined dynamic LVOT obstruction, cautious up-titration of atenolol may be initiated to reduce the gradient *once the cat is completely stable*.

Additional treatments may improve CHF in some cats:

- Pimobendan provides an additional treatment approach for cats with chronic CHF. In the author's opinion, pimobendan should be prescribed immediately for cats with CHF due to DCM, RCM, UCM, or RV cardiomyopathy. In contrast, pimobendan is *not* recommended for the cat with well defined HCM until CHF becomes progressive or unresponsive to furosemide and an ACE inhibitor
- Digoxin is rarely used in cats today
- Rutin (250 mg orally q12h) is prescribed when there is chylothorax associated with CHF
- Famotidine (2.5–5 mg orally q12–24h for 1–2 weeks) represents an empirical treatment for cats with partial anorexia associated with CHF; this drug also can be prescribed long term.

The overall efficacy of heart failure therapy and quality of life can be gauged from owner reports.

Objective measures of CHF control and adverse drug effects can be obtained through physical examination, measurement of blood pressure, evaluation of serum biochemistries, inspection of thoracic radiographs and, perhaps, echocardiography. Furosemide is titrated to effect. In some cats with HCM haemodynamic function stabilizes, allowing diuretic therapy to be withdrawn. In other cases, there is a clear need to tolerate uraemia to prevent discomforting pleural effusion or pulmonary oedema. Lifelong therapy is anticipated for most cats with CHF.

Prevention of thromboembolism

A number of approaches have been advocated for prevention of ATE in cats. These include:

- Aspirin monotherapy (doses range from 5 to 81 mg/cat orally q72h)
- Warfarin (0.5 mg/cat orally q24h)
- Low-molecular-weight heparins, including enoxaparin (1 mg/kg s.c. q12–24h) and dalteparin (100 IU/kg s.c. q12–24h)
- Clopidogrel (75 mg tablets, ¼ tablet – or 18.75 mg/cat – orally q24h).

Aside from an ongoing clinical trial evaluating clopidogrel *versus* aspirin, and a number of retrospective reports indicating apparently safe dosages of these drugs and effects on *in vitro* coagulation tests, there are no prospective trial data demonstrating efficacy for any prevention of ATE in cats with cardiomyopathy.

In terms of specific recommendations, the author does not routinely prescribe antithrombotic therapy in asymptomatic cats with a normal or minimally dilated LA and auricular emptying velocities >20 cm/s. Clopidogrel (¼ of a 75 mg tablet) is prescribed for the cat with a moderate (≥20 mm) to severely dilated LA, or when auricular emptying velocities are <20 cm/s. Adult-regimen 75 mg aspirin dosed at one tablet orally q72h is an alternative to clopidogrel, but is often ineffective.

In cats at high risk for ATE (LA dilatation ≥25 mm, echogenic smoke in LA, auricular emptying velocities <10 cm/s, or a history of prior ATE) more

aggressive therapy is recommended. The author typically prescribes clopidogrel (¼ of a 75 mg tablet q24h) along with low-dose daily aspirin (compounded or 'crumbled' to a dose of 5–10 mg). The risk of gastric ulceration must be appreciated with these treatments and managed if anorexia, vomiting, or anaemia becomes evident.

An alternative for cats at high risk of ATE is once- or twice-daily administration of a low-molecular-weight heparin preparation. There is some controversy about the efficacy of this treatment and the best manner of monitoring therapy of these heparins in cats. Clinical trials in cats with spontaneous disease are needed to settle the issues. Practically, since the drugs are prohibitively expensive for most clients and require one or two daily injections, the treatment holds a low acceptability to clients. Some clinicians use low-molecular-weight heparin as a bridge therapy for a few weeks following recovery of aortic ATE.

Warfarin therapy is difficult to control in cats and rarely prescribed.

Management of arterial thromboembolism

The medical management of an acute thromboembolic event (Figure 25.11) demands high-quality critical and nursing care.

The client should be advised about:

- Need for intensive therapy (typically 2–3 days in the hospital)
- Risk of ATE recurrence (high)
- Need for future daily home medical care
- Likely presence of underlying cardiomyopathy
- Attendant costs of managing the condition
- Potential for sudden death during hospitalization (or thereafter).

Experience and published retrospective reports suggest a 40–50% chance for functional limb recovery if treatment is administered. In a retrospective study (Smith *et al.*, 2003) the median survival time was 223 days for cats not presenting in CHF (median survival for those with CHF was 77 days). It is emphasized that there are no *prospective* trials of

Disease stage	Standard treatment	Optional use
Normal or minimal LA enlargement	No treatment	
Moderate LA enlargement (normal atrial systolic function; no spontaneous echo-contrast)	Clopidogrel or aspirin	
ATE: initial management	Analgesia with mu agonist (e.g. intravenous fentanyl) Passive warming Heparin	Morphine, buprenorphine if intravenous fentanyl not available Cautious fluid therapy if **hypotensive and no CHF** Dobutamine if **hypotensive with CHF**
ATE: care after discharge	Protect limbs: scrupulous hygiene; soft bedding Physiotherapy	Stool softeners if constipated
Previous ATE or high risk of ATE (spontaneous echo-contrast; poor LA systolic function)	Clopidogrel plus aspirin	Low-molecular-weight heparins

25.11 Management of ATE (see text for dosage information).

therapy. Retrospective data probably represent less than optimal outcomes, since care is not standardized in these observational studies and many cats are euthanased at admission.

Analgesia

If the client decides to proceed, the first treatment is analgesia with a mu agonist for the first 24–48 hours following an event. While there are no comparative studies of pain control in this condition, fentanyl is most commonly used in the author's practice and provides good to excellent analgesia. Transdermal therapy is too slow in onset for management of this severe pain and intravenous administration is needed.

- The author initiates fentanyl therapy with a low dose of 3 µg/kg (very slow intravenous bolus) followed by an intravenous maintenance infusion of 1–5 µg/kg per *hour* (not per minute).
- Morphine (0.1–0.2 mg/kg i.m. or s.c. q6h) or buprenorphine (0.005–0.01 mg/kg i.m. or s.c. q6h) represent other options.
- Buprenorphine can also provide some analgesia when administered at 0.01–0.02 mg/kg (10–20 µg/kg) on the buccal (oral) mucosa, and it may be useful to dispense one or two doses to the client for immediate administration should an ATE occur at home.
- In the absence of hypothermia or hypotension, acepromazine (0.025 mg/kg s.c.) will sedate the cat further.
- Pain in most cats is markedly diminished by 48 hours, allowing for less aggressive analgesia.

Thrombolytic therapy and surgery

Neither thrombolytic therapy nor a surgical approach to thrombus removal is recommended, as the risks of reperfusion injury outweigh any possible benefit. Heparin is administered in the case of acute ATE to prevent further thrombosis (300 units/kg i.v., then 150–250 IU/kg s.c. q8h for 48–72 hours).

Hypo/hyperthermia and hypotension

- Passive warming is undertaken. Some cats are profoundly hypothermic, and these cats have a poorer prognosis. This finding may indicate shock accompanied by severe metabolic acidosis.
- Hypotension in the absence of CHF should be treated with cautious fluid therapy initially. When associated with CHF, dobutamine at low infusion rates (2.5 µg/kg/min) is preferred.
- Cats on opiates may pant in a heated environment, creating a situation that can be confused with CHF. This sign will abate once the external environmental temperature and humidity are lowered.
- If true fever occurs following an ATE, intravenous cefazolin or oral amoxicillin/clavulanic acid are usually effective.

Hyperkalaemia

The patient should be monitored for potentially fatal hyperkalaemia from potassium leaked from necrotic muscles during the first 48–72 hours of treatment.

Most cats that do improve are better within 72 hours of admission and can be released for homecare.

Limb function

There is often asymmetry noted between the limbs. With revascularization, tail function returns and limb function is reinstated from proximal to distal. Reassessment every 2–3 days is recommended following release until the status of ischaemic tissues is determined.

Homecare

Homecare includes:

- Protecting the limbs
- Daily inspection for subcutaneous or muscle oedema (a poor prognostic sign)
- Cleaning urine-soaked hair and bedding
- Providing a soft bed
- Encouragement to eat
- A low-stress area for convalescence.

Physiotherapy in the form of passive flexion of the limbs is encouraged. Additional consideration should be given to soft dressings to encourage a functional limb position. If constipation becomes a problem, stool softeners can be used.

Cardiac arrhythmias

Heart rhythm disturbances can complicate cardiomyopathies in some cats.

- Isolated atrial or ventricular premature complexes are not treated.
- Ventricular tachycardia is managed in hospital with lidocaine (0.5–1 mg/kg i.v.); esmolol (50–500 µg/kg i.v. over 5 minutes, followed by 50–100 µg/kg/min); atenolol (6.25–12.5 mg orally q12h); or sotalol (1–2 mg/kg orally q12h).
- Sustained, regular supraventricular tachycardia also may respond to beta-blockade, or to intravenous diltiazem (0.1 mg/kg i.v., repeated to a cumulative dosage of 0.5 mg/kg with BP monitoring).
- The negative inotropic effects of beta-blockers and of diltiazem may limit usage, especially in cats with LV dysfunction or CHF.

Diltiazem is an effective blocker of AV nodal conduction and represents an excellent choice for heart rate control in cats with atrial fibrillation or sustained SVT. Atrial fibrillation is most often – though not always – associated with severe LA or RA dilatation in cats. Atenolol represents an alternative therapy for heart rate control. Digoxin is rarely used by the author in cats.

Circulatory volume overload

Fluid therapy in cats with common medical conditions can lead to cardiovascular complications that can mimic or precipitate CHF. Conditions likely to lead to volume retention include moderate to severe anaemia (PCV <20%), thyrotoxicosis, some forms of chronic renal disease and possibly glucocorticoid administration. Often these cats receive appropriate crystalloid therapy for their medical disease at one to two times 'maintenance' requirements but develop respiratory problems related to volume overload of the circulation. Most of these cats have evidence of cardiac dysfunction on examination.

Clinical examination and diagnostic imaging are useful for diagnosis. Most cats develop tachypnoea, jugular venous engorgement and radiographic evidence of pleural effusion or pulmonary infiltration. Echocardiography typically shows dilated atria (moderate), a prominent RV, and variable changes in the LV related to underlying disease (such as HCM, hypertensive heart disease, or thyrotoxic heart disease). Prompt recognition, diuresis, reduction of fluid administration and treatment of the underlying disorder will generally resolve the situation.

References and further reading

Benigni L, Morgan N and Lamb C (2009) Radiographic appearance of cardiogenic pulmonary oedema in 23 cats. *Journal of Small Animal Practice* **50**, 9–14

Connolly DJ, Soares Magalhaes RJ, Luis Fuentes V *et al.* (2009) Assessment of the diagnostic accuracy of circulating natriuretic peptide concentrations to distinguish between cats with cardiac and non-cardiac causes of respiratory distress. *Journal of Veterinary Cardiology* **11**, S41–S50

Connolly DJ, Soares Magalhaes RJ, Syme HM *et al.* (2008) Circulating natriuretic peptides in cats with heart disease. *Journal of Veterinary Internal Medicine* **22**, 96–105

Fox P, Liu S and Maron B (1995) Echocardiographic assessment of spontaneously occurring feline hypertrophic cardiomyopathy. An animal model of human disease. *Circulation* **92**, 2645–2651

Fox P, Maron B, Basso C *et al.* (2000) Spontaneously occurring arrhythmogenic right ventricular cardiomyopathy in the domestic cat: a new animal model similar to the human disease. *Circulation* **102**, 1863–1870

Fox PR, Oyama MA, Reynolds JE *et al.* (2009) Utility of plasma *N*-terminal pro-brain natriuretic peptide (NT-proBNP) to distinguish between congestive heart failure and non-cardiac causes of acute dyspnea in cats. *Journal of Veterinary Cardiology* **11**, S51–S61

MacDonald KA, Kittleson MD, Kass PH and White SD (2008) Effect of spironolactone on diastolic function and left ventricular mass in Maine Coon cats with familial hypertrophic cardiomyopathy. *Journal of Veterinary Internal Medicine* **22**, 335–341

MacDonald K, Kittleson M, Larson R *et al.* (2006) The effect of ramipril on left ventricular mass, myocardial fibrosis, diastolic function, and plasma neurohormones in Maine Coon cats with familial hypertrophic cardiomyopathy without heart failure. *Journal of Veterinary Internal Medicine* **20**, 1093–1105

Peterson M, Taylor R, Greco D *et al.* (1990) Acromegaly in 14 cats. *Journal of Veterinary Internal Medicine* **4**, 192–201

Pion P, Kittleson M, Rogers Q and Morris J (1987) Myocardial failure in cats associated with low plasma taurine: a reversible cardiomyopathy. *Science* **237**, 764–768

Smith S, Tobias A, Jacob K *et al.* (2003) Arterial thromboembolism in cats: acute crisis in 127 cases (1992–2001) and long-term management with low-dose aspirin in 24 cases. *Journal of Veterinary Internal Medicine* **17**, 73–83

26

Congenital heart disease

Mike Martin and Joanna Dukes-McEwan

Introduction

The vast majority of animals with congenital heart disease present with an audible murmur; thus, auscultation is the initial key diagnostic test (see Chapter 4). Nearly all congenital defects have a systolic murmur – except most notably a patent ductus arteriosus (PDA), which has a characteristic continuous murmur (Figure 26.1). However, some rare defects may have no murmur, such as a reversed/balanced shunt. Recent reviews of congenital heart disease are available (Oyama *et al.*, 2005; MacDonald, 2006).

In very young puppies and kittens, flow murmurs are common. They are difficult to differentiate from a congenital defect on auscultation alone and thus create a diagnostic dilemma for the clinician when a murmur is discovered, and cause problems on how best to advise the owner.

In addition to auscultation, it is important to determine whether there are any signs of congestive heart failure (CHF), thus requiring more immediate attention. Mucosal colour (both cranial and caudal) should be checked for cyanosis at rest and, if indicated, following exertion. Pulse quality should also be assessed: if it is weak or hyperkinetic, this can guide the differential diagnosis.

Finally, it is important to be aware of breed predispositions for various congenital defects.

Murmurs in puppies and kittens

Auscultation of very young puppies may be requested by a breeder prior to selling, or by the new owner at first vaccination. The former poses greater problems. In animals under 6–7 weeks of age the heart rates are fairly rapid, there are often extraneous respiratory (or sniffing) noises, and keeping the puppy or kitten still for long enough is difficult. A reliable and accurate assessment of the heart is close to impossible and even an experienced person may miss a murmur in this situation.

Puppies and kittens presented at first vaccination may have *innocent flow murmurs*, which tend to be of low grade and usually disappear by 14–16 weeks of age (though flow murmurs may persist in some adults). These murmurs are brief, systolic and tend to vary in intensity with heart rate, becoming louder with faster rates. This variation can be useful in identification, but these murmurs cannot be distinguished from those of congenital defects on auscultation alone. The diagnosis is therefore often made retrospectively, i.e. after the murmur disappears in a few weeks or months.

Procedures on discovery of a systolic murmur

In the animal with no clinical signs and a low-grade systolic murmur, it is often reasonable and pragmatic to reassess at the second vaccination rather than to pursue further diagnostics immediately, although the owners should be given the choice. It is uncommon for owners to return a puppy or kitten with a murmur, as they have usually bonded in a short time. Further investigations should always be offered, particularly if the murmur is continuous (see PDA, below), associated with a palpable thrill, or if the animal is stunted or showing clinical signs.

Condition	Murmur characteristics		
	Timing	Point of maximum intensity (PMI)	Radiation
Patent ductus arteriosus (PDA)	Continuous	Dorsal left base	Dorsally and cranially
Aortic stenosis (AS)	Systolic	Left base	To right and carotids
Pulmonic stenosis (PS)	Systolic	Left base	Dorsally and cranially
Ventricular septal defect (VSD)	Systolic	Right cranial parasternal	To left base
Mitral dysplasia	Systolic	Left apex	Apex and to right
Tricuspid dysplasia	Systolic	Right apex	To left side
Tetralogy of Fallot	Systolic	Left base	Dorsally and apex

26.1 Murmurs in congenital heart disease (see also Chapter 4).

Electrocardiography
Electrocardiography provides little useful information in the young animal with a murmur and no arrhythmia. If there is right heart enlargement, this may be evident on an electrocardiogram (ECG), but this is insufficient alone to provide a diagnosis. If an arrhythmia is present, an ECG is indicated as part of the diagnostic assessment.

Thoracic radiography
Radiographs can demonstrate the presence of cardiomegaly, but the accuracy is reduced in young animals. If cardiomegaly is present radiography may suggest left heart enlargement, or a bulge in the aorta or pulmonary artery, which can help to narrow the list of differential diagnoses, but this does not provide a definitive diagnosis. It should be noted that very young animals without cardiac disease may have a degree of right-sided cardiomegaly associated with the transition from neonatal to adult cardiac anatomy.

Radiographs are important to screen for signs of congestion (pulmonary oedema, pleural effusion) that would warrant medical treatment.

Echocardiography
Echocardiography is now the key diagnostic test for animals with murmurs, but requires more advanced training and knowledge to perform reliably. Two-dimensional (2D) echocardiography assesses changes in chamber dimensions and lesion morphology. Colour Doppler usually demonstrates the turbulent high-velocity flow of the blood that creates the murmur; and spectral Doppler studies can often assess the severity of defects to provide a prognosis.

Patent ductus arteriosus

Incidence
PDA is one of the three most common congenital cardiac defects seen in dogs (Patterson, 1971). It is the only congenital cardiac defect where there is a distinct sex predisposition for females (3:1), regardless of breed (Buchanan *et al.*, 1992). An autosomal dominant mode of inheritance has been suggested (Patterson, 1968).

Predisposed breeds include Maltese Terrier, Pomeranian, Shetland Sheepdog, English Springer Spaniel, Bichon Frisé, Poodle, Yorkshire Terrier, collies and German Shepherd Dog (Patterson, 1971; Buchanan *et al.*, 1992). Cats also may have PDA, though it is less common in this species.

Pathophysiology
PDA is a condition where the normal ductus arteriosus of the fetus fails to close after birth because of a reduction in, or absence of, vascular smooth muscle (Buchanan, 2001a). There is therefore a vascular conduit between the descending aorta and the pulmonary trunk (Figure 26.2ab). The pressure in the aorta is greater than in the pulmonary artery throughout the cardiac cycle and blood shunts continuously from the aorta into the pulmonary artery (*left to right*).

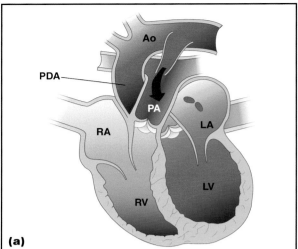

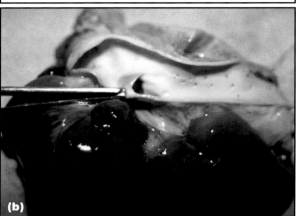

26.2 PDA. **(a)** The ductus remains as a vascular connection between the descending aorta (Ao) and the main pulmonary artery (PA). There is a continuous left-to-right shunt of blood throughout systole and diastole, giving the characteristic waxing and waning continuous murmur, as aortic pressures exceed pulmonary artery pressures throughout the cardiac cycle. **(b)** Post-mortem appearance of the heart of a dog with PDA, showing the aorta opened along its length. The forceps point to the duct. LA = Left atrium; LV = Left ventricle; RA = Right atrium; RV = Right ventricle.

This results in over-circulation of the pulmonary vasculature and lung fields, and volume overload of the left atrium (LA) and left ventricle (LV). This may progress to left-sided heart failure. Secondary mitral regurgitation sometimes develops as a result of the left ventricular dilatation. In some cases of untreated long-standing PDA, left ventricular myocardial failure develops secondary to the chronic volume overload. The LA may become very enlarged, predisposing to atrial fibrillation.

Right-to-left shunting PDAs
In rare circumstances, pulmonary hypertension can develop as a response to the over-circulation of the pulmonary vasculature or to retention of fetal vasculature. If the pulmonary artery pressure becomes so high as to match or exceed the aortic pressure, then flow in the PDA shunts *from right to left*. This right-to-left shunting results in deoxygenated blood passing to the caudal parts of the body only, as the

brachiocephalic trunk and left subclavian artery arise from the ascending aorta, prior to the ductus. This can result in differential cyanosis; the caudal mucous membranes of the vulva or prepuce should be checked if this is suspected. It is often not easily appreciated and may only be evident after exertion.

Actual change from left-to-right to right-to-left shunting is not well documented in dogs. It is more likely that the right-to-left shunting PDA is a separate form with associated pulmonary hypertension, perhaps secondary to prematurity or neonatal hypoxia with retained fetal vasculature (Oyama *et al.*, 2005). It must be emphasized that right-to-left shunting PDAs are extremely rare but may be seen most frequently with a very large (tubular-type) ductus (Patterson *et al.*, 1971).

Cats are more likely than dogs to develop pulmonary hypertension over time with PDA and will sometimes present with bidirectional shunting.

History

In left-to-right shunting PDA, the murmur is usually detected at initial vaccination. Some puppies are presented with left-sided heart failure with pulmonary oedema. Occasionally, observant owners will detect the precordial thrill themselves. In some animals, the murmurs may go undetected until adulthood, especially if the murmur is quite localized. Dogs with right-to-left shunting PDAs may be stunted and present with pelvic limb weakness exacerbated by exercise.

Physical examination

A loud continuous murmur (grade 5 or 6; see Chapter 4) is heard with maximal intensity at the dorsal left heart base (under the triceps muscle). It is a characteristic continuous murmur that waxes in systole and wanes through diastole. It is usually very loud and associated with a precordial thrill that radiates widely. The femoral pulses are usually hyperdynamic. Signs of left-sided heart failure may be detected with breathlessness and coughing. Many dogs with heart failure are cachexic.

In the very rare right-to-left shunting PDA, there is caudal cyanosis but often no murmur. A loud second heart sound may provide some clinical evidence of pulmonary hypertension to the trained examiner (auscultating at the left heart base). Pelvic limb weakness (due to the caudal cyanosis) can mimic neuromuscular disease (e.g. myasthenia gravis). Polycythaemia is common and may be severe.

Cats with a left-to-right PDA have a typical continuous murmur, but cats with pulmonary hypertension may have a systolic murmur without a prominent diastolic component (Connolly *et al.*, 2003).

Establishing the diagnosis

A continuous murmur is almost pathognomonic for PDA, especially in a predisposed breed. However, it is essential to confirm the diagnosis and to exclude other congenital defects prior to attempting closure. Continuous murmurs may also be present with aorticopulmonary windows and aberrant broncho-oesophageal arteries (Yamane *et al.*, 2001). Ancillary investigations are therefore required (Figure 26.3).

Technique	Findings
Radiography (Figure 26.4)	LA enlargement common Dilated pulmonic trunk on dorsoventral (DV) view (1–2 o'clock) Dilated descending aorta (12–1 o'clock) Left auricular appendage enlargement gives a bulge at 2–3 o'clock on the DV view (All three bulges on the DV view occur in only ~25% of cases) LV enlargement Pulmonary over-circulation, leading to pulmonary oedema
Electrocardiography	Not specific Tall R waves (>4.0 mV in dogs) Wide P waves (P mitrale) due to LA enlargement Arrhythmias possible – most commonly atrial fibrillation and supraventricular arrhythmias
2D and M-mode echocardiography (Figure 26.5ad)	LA dilatation common LV rounded and dilated with eccentric LV hypertrophy Dilated main pulmonary trunk Normal LV function initially; subsequent myocardial failure in long-standing cases with reduced fractional shortening Ductus may be imaged with difficulty between main pulmonary arteries and descending aorta (best from left cranial position)
Doppler echocardiography (Figure 26.5bc)	Continuous retrograde systolic and diastolic flow in main pulmonary artery, arising from ductus Ductus may be imaged with colour flow mapping Secondary mitral regurgitation common

26.3 Ancillary investigations in PDA.

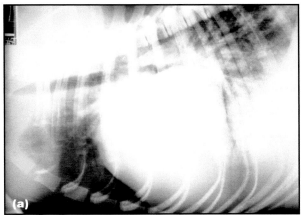

26.4 Radiographs of a mature German Shepherd Dog with PDA and clinical signs of left-sided CHF. **(a)** Lateral view showing marked LA and LV enlargement. The lung fields appear hypervascular. Cranial lobar pulmonary arteries and veins are both enlarged, and pulmonary venous distension is most marked. There is a generalized mixed (interstitial and alveolar) pulmonary infiltrate, consistent with pulmonary oedema, which is predominantly perihilar, although the alveolar infiltrate is well illustrated by the presence of air bronchograms in the cranial lobes. (continues) ▶

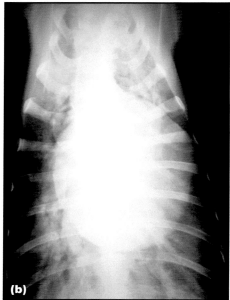

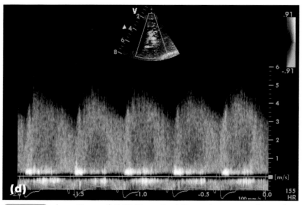

26.4 (continued) Radiographs of a mature German Shepherd Dog with PDA and clinical signs of left-sided CHF. **(b)** The DV view confirms the LA and LV enlargement and the pulmonary changes. Additionally, the classic 'triple knuckle' is seen between 12 and 3 o'clock, with a bulge on the descending aorta (12–1 o'clock), a pulmonary artery bulge (1–2 o'clock) and a left auricular appendage bulge (2–3 o'clock).

26.5 (continued) **(d)** Spectral Doppler recording of flow arising from the pulmonary ostium within the pulmonary trunk. The flow is continuous: waxes in systole (QRS complex to T wave) and wanes in diastole (T wave to QRS complex).

Management options

The prognosis for dogs with an uncorrected PDA is poor, with an estimated 50% 1-year survival rate (Eyster *et al.*, 1976). Closure of the PDA is indicated and typically provides an excellent prognosis, with most animals living a full and normal life. If the animal presents in CHF with left ventricular myocardial failure, however, the prognosis is more guarded and difficult to predict. In such cases treatment for the CHF is also required prior to considering anaesthesia. Closure is contraindicated when severe pulmonary hypertension develops and shunting is right to left.

The PDA can be surgically ligated, or closed using a coil or occluder via a transcatheter closure technique. An experienced cardiothoracic surgeon operating on uncomplicated cases can achieve a high success rate and very low mortality (Buchanan, 1994). Surgery in older dogs carries a higher risk, as the ductus and dilated pulmonary arteries are more friable. Transcatheter closure techniques have developed since the late 1990s and now are considered reliable and successful, with an increasing number of centres opting for this as their treatment of choice. The main two closure devices are coils (Saunders *et al.*, 2004; Campbell *et al.*, 2006) and occlusion devices such as the Amplatz Canine Duct Occluder™ (ACDO; Figure 26.6) (Nguyenba and Tobias, 2008).

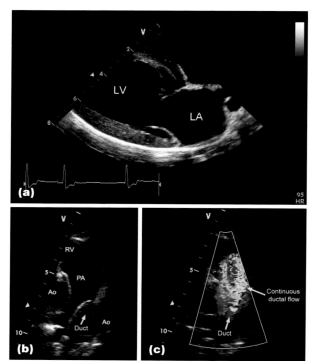

26.5 **(a)** Right parasternal long-axis view of a dog with a PDA, demonstrating mild LA and LV dilatation. **(b)** Left cranial parasternal view of a dog showing the duct between the aorta and pulmonary artery. **(c)** Colour flow mapping of (b) showing laminar (red) flow within the ampulla of the duct and the turbulent jet of flow towards the transducer, arising from the ostium of the duct within the pulmonary trunk. Ao = Aorta; LA = Left atrium; LV = Left ventricle; PA = Pulmonary artery; RV = Right ventricle. (continues) ▶

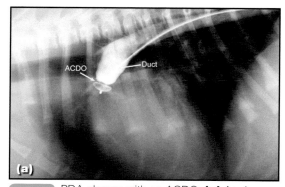

26.6 PDA closure with an ACDO. **(a)** Angiogram taken following positioning of the ACDO, showing contrast medium in the aorta and duct, but none in the pulmonary artery, indicating absence of ductal flow. (continues) ▶

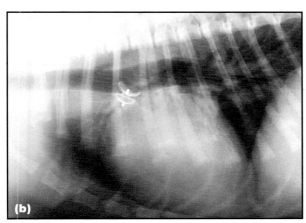

26.6 (continued) PDA closure with an ACDO. **(b)** Radiograph showing the ACDO after release. Note the pre-existing cardiomegaly and pulmonary vascular pattern.

Aortic stenosis

Incidence

Aortic stenosis (AS) is one of the three most common congenital cardiac defects seen in dogs. It is particularly prevalent in Boxers, Golden Retrievers, German Shepherd Dogs and Newfoundlands (Kienle *et al.*, 1994; Buchanan *et al.*, 1999). It is a condition with a broad spectrum of severity, from the severely incapacitated dog, to the dog that is essentially normal and active with a low grade murmur. An autosomal dominant mode of inheritance has been proposed in Newfoundlands (Pyle *et al.*, 1976).

AS is uncommon in cats and a more uniform severity is recognized (Stepien and Bonagura, 1991).

Pathophysiology

AS may be valvular, subvalvular or, more rarely, supravalvular. The commonest form in dogs is subvalvular (subaortic stenosis), where the lesions usually consist of fibrous bands (Pyle *et al.*, 1976) (Figure 26.7). These may range from a complete circumferential band (resulting in severe stenosis) to a small crescentic area in the left ventricular outflow tract (LVOT), which may not cause any clinical problems. These mild lesions may be difficult to detect on 2D echocardiography, but Doppler echocardiography demonstrates turbulent flow in the LVOT, with elevated blood flow velocities. Subaortic stenosis is unusual in that the lesions may not be present at birth, and may progress as the animal matures (Pyle *et al.*, 1976). Subvalvular lesions do not generally progress beyond early adulthood, though the less common valvular lesions may continue to become more stenotic with age.

A dynamic form of subaortic stenosis has also been described, perhaps similar to hypertrophic (obstructive) cardiomyopathy (Connolly and Boswood, 2003). It has also been suggested that some breeds of dog (e.g. Boxers, Bull Terriers) have an inappropriately narrow aortic diameter for their size, perhaps representing some form of aortic hypoplasia (Bussadori *et al.*, 2000). This results in increased velocity of flow from the LVOT to the aorta and a

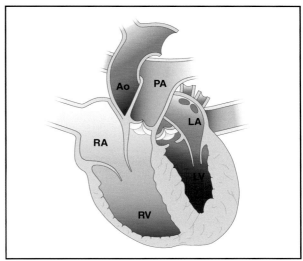

26.7 AS is usually in the form of a fibrous ring or crescent in the LVOT below the aortic valve (subaortic stenosis). This causes increased impedance to LV ejection (increased afterload). Compensatory concentric LV hypertrophy occurs to minimize LV wall stress.

systolic murmur, even without distinct lesions of the aortic valves or the LVOT.

The lesion in some dogs with subaortic stenosis extends to involve the mitral valve apparatus (mitral dysplasia).

The AS lesion increases impedance to LV ejection. The resultant increased afterload results in concentric myocardial hypertrophy, generally in proportion to the pressure overload and the degree of stenosis. Unfortunately, the coronary capillary vascular bed is unable to compensate for the degree of hypertrophy. The increased wall stress also compromises coronary perfusion (particularly of the subendocardium), and the resulting myocardial ischaemia can lead to ventricular arrhythmias. Exertional syncope may result, and there is also a risk of sudden death, particularly in those with more severe AS. Myocardial failure and/or CHF may occur in long-standing cases of severe AS (Kienle *et al.*, 1994).

History

The murmur should be audible at initial veterinary examination. Patients may be presented with a history of exercise intolerance or syncope. Sometimes sudden death is the only indication of the problem, and diagnosis is made at post-mortem examination.

Physical examination

The classic signs of AS are a left-sided systolic murmur at the left base, radiating to the right base and thoracic inlet. The grade of the murmur usually correlates with the severity of the stenosis in fixed obstructions. There is a spectrum of severity, and some dogs will have a very localized low-grade systolic murmur audible cranially at the left base without any radiation. Such low-grade murmurs may be indistinguishable from innocent 'puppy murmurs' on auscultation and the distinction between functional flow murmurs and mild AS is blurred (Koplitz *et al.*, 2003). The femoral pulse may be weak in severe cases.

Establishing the diagnosis

Figure 26.8 lists pertinent findings from ancillary investigations.

Technique	Findings
Radiography	Cardiac silhouette often unremarkable LV enlargement may be recognized Post-stenotic dilatation of aorta on DV view
Electrocardiography	Often unremarkable Tall R waves ± prolonged QRS complex duration ± ST segment changes indicating myocardial hypoxia ± Notched QRS complexes ± Ventricular premature complexes (due to myocardial hypoxia/ischaemia)
2D and M-mode echocardiography (Figure 26.9)	May find no abnormality in mild cases Concentric LV hypertrophy in more severe cases Anatomical abnormalities of LVOT and aortic valve may be recognized (e.g. fibrous ridge in LVOT) ± Post-stenotic dilatation of ascending aorta
Doppler echocardiography (Figure 26.10)	Maximal aortic velocities >2.25 m/s arbitrarily defined as AS Turbulent high-velocity aortic flow Aortic insufficiency common

26.8 Ancillary investigations in AS.

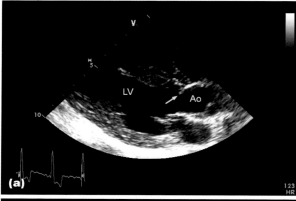

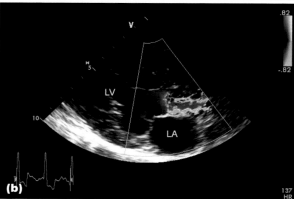

26.9 Echocardiography of AS. **(a)** LVOT and aortic valve. There is a visible subaortic lesion (arrowed). **(b)** Colour flow mapping shows laminar (blue) flow proximal to the subaortic lesion and a turbulent jet of flow arising from the stenosis and continuing into the ascending aorta. Ao = Aorta; LA = Left atrium; LV = Left ventricle.

Management options

The requirement for treatment is dictated by clinical signs and/or the severity of the stenosis. Doppler echocardiographic studies (Figure 26.10) can assess the trans-stenotic pressure gradient: mild <50 mmHg and severe >80 mmHg (Oyama *et al.*, 2005).

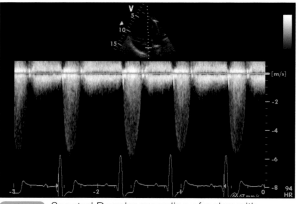

26.10 Spectral Doppler recording of a dog with subaortic stenosis. The peak velocity approaches 6 m/s, which equates to a trans-stenotic pressure gradient of 140 mmHg, classifying this as a severe stenosis.

The majority of cases are mild, do not require treatment and are likely to live a full and normal life, but the animals should not be used for breeding. Most cases with clinical signs or severe AS are managed medically, as there is no clear advantage to balloon valve dilation over medical management with subaortic stenosis (Meurs *et al.*, 2005). Medical management is based on beta-adrenergic antagonists (beta-blockers). Surgical correction has been described, but does not offer clear survival advantages (Monnet *et al.*, 1996). Exertion should be avoided in severe cases.

Pulmonic stenosis

Incidence

Pulmonic stenosis (PS) is one of the three most common congenital cardiac defects seen in dogs (Buchanan *et al.*, 1999). Predisposed breeds include Cocker Spaniel, Miniature Schnauzer, Boxer, English Bulldog, terriers and Samoyed. An autosomal dominant mode of inheritance has been reported in Beagles (Patterson *et al.*, 1981). The prognosis is poorer in the 10–20% of dogs that may have concurrent tricuspid dysplasia. In Bulldogs (and other 'bull' breeds), PS may be complicated by (or caused by) an aberrant single right coronary artery, giving a left branch encompassing the pulmonary annulus (Buchanan, 2001b).

PS is not common in cats, although it is recognized in association with other congenital cardiac defects.

Pathophysiology

PS in dogs is usually caused by stenosis of the pulmonic valve, but subvalvular and supravalvular lesions are also described. The obstruction to outflow causes pressure overload of the right ventricle (RV), resulting in RV hypertrophy (Figure 26.11). RV hypertrophy may cause infundibular narrowing of the right ventricular outflow tract (RVOT), exacerbating the stenosis, and sometimes resulting in a dynamic component to obstruction. The higher the pressure gradient across the stenotic area, the worse the prognosis (Fingland *et al.*, 1986). Severe or long-standing cases may progress to right-sided heart failure. PS can be classified based on whether the pulmonary annulus diameter is normal (Type A) or narrow (Type B). Type B cases often have hypoplasia of the pulmonary trunk and are less likely to show post-stenotic dilatation (Bussadori *et al.*, 2000).

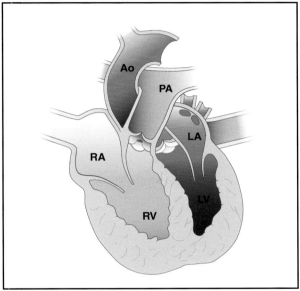

26.11 PS. There is increased afterload on the RV due to the stenotic pulmonic valve. Secondary RV hypertrophy occurs, which may cause further dynamic RVOT (infundibular) obstruction, exacerbating the pressure gradient across this area.

History
A murmur is usually detected at initial vaccination. Affected animals may have no clinical signs, or be presented for exercise intolerance, after syncopal episodes, or with right-sided CHF.

Physical examination
The classic finding in PS is a left-sided systolic murmur at the heart base. The grade of the murmur usually correlates with the severity of the stenosis in fixed obstructions. If there is significant RV hypertrophy, the precordial impulse in thin deep-chested breeds may be more pronounced over the right hemithorax. Pulse quality is usually good. If right-sided heart failure has developed, there may be distended jugular veins, hepatomegaly, ascites and/or positive hepatojugular reflux.

Establishing the diagnosis
Figure 26.12 lists pertinent findings from ancillary investigations.

Technique	Findings
Radiography	RV enlargement with apex tipping on the lateral view Post-stenotic dilatation of the pulmonary trunk (may appear as a 'cap' overlying trachea on lateral view) Normal/underperfused pulmonary vasculature May appear normal if mild lesion Angiography (Figure 26.13) will confirm diagnosis
Electrocardiography	Deep S waves in leads I, II, III and aVF Right axis deviation (> +100° dogs or > +160° cats) in frontal plane ± Ventricular premature complexes (RV origin)
2D and M-mode echocardiography (Figure 26.14)	RV hypertrophy in moderate to severe cases Interventricular septum has flat or paradoxical motion Abnormal pulmonic valve leaflets (often fused and/or thickened) Annular hypoplasia may be present in some cases Post-stenotic dilatation of pulmonary trunk often present
Doppler echocardiography (Figure 26.15)	High velocity and turbulent flow across pulmonic valve Dynamic outflow tract obstruction common in moderate to severe cases Pulmonic regurgitation common ± Tricuspid regurgitation

26.12 Ancillary investigations in PS.

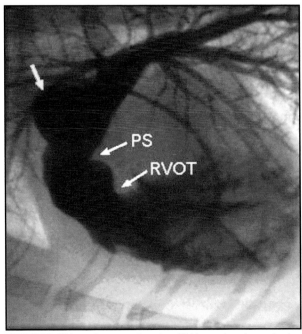

26.13 RV angiogram showing RV hypertrophy, valvular PS (arrowed) and a post-stenotic dilatation (yellow arrow). The RVOT is also shown (arrowed). Note the absence of tricuspid regurgitation in this case.

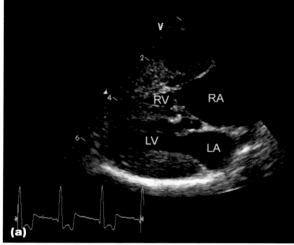

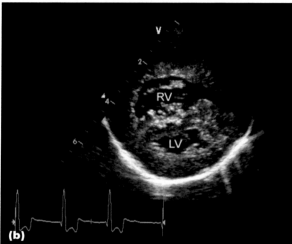

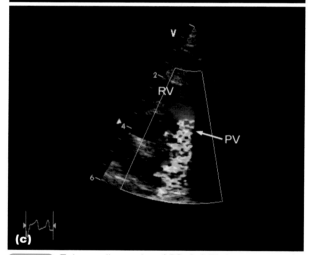

26.14 Echocardiography of PS. **(a)** Right parasternal long-axis view of a dog with a PS, demonstrating RV hypertrophy. The RA is also dilated, which was associated with a concurrent tricuspid dysplasia in this case. **(b)** Right parasternal short-axis view of the LV and RV. Note the marked RV hypertrophy and mild flattening of the ventricular septum associated with the higher RV pressure. **(c)** Right parasternal short-axis view with colour flow mapping recorded during systole, showing laminar (blue) flow approaching the stenosis and turbulent (mixed mosaic colours) flow distal to the stenosis. LA = Left atrium; LV = Left ventricle; PV = Pulmonic valve; RA = Right atrium; RV = Right ventricle.

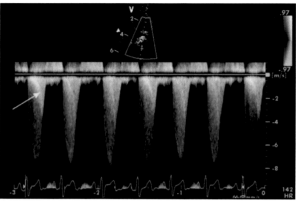

26.15 Spectral Doppler recording of a dog with PS. The peak velocity approaches 8 m/s, which equates to a trans-stenotic pressure gradient of 250 mmHg, classifying this as a very severe stenosis. Within the spectral trace a second signal can be seen, with slower acceleration and lower peak velocity (arrowed). This appearance is typical of concurrent dynamic (infundibular) obstruction.

Management options

Balloon valvuloplasty (Figure 26.16) is considered the treatment of choice (Stafford Johnson *et al.*, 2004b). Various surgical techniques have also been described,

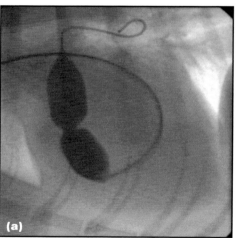

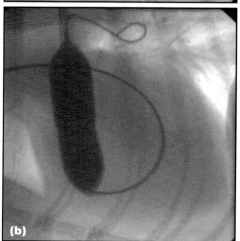

26.16 Fluoroscopic images showing balloon dilation of a PS. **(a)** The indent in the balloon is associated with the stenosis. **(b)** The balloon has been fully inflated to alleviate the stenosis.

from manually dilating the affected area, to patch graft techniques (Orton and Monnet, 1994). Balloon valvuloplasty is most effective when the cause of the stenosis is commissural fusion of the valve cusps, and least effective when there is annular hypoplasia. Indications for balloon valvuloplasty include:

- The PS is causing clinical signs (e.g. exercise intolerance, syncope)
- Doppler pressure gradient >80 mmHg.

Intervention typically results in a reduction in the trans-stenotic pressure gradient by 50% and provides a good long-term clinical outcome (improvement in exercise tolerance and in life expectancy) in 85% of cases (Stafford Johnson et al., 2004b). The operative mortality is much lower than for surgical techniques, but can still be up to 7% (Stafford Johnson and Martin, 2004). Intervention is less successful when there is concurrent tricuspid regurgitation and moderate to severe right atrium (RA) dilatation – this is likely with concurrent tricuspid dysplasia.

Dogs that present with right-sided CHF (e.g. ascites) are less likely to benefit from balloon valvuloplasty, though it is still the most useful therapeutic option in these cases. Beta-blockers appear to be beneficial in dogs with dynamic outflow tract obstruction and are often used as medical management in these cases, or prior to intervention. Surgical intervention is contraindicated if the stenosis is caused by a single aberrant coronary artery, as there is a risk of rupturing the artery, resulting in death.

Double-chambered right ventricle

This is included within PS, as it results in similar pathophysiology (Figure 26.17). It can be regarded as a form of 'subvalvular' PS and is sometimes termed primary infundibular stenosis. A fibrous, fibromuscular or muscular circumferential ridge is present within the RVOT, resulting in stenosis of this region (Martin et al., 2002). There is marked concentric RV hypertrophy proximal to this obstruction, but a normal RV wall in the distal RVOT, leading to the pulmonary

trunk. Pulmonic valves are usually structurally normal, but turbulent flow continues past the valve into the main pulmonary artery. Golden Retrievers appear to be predisposed, and feline cases have also been reported (Koffas et al., 2007). Balloon valvuloplasty is often not successful for this lesion, but may be worth attempting prior to considering surgical correction (preferably with cardiopulmonary bypass facilities).

Ventricular septal defect

Incidence

Ventricular septal defects (VSDs) are common in cats but not common in dogs. Bulldogs, West Highland White Terriers and Cocker Spaniels have been reported as predisposed breeds (Oyama et al., 2005).

Pathophysiology

The lesion is usually in the membranous part of the interventricular septum just below the aortic valve and the septal tricuspid leaflet (Figure 26.18a). Because of the systolic pressure difference between the left and right ventricles, left-to-right shunting of blood occurs through systole, though some degree of right-to-left shunting can occur with very large defects. Small defects offer high resistance to left-to-right flow (high pressure gradients maintained between the left and right ventricles) and loud murmurs are generated. These are called *restrictive* (or *resistive*) VSDs, and are unlikely to become haemodynamically significant. Larger defects offer less resistance to the shunt; these are haemodynamically significant and are associated with quieter murmurs. With significant left-to-right shunting, volume overload of the pulmonary circulation occurs. Increased pulmonary venous blood returns to the LA and LV, so these chambers become volume overloaded as well (Figure 26.18b).

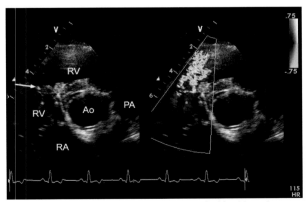

26.17 Left cranial parasternal view (left) with colour flow mapping (right) of a young Labrador Retriever with a double-chambered RV. The arrow points to the obstruction which divides the RV. The image on the right shows the turbulent systolic flow through the defect. Ao = Aorta; PA = Pulmonary artery; RA = Right atrium; RV = Right ventricle.

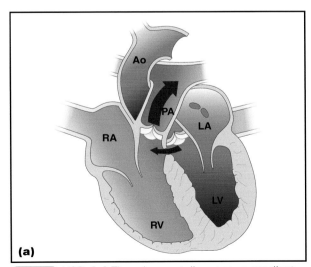

26.18 VSD. **(a)** There is a systolic pressure gradient between the LV and RV, allowing left-to-right shunting across the defect. The RV and pulmonary vasculature, LA and LV are therefore volume overloaded. LA = Left atrium; LV = Left ventricle; RA = Right atrium; RV = Right ventricle. (continues) ▶

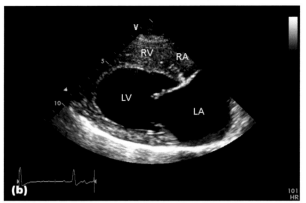

26.18 (continued) VSD. **(b)** Right parasternal long-axis view of a dog with a VSD, showing moderate LA and LV dilatation. Note that the VSD is not evident in this plane. LA = Left atrium; LV = Left ventricle; RA = Right atrium; RV = Right ventricle.

Various sequelae are described:

- Left-sided heart failure may result from the left-sided volume overload
- Eisenmenger's physiology may develop, where chronic over-circulation of the pulmonary vasculature results in pulmonary hypertension. It is not clear whether the increased pulmonary vascular resistance is reactive, or present from birth in dogs (retained fetal type vasculature). Whatever the mechanism of pulmonary hypertension, the resulting increased RV systolic pressures cause right-to-left shunting, and cyanosis may become evident. Eisenmenger's syndrome is usually evident before the age of 6 months (Bonagura *et al.*, 1995)
- Aortic regurgitation can occur because of prolapse of the right aortic valve cusp into the VSD during diastole. This can increase LV wall stress.

History

A murmur is usually detected at primary vaccination. Most affected animals do not have clinical signs. Left-sided heart failure may occur with large defects, and right-to-left shunting may cause stunting and signs of exercise intolerance.

Physical examination

The murmur is systolic and is louder on the right craniosternal hemithorax (as the blood shunts to the right side). The murmur is also heard on the left side – due either to radiation of the primary murmur or to a relative PS (caused by increased blood flow across a normal pulmonic valve). The grade of the murmur is often inversely proportional to the size of the defect; louder murmurs, possibly with precordial thrills, are associated with smaller defects and a better prognosis.

Establishing the diagnosis

Figures 26.19 lists typical results from ancillary investigations.

Technique	Findings
Radiography	LV enlargement LA enlargement RV enlargement Pulmonary over-circulation if significant left-to-right shunting
Electrocardiography	May be unremarkable Tall R waves Wide P waves (P mitrale)
2D and M-mode echocardiography (Figure 26.20a)	LA dilatation LV dilatation (eccentric hypertrophy) Hyperkinetic LV May image VSD in membranous part of septum below aortic valve and septal leaflet of tricuspid valve VSDs <2 mm can be difficult to visualize without colour Doppler
Doppler echocardiography (Figure 26.20bc)	Spectral or colour flow Doppler should be used to interrogate the RV side of the VSD Turbulent high velocity left-to-right flow is identified Velocity of blood flow across the VSD should be measured to assess pressure gradient; the higher the velocity, the better the prognosis Mitral regurgitation common Aortic regurgitation if aortic valve prolapse into the VSD

26.19 Ancillary investigations in typical left-to-right shunting VSDs.

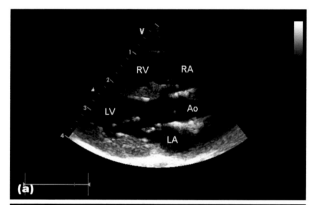

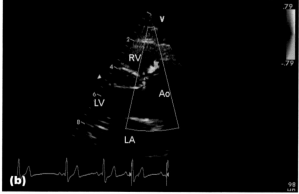

26.20 Echocardiography of feline VSDs. **(a)** Right parasternal long-axis view showing a reasonably large VSD. Note: small VSDs can be difficult to see on 2D echocardiography. **(b)** Colour flow mapping recorded in systole. Note the left-to-right flow through the VSD from just ventral to the aortic valve. Ao = Aorta; LA = Left atrium; LV = Left ventricle; RA = Right atrium; RV = Right ventricle. (continues) ▶

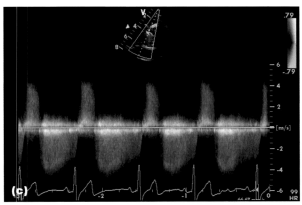

26.20 (continued) Echocardiography of feline VSDs. **(c)** Spectral Doppler recording through the VSD, showing flow towards the transducer in systole (QRS complex to T wave). The flow away from the transducer in diastole (T wave to QRS complex) is due to aortic regurgitation, which is common with a VSD, due to prolapse of the right coronary cusp of the aortic valve into the VSD.

Management options

The principal palliative surgical technique described is pulmonary artery banding to protect the pulmonary vascular bed.

- Some small VSDs may close spontaneously with growth to adulthood (Breznock, 1973).
- Most cases of uncomplicated VSDs are small resistive defects that need no special management or treatment.
- Diuretics and angiotensin-converting enzyme (ACE) inhibitors are indicated with left-sided heart failure. Transcatheter closure of VSDs is possible in children with an Amplatzer device and there has been a report of closure of a perimembranous VSD in a dog (Bussadori *et al.*, 2007).
- If significant right-to-left shunting and polycythaemia are present, phlebotomy may be required and occlusion of the defect is contraindicated.

Mitral dysplasia

Incidence

There appears to be a breed predisposition to mitral dysplasia in Bull Terriers (Malik and Church, 1988).

Pathophysiology

The defect (Figure 26.21) is usually associated with mitral regurgitation, causing volume overload of the LA and LV, as in acquired mitral valve disease. Left-sided heart failure usually results. Occasionally (especially in Bull Terriers) the dysplastic mitral valve apparatus is also stenotic (Lehmkuhl *et al.*, 1994; Dukes McEwan, 1995).

History

A systolic murmur should be recognized at initial vaccination. Coughing (dogs only), respiratory distress and exercise intolerance may be the presenting signs reported by the owner.

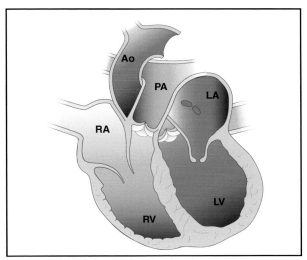

26.21 Mitral dysplasia. The dysplastic changes affecting the mitral valve may also affect the papillary muscles and the chordae tendineae and typically result in mitral incompetence. Mitral regurgitation causes LA and LV volume overload.

Physical examination

The systolic murmur is typically most intense over the mitral valve area. It may be of variable grade and radiate extensively if loud; the murmur does not correlate well with the severity of the lesion. In rare cases with mitral stenosis, a diastolic murmur may also be evident. Arrhythmias such as atrial fibrillation, other supraventricular arrhythmias and sinus tachycardia may be present. Adventitious respiratory sounds may be identified if the patient is in left-sided heart failure.

Establishing the diagnosis

Figure 26.22 lists typical results from ancillary investigations.

Technique	Findings
Radiography	LA enlargement LV enlargement Pulmonary venous congestion and pulmonary oedema if left-sided heart failure
Electrocardiography	Wide P waves ± Tall R waves ± Arrhythmias such as atrial fibrillation
2D and M-mode echocardiography (Figures 26.23 and 26.24)	LA dilatation LV dilatation Dysplastic mitral valve apparatus may be recognized (e.g. thick mitral valve leaflets, short chordae tendineae, large papillary muscles) Abnormal mitral valve motion may be appreciated if mitral stenosis present
Doppler echocardiography (Figure 26.24c)	Mitral regurgitation common Increased velocity mitral inflow ± Abnormal mitral inflow spectral signal with mitral stenosis (rare)

26.22 Ancillary investigations in mitral dysplasia.

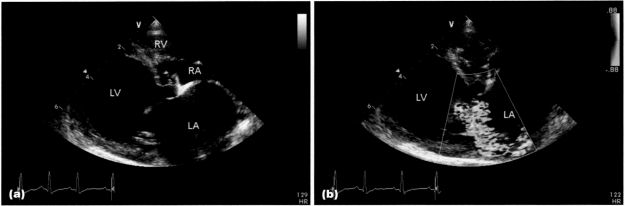

26.23 Mitral dysplasia results in volume loading of the left heart and therefore the LA and LV are seen to be dilated on echocardiography. **(a)** Right parasternal long-axis view of a dog with mitral dysplasia, demonstrating mild LA and LV dilatation. It can be difficult to appreciate specific abnormalities of the mitral apparatus. **(b)** Colour flow mapping recorded in systole, showing a large volume mitral regurgitation back into the LA. LA = Left atrium; LV = Left ventricle; RA = Right atrium; RV = Right ventricle.

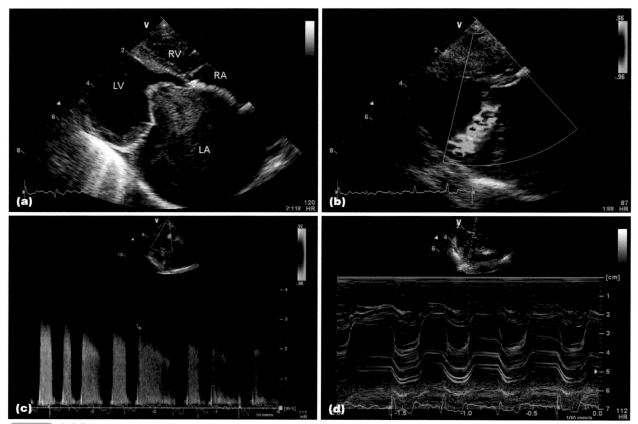

26.24 **(a)** Right parasternal long-axis view showing massive LA dilatation and a dysplastic, stenotic mitral valve in a Border Terrier with mitral dysplasia. This end-diastolic image shows the extent of opening of the mitral valve. The dog had atrial flutter as a consequence of severe atrial stretch. There is spontaneous echocontrast ('smoke') within the LA due to stasis of atrial flow. **(b)** Colour flow mapping (diastolic image) shows high-velocity turbulent flow into the LV, corresponding to the diastolic murmur detected. **(c)** Left apical four-chamber view with spectral Doppler recording showing mitral inflow. This view confirms the high-velocity, slowly decelerating mitral inflow typical of mitral stenosis. **(d)** M-mode echocardiogram of the mitral valve. The anterior leaflet has an abnormal 'box-shaped' motion towards the septum; and the posterior leaflet motion parallels this, rather than moving towards the posterior wall. LA = Left atrium; LV = Left ventricle; RA = Right atrium; RV = Right ventricle.

Management options

The condition is usually managed as for CHF due to acquired mitral regurgitation associated with myxomatous degenerative mitral valve disease, with diuretics, ACE inhibitors and pimobendan. The prog- nosis for dogs with moderate to severe mitral dysplasia is generally poor. Heart rate control is important in dogs with mitral stenosis, particularly if atrial fibrillation is present.

Atrial septal defect

Atrial septal defects (ASDs) are uncommon in cats and dogs, and isolated defects are not usually haemodynamically significant. They may be identified in association with other congenital defects. The defects are classified depending on the embryological development of the septum. Because the pressures between the two atria are similar, shunting is of low velocity and no murmur is heard. Shunting is usually left to right.

Tricuspid dysplasia

Tricuspid dysplasia (Figure 26.25) has been reported in the literature in Labrador Retrievers, Weimaraners and other large breeds of dog (Buchanan *et al.*, 1999). The condition is associated with tricuspid regurgitation and may progress to right-sided heart failure. A genetic basis for tricuspid dysplasia has

been reported for Labrador Retrievers (Famula *et al.*, 2002), with a locus identified on canine chromosome 9 (Andelfinger *et al.*, 2003). Figures 26.26 lists the typical findings in tricuspid dysplasia.

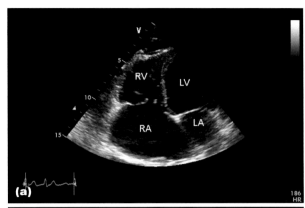

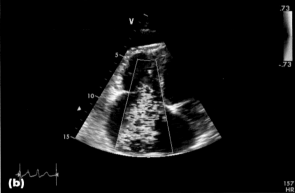

26.27 Tricuspid dysplasia results in volume loading of the right heart and therefore the RA and RV are seen to be dilated on echocardiography; the RA is often much more dilated than the RV. **(a)** Left apical four-chamber view of a dog with tricuspid dysplasia, demonstrating marked RA dilatation and mild to moderate RV dilatation. It can be difficult to appreciate specific abnormalities of the tricuspid apparatus. Note that there is also some pleural effusion, seen between the probe and the apex of the heart. **(b)** Colour flow mapping shows a turbulent jet of flow back into the RA during systole. LA = Left atrium; LV = Left ventricle; RA = Right atrium; RV = Right ventricle.

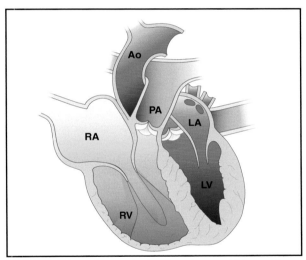

26.25 Tricuspid dysplasia. The abnormal tricuspid valves are incompetent and tricuspid regurgitation results in volume overload of the RA and RV.

Technique	Findings
Radiography	RA enlargement RV enlargement
Electrocardiography	Tall P waves Deep Q waves in leads I, II, III and aVF ± Right-axis deviation Splintered QRS complexes in some cases ± Supraventricular arrhythmias
2D and M-mode echocardiography (Figure 26.27)	RA dilatation RV dilatation Abnormal appearance of tricuspid valve apparatus
Doppler echocardiography	Tricuspid regurgitation

26.26 Ancillary investigations in tricuspid dysplasia.

Tetralogy of Fallot

Although it is uncommon in small animals, tetralogy of Fallot (Figure 26.28) is the most common of the cyanotic congenital defects. PS, aortic malalignment and VSD are present due to abnormal development of the conotruncal system (Patterson *et al.*, 1974). RV hypertrophy is secondary to the PS, often with a hypoplastic pulmonary trunk. Patients are usually presented with stunting, cyanosis and severe exercise intolerance. It is most commonly reported in Golden Retrievers, Wire-haired Fox Terriers, Labrador Retrievers, Siberian Huskies and Toy Poodles (Ringwald and Bonagura, 1988). Typical findings are listed in Figure 26.29.

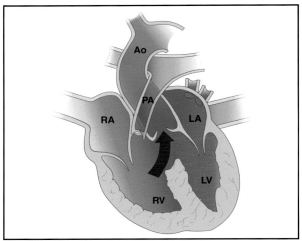

26.28 Tetralogy of Fallot consists of PS with concentric RV hypertrophy. There is also a subaortic VSD, which is usually large, and a malaligned (over-riding) aorta. The pulmonary trunk is usually also hypoplastic. Right-to-left flow across the VSD, due to the high RV pressure associated with PS, results in desaturated blood entering the aorta, with cyanosis, hypoxaemia and polycythaemia.

Technique	Findings
Radiography	RV enlargement Hypovascular lung fields
Electrocardiography	Deep S waves in leads I, II, III and aVF Right-axis deviation
2D and M-mode echocardiography (Figure 26.30)	RV hypertrophy Flat interventricular septum or paradoxical septal motion VSD visible if large enough Aortic malalignment (overlying VSD) Pulmonary trunk often hypoplastic – can be difficult to locate
Doppler echocardiography	PS – high-velocity and turbulent pulmonic flow VSD – low-velocity flow shunting right to left

26.29 Ancillary investigations in tetralogy of Fallot.

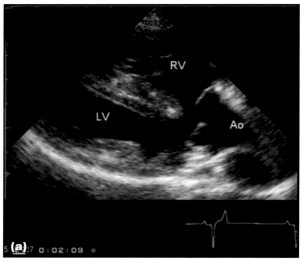

26.30 Echocardiography of tetralogy of Fallot. **(a)** Right parasternal long-axis five-chamber view of a Border Collie. The aorta is malaligned, over-riding the septum, and a high VSD is present. Ao = Aorta; LV = Left ventricle; RV = Right ventricle. (continues) ▶

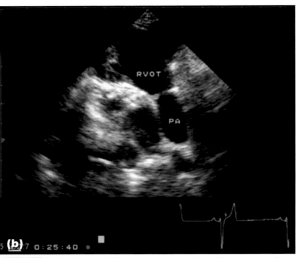

26.30 (continued) Echocardiography of tetralogy of Fallot. **(b)** Right parasternal short-axis view obtained at the level of the heart base and optimized for the RVOT. The pulmonic valves are thickened and stenotic, and the main pulmonary artery is hypoplastic. PA = Pulmonary artery; RVOT = Right ventricular outflow tract.

Atrioventricular septal defect

Also known as 'endocardial cushion defect' (Figure 26.31) or 'persistent common atrioventricular canal', this is a relatively common congenital defect in cats. It is an embryological developmental defect of the endocardial cushions, resulting in a low ASD, a high VSD and atrioventricular valvular abnormalities. A spectrum of haemodynamic effects can be seen, from cyanosis with pulmonary hypertension and right-to-left shunting, to left-sided congestive failure associated with mitral regurgitation and left-to-right shunting.

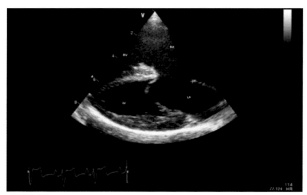

26.31 Right parasternal four-chamber view of a Weimaraner with an endocardial cushion defect. There is a primum-type ASD (measuring >2.3 cm) over the atrioventricular annuli. The atrioventricular valves are in the same plane. Concurrent pulmonary hypertension also exacerbates the right heart enlargement.

Cor triatriatum dexter

This rare congenital heart defect has been reported in dogs, but not in cats. Rottweilers may be predisposed. It is not associated with an audible heart murmur, unless complicated by other congenital cardiac lesions. The RA is separated by a diaphragm or membrane, resulting in a caudal high-pressure chamber into which the caudal vena cava drains. The cranial chamber receives cranial vena cava drainage from the head and neck. Consequently, patients with clinical signs referable to the condition will usually present with signs of caudal right-sided CHF (i.e. ascites), while jugular veins are not distended. There is normally a perforation in the membrane, allowing flow into the normal RA.

Minimally invasive correction has been described with balloon dilation of this perforation (Stafford Johnson *et al.*, 2004a) to improve RA flow, reduce the caudal chamber pressure and thus alleviate right-sided CHF signs. Surgical correction has also been reported (Chanoit *et al.*, 2009).

Cor triatriatum sinister (CTS) and supravalvular mitral stenosis (SMS)

These have been reported in cats, but not dogs. The LA is partitioned into a proximal and distal (nearest the mitral valve) chamber by a fibromuscular diaphragm with a perforation, leading to a high-pressure proximal (dorsal) chamber, into which the pulmonary veins drain. Cats with clinical signs referable to the condition typically present with pulmonary venous congestion and pulmonary oedema. Some cats develop pulmonary hypertension secondary to pulmonary venous hypertension. The position of the left auricular appendage distinguishes between CTS and SMS: in CTS, the auricular appendage is distal to the membrane and therefore is not dilated; in SMS, the auricular appendage is connected to the dilated proximal chamber (Fine *et al.*, 2002). Successful surgical correction has been reported in a cat (Wander *et al.*, 1998).

Other congenital defects

Vascular ring anomalies
Vascular ring anomalies (Figure 26.32) usually result in regurgitation of food immediately after eating, usually at the time of weaning on to solid foods. These puppies are usually markedly stunted compared with littermates. A persistent right aortic arch (PRAA) is the most common cause and surgical correction is possible.

Congenital venous abnormalities
A persistent left cranial vena cava (PLCVC) (Figure 26.33) may be recognized as an incidental echocardiographic finding, possibly in association with other congenital defects. It is not of clinical significance, but it is important to note prior to cardiac catheterization procedures.

Pericardial defects
Pericardial defects such as peritoneal–pericardial–diaphragmatic hernias (PPDHs) (Figure 26.34) may result in gastrointestinal disturbance, without the presence of heart murmurs.

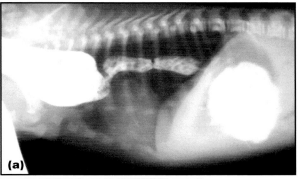

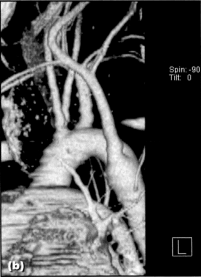

26.32 Vascular ring anomalies. **(a)** Lateral thoracic radiograph of a 6-week-old Jack Russell Terrier with regurgitation of solid foods since weaning. Barium sulphate mixed with canned food was fed. Megaoesophagus cranial to the heart base, with a relatively normal oesophagus coursing caudally from the heart to the stomach, was identified. A PRAA was confirmed at thoracotomy, with oesophageal entrapment between the heart base, pulmonary trunk on the left, and the ligamentum arteriosum. **(b)** 3D reconstruction from a CT angiographic study in a dog with an unusual vascular ring anomaly (PRAA with retroesophageal left subclavian artery). This is a view from the left, showing the PRAA, but with the left subclavian artery also resulting in partial oesophageal obstruction. Additional vascular abnormalities are evident, with the carotids arising directly off the aortic arch. (Courtesy of F. McConnell.)

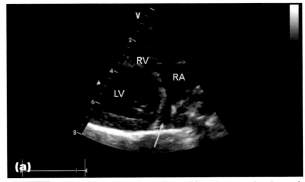

26.33 **(a)** Right parasternal modified long-axis view of a dog with a PLCVC (arrowed). LV = Left ventricle; RA = Right atrium; RV = Right ventricle. (continues) ▶

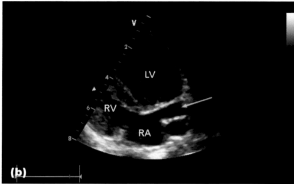

26.33 (continued) **(b)** Left apical four-chamber view. The left cranial vena cava (arrowed) normally enters into the coronary sinus; the dilated coronary sinus courses around the left atrioventricular groove and enters the RA. LV = Left ventricle; RA = Right atrium; RV = Right ventricle.

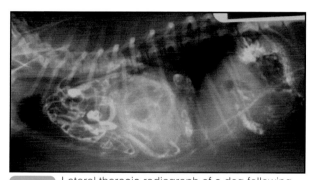

26.34 Lateral thoracic radiograph of a dog following oral administration of barium liquid. Note that much of the intestines are visible within the pericardium.

References and further reading

Andelfinger G, Wright KN, Lee HS, Siemens LM and Benson DW (2003) Canine tricuspid valve malformation, a model of human Ebstein anomaly, maps to dog chromosome 9. *Journal of Medical Genetics* **40**, 320–324

Bonagura JD, Darke PGG, Ettinger SJ and Feldman EC (1995) Congenital heart disease. In: *Textbook of Veterinary Internal Medicine*, ed. SJ Ettinger and EC Feldman, pp. 892–943. WB Saunders, Philadelphia

Breznock EM (1973) Spontaneous closure of ventricular septal defects in the dog. *Journal of the American Veterinary Medical Association* **162**, 399–399

Buchanan JW (1994) Patent ductus arteriosus. [Review] [16 refs]. *Seminars in Veterinary Medicine & Surgery (Small Animal)* **9**, 168–176

Buchanan JW (2001a) Patent ductus arteriousus morphology, pathogenesis, types and treatment. *Journal of Veterinary Cardiology* **3**, 7–16

Buchanan JW (2001b) Pathogenesis of single right coronary artery and pulmonic stenosis in English Bulldogs. *Journal of Veterinary Internal Medicine* **15**, 101–104

Buchanan JW, Fox PR, Sisson D and Moïse NS (1999) Prevalence of cardiovascular disorders. In: *Textbook of Canine and Feline Cardiology: Principles and Clinical Practice*, ed. PR Fox *et al.*, pp. 457–470. WB Saunders, Philadelphia

Buchanan JW, Kirk RW and Bonagura JD (1992) Causes and prevalence of cardiovascular disease. In: *Current Veterinary Therapy XI*, pp 647–655. WB Saunders, Philadelphia

Bussadori C, Amberger C, Le Bobinnec G and Lombard CW (2000) Guidelines for the echocardiographic studies of suspected subaortic and pulmonic stenosis. *Journal of Veterinary Cardiology* **2**, 17–24

Bussadori C, Carminati M and Domenech O (2007) Transcatheter closure of a perimembranous ventricular septal defect in a dog. *Journal of Veterinary Internal Medicine* **21**, 1396–1400

Campbell FE, Thomas WP, Miller SJ, Berger D and Kittleson MD (2006) Immediate and late outcomes of transarterial coil occlusion of

patent ductus arteriosus in dogs. *Journal of Veterinary Internal Medicine* **20**, 83–96

Chanoit G, Bublot I and Viguier E (2009) Transient tricuspid valve regurgitation following surgical treatment of cor triatriatum dexter in a dog. *Journal of Small Animal Practice* **50**, 241–245

Connolly DJ and Boswood A (2003) Dynamic obstruction of the left ventricular outflow tract in four young dogs. *Journal of Small Animal Practice* **44**, 319–325

Connolly DJ, Lamb CR and Boswood A (2003) Right-to-left shunting patent ductus arteriosus with pulmonary hypertension in a cat. *Journal of Small Animal Practice* **44**, 184–188

Dukes McEwan J (1995) Mitral dysplasia in Bull Terriers. *The Veterinary Annual* **35**, 130–146

Eyster GE, Eupler JT, Cords GB and Johnston J (1976) Patent ductus arteriosus in the dog: characteristics of occurrence and results of surgery in one hundred consecutive cases. *Journal of the American Veterinary Medical Association* **168**, 435–438

Famula TR, Siemens LM, Davidson AP and Packard M (2002) Evaluation of the genetic basis of tricuspid valve dysplasia in Labrador Retrievers. *American Journal of Veterinary Research* **63**, 816–820

Fine DM, Tobias AH and Jacob KA (2002) Supravalvular mitral stenosis in a cat. *Journal of the American Animal Hospital Association* **38**, 403–406

Fingland RB, Bonagura JD and Myer CW (1986) Pulmonic stenosis in the dog: 29 cases (1975–1984). *Journal of the American Veterinary Medical Association* **189**, 218–226

Kienle RD, Thomas WP and Pion PD (1994) The natural clinical history of canine congenital subaortic stenosis. *Journal of Veterinary Internal Medicine* **8**, 423–431

Koffas H, Fuentes VL, Boswood A *et al.* (2007) Double chambered right ventricle in 9 cats. *Journal of Veterinary Internal Medicine* **21**, 76–80

Koplitz SL, Meurs KM, Spier AW *et al.* (2003) Aortic ejection velocity in healthy Boxers with soft cardiac murmurs and Boxers without cardiac murmurs: 201 cases (1997–2001). *Journal of the American Veterinary Medical Association* **222**, 770–774

Lehmkuhl LB, Ware WA and Bonagura JD (1994) Mitral stenosis in 15 dogs. *Journal of Veterinary Internal Medicine* **8**, 2–17

MacDonald KA (2006) Congenital heart diseases of puppies and kittens. *Veterinary Clinics of North America: Small Animal Practise* **36**, 503–531, vi

Malik R and Church DB (1988) Congenital mitral insufficiency in bull terriers. *Journal of Small Animal Practice* **29**, 549–557

Martin JM, Orton EC, Boon JA *et al.* (2002) Surgical correction of double-chambered right ventricle in dogs. *Journal of the American Veterinary Medical Association* **220**, 770–774

Meurs KM, Lehmkuhl LB and Bonagura JD (2005) Survival times in dogs with severe subvalvular aortic stenosis treated with balloon valvuloplasty or atenolol. *Journal of the American Veterinary Medical Association* **227**, 420–424

Monnet E, Orton EC, Gaynor JS *et al.* (1996) Open resection for subvalvular aortic-stenosis in dogs. *Journal of the American Veterinary Medical Association* **209**, 1255–1261

Nguyenba TP and Tobias AH (2008) Minimally invasive per-catheter patent ductus arteriosus occlusion in dogs using a prototype duct occluder. *Journal of Veterinary Internal Medicine* **22**, 129–134

Orton EC and Monnet E (1994) Pulmonic stenosis and subvalvular aortic stenosis: surgical options. *Seminars Veterinary Medicine and Surgery (Small Animals)* **9**, 221–226

Oyama MA, Sisson DD, Thomas WP and Bonagura JD (2005) Congenital heart disease. In: *Textbook of Veterinary Internal Medicine, 6th edn*, ed. SJ Ettinger and EC Feldman, pp. 972–1021. Elsevier Saunders, St Louis

Patterson DF (1968) Epidemiologic and genetic studies of congenital heart disease in the dog. *Circulation Research* **23**, 171–202

Patterson DF (1971) Canine congenital heart disease: epidemiology and etiological hypotheses. *Journal of Small Animal Practice* **12**, 263–287

Patterson DF, Haskins ME and Schnarr WR (1981) Hereditary dysplasia of the pulmonary valve in beagle dog. *American Journal of Cardiology* **47**, 631–641

Patterson DF, Pyle RL, Buchanan JW, Trautvetter E and Abt DA (1971) Hereditary patent ductus arteriosus and its sequelae in the dog. *Circulation Research* **29**, 1–13

Patterson DF, Pyle RL, Van ML, Melbin J and Olson M (1974) Hereditary defects of the conotruncal septum in Keeshond dogs: pathologic and genetic studies. *American Journal of Cardiology* **34**, 187–205

Pyle RL, Patterson DF and Chacko S (1976) The genetics and pathology of discrete subaortic stenosis in the Newfoundland dog. *American Heart Journal* **92**, 324–334

Ringwald RJ and Bonagura JD (1988) Tetralogy of Fallot in the dog: clinical findings in 13 cases. *Journal of the American Animal Hospital Association* **24**, 33–43

Saunders AB, Miller MW, Gordon SG and Bahr A (2004) Pulmonary embolization of vascular occlusion coils in dogs with patent ductus arteriosus. *Journal of Veterinary Internal Medicine* **18**, 663–666

Stafford Johnson M and Martin M (2004) Results of balloon

valvuloplasty in 40 dogs with pulmonic stenosis. *Journal of Small Animal Practice* **45**, 148–153

Stafford Johnson MS, Martin M, De Giovanni JV, Boswood A and Swift S (2004a) Management of cor triatriatum dexter by balloon dilatation in three dogs. *Journal of Small Animal Practice* **45**, 16–20

Stafford Johnson MS, Martin M, Edwards D, French A and Henley W (2004b) Pulmonic stenosis in dogs: balloon dilation improves clinical outcome. *Journal of Veterinary Internal Medicine* **18**, 656–662

Stepien RL and Bonagura JD (1991) Aortic stenosis clinical findings in six cats. *Journal of Small Animal Practice* **32**, 341–350

Wander KW, Monnet E and Orton EC (1998) Surgical correction of cor triatriatum sinister in a kitten. *Journal of the American Animal Hospital Association* **34**, 383–386

Yamane T, Awazu T, Fujii Y *et al.* (2001) Aberrant branch of the bronchoesophageal artery resembling patent ductus arteriosus in a dog. *Journal of Veterinary Medical Science* **63**, 819–822

27

Systemic hypertension

Rosanne Jepson and Harriet Syme

Introduction

Systemic hypertension is increasingly recognized within the canine and feline population, particularly in older patients. Blood pressure (BP) is the product of cardiac output and total peripheral resistance, and cardiac output in turn is determined by the heart rate and stroke volume.

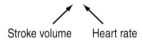

In health, the baroreceptor reflex interacts with the autonomic nervous system and both local and systemic vasoactive agents to regulate the heart, peripheral vasculature and the renin–angiotensin–aldosterone system (RAAS), keeping BP tightly controlled. Systemic vascular resistance is maintained partly through peripheral vascular compliance and elasticity, particularly of the arteriolar beds (Figure 27.1).

Pathophysiological mechanisms contributing to the development of hypertension are presented in Figure 27.2.

In human medicine the diagnosis of systemic hypertension is sub-classified according to whether a patient has isolated or combined, systolic or diastolic hypertension. Currently in veterinary medicine little emphasis is placed on diastolic blood pressure (DBP), due to the inaccuracy of indirect techniques for determining DBP and also because clinical studies demonstrating target organ damage in association with isolated diastolic hypertension are lacking. This chapter therefore focuses on the diagnosis and management of systolic hypertension.

Factors	Vasoconstrictors	Vasodilators
Neurotransmitters	Sympathetic nervous system – noradrenaline	Parasympathetic nervous system – acetylcholine via nitric oxide
Endothelium-derived and locally produced factors	Prostaglandin F2; thromboxane	Prostaglandin E2; bradykinin; nitric oxide; endothelial-derived hyperpolarizing factor
Hormones	Adrenaline; angiotensin II; vasopressin; endothelin-1	Atrial naturetic peptide
Hypoxia	Pulmonary vasoconstrictor	Systemic vasodilator

27.1 Factors influencing total peripheral resistance.

Disease condition	Potential pathophysiological mechanisms underlying hypertension	Reported prevalence of hypertension with underlying disease condition	
		Dogs	**Cats**
Chronic kidney disease (CKD)	Reduced sodium excretion with subsequent plasma volume expansion and increased cardiac output Activation of RAAS influencing both cardiac output and total peripheral resistance (TPR) (angiotensin II) Aldosterone may play an important role, particularly in cats	10–80%	20–65%
Hyperthyroidism	Activation of RAAS, sodium retention and expansion of plasma volume increasing cardiac output Increased cardiac output due to tachycardia and increased stroke volume, though this is offset by a reduction in TPR Hypertension developing with treatment may be associated with the resulting fall in glomerular filtration rate	N/A	Pre-treatment: 10–25% Post-treatment: 20%

27.2 Clinical conditions associated with the development of secondary hypertension. (continues) ▶

Disease condition	Potential pathophysiological mechanisms underlying hypertension	Reported prevalence of hypertension with underlying disease condition	
		Dogs	**Cats**
Hyperadrenocorticism	Increased sensitivity to vasoactive agents such as noradrenaline and angiotensin II, increasing TPR Increased myocardial sensitivity to catecholamines, increasing cardiac output Saturation of 11-β-hydroxysteroid dehydrogenase (enzyme responsible for deactivation of cortisol in mineralocorticoid target tissues), resulting in mineralocortiocoid effects Chronic vascular changes leading to reduced vascular compliance and elasticity, resulting in increased TPR	Pre-treatment: 60–85% Post-treatment: 40%	N/A
Diabetes mellitus	Poorly defined in cats and dogs; in humans, vascular disease and diabetic nephropathy contribute Disturbances in lipid profile and disturbances in vascular compliance affecting TPR	25–50%	No association made
Primary hyperaldosteronism	Retention of sodium, plasma volume expansion and subsequent increase in cardiac output Central actions of aldosterone	Unknown	50–100% Uncommon condition
Phaeochromocytoma	Adrenergic stimulation by products from tumour (chromaffin cells of adrenal medulla) e.g. noradrenaline, adrenaline and dopamine Some cases may have concurrent disease predisposing to systemic hypertension Can be episodic	40–85% Rare condition	Unknown Extremely rare condition

27.2 (continued) Clinical conditions associated with the development of secondary hypertension.

Target organ damage

Persistent systemic hypertension can lead to target organ damage (TOD), particularly in organs that are highly vascularized or are dependent on an autoregulatory mechanism to control blood flow, such as the eye, kidney, cardiovascular and central nervous systems (Figure 27.3).

Ocular damage

One of the most common manifestations of hypertensive TOD in the cat is a hypertensive retinopathy/choroidopathy, which can be identified by performing a fundic examination (Figure 27.4). Ocular changes are reported to occur in 60–100% of cats with systemic hypertension (Sansom *et al.*, 1994; Stiles *et al.*, 1994; Maggio *et al.*, 2000; Syme *et al.*, 2002). In clinical studies hypertensive retinopathy/choroidopathy

has rarely been reported in cats with systolic blood pressure (SBP) <170 mmHg. However, in experimentally induced renal hypertension, where sudden fluctuations in systemic pressures are seen, hypertensive ocular changes have been reported with SBP as low as 160 mmHg (Mathur *et al.*, 2004). Hypertensive ocular changes are less frequently reported in the dog, with a prevalence of just 5–20% (Jacob *et al.*, 2003; Cortadellas *et al.*, 2006).

Left ventricular hypertrophy

Left ventricular hypertrophy (LVH) and associated murmurs, arrhythmias and gallop rhythms have been reported in up to 85% of cats with systemic hypertension (Snyder *et al.*, 2001; Chetboul *et al.*, 2003; Henik *et al.*, 2004). Similarly in dogs, the prevalence of LVH associated with hypertension is reported to be high (up to 90%) (Cortadellas *et al.*, 2006).

Target organ	Pathological damage	Clinical findings
Eye	Hypertensive retinopathy/choroidopathy	Acute-onset blindness; multifocal bullous retinal detachments; fresh/resolving retinal haemorrhages; exudative retinal detachment; hyphaema; retinal vessel tortuosity/perivascular oedema creating impression of vessel narrowing; papilloedema (difficult to discern in cats); secondary glaucoma
Kidneys	Glomerular hypertension and glomerulosclerosis with potential for progression of pre-existing kidney disease in rodent studies	Increase in plasma creatinine/blood urea nitrogen (BUN); serial decline in glomerular filtration rate; exacerbation or development of proteinuria/microalbuminuria
Cardiovascular system	Left ventricular hypertrophy and damage to vessels	Left ventricular hypertrophy; gallop sounds; arrhythmias; heart murmurs; epistaxis
Central nervous system (brain)	Cerebral white matter oedema, cerebrovascular lesions, arteriolar hyalinosis, hyperplastic arteriosclerosis and parenchymal microhaemorrhages	Seizures; lethargy; altered mentation or behavioural change; disorientation; ataxia; vestibular signs; head tilt or nystagmus; focal neurological deficits

27.3 Pathological and clinical consequences of target organ damage secondary to hypertension.

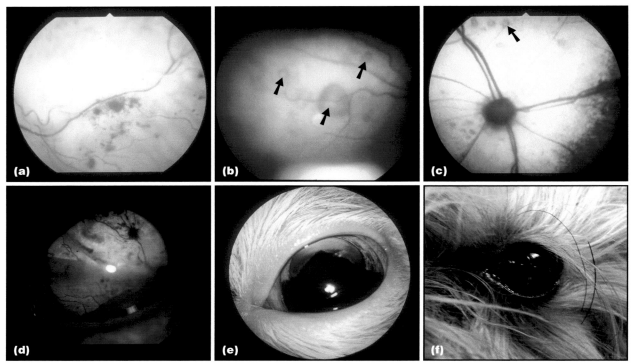

27.4 Ocular lesions secondary to systemic hypertension. **(a)** Feline fundus with evidence of multifocal intraretinal haemorrhages, large bullous retinal detachment and oedema. Marked variation in vessel calibre, with marked apparent loss/attenuation of retinal arterioles, is present (likely due to detachment/oedema). **(b)** Feline fundus with central focal bullous retinal detachment; peripherally similar smaller circular lesions can also be identified. There is also generalized oedema. Note how the blood vessel is raised by the bullous detachment (arrowed). **(c)** Feline fundus with multifocal areas of pigmentary disturbance. These represent old/inactive lesions likely to be secondary to small bullous detachment in the past (for example, that indicated by arrow). This cat did not have any detectable visual problem. **(d)** Feline eye demonstrating an area of total bullous retinal detachment, with large folds of retina displaced anteriorly within the vitreous and therefore now visible directly via the pupil with a focal light source (optic disc more posterior and obscured by retinal folds in this image). Multifocal intraretinal haemorrhages are present. Note also the marked mydriasis. This cat was clinically blind on presentation with similar changes observed bilaterally. **(e)** Feline eye with evidence of gross hyphaema (blood in anterior chamber). The blood has formed a solid clot. Also note the mydriasis, which is suggestive of concurrent fundic damage. **(f)** Canine eye with evidence of gross hyphaema. ((a)–(e) courtesy of R. Elks.)

Renal damage

Experimental evidence would suggest that hypertension can damage the kidney directly by overriding the autoregulatory mechanism at the afferent arteriole, which controls glomerular capillary pressure. Unchecked, this can lead to glomerular hypertension, glomerulosclerosis and proteinuria. If there is stimulation of the RAAS as a causal factor in the development of hypertension, there is concern that this may also have a detrimental effect on the kidney. Evidence from experimental studies would suggest that hypertension is damaging to the canine kidney (Brown *et al.*, 2000), and a recent clinical study showed that dogs with SBP >160 mmHg were at risk of more rapidly progressive kidney disease (Jacob *et al.*, 2003). The majority of hypertensive cats are reported to have some degree of renal impairment. Further study is necessary to define fully the relationship between hypertension, proteinuria and kidney disease in cats and dogs.

Neurological complications

Neurological complications associated with hypertension are infrequently documented in spontaneous hypertension but have been reported in association with experimental models of hypertension and following renal transplantation. Neurological complications of hypertension may be under-recognized.

Classification of systolic hypertension

Systolic hypertension is usually categorized into one of three classes, depending on underlying aetiology.

Secondary hypertension

This is where hypertension is thought to result from an underlying disease process. Renal disease is the most important cause of secondary hypertension in humans and cats. In dogs, the significance of renal disease as a cause of hypertension is more controversial but it is certainly one of the leading causes. For disease conditions that have been associated with hypertension and reported prevalence, see Figure 27.2. Variation in prevalence can be attributed to differences in populations studied, criteria for inclusion and the techniques used for assessment of BP.

Secondary hypertension may also be iatrogenic from the administration of therapeutic agents that can result in increased BP, e.g. phenylpropanolamine, glucocorticoids, mineralocorticoids and erythropoietin.

Idiopathic hypertension

In human medicine the terms idiopathic, primary and essential are used to describe hypertension where no underlying disease state can be identified. This requires a full diagnostic evaluation, including, for example, direct assessment of glomerular filtration rate (GFR) to exclude the possibility of subclinical kidney disease. In veterinary medicine this is rarely performed. The term 'idiopathic' hypertension is therefore preferred to primary or essential hypertension and the diagnosis is often made on the basis of persistent hypertension, perhaps with evidence of hypertensive ocular changes in combination with an unremarkable diagnostic evaluation. Studies suggest that, in cats, approximately 20% of hypertensive cases may be idiopathic (Elliott *et al.*, 2003). Reports of idiopathic hypertension in dogs are rare. With systemic hypertension and no biochemical evidence of persistently elevated plasma creatinine, care must be taken in interpreting a seemingly reduced urine concentrating ability (urine specific gravity (USG) <1.030). In certain situations, such as hypertension-induced pressure diuresis, a USG <1.030 does not imply that kidney disease is present.

'White coat' hypertension

'White coat' hypertension is a physiological response to the clinic situation where SBP measurements are transiently elevated due to activation of the sympathetic nervous system by anxiety or excitement. It can be difficult to distinguish 'white coat' hypertension from idiopathic hypertension, as it is unpredictable and varies widely between individuals.

'White coat' hypertension can be minimized by ensuring an adequate acclimatization period. However, there may be huge variability in response of BP to the clinic situation, and the demeanour of the cat or dog can be an unreliable predictor of fluctuations in BP. A diagnosis of 'white coat' hypertension should only be made where:

- High BP measurements have been recorded on multiple occasions in the absence of clinical signs
- There is no evidence of TOD or underlying disease conditions
- The individual is considered to be at low risk of systemic hypertension
- The clinician is sufficiently convinced that the elevation in BP can be attributed to the clinic situation.

In human patients 24-hour BP measurement is used to confirm a diagnosis of 'white coat' hypertension. Whilst this is not feasible in most clinical veterinary situations, it may be possible to measure BP in more comfortable surroundings to which the animal has been habituated. There is some evidence that human patients with 'white coat' hypertension demonstrate more labile BP and may actually be at increased risk for the development of hypertensive TOD. However, to date there is no indication in veterinary medicine that animals with 'white coat'

hypertension should be treated, although longitudinal intermittent monitoring of BP and animals should be monitored for disease processes that cause secondary hypertension.

Indications for measuring blood pressure

Blood pressure should be measured in patients presenting with evidence of TOD that may be associated with hypertension (e.g. LVH, gallop rhythms, arrhythmias, systolic murmurs). It should always be assessed in cases presenting with ocular changes (e.g. sudden-onset blindness, retinal detachment, hyphaema, retinal haemorrhage), neurological signs (e.g. seizures, altered mentation, ataxia, focal neurological deficits) or epistaxis which could represent severe hypertensive vascular damage and which would indicate that immediate antihypertensive treatment is required.

Routine evaluation of SBP should be performed in patients that have been diagnosed with clinical conditions that are associated with secondary hypertension (see Figure 27.2). Even if a patient is initially considered normotensive, continued monitoring may be required since hypertension that develops in hyperadrenocorticism does not necessarily resolve with treatment, and BP in hyperthyroidism may increase following successful treatment.

Assessment of BP should also be performed if clinical manifestations of hypertensive TOD are suspected following the administration of therapeutic agents that may increase BP. However, it should also be appreciated that the clinical signs of hypertension can be minimal and TOD incipient. An astute owner may report vague behavioural changes and in such cases BP measurement should be considered.

Routine monitoring of BP is advocated for geriatric cats and dogs (>9 years) as many of the disease conditions that have been associated with secondary hypertension are most prevalent in this age group (Brown *et al.*, 2007).

Diagnosis of systemic hypertension

In both dogs and cats the diagnosis of hypertension should be made in light of the clinical status of the patient, considering the following factors:

- Method used for BP measurement
- Historical and physical examination findings and results of a minimum diagnostic work up (Figure 27.5)
- Concurrent disease conditions
- Current medications being administered
- Hydration status/fluid therapy administration
- Attitude and temperament of patient in the clinic situation
- Age – Small increases of 1–3 mmHg/year have been demonstrated in dogs in some but not all studies. Similarly some studies in cats suggest an age-related increase in BP while others show no effect of age. However, most cats diagnosed with hypertension and TOD are >10 years

Minimum diagnostic work up
Full history
Physical examination
Blood pressure measurement
Ophthalmological examination
Biochemistry
Packed cell volume
Urinalysis including measurement of specific gravity, dipstick analysis and sediment examination

Additional diagnostic tests
Haematology
Assessment for hyperthyroidism (Total T4 concentration) [a] (cats)
Quantification of proteinuria, e.g. urine protein to creatinine ratio or assessment of microalbuminuria
Assessment for hyperadrenocorticism [a] (dogs)
Assessment for hypothyroidism [a] (dogs)
Abdominal ultrasonography with particular reference to kidney and adrenal gland
Urinary and plasma aldosterone concentration [a]

27.5 Minimum and extended diagnostic work up for the evaluation of cases of systemic hypertension. [a] These tests should be considered where there is clinical evidence or suspicion of underlying disease process.

- Gender – There is some evidence that male dogs may have slightly higher (<10 mmHg) and entire females lower BP. There is no evidence for gender association in cats
- Breed – Sight-hounds (e.g. Greyhounds), can have systemic pressure 10–20 mmHg higher than other breeds. The exception to this rule is the Irish Wolfhound, which reportedly has low systemic pressures compared with other sight-hounds. Currently no breed predispositions have been established in cats
- Obesity – Possible association of hypertension with obesity reported in the dog but no evidence for this in the cat.

Risk levels
Guidelines were recently formulated by the American College of Veterinary Internal Medicine (ACVIM) hypertension consensus panel; an international group of clinicians working in the hypertension field (Brown *et al.*, 2007). These recommendations consider SBP and DBP as continuous variables and categorize them in terms of the risk of development or progression of TOD. Broadly they indicate that, for both cats and dogs, the risk of hypertensive TOD increases at SBP >160 mmHg and DBP >95 mmHg, and, if persistent, may require antihypertensive intervention. However, it should be appreciated that these guidelines have yet to be validated by independent clinical studies.

The risk levels are:

- Minimal risk: BP <150/95 mmHg
- Mild risk: BP 150/95–159/99 mmHg
- Moderate risk: BP 160/100–179/119 mmHg
- Severe risk: BP >180/120 mmHg.

Minimal and mild risk
Patients in these categories have a minimal to mild risk of developing TOD. There is limited evidence that

antihypertensive medication is required with SBP <160 mmHg. Some patients in this category may be demonstrating 'white coat' hypertension. However, antihypertensive medication should be considered if ocular or central nervous system (CNS) TOD can be attributed to hypertension and other potential causes of the lesions have been excluded. Intermittent re-evaluation of BP should be performed in patients with evidence of TOD, in geriatric patients or those with clinical conditions that have been associated with secondary hypertension. This represents the ideal target for patients treated with antihypertensive drugs.

Moderate risk
Patients in this category have a moderate risk for the development or progression of TOD. Antihypertensive treatment is indicated for patients in this category where there is evidence of TOD or where concurrent clinical conditions that may be associated with the development of hypertension have been identified. Confirmation of category status should be made by performing BP measurements on at least two occasions, unless there is evidence of ocular or CNS TOD that requires immediate antihypertensive therapy. Patients with no evidence of TOD and no secondary disease associations, and where 'white coat' hypertension cannot be excluded, should be monitored further before a diagnosis of idiopathic hypertension is made and long-term antihypertensive medication instigated.

Severe risk
The risk of both developing TOD or of progression of pre-existing TOD is high where BP is >180/120 mmHg. 'White coat' hypertension is less commonly identified in this category. Evidence of ocular or neurological hypertensive TOD indicates a need for immediate antihypertensive medication. Otherwise, confirmation of BP status should be made by performing BP assessment on at least two occasions before starting antihypertensive treatment.

Treatment and management of systemic hypertension

The primary aim of antihypertensive medication should be a gradual persistent reduction in systemic pressures to a level at which severe hypertensive ocular or CNS damage is prevented and the effects of chronic vascular damage (e.g. kidney damage) and adaptive mechanisms (e.g. LVH) are minimized. Sudden fluctuations and precipitous drops in blood pressure should be avoided.

In human patients, BP goals are currently 140/85 mmHg but lower targets are recommended for patients with concurrent disease, e.g. chronic kidney disease (CKD) or diabetes mellitus (Williams *et al.*, 2004). No such disease-stratified guidelines currently exist in veterinary medicine, although the ACVIM guidelines now provide a framework for antihypertensive therapy. From current evidence a reasonable target of antihypertensive medication in both dogs and cats is to reduce SBP to <160 mmHg.

Figures 27.6 to 27.8 demonstrate suggested management protocols for starting antihypertensive therapy after a diagnosis of systemic hypertension for dogs and cats. BP should be re-evaluated 7–14 days after initiating or modifying antihypertensive treatment, or with any change in underlying disease status or concurrent medication.

Antihypertensive drugs

Antihypertensive agents (Figure 27.9) should be started at the lowest therapeutic dose. Failure of a single agent to reduce BP adequately should trigger either an increase in dosage of the primary agent or the addition of a second therapeutic agent in order to maintain SBP at <160 mmHg.

In human medicine multimodal antihypertensive medication is often advocated for the control of BP and proteinuria in hypertension associated with renal disease. Preliminary evidence suggests that the magnitude of proteinuria is inversely associated with survival in dogs and cats with hypertension but further clinical studies are necessary before treatment protocols based on both BP and proteinuria can be advocated.

Once BP has been stabilized, long-term monitoring every 2–3 months is usually adequate, provided that underlying disease conditions and other therapeutic regimes remain constant. Any underlying disease conditions that may be contributing to the increase in BP and pre-existing TOD (e.g. kidney or cardiovascular disease) should be identified and treated. Discontinuation of medications that may be elevating BP (e.g. phenylpropanolamine,

corticosteroids) should also be considered. Certain disease conditions may necessitate the use of specific therapies, such as the use of aldosterone antagonists (e.g. spironolactone) and surgical management for aldosterone-secreting adrenal tumours, and alpha-blockers (e.g. phenoxybenzamine), beta-blockers (e.g. atenolol) and surgical management for phaeochromocytomas (see Figure 27.9).

Other therapies

Disease- or target organ-specific therapies may lead to the complete or partial resolution of hypertension in some cases (e.g. hyperadrenocorticism) but more frequently additional antihypertensive medications will be required. One notable exception is feline hyperthyroidism, where the untreated hyperthyroid state is associated with hypertension in 9–23% of cases but a further 20% of cats may develop hypertension after successful treatment and return to euthyroidism (Stiles *et al.*, 1994; Syme, 2007).

Diet

Although widely discussed in human medicine, the evidence for salt-restricted diets in hypertensive dogs and cats is controversial and is unlikely to modify BP. Salt restriction may in fact lead to stimulation of the RAAS with detrimental effects on both the cardiovascular system and the kidney. In general, whilst high-salt diets should be avoided, there is limited evidence to instigate a salt-restricted diet. However, dietary therapy targeted at any underlying disease process (e.g. kidney disease) should be prescribed.

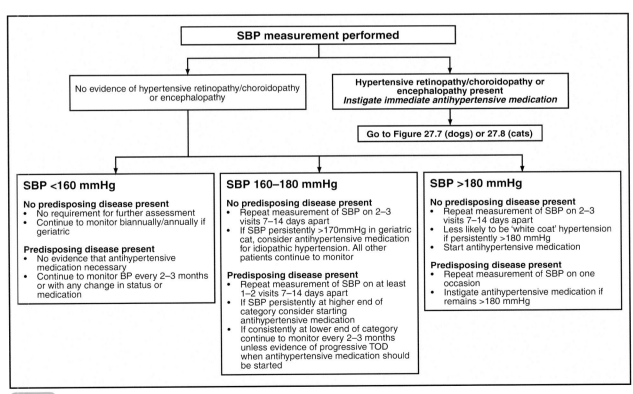

27.6 Protocol for the management of systemic hypertension in the cat and dog.

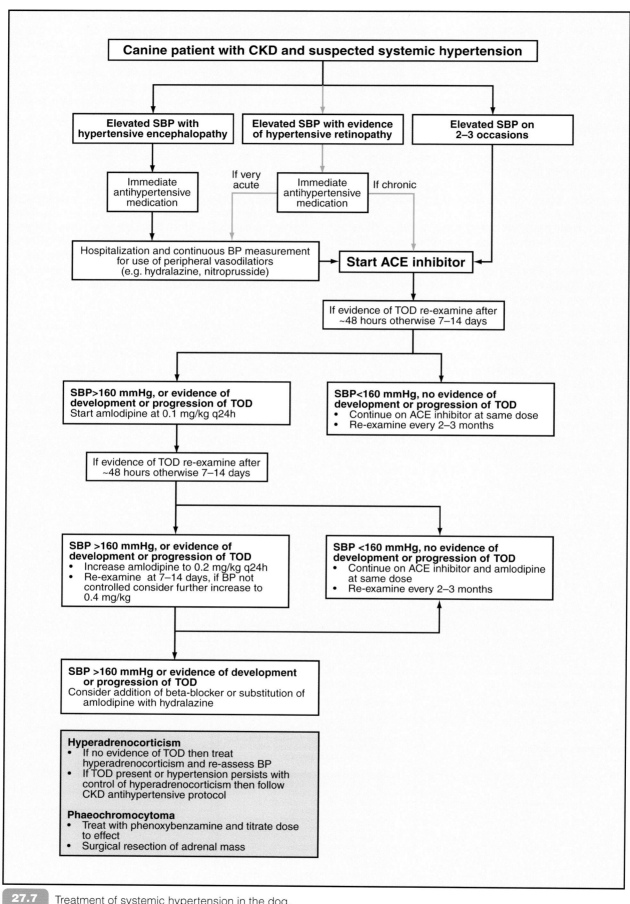

27.7 Treatment of systemic hypertension in the dog.

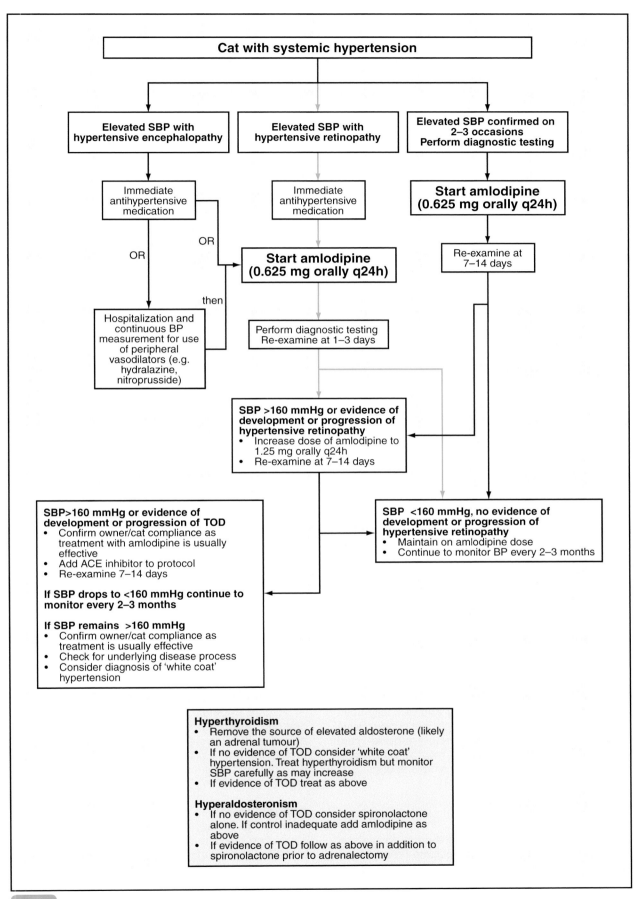

27.8 Treatment of systemic hypertension in the cat.

Antihypertensive medication	Dosage	Comments
Calcium-channel blocker		
Amlodipine	Cats: 0.625–1.25 mg/cat orally q24h Dogs: 0.1–0.4 mg/kg orally q24h	Primary antihypertensive agent for cats but usually second-line agent in dogs. In cats expect 30–50 mmHg decrease in SBP with adequate therapy
Angiotensin-converting enzyme inhibitors		
Benazepril	Cats: 0.5–1.0 mg/kg orally q24h Dogs: 0.25–0.5 mg/kg orally q24h	Primary antihypertensive agent in dogs but second-line therapy in cats. Care with administration if moderate to severe kidney disease or dehydration. Expect only small decline in SBP (5–10 mmHg), if any. Additional benefits/indication in cases of protein-losing nephropathy or concurrent LVH
Enalapril	Cats: 0.25–0.5 mg/kg orally q12–24h Dogs: 0.25–0.5 mg/kg orally q12–24h	
Beta-blockers		
Atenolol	Cats: 6.25–12.5 mg/cat orally q12–24h Dogs: 0.5–2 mg/kg orally q12h	Consider in cats with tachycardia and arrhythmia associated with hyperthyroidism. Limited antihypertensive effect reported
Propranolol	Cats: 2.5–5 mg/cat orally q8h Dogs: 0.2–1 mg/kg orally q8h	
Aldosterone antagonist		
Spironolactone	Cats/dogs: 2–4 mg/kg orally q24h	Consider with evidence of hypertension associated with primary hyperaldosteronism or in cats where combined antihypertensive therapy with other agents has failed
Direct peripheral vasodilators		
Hydralazine	Cats: 1.0–2.5 mg/cat s.c. has been used to treat severe hypertension after kidney transplantation due to its rapid onset of action (<15 min). Alternatively, 2.5–10 mg/cat orally q12h. Start at lowest dose, titrate to effect Dogs: 0.5–3 mg/kg orally q8–12h. Start at lowest dose, titrate to effect	Potent direct vasodilators with rapid-onset reduction in BP. Use both with extreme care. Should be used only in conjunction with continuous measurement of BP, ideally direct. Infusion device required for accurate administration of nitroprusside. Solution and infusion set require protection from light
Nitroprusside	Cat/dog: 0.5–5µg/kg/min given as a continuous i.v. infusion. Start at lowest dose and titrate to effect	
Alpha-blocker		
Phenoxybenzamine	Variable and unpredictable effect. Start at 0.25 mg/kg orally q12h and gradually up-titrate dose towards 2.5 mg/kg orally q12h; do not increase further if clinical signs of hypotension seen (e.g. lethargy, weakness, syncope) or adverse reactions (e.g. vomiting) develop or until maximal dose is reached (2.5 mg/kg orally q12h)	Primarily used in the chronic and presurgical management of phaeochromocytoma in dogs. Other alpha-blockers are also available

27.9 Medications commonly used to treat hypertension in dogs and cats.

Client education

Clients should be educated to ensure that they understand the underlying principles of antihypertensive treatment and the necessity for lifelong medication for the prevention of TOD, particularly as these benefits may not be immediately and clinically obvious. In an ideal situation a single antihypertensive agent administered once daily would provide good long-term BP control. Whilst this may be possible in cats, control of SBP is rarely that simple in dogs.

Cats

Amlodipine

The first line in antihypertensive therapy for cats is the calcium-channel blocker amlodipine (see Figures 27.8 and 27.9). Both clinical and experimental studies have demonstrated that amlodipine is a well tolerated and extremely efficacious antihypertensive agent with a therapeutic action of at least 24 hours in

cats. Reductions in SBP of 30–50 mmHg can be expected with amlodipine monotherapy, but an increase in dose (from 0.625 mg to 1.25 mg q24h) is likely to be required in approximately 50% of cats (Jepson *et al.*, 2007).

Recent evidence suggests that amlodipine therapy can result in a significant decline in proteinuria as well as SBP in cats that are considered borderline proteinuric (urine protein (UP) to creatinine (C) ratio 0.2–0.4) or proteinuric (UP:C > 0.4) (Elliott, 2007; Jepson *et al.*, 2007).

ACE inhibitors

Second-line therapy in cats is often an angiotensin-converting enzyme (ACE) inhibitor (see Figures 27.8 and 27.9) but this class of drug has limited antihypertensive action in the cat and decreases of only ~5–10 mmHg should be expected. Activation of the RAAS would suggest a useful role for combination therapy with either an ACE inhibitor or angiotensin receptor blocker (ARB) in hypertensive cats with evidence of kidney disease. However, a small placebo-controlled study failed to show any significant benefit on BP or proteinuria with the combined administration of amlodipine and benazepril (Elliott *et al.*, 2004) over the use of amlodipine monotherapy.

Care should be taken with the administration of ACE inhibitors to cats with moderate to severe CKD and dehydration, where a sudden decline in GFR may be detrimental, resulting in a rapid decline in renal function and increase in serum creatinine. In cats with uncontrolled hyperthyroidism, beta adrenergic receptor blockers (e.g. atenolol) may be useful but are unlikely to reduce SBP dramatically.

Dogs

ACE inhibitors

In dogs with hypertension secondary to CKD, an ACE inhibitor is usually the first line of treatment although efficacy is variable (see Figures 27.7 and 27.9). There is evidence that ACE inhibitors have additional benefits in the treatment of canine hypertension associated with CKD where preferential reduction in efferent renal arteriolar tone may reduce glomerular pressures and contribute to a reduction in proteinuria (Grauer *et al.*, 2000; Brown *et al.*, 2003). These benefits are likely to be most evident in patients with glomerular disease. ACE inhibitors may help limit the adverse cardiovascular and renal effects of angiotensin II and aldosterone.

Care must be taken when administering ACE inhibitors to dogs with evidence of moderate to severe CKD and where dehydration is suspected, because efferent arteriolar vasodilatation may lead to an effective reduction in GFR and exacerbation of azotaemia.

Combined therapies

Amlodipine is often added to the regime if monotherapy with ACE inhibitors does not adequately reduce SBP. Beta-blockers, hydralazine or aldosterone antagonists may be added if combined ACE inhibitor and amlodipine therapy is ineffective. The use of diuretic agents is rarely indicated. Great care should be taken when combining multiple therapeutic agents to ensure that hypotension (SBP <120 mmHg) does not occur. Owner and patient compliance in administering tablets should always be confirmed before additional medications are introduced.

Treatment protocols for hypertension in secondary disease processes other than CKD are suggested in Figure 27.7.

Emergency therapy

Patients with hypertensive retinopathy/choroidopathy or encephalopathy are candidates for more immediate and aggressive antihypertensive therapy. Various parenteral antihypertensive agents with a rapid onset of action are available (e.g. nitroprusside; see Figure 27.9). However, hospitalization is essential with the use of such agents, which should be restricted to situations where continuous BP monitoring is available (preferably by direct arterial catheterization), or at least an intensive care environment that allows frequent BP assessment.

In cats presenting with hypertensive retinopathy/choroidopathy, immediate treatment with oral amlodipine is usually sufficient to reduce SBP substantially and to prevent exacerbation of TOD. In such cases hospitalization is not an absolute requirement but SBP and efficacy of treatment should be reassessed sooner than in patients without such lesions (see Figures 27.7 and 27.8).

References and further reading

Brown SA, Atkins CE, Bagley R *et al.* (2007) Guidelines for the identification, evaluation and management of systemic hypertension in dogs and cats. *Journal of Veterinary Internal Medicine* **21**, 542–558

Brown SA, Brown CA and Hendi R (2000) Does systemic hypertension damage the canine kidney? (abstract). *Journal of Veterinary Internal Medicine* **14**, 351

Brown SA, Finco DR, Brown CA *et al.* (2003) Evaluation of the effects of inhibition of angiotensin converting enzyme with enalapril in dogs with induced chronic renal insufficiency. *American Journal of Veterinary Research* **64**, 321–327

Chetboul V, Lefebvre HP, Pinhas C *et al.* (2003) Spontaneous feline hypertension: clinical and echocardiographic abnormalities and survival rate. *Journal of Veterinary Internal Medicine* **17**, 89–95

Cortadellas O, del Palacio MJ, Bayon A, Albert A and Talavera J (2006) Systemic hypertension in dogs with leishmaniasis: prevalence and clinical consequences. *Journal of Veterinary Internal Medicine* **20**, 941–947

Elliott J (2007) Staging chronic kidney disease. In: *BSAVA Manual of Canine and Feline Nephrology and Urology, 2nd edn*, ed. J Elliott and GF Grauer, p. 159–166. BSAVA Publications, Gloucester

Elliott J, Fletcher M, Souttar K *et al.* (2004) Effect of concomitant amlodipine and benazepril therapy in the management of feline hypertension (abstract). *Journal of Veterinary Internal Medicine* **18**, 788

Elliott J, Fletcher M and Syme H (2003) Idiopathic feline hypertension: epidemiological study (abstract). *Journal of Veterinary Internal Medicine* **17**, 754

Grauer GF, Greco DS, Getzy DM *et al.* (2000) Effects of enalapril versus placebo as a treatment for canine idiopathic glomerulonephritis. *Journal of Veterinary Internal Medicine* **14**, 526–533

Henik RA, Stepien R and Bortnowski HB (2004) Spectrum of M-mode echocardiographic abnormalities in 75 cats with systemic hypertension. *Journal of the American Animal Hospital Association* **40**, 359–363

Jacob F, Polzin DJ, Osborne CA *et al.* (2003) Association between initial systolic blood pressure and risk of developing a uremic crisis or of dying in dogs with chronic renal failure. *Journal of the American Veterinary Medical Association* **222**, 322–329

Jepson RE, Elliott J, Brodbelt D and Syme H (2007) Evaluation of the effects of control of systolic blood pressure on survival in cats with systemic hypertension. *Journal of Veterinary Internal Medicine* **21**, 402–409

Maggio F, Defrancesco TC, Atkins CE *et al.* (2000) Ocular lesions associated with systemic hypertension in cats: 69 cases (1985–1998). *Journal of the American Veterinary Medical Association* **217**, 695–702

Mathur S, Brown CA, Dietrich UM *et al.* (2004) Evaluation of a technique of inducing hypertensive renal insufficiency in cats. *American Journal of Veterinary Research* **65**, 1006–1013

Sansom J, Barnett KC, Dunn KA, Smith KC and Dennis R (1994) Ocular disease associated with hypertension in 16 cats. *Journal of Small Animal Practice* **35**, 604–611

Snyder PS. Sadek D and Jones GL (2001) Effect of amlodipine on echocardiographic variables in cats with systemic hypertension. *Journal of Veterinary Internal Medicine* **15**, 52–56

Stiles J, Polzin DJ and Bistner DI (1994) The prevalence of retinopathy in cats with systemic hypertension and chronic renal failure or hyperthyroidsim. *Journal of the American Animal Hospital Association* **30**, 564–572

Syme HM (2007) Cardiovascular and renal manifestations of hyperthyroidism. *Veterinary Clinics of North America: Small Animal Practice* **37**, 723–743

Syme HM, Barber PJ, Markwell PJ and Elliott J (2002) Prevalence of systolic hypertension in cats with chronic renal failure at initial evaluation. *Journal of the American Veterinary Medical Association* **220**, 1799–1804

Williams B, Poulter NR, Brown MJ *et al.* (2004) British Hypertension Society guidelines for hypertension management 2004 (BHS-IV) summary. *British Medical Journal* **328**, 634–640

28

Pulmonary hypertension

Lynelle R. Johnson

Introduction

Pulmonary hypertension (PH) is defined by a systolic pulmonary artery pressure exceeding 32 (or up to 45) mmHg, or a diastolic pressure that exceeds 20 mmHg (Berger *et al.*, 1985; Schober and Baade, 2006). The most recent clinical classification scheme for PH in human medicine utilizes pathophysiological characteristics and response to therapy (McLaughlin *et al.*, 2009). This scheme defines the following:

- Pulmonary arterial hypertension
- PH with left heart disease
- PH associated with lung diseases and/or hypoxaemia
- PH due to thrombotic and/or embolic disease.

This classification replaces the previous designation of primary *versus* secondary PH. Application of the new classification to two retrospective studies of PH in dogs (Johnson *et al.*, 1999; Pyle *et al.*, 2004) reveals that the most common is PH with left heart disease, while the second most common is PH associated with lung diseases and/or hypoxaemia (Figure 28.1). Primary (idiopathic) pulmonary arterial hypertension has been reported in dogs (Glaus *et al.*, 2004; Zabka *et al.*, 2006) but is the least likely. PH as a complication of cardiopulmonary disease seems to be reported more commonly in dogs than in cats.

Physiology

In the normal dog and cat, pulmonary circulatory pressures are maintained at a level much lower than systemic pressures, in order to reduce the workload on the thin-walled right ventricle. Normal systolic pulmonary artery (PA) pressure is 15–25 mmHg, end-diastolic PA pressure is 5–10 mmHg, and the mean PA pressure is 10–15 mmHg.

Local pulmonary blood flow is controlled by the partial pressure of oxygen in the alveolus through hypoxic pulmonary vasoconstriction (HPV), and more globally by the balance of endothelium-derived vasoconstrictors and vasodilators. The most potent vasoconstrictor is endothelin-1; thromboxane A2 and superoxide also mediate vasoconstriction. Vasodilators produced by the endothelium include nitric oxide and prostacyclin. Release and activity of these vasoreactive mediators are altered in disease states, and imbalance among the various mediators can initiate or perpetuate a rise in PA pressure.

History and physical examination

Dogs or cats with PH can be of any age, sex or breed, depending on the underlying aetiology of elevated pulmonary artery pressures. Presenting complaints are usually related to underlying cardiopulmonary disease. Acute or chronic respiratory disease (infectious pneumonia in the young animal, interstitial pneumonia or tracheobronchial disease in the older animal) and congestive heart failure (CHF) are the most commonly identified disorders. Therefore, animals can display any combination of signs, including lethargy, weakness, cough, respiratory distress, tachypnoea, abdominal distension and collapse. Syncope in a dog with cardiopulmonary disease should prompt consideration of PH as a complication of disease (see Chapter 3).

Pathophysiology	Veterinary conditions	Johnson (1999)	Pyle *et al.* (2004)	Total
Pulmonary arterial hypertension	Congenital left-to-right shunts; idiopathic	2/53	1/54	3/107 (3%)
Pulmonary hypertension with left heart disease	Mitral valve disease; dilated cardiomyopathy; hypertrophic cardiomyopathy	23/53	24/54	47/107 (44%)
Pulmonary hypertension associated with lung diseases and/or hypoxaemia	Idiopathic pulmonary fibrosis; chronic tracheobronchial disease; interstitial fibrosis or pneumonia	12/53	21/54	33/107 (31%)
Pulmonary hypertension due to chronic thrombotic and/or embolic disease	Pulmonary thromboembolism; *Dirofilaria immitis*; *Angiostrongylus vasorum*; pulmonary endarteritis	11/53	5/54	16/107 (15%)
Miscellaneous	Pulmonary venous obstruction (e.g. by tumours), other	5/53	3/54	8/107 (8%)

28.1 Current classification of pulmonary hypertension.

Animals with PH generally display signs typical of the underlying aetiology:

- Tachypnoea and fine crackles are anticipated in an animal with pulmonary oedema associated with heart failure
- Harsher crackles, wheezes and abdominal effort on expiration suggest chronic tracheobronchial disease
- A systolic heart murmur due to mitral or tricuspid regurgitation is found in the majority (up to 83%) of dogs (Johnson *et al.*, 1999; Pyle *et al.*, 2004)
- A very loud or split-second heart sound resulting from high pulmonary artery pressure might also be detected
- Animals that develop right heart failure will display jugular venous distention, ascites, or rarely, subcutaneous oedema.

Diagnosis

Clinical pathology

Basic laboratory tests generally reflect the underlying disease and do not add to the diagnosis of PH. Neutrophilia associated with a stress response could be anticipated, while a biochemistry profile may show elevated liver leakage enzymes, suggestive of a hypoxic insult to the liver or right-sided CHF.

Tests to determine the severity of gas exchange abnormalities should be performed. Haemoglobin saturation determined through pulse oximetry is reflected by the peripheral oxygen saturation (S_pO_2) and is related to oxygen content by a sigmoidal relationship, with values >95% indicating normoxaemia. Below 95–96%, values for S_pO_2 lie on the exponential part of the curve, and small changes in S_pO_2 reflect very large changes in arterial oxygen concentration. Thus, pulse oximetry provides only a crude estimate of lung function, and values <95% indicate the need to perform an arterial blood gas for more accurate assessment of arterial oxygenation. An arterial blood gas analysis can also be used to follow response to therapy (see Chapter 12).

In addition, it should be noted that PH can be a cause for elevated plasma B-type natriuretic peptide (BNP) concentrations (DeFrancesco *et al.*, 2007).

Thoracic radiography

Thoracic radiographs are typically abnormal in dogs with moderate to severe PH and demonstrate right ventricular enlargement or generalized cardiomegaly, as well as enlarged pulmonary arteries and any underlying cardiac or respiratory disease (Figure 28.2).

Mild PH may not result in detectable radiographic abnormalities, apart from any underlying cardiac or respiratory disease. Radiographic abnormalities associated with the cardiac silhouette are usually more obvious in dogs than in cats, although large pulmonary arteries in the cat should prompt consideration of PH or heartworm disease. Pulmonary infiltrative patterns reflect the underlying disease process, and pleural effusion can be present if cor pulmonale develops or if concurrent pulmonary thromboembolism is present.

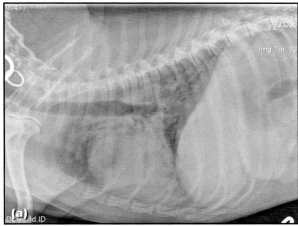
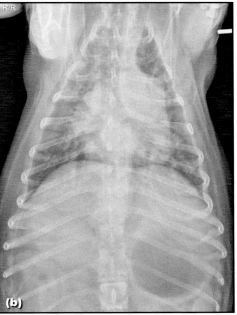

28.2 Radiographs of a 10-year-old Boston Terrier with pulmonary hypertension due to chronic tracheobronchial disease. **(a)** The lateral radiograph demonstrates increased sternal contact due to right ventricular enlargement. **(b)** The dorsoventral radiograph reveals rounding of the right heart and an enlarged main pulmonary artery. The pulmonary infiltrative pattern obscures visualization of the pulmonary arteries.

Electrocardiography

Reported electrocardiogram (ECG) abnormalities with right ventricular enlargement include deep S waves in leads II and aVF, and a right axis deviation. Right atrial enlargement is supported by tall or peaked P waves, but ECG evaluation of right heart enlargement is insensitive and abnormalities may not develop unless severe right ventricular enlargement is present. The ECG should be examined for rhythm disturbances (particularly in animals presenting with syncope); however, sinus tachycardia is a common rhythm finding.

Echocardiography

Two-dimensional echocardiography can provide subjective evidence of PH. Pulmonic stenosis must be ruled out at the beginning of the examination by visualizing a normal pulmonary valvular structure, right ventricular outflow tract and PA velocities with spectral Doppler. Subjective evidence of PH and right ventricular overload includes:

- Right ventricular dilatation with or without concentric hypertrophy
- Dilatation of the main pulmonary artery and branches
- Systolic flattening of the interventricular septum
- Paradoxical septal motion.

Doppler echocardiography can be used to estimate pulmonary artery pressure when tricuspid or pulmonic regurgitation is present (Berger *et al.*, 1985). Right ventricular systolic pressure equals pulmonary artery systolic pressure and is approximated by the right ventricular to right atrial pressure gradient (see Chapter 11). Application of the modified Bernoulli equation (pressure gradient = $4 \times$ velocity^2) to the velocity of a tricuspid regurgitant jet provides a reasonably accurate estimate of the right ventricular to right atrial pressure gradient, which correlates with right ventricular systolic pressure (Figure 28.3).

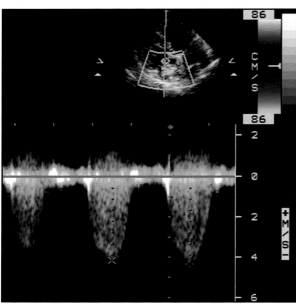

28.3 Doppler echocardiography reveals a regurgitant velocity across the tricuspid valve of 4.2 m/s, which correlates with a right ventricular to right atrial pressure gradient of 71 mmHg.

A closer estimate of systolic pulmonary artery pressure can be obtained by addition of right atrial pressure to the Doppler-derived pressure gradient:

- In the animal without right heart failure, right atrial pressure is estimated at 5 mmHg
- The animal in heart failure is expected to have an approximate right atrial pressure of 10–15 mmHg.

Pulmonary artery diastolic pressure is estimated by measurement of the pulmonic insufficiency velocity and calculation of the pressure gradient between the pulmonary artery and right ventricle. Therefore, PH is documented by a tricuspid regurgitant jet >2.8 m/s or a pulmonic insufficiency jet >2.2 m/s.

One drawback of Doppler assessment of PA pressure is that it requires the detection of a velocity jet of tricuspid or pulmonic regurgitation, and this may not be present or reliably measured in every animal with PH. Recently, Doppler-derived systolic time intervals of pulmonary artery flow have been evaluated as a means for documenting PH in dogs that lack a detectable regurgitant jet on the right side of the heart. Reduced acceleration time and the ratio of acceleration time to ejection time could be documented in dogs with PH associated with chronic pulmonary disease, and a good correlation with the Doppler-derived pressure gradient has been reported (Schober and Baade, 2006).

Tissue Doppler imaging, which can quantitate regional myocardial movement, has also been evaluated as a means to predict pulmonary hypertension, and multiple variables correlated with echo-Doppler estimates of systolic PA pressure (Serres *et al.*, 2007). There are as yet no firm guidelines for the use of these indices for the reliable detection of PH in patients without tricuspid or pulmonic regurgitation.

Treatment

Therapy for PH has not been well defined in veterinary medicine. Standard treatment of the underlying cardiopulmonary condition may lessen PH, and such therapy should be aggressively instituted on diagnosis (see Chapters 18, 19 and 30).

Drugs that mimic the effects of endothelium-derived vasodilators have been investigated. Sildenafil is a phosphodiesterase type V (PDE-5) inhibitor that increases concentrations of cyclic GMP in vascular smooth muscle cells, resulting in pulmonary vasodilation. Two retrospective studies evaluated the use of sildenafil in dogs with naturally occurring PH (Bach *et al.*, 2006; Kellum and Stepien, 2007); both described clinical improvements and better quality of life, but only one study (Bach *et al.*, 2006) reported lowering of pulmonary arterial pressures. Neither study compared treated with untreated groups to determine whether the effects observed were the result of the drug, natural disease variability, or placebo effect. Reported doses range from 0.5 mg to 2.5 mg/kg orally q8–24h, but additional studies are required to determine appropriate dosing regimens. Sildenafil therapy can result in systemic hypotension and clinical monitoring is required.

Tadalafil, a longer-acting PDE-5 inhibitor, has also been used in management of PH in dogs (Serres *et al.*, 2006). Little information is available on use of PDE-5 inhibitors in cats with PH.

Adjunctive therapy with other phosphodiesterase inhibitors could be considered for their different effects within the respiratory tract. Caution is recommended to avoid unwanted side effects when combining these drugs with sildenafil, though anecdotally few problems have been seen. Pentoxifylline may reduce blood viscosity, improving capillary blood flow and delivery of nitric oxide. Theophylline is purported to improve global cardiac function through pulmonary vasodilatory effects and might be indicated for concurrent treatment of an airway disorder.

Anticoagulants might be useful in treatment of dogs with PH through reduction of *in situ* thrombosis, progressive vascular occlusion and proliferative vascular disease. The utility of this therapy in dogs is unclear, but low-dose aspirin therapy can be employed at 1–3 mg/kg orally q12h. Alternatively, heparin or low-molecular-weight heparin could be considered.

Other management strategies used in human pulmonary arterial hypertension patients, but not yet reported in dogs or cats, include intravenous prostanoids and endothelin receptor antagonists (McLaughlin *et al.*, 2009).

Prognosis

It is unclear whether the development of PH in conjunction with a primary cardiopulmonary disease results in a worsened prognosis. Clinically, it seems that dogs with sustained and severe elevations of pulmonary artery pressure do not have as good a prognosis as dogs without PH, but the severity of PH was not associated with outcome in an early study (Johnson *et al.*, 1999). Certainly, documentation of PH would suggest a need for more intensive therapy and more frequent monitoring. Development of right-sided heart failure in association with PH would necessitate further therapeutic considerations (see Chapter 18).

References and further reading

Bach JF, Rozanski EA, MacGregor J *et al.* (2006) Retrospective evaluation of sildenafil citrate as a therapy for pulmonary hypertension in dogs. *Journal of Veterinary Internal Medicine* **20**, 1132–1135

Berger M, Hamowitz A, VanTosh A *et al.* (1985) Quantitative assessment of pulmonary hypertension in patients with tricuspid regurgitation using continuous wave Doppler ultrasound. *Journal of the American College of Cardiology* **6**, 359–365

DeFrancesco TC, Rush JE, Rozanski EA *et al.* (2007) Prospective clinical evaluation of an ELISA B-type natriuretic peptide assay in the diagnosis of congestive heart failure in dogs presenting with cough or dyspnea. *Journal of Veterinary Internal Medicine* **21**, 243–250

Glaus TM, Soldati G, Maurer R *et al.* (2004) Clinical and pathological characterisation of primary pulmonary hypertension in a dog. *Veterinary Record* **154**, 786–789

Johnson L (1999) Diagnosis of pulmonary hypertension. *Clinical Techniques in Small Animal Practice* **14**, 231–236

Johnson L, Boon J and Orton EC (1999) Clinical characteristics of 53 dogs with Doppler derived evidence of pulmonary hypertension: 1992–1996. *Journal of Veterinary Internal Medicine* **13**, 440–447

Kellum HB and Stepien RL (2007) Sildenafil citrate therapy in 22 dogs with pulmonary hypertension. *Journal of Veterinary Internal Medicine* **21**, 1258–1264

McLaughlin VV, Archer SL, Badesch DB *et al.* (2009) ACCF/AHA 2009 Expert Consensus Document on Pulmonary Hypertension: a report of the American College of Cardiology Foundation Task Force on Expert Consensus Documents and the American Heart Association: Developed in collaboration with the American College of Chest Physicians, American Thoracic Society, Inc., and the Pulmonary Hypertension Association. *Circulation* **119**, 2250–2294

Pyle RL, Abbott J and MacLean H (2004) Pulmonary hypertension and cardiovascular sequelae in 54 dogs. *International Journal of Applied Research in Veterinary Medicine* **2**, 99–109

Schober KE and Baade H (2006) Doppler echocardiographic prediction of pulmonary hypertension in West Highland White Terriers with chronic pulmonary disease. *Journal of Veterinary Internal Medicine* **20**, 912–920

Serres F, Chetboul V, Gouni V *et al.* (2007) Diagnostic value of echo-Doppler and tissue Doppler imaging in dogs with pulmonary arterial hypertension. *Journal of Veterinary Internal Medicine* **21**, 1280–1289

Serres F, Nicolle AP, Tissier R *et al.* (2006) Efficacy of oral tadalafil, a new long-acting phosphodiesterase-5 inhibitor, for the short-term treatment of pulmonary arterial hypertension in a dog. *Journal of Veterinary Medicine Series A – Physiology Pathology Clinical Medicine* **53**, 129–133

Zabka TS, Campbell FE and Wilson DW (2006) Pulmonary arteriopathy and idiopathic pulmonary arterial hypertension in six dogs. *Veterinary Pathology* **43**, 510–522

29

Laryngeal diseases

Richard A.S. White

Anatomy of the larynx

The larynx is a semi-rigid valve comprising three major and two smaller hyaline cartilages and striated muscles that separate the upper and lower respiratory tracts (Figure 29.1). The vocal ligaments in the lumen of the larynx extend from the vocal processes of the arytenoids to the ventral midline, and the vestibular ligaments extend from the cuneiform processes to the ventral midline (Figure 29.2). The larynx is lined with stratified mucosa, folds of which protrude into the lumen of the cylinder over these ligaments; these are the vocal and vestibular folds, respectively. The resultant crypts formed between the two folds are the laryngeal ventricles. The ventricles are absent in cats.

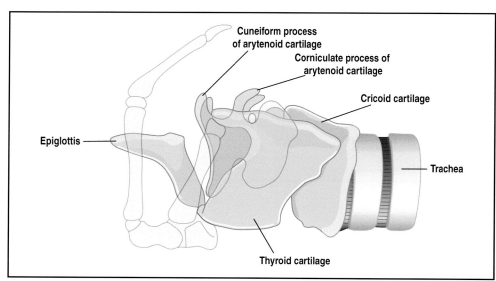

29.1 The cartilages of the canine larynx. (Redrawn after RAS White.)

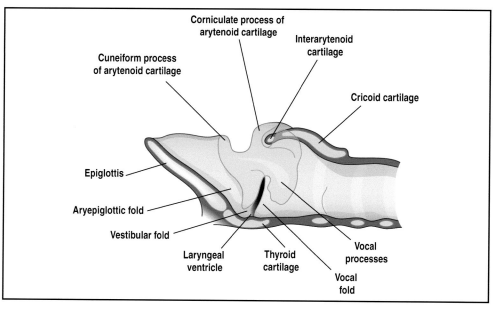

29.2 Sagittal section of the canine larynx. (Redrawn after RAS White.)

The larynx is innervated by the vagus via the cranial and caudal laryngeal nerves. The cranial laryngeal nerves are concerned primarily with sensory function and provide innervation to the mucosal lining of the larynx via internal branches. The caudal (recurrent) laryngeal nerves arise from the vagal branches at the thoracic inlet, the right looping behind the subclavian artery and the left behind the aorta before heading rostrally to the lateral surface of the larynx. The caudal laryngeal nerves provide motor innervation to all the intrinsic muscles of the larynx with the exception of the cricothyroid muscle and, most importantly, innervate the only dilator of the larynx, the dorsal cricoarytenoid muscle.

Laryngeal function

The larynx performs a valve-like role at the junction of the upper and lower respiratory tracts, and its major functions can be summarized as:

- Protection of the lower respiratory tract from inhalation of debris
- Control of airway diameter during the respiratory cycle
- Phonation.

Airway protection
Aspiration of oropharyngeal debris and foreign material into the larynx is prevented by a two-fold reflex mechanism:

- Firstly, during the swallowing phase the epiglottis hinges about its base and is 'flipped' backwards over the aditus to direct food upwards and over the larynx into the lateral food channels, thereby preventing aspiration. The epiglottis provides a tight seal at the level of the aryepiglottic fold, and the process occurs in conjunction with rostral movement of the larynx and caudal movement of the tongue.
- Secondly, glottic protection is provided by the intrinsic muscles of the larynx that adduct the vocal folds and arytenoid cartilages, thus sealing off the rima tightly during swallowing.

Control of airway diameter
Airway diameter is controlled by the position of the arytenoid cartilages and vocal folds. During the resting phase of the respiratory cycle, the arytenoids and vocal folds lie in a passive or 'neutral' midline position, such that the rima is a narrow slit. Contraction of the dorsal cricoarytenoid muscles during inspiration causes the arytenoids to rotate in a dorsolateral direction, dilating the rima to accommodate the inward flow of air. On expiration, the vocal folds move passively towards the midline. During prolonged or heavy exercise, the rima may remain dilated during both the inspiratory and expiratory phases to minimize resistance to air flow.

Phonation
Barking or meowing is a glottic function and is the result of vibration of the vocal folds as air flows over them. The tone and pitch of the bark or meow are determined by the speed and amplitude of the vibrations, which in turn are governed by air flow rate and the length of the vocal cords.

Diseases of the larynx

Laryngeal paralysis

Pathophysiology
Laryngeal paralysis is the failure of arytenoid and vocal fold movement during the respiratory cycle. Both adduction and abduction functions are usually impaired; however, it is the absence of abduction during inspiration that results in increased resistance to air flow through the larynx and in clinical signs. Air flow becomes turbulent due to increased resistance, which necessitates a higher flow rate through the rima, and due to movement of air over the fixed vocal fold(s). The concomitant reduction in intralaryngeal pressure may narrow the rima still further, contributing to additional flow resistance. This airway obstructive disease is encountered most commonly in dogs and is recognized in cats, although with considerably less frequency (Schachter and Norris, 2000).

Aetiology
Arytenoid dysfunction most often results from disease or damage to the innervation of the intrinsic muscles of the larynx. Much less frequently, it may occur as the result of disease or injury involving the dorsal cricoarytenoid muscles or the arytenoid cartilages. The aetiology of laryngeal paralysis in the cat is unclear, although it has been recorded as a consequence of a generalized neuropathy.

Idiopathic laryngeal paralysis: The majority of dogs affected by acquired laryngeal paralysis are grouped in this category. Some studies have suggested that this may be a manifestation of a more generalized neuromuscular disease, and the condition has been reported as part of a laryngeal paralysis–polyneuropathy (LPP) complex in which affected dogs exhibit signs of generalized neuropathy, including motor deficits of the rear limbs (Jeffrey *et al.*, 2006).

Demyelination and remyelination, and axonal degeneration involving the intrinsic laryngeal and appendicular peripheral nerves, have been recorded in dogs with idiopathic laryngeal paralysis (ILP). Although the suggestion that the condition may arise more frequently in hypothyroid dogs remains largely unsubstantiated (Jeffrey *et al.*, 2006), it may well be that there are a number of differing aetiologies underlying this particular presentation of the disease.

Despite the failure to identify a specific aetiology, the idiopathic form has well established epidemiological characteristics with a marked predisposition for medium to large breeds, including Labrador Retrievers, Afghan Hounds, Irish Setters and Pointers. Giant breeds are occasionally presented, whilst toy and miniature breeds are only rarely affected. Males are affected 2–3 times more frequently than bitches, and the average age of affected dogs is usually >10 years old.

Congenital: Laryngeal paralysis has been reported as an inherited congenital disease in the Bouvier des Flandres, Dalmatian, German Shepherd Dog, Leonberger, Pyreneen, Rottweiler and Siberian Husky. The disease is transmitted as an autosomal dominant trait in the Bouvier des Flandres (Venker van-Haagen *et al.*, 1981), affecting the male more frequently, and may be unilateral or bilateral. Degenerative changes are found both peripherally in the laryngeal nerves and centrally in the nucleus ambiguus. Selective breeding has now significantly reduced the incidence of this condition in Europe.

In the Dalmatian, the disease is transmitted as an autosomal recessive gene and affected dogs present at <6 months of age with a diffuse, generalized polyneuropathy distinct from that found in the Bouvier des Flandres and Siberian Husky (Braund *et al.*, 1994). Electromyographic abnormalities are present in the laryngeal, facial, oesophageal and distal appendicular muscles, and axonal degeneration affects the laryngeal and appendicular nerves. A significant number of these dogs also have megaoesophagus.

In the Leonberger, the mode of inheritance is X-linked and recessive with partial penetration (Shelton *et al.*, 2003); a possible autosomal recessive mode of inheritance has been postulated for the disease in Pyreneens (Gabriel *et al.*, 2006). A possible association between white coat colour and a heritable form of congenital laryngeal paralysis has been reported in juvenile German Shepherd Dogs (Ridyard *et al.*, 2000). Most dogs with congenital laryngeal paralysis are presented as young puppies and are rarely suitable for treatment.

Traumatic: Injuries to the neck or cranial thorax may bruise or even sever laryngeal innervation. Pharyngo-oesophageal trauma and 'big dog/little dog' confrontations, resulting in crush injuries to the cervical region, are probably the most important causes of this presentation.

Neoplastic: Tumour infiltration or impingement of the caudal laryngeal nerve may disrupt normal nerve conduction. Amongst the more common tumours causing this presentation are malignancies of the thyroid gland and cranial mediastinal masses such as lymphomas and thymomas.

Iatrogenic: Any surgical intervention in the cervical region or cranial thorax which involves dissection of the caudal laryngeal nerves may potentially result in temporary dysfunction or in permanent paralysis. The recent decline in the popularity of tracheal reconstruction procedures using external prostheses has reduced this presentation somewhat; the most notable procedure in this category is now resection of thyroid adenoma in the cat.

Clinical presentation

ILP typically has a prolonged and insidious course, and the onset of clinical signs may pre-date presentation by months or even years.

- *Inspiratory stridor* is the major and consistent finding in all patients and results from accelerated, turbulent air flow over fixed vocal folds. *Whistling inspiratory stridor* is a consistent presenting sign in cats with laryngeal paralysis (Schachter and Norris, 2000).
- *Exercise intolerance* occurs frequently, although this sign may be less obvious in some dogs that appear to limit their own exercise.
- *Cyanosis* is common, particularly during exercise; *syncope*, possibly progressing to asphyxiation, is seen in severely affected cases.
- *Dysphonia* (change in the character of the bark) is a very useful diagnostic finding, but is only present in approximately half of dogs with ILP.
- *Dysphagia or cough* whilst eating or drinking is occasionally encountered, although aspiration leading to lower respiratory infection and coughing is probably less common than previously suggested.

All clinical signs are exacerbated by exercise and a warm environment; therefore, many patients are presented during the summer months or, paradoxically, during the winter months if housed in a heated environment. Excitement, car travel, anxiety, stress and the presence of coexisting respiratory disease also tend to promote signs.

Diagnosis

Signalment: The presenting signalment often helps the clinician reach a presumptive diagnosis. For example, a 10 year-old male Labrador Retriever with a prolonged history of exercise intolerance and stridorous breathing should raise a significant index of suspicion for laryngeal paralysis.

Auscultation: The earliest signs of inspiratory stridor can be detected by careful auscultation over the larynx in the resting dog. The presence of any respiratory noise during the respiratory cycle is abnormal and deserves further investigation. This high-pitched, whistling respiratory noise becomes more audible with exercise, but care should be taken not to overstress the patient and precipitate an obstructive crisis merely for the purposes of diagnosis. Common signs in cats with laryngeal paralysis include respiratory difficulty, whistling stridor, dysphonia, weight loss and cough (Schachter and Norris, 2000).

Radiography: Thoracic radiographs should be taken to search for possible underlying causes (e.g. thoracic mass) and to determine whether aspiration pneumonia is present, which may temporarily preclude progression to the next diagnostic step.

Laryngoscopy: Laryngeal paralysis is the failure of dynamic function and hence a definitive diagnosis can only be made by observation. In most instances this is undertaken by laryngoscopy. In some dogs, it may be possible to inspect laryngeal function under sedation but in most, a light plane of anaesthesia is more satisfactory. A deep plane of anaesthesia will paralyse the intrinsic laryngeal muscles and remove all laryngeal movement, preventing a meaningful assessment of function. Laryngoscopy may also be performed via a transnasal approach (Radlinksy *et al.*, 2004). Although this can be performed in the sedated rather than unconscious patient, it does not appear to increase the accuracy of diagnosis.

Arytenoid abduction is reduced or absent during the inspiratory phase in dogs with laryngeal paralysis. Most patients with ILP are affected bilaterally; however, it is common for one side to be more severely affected than the other, resulting in asymmetrical abduction. Care should be exercised when evaluating arytenoid movement since paralysed vocal folds often show paradoxical movement (i.e. move apart passively due to the expiratory air flow). Therefore, it is essential that an assistant identifies each phase of the respiratory cycle whilst the larynx is observed. The use of doxapram hydrochloride at 1–2 mg/kg intravenously has been advocated to assist in recognizing abnormal function. In some dogs the mucosa overlying the corniculate process of the paralysed arytenoid cartilage(s) is hyperaemic due to the turbulent air flow over the mucosal surface (Figure 29.3).

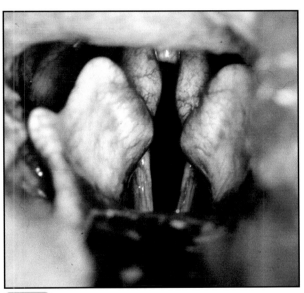

29.3 Oral view of a hyperaemic canine larynx.

Ultrasonography: Ultrasound examination of the larynx may be suitable for some dogs. Movement of the arytenoid and vocal folds during the respiratory cycle can be identified and allows laryngeal dysfunction to be recognized (Rudorf *et al.*, 2001). The non-invasive nature of echolaryngography and its application in non-sedated patients are useful advantages, although it does not appear to provide the same accuracy of diagnosis as laryngoscopy.

Electromyography, nerve conduction velocity studies and histological studies: These have been used to demonstrate abnormalities in the laryngeal and peripheral nerves and the intrinsic muscles. Although helpful in establishing the underlying pathological changes in some cases of laryngeal paralysis, they rarely contribute to the initial diagnostic steps.

Respiratory function measurements: Respiratory function measurements (e.g. blood gas analysis, tidal breathing flow volume loop) can provide objective confirmatory measurement of the pathophysiological consequences of laryngeal paralysis, but are rarely performed clinically.

Laryngeal eversion and collapse syndrome

Pathophysiology
Chronic respiratory diseases, resulting in turbulent air flow and abnormal negative pressures in the upper respiratory tract or abnormal cartilage, can initiate progressive degeneration within the upper airway that eventually results in obstruction of the rima. In early stages, the mucosal lining of the larynx and pharynx become oedematous and chronically thickened. This process also involves the mucosa within the laryngeal ventricle, and the saccules are everted into the ventral rima.

As the condition progresses, laryngeal cartilages begin to lose their rigidity and collapse towards the rima. The leading and lateral edges of the epiglottis roll inward and the cartilage folds dorsally towards the glottic opening. The weaker regions of the arytenoids, including the cuneiform processes, collapse medially drawing the corniculate processes with them (Figure 29.4). The rima is progressively narrowed by these processes and in the final stages is completely occluded.

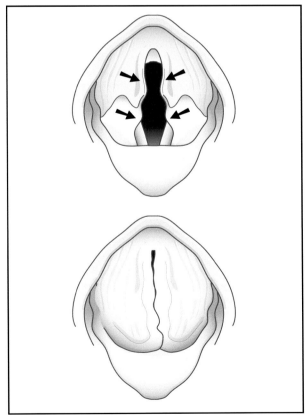

29.4 Laryngeal collapse. The rima is progressively obscured by the collapsing corniculate (upper arrows) and cuneiform (lower arrows) processes of the arytenoid cartilages. The epiglottis may also collapse towards the rima. (Redrawn after RAS White.)

The early changes involving the saccules and pharyngeal tissue are often reversible and may be resolved by prompt management of the underlying problem. However, changes involving the cartilages are more permanent and once clinically evident, laryngeal collapse is a difficult condition to manage.

Aetiology

Airway obstruction syndromes: The development of eversion/collapse is most often associated with concurrent upper airway obstruction. It is frequently encountered in brachycephalic dogs in which the abnormal nasal turbinates, stenotic nares and over large soft palate are responsible for upper airway turbulence. However, it is unclear whether the collapse is due to airway turbulence during the inspiratory phase or due to the presence of weak laryngeal cartilages. Eversion/collapse may also be encountered as a sequel to other obstructive airway conditions such as tracheal collapse and hypoplasia.

Congenital: Laryngeal collapse is seen as an infrequent presentation in English and Staffordshire Bull Terriers during the first year of life. There is some indication that a congenital cartilaginous anomaly, resulting in a weak, non-rigid larynx, may underlie the condition (Hedlund and Taboada, 2002; Torrez and Hunt, 2006).

Clinical presentation
Laryngeal collapse results in stridorous breathing and severely restricted exercise ability. In the brachycephalic dog, the onset of these signs is insidious and often difficult to differentiate from those caused by the remainder of the obstructive airway syndrome. Ongoing exercise intolerance following surgical management of the over large soft palate, tonsils and stenotic nostrils should alert the clinician to the possibility of degenerative laryngeal changes.

Diagnosis
Dogs with laryngeal collapse have severely obstructed upper airway function. Auscultation directly over the larynx should enable the stridorous turbulence to be detected, but in brachycephalic dogs it may be difficult to distinguish this from the accompanying stertor. Echolaryngography may be useful for identifying intralaryngeal changes without general anaesthesia. Laryngoscopy in mildly affected dogs will reveal the glistening pea-like, everted laryngeal saccules immediately in front of the vocal folds, whilst in more advanced cases the rima will be obscured by the inverting epiglottis and arytenoids.

Laryngeal trauma

Pathophysiology and aetiology
Laryngeal trauma is uncommon in small animals because of the relatively protected position of the larynx. External trauma may result from bite wounds and choke chain injuries. Occasionally, crush injuries from road accidents and foreign body perforation will fracture or dislocate the laryngeal cartilages and hyoid bones, resulting in obstruction of the airway. In addition, neurogenic damage (particularly with cervical bite wounds) may result in paralysis of the vocal folds. Internal trauma direct to the laryngeal mucosa, epiglottis and arytenoids can be seen with stick penetration injuries. In the acute phase of laryngeal trauma, the airway may be obstructed due to haemorrhage, oedema and dislocations or fractures of the cartilages. More long-term complications include fibrosis of the cartilage articulations and glottic stenosis due to development of intralaryngeal scar tissue.

Clinical presentation
Injuries involving the larynx are clinically evident due to obstruction of the airway. Patients may have laboured respiratory patterns, stridor, cyanosis and asphyxiating syncope. Occasionally, there may be subcutaneous emphysema due to air leaking into the perilaryngeal tissues.

Diagnosis
Inspection of the cervical region may reveal obvious penetrating wounds, or cervical swelling may be evident on palpation. Auscultation will reveal stridorous laryngeal sounds. Radiography may demonstrate hyoid fractures or variations in the normal relationship of the laryngeal cartilages. Air may be present in the perilaryngeal tissues. Laryngoscopy should be performed to assess the severity of airway obstruction and detect the presence of paralysis.

Laryngeal stenosis

Pathophysiology and aetiology
Disease or injury involving the mucosal lining of the larynx may result in the development of either scar tissue or proliferating granulation tissue that narrows the glottic opening. Intralaryngeal surgical interventions are particularly implicated in the development of scar tissue, and occasionally stenosis may result from traumatic endotracheal intubation. A proliferating granulomatous form of laryngitis has also been recorded as a cause of stenosis.

Clinical presentation
Dogs with laryngeal stenosis will have reduced exercise tolerance and stridorous breathing.

Diagnosis
Laryngeal auscultation will confirm the presence of stridor. Laryngoscopy allows inspection of the scar or proliferating tissue within the rima. Iatrogenic lesions most often involve the vocal fold sites whereas granulomatous lesions may affect the arytenoid cartilages. Histopathology is needed to differentiate inflammatory from neoplastic lesions.

Laryngeal neoplasia

Epidemiology and incidence
Tumours of the larynx are rare in the dog and cat but a variety of histological types have been reported. Benign tumours in the dog include chondroma, plasmacytoma and the previously termed oncocytoma; many of which have now been more accurately

redefined as rhabdomyoma on the basis of immuno-histochemical staining for myoglobin and desmin. Malignant forms include squamous cell carcinoma, lymphoma, adenocarcinoma and various sarcomas. Little is known of the epidemiology of tumours at this site, although lymphoma seems to be common in the cat. There is no apparent breed predilection, but males may be at greater risk. Secondary tumours or local extension of other primary tumours, most notably thyroid carcinomas, are occasionally seen.

Clinical presentation

Clinical signs result from upper airway obstruction and failure of laryngeal function, as is found with laryngeal paralysis. Early signs include respiratory stridor, exercise intolerance, dysphonia and hoarseness, dysphagia and cough. More advanced lesions cause serious respiratory obstruction with episodes of cyanosis and syncope.

Diagnosis

Auscultation over the laryngeal region may localize the source of the respiratory stridor, and echo-laryngography may permit needle aspirate biopsy. Radiography plays little role in the diagnosis of the primary tumour, but does allow a search for metastasis. Direct inspection under general anaesthesia is the primary means of confirming the presence of the lesion. This should be undertaken with great care since the upper airway may be obstructed to a considerable degree by the tumour, and preparation should be made to pass a narrow endotracheal tube or if necessary to perform tracheostomy intubation. Biopsy (e.g. grab, brush) should be performed with caution because of the risk of aspirating any resulting haemorrhage.

Treatment

For details on the treatment laryngeal diseases, see the *BSAVA Manual of Canine and Feline Head, Neck and Thoracic Surgery*.

References and further reading

Braund KG, Shores A, Cochrane S, Forrester D, Kwiecien JM and Steiss JE (1994) Laryngeal paralysis–polyneuropathy complex in young Dalmatians. *American Journal of Veterinary Research* **55**, 534–542

Gabriel A, Poncelet L, Van Ham L, Clercx C, Braund KG, Bhatti S, Detilleux J and Peeters D (2006) Laryngeal paralysis–polyneuropathy in young related Pyrenean mountain dogs. *Journal of Small Animal Practice* **47**, 144–149

Hedlund C and Taboada J (2002) *Clinical Atlas of Ear, Nose and Throat Diseases in Small Animals.* Schlutersche, Hannover

Jeffrey ND, Talbot CE, Smith PM and Bacon NJ (2006) Acquired idiopathic laryngeal paralysis as a prominent feature of generalised neuromuscular disease in 39 dogs. *Veterinary Record* **158(1)**, 17–20

Radlinksy MA, Mason DE and Hodgson D (2004) Transnasal laryngoscopy for the diagnosis of laryngeal paralysis in dogs. *Journal of the American Animal Hospital Association* **40**, 211–215

Ridyard AE, Corcoran BM, Tasker S, Willis R, Welsh EM, Demetriou JL and Griffiths LG (2000) Spontaneous laryngeal paralysis in four white-coated German Shepherd Dogs. *Journal of Small Animal Practice* **41**, 558–561

Rudorf H, Barr FJ and Lane JG (2001) The role of ultrasound in the assessment of laryngeal paralysis in the dog. *Veterinary Radiology and Ultrasound* **42**, 338–343

Schachter S and Norris CR (2000) Laryngeal paralysis in cats: 16 cases (1990–1999). *Journal of the American Veterinary Medical Association* **216**, 1100–1103

Shelton GD, Podell M, Poncelet L, Schatzberg S, Patterson E, Powell HC and Mizisin AP (2003) Inherited polyneuropathy in Leonberger dogs: a mixed or intermediate form of Charcot-Marie-Tooth disease? *Muscle Nerve* **27(4)**, 471–477

Torrez CV and Hunt GB (2006) Results of surgical correction of abnormalities associated with brachycephalic airway obstruction in dogs in Australia. *Journal of Small Animal Practice* **47**, 150–157

Venker van-Haagen AJ, Bouw J and Hartmann W (1981) Hereditary transmission of laryngeal paralysis in Bouviers. *Journal of the American Animal Hospital Association* **17**, 75–76

30

Canine tracheobronchial disease

Lynelle R. Johnson and Brendan C. McKiernan

Introduction

Chronic cough in the dog is most commonly related to: inflammation in the airways, resulting in mucus accumulation; and/or structural disease of the airways, caused by weakening of the cartilaginous support system. Chronic bronchitis is usually of unknown aetiology in the dog but may be related to environmental irritants. Airway collapse (also referred to as airway malacia) can affect the cervical trachea, intrathoracic trachea or primary bronchi, or a diffuse generalized collapse of small airways can be seen. In some cases, multiple abnormalities may be present that contribute to chronic or recurrent signs. Because many characteristics of the history, signalment and physical examination are similar in these disorders and because concurrent disease is common, a step-wise approach to diagnosis and therapy is required to provide optimal control of clinical signs.

Signalment

Dogs of any age can present with clinical signs related to tracheal disease. Dogs with airway collapse can show signs at a very young age that may resolve, remain static, or progress in severity over time. Because some dogs are puppies at the time of initial clinical presentation, investigators have theorized that weakness in the cartilage is an inherited or congenital defect. Histological studies have demonstrated lack of chondrocytes in cartilage from the cervical tracheal of affected dogs (Dallman et al., 1988), suggesting an error in metabolism. However, affected dogs can range from <1 to 15 years of age at the onset of signs, and it is likely that multiple factors play a role in the development of signs related to airway collapse.

Dogs with lower airway or bronchial collapse tend to be older when clinical signs worsen to the point where veterinary care is sought. Chronic bronchitis most commonly affects middle-aged to older dogs (>8 years of age) that appear relatively healthy other than the persistent cough. Chronic bronchitis has been defined in the dog as coughing for more than 2 months of the preceding year and not attributable to another disease process (Wheeldon et al., 1974).

Tracheal collapse is most commonly recognized in small or toy breeds, such as Chihuahua, Pomeranian, Toy and Miniature Poodles and Yorkshire Terrier.

While cervical tracheal collapse is diagnosed rarely in large breeds, chronic bronchitis with or without lower airway collapse is diagnosed frequently in retrievers, German Shepherd Dog, Dobermann and Sheltie or mix-breed larger dogs.

Presenting signs

Dogs with tracheobronchial disease are most commonly presented for evaluation of cough. Those with tracheal or bronchial collapse typically present with a dry 'honking' cough that may be paroxysmal in nature. Owners may describe vomiting, gagging, or retching in association with the cough. Signs commonly worsen after eating or drinking, with activity, or in hot or humid conditions. Intractable cough, respiratory distress, cyanosis or collapse can also be seen in dogs with airway collapse that become overly agitated or stressed.

Cough is the most common presenting complaint in dogs with chronic bronchitis. Many dogs have been coughing for years before presentation. To owners, the cough may sound harsh or productive. Over time, owners may also note exercise intolerance, marked expiratory effort or an abdominal push, or loud respiratory sounds. Cyanosis generally occurs late in disease; syncope may be a presenting complaint in severely affected animals that secondarily develop pulmonary hypertension.

Physical examination

Dogs with tracheobronchial disease are usually systemically well unless severe disease is present, or if disease is severe enough to result in hypoxaemia or cyanosis. Infection is not a common component of chronic airway disease, and body temperature will be normal unless the work of breathing or agitation results in hyperthermia. Heart rate is also generally normal, except during episodes of cough or excitement. Augmented vagal tone associated with respiratory disease can result in a slowing of the heart rate or an exaggerated sinus (respiratory) arrhythmia. Many dogs are obese because of lack of ability to exercise, and recent weight gain may be discovered as a cause for exacerbation of clinical signs.

A common feature in dogs with airway collapse or chronic bronchitis is the presence of increased tracheal sensitivity, which is a non-specific indicator of inflamed or irritated airways. This is detected by gently pinching or strumming the cervical trachea. Gentle palpation of the trachea will generally induce a severe cough in dogs with airway collapse, and caution is advised to avoid overstimulation of the cough response. Dogs with bronchitis will generally also cough readily on tracheal palpation, though paroxysms of coughing are less common.

Respiratory pattern
Respiratory rate and effort can be abnormal in dogs with chronic bronchitis, but dogs with tracheal collapse may appear relatively normal at rest. Chronic bronchitis is a disease of small airways. Mucus accumulation causing a reduction in airway diameter results in expiratory flow limitation. Dogs gradually develop prolonged expiratory time and expiratory effort. Animals that have intrathoracic airway collapse often have severe expiratory effort and will show an abdominal push during exhalation. In severe cases there may be a ballooning noted at the thoracic inlet as cranial lungs are 'herniated' into the cervical region (Guglielmini *et al.*, 2007).

Auscultation
Upper airway auscultation may reveal abnormalities in dogs with tracheobronchial disease due to inflammation or oedema of the larynx or eversion of laryngeal saccules. Dramatic stridor over the upper airway is suggestive of concurrent laryngeal paresis or paralysis, which has been reported in 30–60% of dogs with tracheal collapse (Tangner and Hobson, 1982; Buback *et al.*, 1996). Dogs with tracheal collapse often have musical or wheezing sounds on tracheal auscultation, due to turbulent airflow.

Pulmonary auscultation can be difficult, due to tachypnoea, obesity, referred upper airway sounds, or severe coughing. Lung sounds in dogs with cervical tracheal collapse are often normal, but dogs with lower airway collapse and chronic bronchitis generally have adventitious lung sounds. It is valuable to listen to the lungs both at rest and after induction of a cough, as the deep inspirations associated with coughing will augment lung sounds. Airway collapse of large intrathoracic airways may be associated with a snapping sound over the thorax at the end of expiration, when airways collapse and open rapidly with pressure equilibration along the airway. With generalized collapse of small airways, diffuse loud crackles can sometimes be heard during airway opening. Dogs with chronic bronchitis would be expected to display expiratory wheezes as airflow progresses from the alveoli to the mouth and passes through narrowed airways lined by mucus. Crackles can also be heard on either inspiration or expiration and are usually harsh or coarse.

Diagnosis

Tracheal collapse and chronic bronchitis are the most common causes of cough in the dog, and the diagnosis is generally suspected based on history, signalment and physical examination. Radiographs and airway sampling are required to confirm the diagnosis and, importantly, to exclude other diseases that can result in cough or to reveal concurrent disease syndromes. Infectious tracheobronchitis caused by *Bordetella* or *Mycoplasma* spp. causes similar clinical signs or may complicate either airway collapse or chronic bronchitis. Airway parasites such as *Filaroides hirthi* or *Oslerus osleri* may be found in specific geographical regions. Bronchiectasis (permanent dilatation of the airways) can develop as a sequel to chronic bronchitis and will complicate therapy.

Diagnostic testing will confirm the diagnosis, allowing for more accurate prognostication. Dogs with airway collapse usually have chronic, recurrent signs that require continual management or more aggressive intervention. Chronic bronchitis generally requires lifelong therapy with glucocorticoids with their attendant side effects. Therefore obtaining an accurate diagnosis in dogs with cough is most beneficial to the patient, client and attending veterinary surgeon.

Diagnostic imaging
Cervical and two- or (best) three-view thoracic radiographs should be obtained in dogs with chronic cough. When airway collapse is suspected, it is valuable to obtain dynamic radiographs during different phases of respiration. The cervical trachea collapses on inspiration and often balloons on expiration, while intrathoracic airways collapse on expiration and may balloon open on inspiration (Figure 30.1). In dogs with lower airway collapse, the principal bronchi may also be affected, but radiographs are relatively insensitive for detecting intrathoracic collapse. Inducing a cough during radiography may enhance the likelihood of making a diagnosis.

A recent comparison of radiography with fluoroscopy in the diagnosis of tracheal collapse presented encouraging results: most dogs with fluoroscopic evidence of collapse also had radiographically apparent collapse (Macready *et al.*, 2007). However, close inspection of the results revealed that the site of collapse determined by fluoroscopy matched the site visible radiographically in just over 50% of cases,

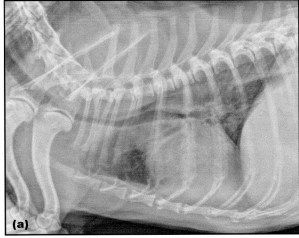

30.1 Lateral radiographs of dogs with tracheal collapse: **(a)** inspiratory film showing collapse at the thoracic inlet. (continues) ▶

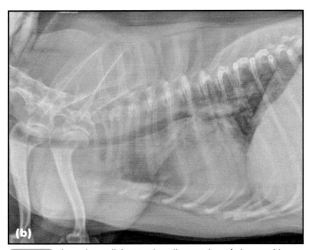

30.1 (continued) Lateral radiographs of dogs with tracheal collapse: **(b)** expiratory film showing collapse of the mainstem bronchus.

indicating that radiographs often result in an inaccurate diagnosis of tracheal/bronchial collapse. Also, radiographs were poor at identifying collapse of the carina and mainstem bronchi, which displayed a greater degree of collapse than the cervical trachea in affected dogs. Thus static radiography cannot provide a definitive diagnosis of tracheobronchial collapse or exclude it as a diagnosis.

Skyline radiography has been used in selected cases to document cervical tracheal collapse. This technique requires parallel alignment of the radiographic beam with the trachea. An X-ray machine with a moveable arm is required and the animal must be restrained manually to ensure perfect alignment. Because of these requirements, this view is rarely obtained clinically.

Cervical ultrasonography has also been reported as a means for documenting cervical tracheal collapse (Rudorf *et al.*, 1997). The cross-sectional beam allows delineation of deformed cartilage ring structures and of prolapse of the dorsal tracheal membrane into the tracheal lumen. This technique is difficult because of air interference with the ultrasound beam as it passes through the trachea. In addition, the intrathoracic trachea and mainstem bronchi cannot be imaged.

Thoracic radiography can be helpful in documenting bronchial or interstitial infiltrates consistent with chronic bronchitis, but findings are often subtle. In a case-controlled study, dogs with bronchitis shared many radiographic findings with age-matched healthy dogs, including interstitial bronchial calcification, or dilatation and interstitial infiltrates (Mantis *et al.*, 1998). Only visible airway walls and thickened airway walls were found significantly more commonly in dogs with bronchitis than in healthy dogs, indicating that radiographs have poor sensitivity for detection of airway pathology.

Pulmonary infiltrates may be difficult to distinguish in extremely obese dogs, due to superimposition of fat over the thorax and within the mediastinum. Ventrodorsal radiographs are helpful in documenting the degree of obesity. The depth of fat present between the thoracic cage and the skin should be noted for client communication on obesity control and for follow-up comparisons. Cautious interpretation of the cardiac silhouette is warranted in obese dogs with tracheal collapse or chronic bronchitis. Failure to obtain full inspiratory radiographs increases interstitial lung density. Hepatomegaly, fat in and around the heart and reduced lung volume in obese dogs can lead to the impression of cardiomegaly. This should be distinguished from right-sided heart enlargement that may be present in dogs with severe tracheal collapse, pulmonary disease, or other factors that predispose to the development of pulmonary hypertension.

Airway sampling

Airway sampling (see Chapter 10) should be performed in all dogs with chronic cough, to define the disease process more accurately. Laryngeal structure and function should be evaluated concurrently to detect upper airway disease. A transoral tracheal wash can be useful for sampling bronchial cytology and performing aerobic and *Mycoplasma* cultures. A transtracheal approach is rarely used in small breeds suspected of airway collapse, because trauma through tracheal puncture could exacerbate clinical signs. In addition, caution is warranted when anaesthetizing a dog with airway collapse, especially when the dog is obese and displays marked expiratory effort, because excitement during recovery from anaesthesia can worsen airway collapse, cough and hypoxaemia. A slow recovery from anaesthesia is advisable to minimize stress, and an oxygen-enriched environment should be available. One millilitre of 1% lidocaine sprayed into the distal trachea at the end of the procedure may help to decrease the cough reflex.

Airway cytology in dogs with tracheal or airway collapse is generally normal, but samples from dogs with chronic bronchitis demonstrate neutrophilic inflammation. Occasionally, samples will show primarily eosinophilic inflammation or a preponderance of lymphocytes, though the significance of this is unknown. To rule out infection, bacterial cultures are warranted in all animals with cough but it is rare for significant numbers or types of organisms to be obtained on culture (Peeters *et al.*, 2000; Johnson and Fales, 2001). Isolation of *Bordetella* or *Mycoplasma* spp. always warrants therapy; however, small numbers of aerobic bacteria can be isolated from many animals because the lower airway is not always sterile. True bacterial infection is characterized by significant growth of >1.7 × 10³ colony-forming units/ml on quantitative culture and septic, suppurative inflammation on cytology (Peeters *et al.*, 2000). In general, airway cultures reporting 'light' or '1+' bacterial growth should be interpreted cautiously, as these results may represent airway colonization rather than actual airway infection. Simultaneous cytology interpretation will help with the assessment.

Bronchoscopy

Bronchoscopy (see Chapter 10 for techniques) is sometimes required to document tracheal collapse when radiography or fluoroscopy are inconclusive.

Bronchoscopy also allows grading of the degree of tracheal ring flattening in dogs with airway collapse (Figure 30.2), documents protrusion of the dorsal tracheal membrane into the tracheal lumen, identifies mucosal inflammation or irregularity, defines the extent and location of tracheal collapse for possible surgical intervention, and confirms or rules out intrathoracic airway collapse (Figure 30.3). This tool can also provide both diagnostic and prognostic information in dogs with chronic bronchitis. Coughing dogs that do not have apparent radiographic evidence of disease

Grade I	The cartilage ring structure of the trachea remains circular and is almost normal. Slight protrusion of the dorsal tracheal membrane into the lumen reduces the diameter by < 25%
Grade II	Flattening of the tracheal cartilage leads to lengthening of the dorsal tracheal membrane and further reduces the luminal diameter to approximately 50%
Grade III	The tracheal cartilage rings are severely flattened and the trachealis muscle contacts the inner surface of the tracheal cartilage. The lumen is reduced by 75%
Grade IV	The trachealis muscle is collapsed on to the inner surface of the cartilage leading to complete obstruction of the lumen. A double lumen may be seen in some cases

30.2 Grades of tracheal collapse. (After Tangner and Hobson, 1982)

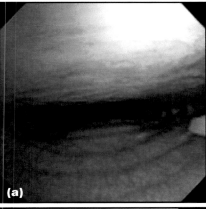
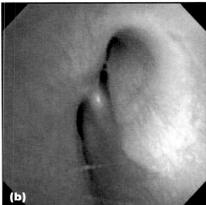

30.3 Bronchoscopic images from dogs with airway collapse. **(a)** Grade IV/IV cervical tracheal collapse. **(b)** There is 90% collapse of the bronchi to the left cranial lung lobe; the cranial and caudal segments are both collapsed.

will generally show obvious airway pathology on bronchoscopy, such as mucosal hyperaemia, increased mucus secretions, bronchitic nodules and irregular mucosa (Figure 30.4). When performed by an experienced endoscopist, bronchoscopy is the single best diagnostic test in these cases.

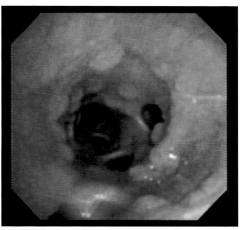

30.4 Bronchoscopic image of nodular and hyperaemic bronchitic epithelium.

Medical and surgical management

Airway collapse
Occasionally, dogs with tracheal collapse will present in an acute crisis of uncontrollable cough and respiratory distress. This is often associated with excessive excitement, heat, humidity or stress. In these situations, aggressive supportive care should be instituted and every effort made to minimize stress.

Placing the dog in a cool or temperature-controlled oxygen cage and limiting intervention will often resolve respiratory distress. Cough suppression and sedation can be achieved by using a combination of acepromazine (0.01–0.1 mg/kg) and butorphanol (0.05–0.1 mg/kg) given subcutaneously every 2–6 hours as needed. Over-sedation should be avoided to ensure that spontaneous respiration is maintained. Intubation of dogs with tracheal collapse can lead to worsening airway inflammation, activation of irritant receptors and loss of ventilatory drive. If needed, a short-acting steroid such as dexamethasone-SP (0.10–0.5 mg/kg i.v.) can be used to reduce laryngeal and tracheal inflammation.

Management of airway collapse generally relies on treatment of any concurrent diseases identified during the diagnostic work up and controlling factors that stimulate cough. Obesity is a common complication in dogs with airway collapse, and weight loss alone can result in significant reductions in cough and improvement in overall health.

In the absence of infectious or inflammatory airway disease, narcotic cough suppressants are usually required to control cough. These should be administered often enough to control cough without inducing severe sedation. Suggested drugs include hydrocodone (0.22 mg/kg orally q6–12h) and butorphanol (0.55–1.1 mg/kg orally as required). Dogs are started on a high dose initially and then tapered to the lowest dose that controls clinical signs. Some dogs will respond better to one drug than to the other. Caution is warranted with use of these drugs since tolerance can develop.

Corticosteroids

Increased expiratory effort (abdominal push) and fluctuations in intratracheal pressures cause progressive collapse of the dorsal tracheal membrane into the lumen that can stimulate mucus production or inflammation. Pressure changes can also stimulate upper airway inflammation or oedema. In these situations, a short course of gluocorticoids can be helpful. Prednisolone is used at 0.5 mg/kg divided q12h for 3–5 days and then daily for an additional 3–5 days to control secondary inflammation or oedema. Alternatively, a short course of inhaled steroids can be employed. Airway infection is treated with appropriate antibiotics. Pending culture results, a trial on doxycycline (3–5 mg/kg orally q12h) can be employed to treat potential *Mycoplasma* infection. This antibiotic may be beneficial because it also has mild anti-inflammatory effects.

Bronchodilators

Bronchodilators may be useful in animals with small airway disease or airway collapse. These drugs do not physically dilate the large airways that are visible on fluoroscopy or during bronchoscopy, but instead act on airways in the periphery by improving expiratory airflow and decreasing the likelihood of intrathoracic airway collapse. Some agents may also have mild anti-inflammatory effects. Bronchodilators commonly used include the methylxanthines (extended-release theophylline products at 10 mg/kg q12h), or beta agonists such as terbutaline (0.625–5 mg/dog orally q12h) and salbutamol (20–50 μg/kg orally q8–12h).

Adjunctive interventions

Ancillary measures include avoidance of collars and decreased exposure to heat and humidity. Upper airway surgery (soft palate resection or sacculectomy; see *BSAVA Manual of Canine and Feline Head, Neck and Thoracic Surgery*), if needed, can also improve the dog's presentation (White, 1995). In dogs with cervical tracheal collapse, placement of extraluminal cervical ring prostheses can result in dramatic reduction in clinical signs (Buback *et al.*, 1996). Studies have also shown improved quality of life and good long-term outcome following implantation of intraluminal stenting devices (Moritz *et al.*, 2004; Sura and Krahwinkel, 2008). Fluoroscopically or bronchoscopically placed internal stents are recommended as a salvage procedure for dogs with intractable cough or respiratory difficulty associated with intrathoracic tracheal collapse (Figure 30.5).

Chronic bronchitis

Corticosteroids

Treatment of chronic bronchitis requires anti-inflammatory therapy with corticosteroids to break the cycle of mucosal damage, reduce production of

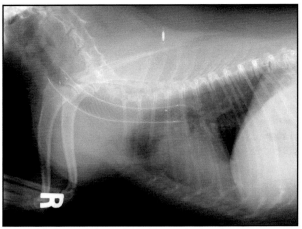

30.5 Lateral thoracic radiograph showing an intraluminal stent supporting the tracheal collapse from distal to the larynx to the carina.

inflammatory mediators by neutrophils, and reduce excessive production of secretions. Prednisolone can be used at relatively high doses initially (0.5–1.0 mg/kg orally q12h for 5–7 days), then the same dosage administered daily for 10–14 days if clinical signs are resolving. The goal is to have dogs on alternate-day therapy as soon as possible in order to normalize the pituitary–hypothalamic axis, but some dogs require therapy for prolonged periods of time. Exacerbations of disease demand an increase to the higher dose that effectively controls clinical signs, a change in drug administration, or addition of another drug.

Dogs with concurrent medical conditions that preclude the use of oral steroids, or those that suffer excessively from side effects associated with steroid use, can be treated with inhaled medications using a facemask and spacing chamber for delivery. A securely fitted facemask is essential for providing drug delivery to the lower airways during tidal breathing. A spacing chamber with nose mask, anaesthetic facemask or human facemask can be used, depending on the facial conformation of the dog. Fluticasone proprionate remains one of the most potent inhaled steroids available and is generally recommended initially. One puff of medication (110 μg/puff) is actuated into the chamber when the facemask is attached to the dog, and 6–8 inhalations are observed to ensure drug delivery into the airways. Twice-daily administration has proved efficacious in alleviating cough in dogs with lower airway inflammation (Bexfield *et al.*, 2006).

Bronchodilators

Dogs with clinical signs that cannot be controlled with glucocorticoids or those that suffer excessively from the common side effects associated with steroid use may benefit from the addition of a bronchodilator. Either an extended-release theophylline or a beta agonist can be used and may help to reduce the dose of steroid required. Side effects may include anorexia, gastrointestinal upset, or restlessness.

Antibiotics

Use of antibiotics should be restricted to those cases in which results of culture/sensitivity and cytology document infection. Antibiotics with good pulmonary penetration, such as doxycycline, chloramphenicol, trimethoprim/sulphonamide and the fluoroquinolones, are likely to be beneficial, although fluoroquinolones are better reserved for significant respiratory infections. Also, caution is warranted when using fluoroquinolones and theophylline in combination, since a drug interaction has been documented (Intorre *et al.*, 1995); at least a 50% reduction in the theophylline dose is recommended.

Adjunctive therapy

When inflammation and infection have resolved, use of cough suppressants should be considered to break the cycle of airway injury. Over-the-counter cough suppressants can be tried initially but are rarely effective. Narcotic agents can be employed judiciously. In some dogs with viscid airway secretions, saline nebulization followed by coupage can be helpful in aiding evacuation of mucus (see Chapter 19). Finally, as with all pulmonary diseases, weight loss is critical in these patients and should be recommended for obese animals.

Prognosis

Owners should be aware that complete abolition of all coughing due to chronic bronchitis or airway collapse is rarely achieved and that variable measures are often required to determine the appropriate regimen of therapy that controls signs in the individual. This is a chronic, ongoing disease, and the goal is simply to control clinical signs and, hopefully, prevent worsening of disease and the onset of cor pulmonale.

Physical examination of the airways through bronchoscopy has been most helpful in allowing discussion of prognosis with owners. The presence of fibrosis, bronchitic nodules and chronic inflammation clearly indicate the irreversibility of the process. When owners realize that the cough of chronic bronchitis may never totally resolve, they find the condition easier to tolerate and treat and understand the importance of environmental and weight management recommendations.

References and further reading

Bexfield NH, Foale RD, Davison LJ *et al.* (2006) Management of 13 cases of canine respiratory disease using inhaled corticosteroids. *Journal of Small Animal Practice* **47**, 377–382

Buback JL, Boothe HW and Hobson HP (1996) Surgical treatment of tracheal collapse in dogs: 90 cases (1983–1993). *Journal of the American Veterinary Medical Association* **208**, 380–384

Dallman MA, McClure RC and Brown EM (1988) Histochemical study of normal and collapsed tracheas in dogs. *American Journal of Veterinary Research* **49**, 2117–2125

Guglielmini C, De Simone A, Valbonetti L and Diana A (2007) Intermittent cranial lung herniation in two dogs. *Veterinary Radiology and Ultrasound* **48**, 227–229

Intorre L, Mengozzi G, Maccheroni M *et al.* (1995) Enrofloxacin–theophylline interaction: influence of enrofloxacin on theophylline steady-state pharmacokinetics in the Beagle dog. *Journal of Veterinary Pharmacology and Therapeutics* **19**, 352–356

Johnson LR and Fales WH (2001) Bacterial cultures in dogs with bronchoscopically diagnosed tracheal collapse. *Journal of the American Veterinary Medical Association* **219**, 1247–1250

Macready DM, Johnson LR and Pollard R (2007) Fluoroscopic and radiographic evaluation of tracheal collapse in 62 dogs. *Journal of the American Veterinary Medical Association* **230**, 1870–1876

Mantis P, Lamb CR and Boswood C (1998) Assessment of the accuracy of thoracic radiography in the diagnosis of canine chronic bronchitis. *Journal of Small Animal Practice* **39**, 518–520

Moritz A, Schneider M and Bauer N (2004) Management of advanced tracheal collapse in dogs using intraluminal self-expanding biliary wallstents. *Journal of Veterinary Internal Medicine* **18**, 31–42

Peeters DE, McKiernan BC, Weisiger RM *et al.* (2000) Quantitative bacterial cultures and cytological examination of bronchoalveolar lavage specimens in dogs. *Journal of Veterinary Internal Medicine* **14**, 534–541

Rudorf H, Herrtage ME and White RAS (1997) Use of ultrasonography in the diagnosis of tracheal collapse. *Journal of Small Animal Practice* **38**, 513–518

Sura PA and Krahwinkel DJ (2008) Self-expanding nitinol stents for treatment of tracheal collapse in dogs: 12 cases (2001–2004). *Journal of the American Veterinary Medical Association* **232**, 228–236

Tangner CH and Hobson HP (1982) A retrospective of 20 surgically managed cases of collapsed trachea. *Veterinary Surgery* **11**, 146–149

Wheeldon EB, Pirie HM, Fisher EW and Lee R (1974) Chronic bronchitis in the dog. *Veterinary Record* **94**, 466–471

White RN (1995) Unilateral arytenoid lateralisation and extra-luminal polypropylene ring prostheses for correction of tracheal collapse in the dog. *Journal of Small Animal Practice* **36**, 151–158

31

Feline tracheobronchial disease

Carol R. Reinero and Amy E. DeClue

Introduction

Inflammatory airway disease is common in cats and primarily includes feline asthma and feline chronic bronchitis. While both are associated with substantial morbidity, feline asthma is associated with occasional acute mortality. This chapter will cover the salient features of both disorders.

Feline asthma

The syndrome of asthma is associated with:

- **Eosinophilic airway inflammation**
- **Airway hyper-responsiveness (the tendency of bronchi to narrow too much and too easily in response to a variety of provocative non-allergenic stimuli)**
- **Bronchoconstriction in response to specific allergen or non-specific stimulant**
- **Airway remodelling (permanent architectural changes in the lung).**

Asthma in humans is often allergic in origin. Because the disorder in cats shares many similarities with the human disease, it is thought that allergy may underlie the feline disorder as well (Corcoran et al., 1995; Norris Reinero et al., 2004). Inhalation of aeroallergens will activate TH_2 helper lymphocytes to produce cytokines that drive the asthmatic response.

Signalment

Most studies in the veterinary literature report asthmatic cats with a median age of 4–5 years at the time of presentation. However, many of the cats had a chronic duration of clinical signs and probably had an onset of disease that could have been months or years earlier. Additionally, since cough is a common clinical sign (see below) and some owners confuse a cat's cough with hacking up hairballs or vomiting, diagnosis could also have been delayed. Overall, it is important to realize that most cats tend to be young when they develop asthma. It would be unlikely for an old cat that had never had clinical signs of asthma to develop the disease suddenly.

There is no clear gender predilection for asthma: some studies have reported this syndrome predominantly in females and others in males, while others have documented no gender predisposition. The Siamese breed has been over-represented in some studies but not in others.

Clinical signs

The most common respiratory abnormalities associated with feline asthma are cough, wheeze and/or respiratory distress. Because of the generally sedentary behaviour of cats, exercise intolerance is not typically reported.

Owners may interpret a cough as attempting to 'hack up a hairball' and further questioning relating to how often a hairball is produced may be relevant. If a cat apparently attempts to bring up hairballs several times in a day, but a hairball is only seen once a week, it is more likely that the hacking behaviour is really a cough. Additionally, vomiting following more violent paroxysmal coughing has been reported in 10–15% of cases.

Physical examination

Findings on physical examination may vary depending on the severity of the asthma.

- Cats that are relatively stable can present with no overt abnormal respiratory signs, though most cats have an easily inducible cough on tracheal palpation.
- Other findings include tachypnoea and an expiratory wheeze heard with or without the aid of a stethoscope.
- Cats presenting in an acute asthmatic crisis ('status asthmaticus') are in visible respiratory distress with a pronounced expiratory component to their breathing. They may exhibit open-mouthed breathing or may be cyanotic.
- Sometimes hypersalivation is seen.
- Cats may appear to be less responsive to external stimuli, as they are focusing intensely on breathing.

Diagnosis

Diagnosis of asthma relies on: identification of compatible clinical signs; thoracic imaging; ruling out other diseases that may mimic asthma; using ancillary tests; and, ultimately, airway lavage cytology. Measurement of airflow limitation is not commonly performed in small animal veterinary patients, primarily due to the need for specialized equipment and training to evaluate pulmonary mechanics.

The decision to perform diagnostics should be based on how stable the cat is at the time of presentation. Cats presenting in status asthmaticus need to be medically stabilized prior to taking thoracic radiographs or anaesthetizing them for bronchoalveolar lavage.

Radiography

Thoracic radiographs are important from the standpoint of ruling out other cardiopulmonary diseases that may lead to cough or respiratory distress. For example, cardiomegaly, pleural effusion, or a heavy interstitial to alveolar pulmonary parenchymal pattern would support a disease other than asthma. For cats with asthma, it is important to note that thoracic radiographs may be completely normal. When pathology is present, findings may include a bronchial or bronchointerstitial pattern, lung lobe collapse (most commonly the right middle lung lobe), or generalized hyperinflation of the lungs. The latter finding is often appreciated as an increased distance between the caudal border of the cardiac silhouette and the diaphragm (Figure 31.1).

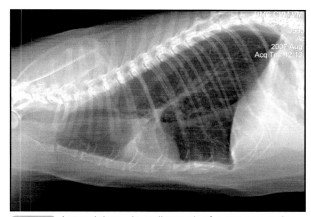

31.1 Lateral thoracic radiograph of a cat presenting in status asthmaticus. Note the hyperinflated lungs, which are indicative of air trapping.

Haematology

A complete blood count is often performed to look for peripheral eosinophilia. Depending on the study, peripheral eosinophilia has been demonstrated in only 17–46% of asthmatic cats. Importantly, it has not been shown to correlate with the degree of airway eosinophilia. Since asthma is not a systemic disease, it is more important to be able to assess local (i.e. airway) inflammation (see below).

Parasitology

In cats presenting with cough (that may or may not have a bronchial or bronchointerstitial pattern) or a peripheral eosinophilia, other differential diagnoses include pulmonary parasites (notably *Aelurostrongylus abstrusus*) or heartworm-associated respiratory disease (HARD). Other relevant diagnostics would include faecal examination and tests for heartworm (*Dirofilaria immitis*) antigen/antibody.

Cytology

Collection of an airway sample can be performed via a transoral tracheal wash, a blind bronchoalveolar

lavage (BAL) technique (Figure 31.2) or using bronchoscopy (Figure 31.3) (see also Chapter 10). Administration of a fast-acting bronchodilator (e.g. salbutamol or terbutaline) 10–15 minutes prior to the procedure may minimize the risk of hypoxaemia associated with bronchoconstriction.

---

1. Lightly anaesthetize the cat and intubate with a sterile endotracheal tube.
2. Advance a 7–8 Fr red rubber feeding tube or polypropylene catheter (open-ended) through the endotracheal tube until slight resistance is met.
3. Instil an aliquot of sterile saline (the authors use 15–20 ml) and retrieve it by gentle hand suction. The presence of a foamy layer (surfactant) on top of the retrieved fluid is indicative of a deep wash of the lung.
4. Remove the catheter and administer oxygen to the cat until it is fully recovered.

31.2 'Blind' bronchoalveolar lavage technique.

---

1. Wedge the bronchoscope into a small airway.
2. Instil saline (3–10 ml) through the biopsy port and retrieve by gentle hand suction.
3. Remove the bronchoscope and intubate the cat in order to provide oxygen supplementation during recovery.

31.3 Bronchoscopic collection of lavage fluid.

The fluid retrieved should be processed efficiently – ideally within 2 hours; if a delay in analysis is anticipated, the sample should be refrigerated or placed on ice. A total nucleated cell count, cellular differential and cytological description should be obtained.

There is variation in the literature about what constitutes a normal cell count and percentage of eosinophils in cats. Various reports on BAL in cats have reported approximately 240–300 cells/µl and 11–25% eosinophils as reference ranges in normal healthy cats. An eosinophilic airway cytology would be considered consistent with the diagnosis of feline asthma. The BAL fluid should also be cultured (including a culture for *Mycoplasma*) to determine whether there is secondary bacterial infection; this, however, is not common in asthmatic cats.

Medical management

Stabilization

Cats presenting in status asthmaticus are very fragile and therefore handling and diagnostic sample collection should be minimal until they are stabilized. They should be given supplemental oxygen by facemask, tent or cage (see Chapter 1). A bronchodilator should also be administered, to alleviate bronchoconstriction that limits airflow. Bronchodilators commonly administered to cats are either in the beta-2 agonist class (e.g. salbutamol, terbutaline) or in the methylxanthine class (e.g. theophylline). Beta-2 bronchodilators such as salbutamol can be administered either via a metered-dose inhalant/spacer or by nebulization (Figure 31.4). Other drugs (e.g. terbutaline) are available in an injectable form. An injectable corticosteroid (e.g. dexamethasone, 0.1–0.25 mg/kg i.v.) should also be administered in crisis situations.

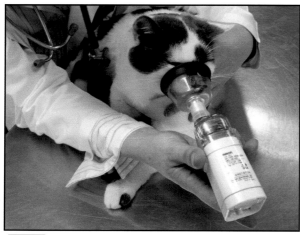

31.4 Use of a nebulizer to deliver an aerosol of salbutamol (0.5% solution) to a cat.

Chronic management

For the stable asthmatic, traditional medical management has consisted of environmental modulation, bronchodilators and glucocorticoids.

Environmental modification: Because cats can react to both allergenic and non-allergenic stimuli in the environment, recommendations to minimize aerosolized allergens and irritants should be made. For example: non-dusty cat litter should be used; exposure to cigarette or other types of smoke should be avoided; the use of aerosols and powders should be minimized; and frequent vacuuming is recommended. For cats spending a large amount of time indoors, using a high-efficiency particulate air (HEPA) filter, which can remove almost 100% of particulate matter smaller than 3 μm, is ideal. If the allergen inducing the asthma can be identified, removing it from the cat's environment or moving the cat to a different environment would be beneficial; however, identification of the underlying allergen(s) is generally difficult.

Bronchodilators: Oral bronchodilators are recommended for chronic management of asthmatic cats, especially those with a history of episodic respiratory distress. There is evidence that chronic administration of inhalant salbutamol (a racemic mixture of *R-* and *S*-salbutamol) can induce inflammation in both healthy and experimentally- induced asthmatic cats, respectively; therefore, it should only be used as 'rescue' therapy. Instead, oral extended release theophylline and terbutaline are reasonable alternatives. Bronchodilators should not be used as monotherapy, because they do not effectively address inflammation.

Glucocorticoids: While bronchodilators are useful in alleviating smooth muscle constriction, administration of glucocorticoids is essential to control the airway inflammation that leads to enhanced airway hyperresponsiveness and airway remodelling. Glucocorticoids are commonly given orally; however, once inflammation is adequately controlled, many cats are changed to inhaled glucocorticoids, which have potent local anti-inflammatory effects in the lung and minimal systemic endocrine and immunological effects. Most cats will need to receive glucocorticoids

for the remainder of their lives, and the goal is to taper to the lowest effective dose to control airway inflammation.

Recent advances: Using an experimental model of feline asthma, multiple drugs and immunomodulatory therapies have been evaluated for the control of clinical signs associated with asthma. Since mediators released or elaborated from mast cells (e.g. serotonin, histamine, cysteinyl leucotrienes) are implicated in the pathogenesis of asthma, use of medications that block the effects of those mediators could have potential benefit.

Cyproheptadine (an antiserotonergic drug), cetirizine (a second-generation histamine-1 receptor antagonist) and zafirlukast (a leucotriene receptor antagonist) were all evaluated for their ability to reduce eosinophilic airway inflammation in experimental feline asthma (Reinero *et al.*, 2005). Compared with placebo, none of the drugs significantly reduced eosinophilic inflammation. Therefore, these treatments cannot be recommended as monotherapy for cats with asthma, and glucocorticoids remain the treatment of choice.

To date, the only curative treatment for allergy in human medicine is allergen-specific immunotherapy ('allergy shots'). While most commonly used in people with allergic rhinitis, allergen-specific immunotherapy has also been used successfully in human asthmatics. A protocol for abbreviated allergen-specific immunotherapy, called rush immunotherapy (RIT), has been developed in cats, with or without an adjuvant, and tested in experimentally-induced asthmatic cats (Reinero *et al.*, 2006). Results are promising and cats receiving RIT had significant decreases in eosinophilic airway inflammation over time compared with cats not receiving RIT; indeed, some cats reverted to being 'non-asthmatic' by the end of the study. In order to maximize the efficacy of this therapy in pet cats with naturally developing asthma, further work must be performed to identify accurately any allergens implicated in an individual cat's disease.

Prognosis

Feline asthma is a chronic disorder, associated with substantial morbidity and occasional mortality. With long-term medical management, overall prognosis is good. Prognosis is more guarded in cats with severe respiratory distress.

Chronic bronchitis

Chronic bronchitis (inflammation of the bronchi/ bronchioles) is an inflammatory airway disease that is characterized by:

- **Neutrophilic inflammation**
- **Mucosal oedema**
- **Mucous gland hypertrophy**
- **Excessive mucus production.**

In humans, chronic bronchitis develops when an insult to the bronchial epithelium, such as inhalation of particulate matter or toxic gases, triggers an inflammatory process. The exact aetiopathogenesis of feline chronic bronchitis is not known, but inhaled bronchial irritants are suspected to play a role. Ultimately, bronchial inflammation can lead to some or all of the following: destruction of the bronchiolar walls; bronchiectasis (abnormal structural widening of the bronchioles); a loss of normal protective mechanisms; and impaired pulmonary gas exchange.

Signalment
Studies in the veterinary literature evaluating client-owned cats have combined data from cats with asthma and chronic bronchitis, despite their varying pathophysiology. Because of this fact, the signalment and breed predisposition in the literature is said to be identical for cats with asthma and chronic bronchitis with a large age range, varying sex predilection and possible over-representation of the Siamese breed. Extrapolating from the pathogenesis of chronic bronchitis in humans, chronic exposure to irritants over the course of years may induce the type of airway inflammation seen in feline chronic bronchitis. In the authors' experience, cats with chronic bronchitis are often older at the time of presentation than are cats with asthma. Further study is needed to determine whether this theory is correct.

Clinical signs
The most common clinical signs of chronic bronchitis are predominantly indistinguishable from those of asthma in cats. Cats with chronic bronchitis may present with cough and expiratory wheeze; when respiratory distress is present it is generally persistent and progressive. Typically, respiratory distress in a cat with chronic bronchitis is either related to a long-term change in pulmonary function associated with chronic airway remodelling, or is due to the development of mucus entrapment within the airways. Nevertheless, cats with chronic bronchitis have been shown to have increased airway hyper-reactivity and thus may have a greater propensity for bronchoconstriction than healthy cats. However, in the authors' experience, cats with bronchitis rarely have the life-threatening bronchoconstriction that is seen in cats with asthma. Similar to cats with asthma, approximately 10–15% of cats with chronic bronchitis will present with vomiting or 'hacking up furballs' as part of their history. Clinical signs may range from mild to severe, with some cats having limited or no clinical signs despite clinically important airway inflammation.

Physical examination
Physical examination findings generally mimic those found in cats with asthma. Depending upon the severity of disease, some cats with chronic bronchitis will have a normal physical examination. Often, cats with chronic bronchitis have a cough that is inducible with tracheal palpation and expiratory wheezes. Cats with end-stage disease have been reported to have a barrel-shaped thorax due to lung hyperinflation, tachypnoea and respiratory compromise.

Diagnosis
The diagnosis of chronic bronchitis in cats is based on appropriate history, physical examination findings, thoracic radiography and BAL fluid cytology. Complete blood count, serum biochemical profile and urinalysis typically reflect non-specific changes or evidence of an unrelated underlying disease process. While these diagnostic tests alone will not lead to the definitive diagnosis of chronic bronchitis, they should be performed to rule out conditions mimicking chronic bronchitis or underlying disease that may alter the management of the patient.

Radiography
Bronchial or bronchointerstitial pattern, collapse of the right middle lung lobe and/or lung hyperinflation may be identified on thoracic radiographs. Radiographic evidence of hyperinflated lungs generally does not resolve with bronchodilator therapy, indicating that there are permanent structural changes in the lungs resulting in air trapping or emphysema. As is true for asthma, cats with chronic bronchitis may lack abnormalities on thoracic radiographs. Hence, normal thoracic radiographs do not rule out clinically important airway inflammation in cats.

Cytology
The diagnostic test of choice for the definitive diagnosis of chronic bronchitis in cats is BAL fluid cytology (see Figures 31.2 and 31.3 and Chapter 10).

- Non-degenerate neutrophils with mucus are the hallmark features of BAL cytology in cats with chronic bronchitis (Figure 31.5).
- In healthy cats, the macrophage is the predominant cell type in BAL fluid, with neutrophils comprising <5% of the total cell population. In cats with chronic bronchitis there should be an increase in the percentage of neutrophils (>5%) in the BAL fluid. In cats with moderate to severe airway inflammation, neutrophils may comprise >50% of the total cells.

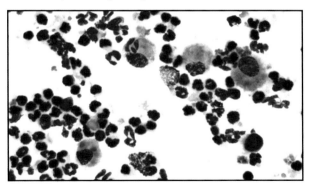

31.5 Neutrophilic airway cytology from a cat with chronic bronchitis. Note the non-degenerate neutrophils admixed with moderately vacuolated macrophages and small lymphocytes. Diff Quick stain; original magnification X40. (Courtesy of L. Johnson.)

Bacteriology
Bacterial pneumonia or bronchitis is uncommon in cats, but care should be taken to differentiate bacterial causes of neutrophilic airway inflammation from sterile causes such as chronic bronchitis. Bacterial culture of BAL fluid is one tool often used to make this differentiation. However, a positive culture result from a cat with airway disease could be

evidence of: a bacterial infection; normal airway bacterial colonization; or contamination of the sample during collection or processing. Aerobic bacteria that are known to colonize normal healthy feline airways include *Pasteurella*, *Pseudomonas*, *Staphylococcus*, *Streptococcus*, *Escherichia coli* and *Micrococcus*. In contrast, *Mycoplasma* spp. have not been cultured from the airways of normal cats, and isolation of these organisms is an indicator of infection.

To differentiate airway colonization or sample contamination from true infection, several criteria should be considered:

- Culture results should be interpreted in light of BAL fluid cytology from the same sample. Degenerate neutrophils or septic suppurative inflammation (i.e. bacteria found within neutrophils) should be evident on cytology if a true bacterial infection is present. A lack of these findings would make a true bacterial infection unlikely
- Whenever possible, quantitative culture should be carried out. In one study of BAL fluid characteristics in normal healthy cats, all positive cultures had $<2 \times 10^3$ colony-forming units (CFU) per ml. Generally, a cat with a true bacterial infection should have $>2 \times 10^3$ CFU/ml
- Care should be taken to avoid oropharyngeal contamination when collecting a lower airway specimen. Culturing multiple bacteria simultaneously in a cat lacking cytological evidence of infection (degenerate neutrophils ± intracellular bacteria) or with cytological evidence of squamous epithelium or *Simonsiella* spp. indicates oropharyngeal contamination, not airway infection.

Medical management
The management of feline chronic bronchitis focuses on controlling airway inflammation.

Glucocorticoids
Traditionally, oral glucocorticoids (prednisolone at 10 mg/cat orally q24h for 2 weeks, then tapered to the lowest effective dose) are used to control inflammation. No studies to date have compared the use of different doses of oral glucocorticoids to determine how high or low a dose will effectively control inflammation. However, in one study of research cats with naturally developing chronic bronchitis, administration of inhaled fluticasone (250 μg q24h via paediatric mask and spacer) significantly decreased airway inflammation (Kirschvink *et al.*, 2006). Therefore, it appears that inhalation is an efficacious method of steroid delivery that may be considered for management of chronic bronchitis. Like asthma, chronic bronchitis is a long-term inflammatory disease, and lifelong therapy with corticosteroids is indicated in almost all cases. Clinical remission (i.e. resolution of clinical signs) and radiographic findings may not correlate with a lack of airway inflammation. Until a less invasive tool for monitoring inflammation is developed, serial BAL cytology can be performed and medications adjusted accordingly to alleviate inflammation.

Bronchodilators
Anecdotally, the use of bronchodilators has been suggested for cats with chronic bronchitis. Most cats with chronic bronchitis will not have severe clinical signs of airway constriction (i.e. episodic respiratory distress) and thus the use of bronchodilators is not clearly indicated. For cats with mild chronic bronchoconstriction, simply controlling inflammation with glucocorticoids will often alleviate the problem. In cases where inflammation control does not alleviate the clinical signs, a trial with bronchodilators such as oral theophylline or terbutaline could be considered.

Recent advances
Although inflammatory bronchial disease (i.e. chronic bronchitis and asthma) has been recognized in cats for several decades, recently the appropriateness of lumping all bronchial diseases under one general classification has been questioned. It is likely that there are marked differences in the aetiopathogenesis of chronic bronchitis and of asthma. Hopefully, as knowledge develops, advances aimed at managing and possibly preventing the development of feline chronic bronchitis will be identified.

Prognosis
Chronic bronchitis is a chronic airway inflammatory disorder associated with substantial morbidity; mortality is rare. Early identification and control of airway inflammation with glucocorticoids are essential to achieve a good long-term outcome for cats with chronic bronchitis. For cats with evidence of moderate to severe airway remodelling or loss of normal gas exchange mechanisms, prognosis is guarded.

References and further reading

Adamama-Moraitou K, Patsikas M and Koutinas A (2004) Feline lower airway disease: a retrospective study of 22 naturally occurring cases from Greece. *Journal of Feline Medicine and Surgery* **6**, 227–233

Corcoran B, Foster D and Luis Fuentes V (1995) Feline asthma syndrome: a retrospective study of the clinical presentation in 29 cats. *Journal of Small Animal Practice* **36**, 481–488

Dye J, McKiernan B, Rozanski E and Hoffmann W (1996) Bronchopulmonary disease in the cat: historical, physical, radiographic, clinicopathologic, and pulmonary functional evaluation of 24 affected and 15 healthy cats. *Journal of Veterinary Internal Medicine* **10**, 385–400

Foster S, Allan G, Martin P, Roberston I and Malik R (2004) Twenty-five cases of feline bronchial disease (1995–2000). *Journal of Feline Medicine and Surgery* **6**, 181–188

Kirschvink N, Leemans J, Delvaux F *et al.* (2006) Inhaled fluticasone reduces bronchial responsiveness and airway inflammation in cats with mild chronic bronchitis. *Journal of Feline Medicine and Surgery* **8**, 45–54

Moise N, Wiedenkeller D and Yeager A (1989) Clinical, radiographic, and bronchial cytologic features of cats with bronchial disease: 65 cases (1980–1986). *Journal of the American Veterinary Medical Association* **194**, 1467–1473

Norris Reinero C, Decile K, Berghaus R *et al.* (2004) An experimental model of allergic asthma in cats sensitized to house dust mite or bermuda grass allergen. *International Archives of Allergy and Immunology* **135**, 117–131

Reinero CR, Byerly JR, Berghaus RD *et al.* (2006) Rush immunotherapy in an experimental model of feline allergic asthma. *Veterinary Immunology and Immunopathology* **110**, 141–153

Reinero CR, Decile KC, Byerly JR *et al.* (2005) Effects of drug treatment on inflammation and hyperreactivity of airways and on immune variables in cats with experimentally induced asthma. *American Journal of Veterinary Research* **66**, 1121–1127

32

Pulmonary parenchymal disease

Gareth Buckley and Elizabeth Rozanski

Introduction

Conditions affecting the pulmonary parenchyma are common in veterinary medicine and include traumatic injuries, pulmonary oedema of both cardiac and non-cardiac origin, primary and/or metastatic neoplasia, pneumonia and interstitial lung disease. The focus of this chapter is on pneumonia and interstitial lung disease.

Clinical signs of lung diseases are similar, despite different causes, and reflect the alterations in lung mechanics that accompany lung pathology. If the lung parenchyma fills with fluid (oedema) or inflammatory cells (pneumonia), the lungs become less compliant and it is more difficult for the patient to breathe. This is recognized as rapid breathing or as an increased effort. Conditions that cause fluid or pus to leak into the airways or cause primary inflammation or infection in the trachea will cause coughing. Thus, clinical signs are not specific for the disease and the clinician should be alert to considering a number of possibilities when initiating diagnostic testing and therapy.

Bacterial pneumonia

Bacterial pneumonia is characterized by bacterial infection with subsequent inflammation and consolidation of lung tissue. The disease process usually results in the classic radiographic appearance of an alveolar pattern (Figure 32.1).

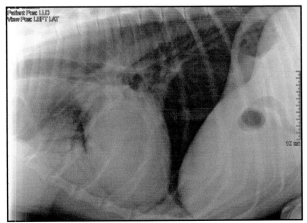

32.1 Lateral thoracic radiograph of a Scottish Deerhound with pneumonia. Note the air bronchograms consistent with alveolar disease in the cranioventral lung fields.

Causes of bacterial pneumonia are numerous. It is important to distinguish between: animals that contract pneumonia spontaneously (usually < 1 year old); animals that have an underlying disease that makes them prone to development of pneumonia; and animals that contract pneumonia whilst hospitalized for another disease.

Bacterial pneumonia is very rare in cats.

Spontaneous (community-acquired) pneumonia

Spontaneous pneumonia, also known as community-acquired pneumonia, is most often seen in young dogs (< 1 year old) that have been acquired recently. One study showed that young dogs presenting with pneumonia had been owned for less than 1 month before presentation to the hospital, with many presenting within a week of ownership. The most common bacterium isolated from this group of puppies is *Bordetella bronchiseptica*. Other common organisms isolated include *Staphylococcus* spp., *Escherichia coli*, *Klebsiella pneumoniae*, *Enterobacter* spp., *Enterococcus faecalis*, *Acinetobacter* and *Pasteurella* spp. (Radhakrishnan *et al.*, 2007).

Underlying disease

Dogs that present with pneumonia secondary to underlying disease are typically older animals and usually present with aspiration pneumonia. They may have a history of gastrointestinal disease (vomiting or regurgitation) or laryngeal dysfunction (Figure 32.2). Oesophageal dysfunction, including megaoesophagus, is associated with significant risk of aspiration pneumonia. Local or generalized myasthenia gravis is also a risk factor for aspiration, as are neurological diseases in general, including lower motor neuron diseases or seizures. Dogs with seizures may also develop non-cardiogenic pulmonary oedema, which can be distinguished from aspiration pneumonia by the location of the pulmonary infiltrates. Non-cardiogenic pulmonary oedema typically has a dorsal–caudal distribution, whilst aspiration pneumonia is more commonly cranial–ventral in distribution. Brachycephalic animals, such as English or French Bulldogs and Pugs, are also predisposed to the development of pneumonia due to poor upper airway conformation and regurgitation, which increase the likelihood for aspiration pneumonia.

Gastrointestinal
Regurgitation: oesophageal dysmotility; megaoesophagus; oesophagitis Vomiting

Neurological
Seizures Intracranial disease (including postoperative craniotomy) Myasthenia gravis (often accompanied by oesophageal dysfunction) Lower motor neuron disease

Upper airway disease
Laryngeal paralysis Brachycephalic airway obstructive syndrome

Multifactorial
Anaesthesia/sedation Recumbency Critical illness

32.2 Risk factors for development of aspiration pneumonia.

Hospitalized patients

Dogs that develop pneumonia in the hospital often have a history of recent anaesthesia or sedation. They may have similar risk factors to older dogs presenting with pneumonia, with the addition of prolonged recumbency or recent surgery. Some surgeries, such as arytenoid lateralization ('tie-back') or craniotomy, can specifically predispose to the development of aspiration pneumonia (Fransson *et al.*, 2001; MacPhail and Monnet, 2001). The main difference between this group of dogs and those presenting with community-acquired pneumonia is that the causative agent is likely to be hospital-acquired, especially in the larger hospitals with high throughput of cases. This results in isolation of a bacterium more resistant to standard antibiotic strategies (see below).

Clinical signs and physical examination

Clinical signs include lethargy, anorexia, tachypnoea, respiratory distress, exercise intolerance, coughing and collapse. Physical examination findings may include increased lung sounds, crackles on auscultation, nasal discharge and fever. All signs are not present in all cases; for example, in a study in puppies with bacterial pneumonia, fever was present in only 48% (Radhakrishnan *et al.*, 2007).

Occasionally animals with pneumonia can present with sepsis or septic shock. Sepsis is defined as an infection with evidence of a systemic inflammatory response, while septic shock is defined as sepsis with hypotension unresponsive to fluid loading.

Diagnosis

Diagnosis of pneumonia typically includes physical examination findings and the results of radiographic imaging of the thorax. On physical examination, most dogs are lethargic and appear quiet. Some, but not all, have a fever, with a rectal temperature in excess of 39.4°C (103°F). The respiratory rate and effort are typically increased, and there may be cough or nasal discharge.

Radiography

Radiographic changes typically reflect alveolar lung disease with evidence of air bronchograms, although marked interstitial patterns are also possible. The distribution of lesions tends to be cranioventral in comparison with: heart failure, which tends to have a more perihilar appearance; or with non-cardiogenic pulmonary oedema, which classically has a dorsocaudal distribution. Aspiration most commonly affects the right middle lung lobe, though other lung lobes can be affected; hence, if aspiration pneumonia is suspected a left lateral recumbent radiograph can be a useful aid to diagnosis. Thoracic radiography can also be useful in diagnosing underlying conditions that predispose animals to development of pneumonia, such as megaoesophagus, or conditions that may masquerade as pneumonia, such as congestive heart failure or pulmonary neoplasia. Two or three views are most helpful in highlighting the abnormalities. Examples of radiographic abnormalities are shown in Figure 32.3.

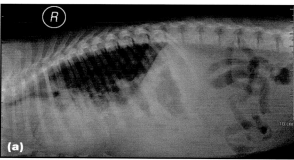
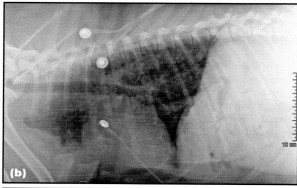
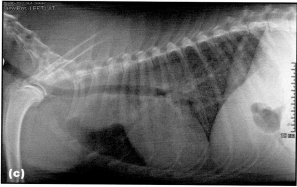

32.3 Thoracic radiographs for a variety of conditions. **(a)** A puppy with severe community-acquired pneumonia. **(b)** An older Retriever with metastatic haemangiosarcoma. **(c)** A young Golden Retriever with disseminated fungal infection due to blastomycosis. (continues) ▶

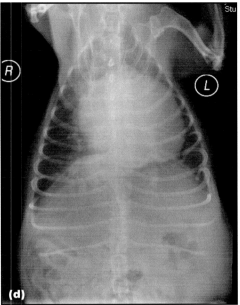

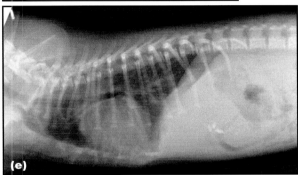

32.3 (continued) Thoracic radiographs for a variety of conditions. **(d)** An older Yorkshire Terrier with chronic valvular disease and community-acquired pneumonia. **(e)** A young Shih Tzu with a patent ductus arteriosus and heart failure.

It is important to note that radiographic changes lag behind clinical signs of disease: it is possible to have severe acute pneumonia with minimal radiographic changes; and during the recovery phase, radiographs may appear static or worse despite marked clinical improvement.

Haematology and blood gases
Changes are usually typical of acute inflammation and infection. In mild cases of disease, a mature neutrophilia is a common finding. In more acute or severe disease, left-shifted neutrophilia or even a degenerative left shift is possible. In puppies or in older dogs with severe disease, hypoglycaemia is a common finding.

Blood gas analysis will often demonstrate hypox-aemia (P_aO_2 <80 mmHg) and hypocarbia (P_aCO_2 <28 mmHg). In severe cases of impending respiratory fail-ure, there will be hypercarbia (P_aCO_2 >45 mmHg), with concurrent respiratory acidosis and hypoxaemia.

The alveolar–arterial (A–a) gradient, which char-acterizes the degree of functional impairment, is best used in a patient that is breathing room air, because supplemental oxygen will increase the A–a gradient.

Calculation of the A–a gradient
The following formula calculates the ideal alveolar oxygen content (A) and then subtracts the actual measured arterial gradient (a):

A–a gradient = {[F_iO_2 × (barometric pressure – water vapour pressure)] – (PCO_2/0.8)} – arterial O_2 content (mmHg)

where A = [fraction inspired oxygen × (barometric pressure – water vapour pressure)] – PCO_2/0.8; and a = measured P_aO_2. Water vapour pressure is 47 mmHg at 37°C and is commonly used in this equation. At normal dog temperature (39°C), water vapour pressure is closer to 53 or 54 mmHg; however, this is commonly ignored as its effect on the A–a gradient is quite limited.

- At sea level with a barometric pressure of 760 mmHg, normal A–a is <15 mmHg.
- In a dog with severe pulmonary disease, at sea level with a body temperature of 39°C, with P_aO_2 = 64 mmHg and P_aCO_2 = 28 mm, the A–a gradient would be [(150 – 28/0.8) – 64] = 51 mmHg, which is markedly elevated.
- Conversely, in a dog showing marked ventilatory failure with P_aO_2 = 58 mmHg and P_aCO_2 = 64 mmHg, the A–a gradient would be [(150 – 64/0.8) – 58] = 12 mmHg, which is within the normal range. This would help the clinician to identify that hypoventilation is the source of the apparent hypoxaemia, rather than lung dysfunction *per se*.

For a dog receiving supplemental oxygen, a good estimate of lung function may be made by calculating the P_aO_2:F_iO_2 ratio, where P_aO_2 is the measured arterial oxygen content (mmHg) and F_iO_2 is the fraction inspired oxygen concentration as a number (e.g. room air = 0.21; 100% oxygen = 1.0). A normal value is >450, while a value of <300 is indicative of acute lung injury and <200 is defined as acute respiratory distress syndrome (see Chapter 1).

Bacteriology
Bacterial culture of a causative agent from an airway sample, coupled with cytological evidence of septic neutrophilic inflammation, is the gold standard for confirming bacterial pneumonia. Accompanying bacterial sensitivity testing is helpful in selection of appropriate antibiotics, although empirically successful antibiotics should be provided pending culture results. Sampling from the airway may be achieved by several techniques (see Chapter 10 for details): transtracheal wash (TTW); endotracheal wash (ETW); guided bronchoalveolar lavage. Bronchoscopic evaluation is also very helpful in visualizing any airway changes.

Cytology
Cytological evaluation of tracheal wash samples may be useful in confirming bacterial infection whilst awaiting culture results. Typically, degenerate neutrophils, foamy macrophages and intracellular

bacteria are observed in the animal with pneumonia. However, if animals have been treated with antibiotics before the sample is collected, it is possible that bacteria will not be seen on cytology. Empirical antimicrobial therapy should be started immediately after sample collection when bacterial pneumonia is suspected; specific treatment is based on culture and sensitivity results when they are available.

Treatment
Treatment should focus on appropriate antimicrobial therapy, fluid therapy, supplemental oxygen and nutritional support. Regular monitoring of blood glucose in anorexic or lethargic puppies is mandatory, and supplementation is often required. For animals that present with bacterial pneumonia secondary to underlying disease, efforts must also be made to diagnose and treat the underlying problem. This can be hampered by the fact that the patient may be oxygen-dependent, may be a poor candidate for anaesthesia, or may have low tolerance for diagnostic procedures such as radiography or other imaging. For dogs with chronic gastrointestinal or neurological disease, failure to diagnose and treat the underlying disease adequately is associated with a grave long-term prognosis.

Clinical improvement is the best guide as to whether or not treatment is successful. It is common for clinical signs to worsen in the first day or two of hospitalization but then to improve rapidly. Persistent fever can be an early warning sign of inappropriate antimicrobial choice.

A full discussion of the treatment of septic shock is outside the scope of this manual (see *BSAVA Manual of Canine and Feline Emergency and Critical Care*) but therapy should concentrate on provision of appropriate antimicrobials, aggressive fluid support, blood pressure support, oxygen supplementation and high-quality nursing care. These animals usually require referral to a facility with 24-hour critical care services, and owners should be counselled as to their guarded prognosis.

Antimicrobials
Appropriate antimicrobial therapy is the basis of treatment for bacterial pneumonia. Ideally, all antimicrobial treatment should be based on results of culture and sensitivity testing, but this is not always practical. In very small puppies or very sick animals,

it is not always possible to perform a tracheal wash safely. When culture and sensitivity testing are performed, it takes several days to obtain results; during this time it is mandatory to begin empirical therapy with antimicrobials if suspicion of bacterial pneumonia is high.

In-hospital treatments commonly use injectable intravenous medications. Broad-spectrum coverage against Gram-positive and Gram-negative bacteria is required, as well as treatment for potential anaerobes and *Mycoplasma*. The correct choice of antimicrobials is essential for a good outcome. Many antibiotic choices are appropriate for pneumonia; the astute clinician should be familiar with several choices. Some recommendations are given in Figure 32.4.

The following classes of antibiotics can be used successfully for treatment of pneumonia.

Penicillins: Ampicillin provides good Gram-positive and anaerobic coverage and has intermediate efficacy against Gram-negative organisms such as *Escherichia coli*. Ampicillin is available as an intravenous preparation and is often combined with either an aminoglycoside antibiotic or a fluoroquinolone to broaden the spectrum of coverage.

Potentiated amoxicillin (amoxicillin/clavulanate) provides relatively broad-spectrum coverage and is widely available as both injectable and oral formulations. It has relatively poor penetration into the airways and so may not reach therapeutic concentrations where it is needed. This class of drug can also cause nausea, vomiting and inappetence and may not be the best choice for very sick pets.

First-generation cephalosporins: These drugs provide mainly Gram-positive coverage. Bacteria show a high level of resistance to these antibiotics in hospital-acquired infection, but most community-acquired infections are sensitive.

Second-generation cephalosporins: These agents provide mainly Gram-negative coverage and may be a good substitute for aminoglycosides when their use is contraindicated (see below).

Fluoroquinolones: These antimicrobials provide excellent Gram-negative coverage and are usually used in combination with ampicillin or other antimicrobials effective against *Streptococcus* spp. and

Patient	Drug and dosage	Notes
Puppy, outpatient	Doxycycline (5–10 mg/kg orally q24h)	Consider nebulized aminoglycosides as an adjuvant therapy
Puppy, inpatient	Ampicillin (22 mg/kg i.v. q8h) and gentamicin (6 mg/kg i.v. 24h)	Ensure adequate hydration before using gentamicin
Adult dog, outpatient	Amoxicillin/clavulanate (12–15 mg/kg orally q12h) or enrofloxacin (10–20 mg/kg orally q24h) and amoxicillin (22 mg/kg orally q12h)	
Adult dog, inpatient	Ampicillin (22 mg/kg i.v. q8h) and gentamicin (6 mg/kg i.v. q24h)	Ensure adequate hydration. Alternative: enrofloxacin may be substituted for gentamacin
Adult dog, hospital-acquired	Often imipenem (3–10 mg/kg i.v. q8h) or ampicillin (22 mg/kg i.v. q8h) plus amikacin (15 mg/kg i.v. q24h) or a third-generation cephalosporin	Choice should reflect in-hospital resistance patterns, which should be recorded

32.4 Recommended antimicrobial treatments.

anaerobes. There is some concern about using these drugs in animals with immature cartilage, because experimental studies have shown deleterious effects on cartilage; however, this has not been recognized as a problem clinically. In cats, use of enrofloxacin has occasionally been associated with acute blindness, but this has not been observed in dogs. The use of fluoroquinolones in hospital-acquired pneumonia is controversial, as rapid development of resistance to these drugs has been demonstrated in hospitalized animals.

Aminoglycosides: These drugs provide excellent Gram-negative coverage, are useful in all types of bacterial pneumonia, and are often used in conjunction with ampicillin or other Gram-positive spectrum antimicrobials. Resistance to these drugs is very rare and they are relatively inexpensive. Once-daily intravenous dosing is preferred.

Due to nephrotoxicity, fluid therapy is mandatory during use and aminogylcosides should not be used in animals with pre-existing renal disease or in dehydrated or hypovolaemic animals without correction of the fluid deficit. They are also relatively contraindicated in neuromuscular disease, due to their effects at the neuromuscular junction. An inexpensive method for monitoring nephrotoxicity is to examine the urine for casts every few days whilst on treatment, because development of casts is an early sign of reversible nephrotoxicity. Should casts be observed, the aminoglycoside should be discontinued promptly. Aminoglycosides are usually restricted to in-hospital use, but short-term use at home is possible if subcutaneous fluids are administered concurrently and the animal is eating and drinking.

Potentiated sulphonamides: Although these antibiotics are often used in treatment of puppy pneumonias, some studies have shown that they are often ineffective against *Bordetella* spp. and so they are not a good choice for young animals with pneumonia. They have also been associated with immune-mediated disease. They are useful in treatment of pneumonia due to meticillin-resistant *Staphylococcus aureus* (MRSA), which has been appreciated as a growing threat in veterinary medicine in recent years (Weese, 2005).

Tetracyclines and doxycycline: Doxycycline has excellent activity *in vitro* against *Bordetella bronchiseptica*. Thus it is a reasonable antibiotic choice for a young dog with pneumonia, particularly since it is also effective against *Mycoplasma* spp., which may complicate *Bordetella* pneumonia.

Metronizadole: This antibiotic is very effective against anaerobes and is advised when anaerobic infections are considered likely. It may also be used in combination with antimicrobials that have poor anaerobic activity, such as the aminoglycosides, fluoroquinolones and most cephalosporins. Caution is warranted since this drug can be associated with neurotoxicity.

Carbapenems: This group of drugs provides excellent four-quadrant antimicrobial activity. These drugs are used as drugs of last resort in humans with severe life-threatening infection. Use should be restricted to situations where a life-threatening infection has been demonstrated and alternative antimicrobials are not practical due to either resistance patterns or contraindications; they are also very expensive.

Adjunctive therapies

Intravenous fluids: Fluid therapy is often essential in managing cases of pneumonia, especially in young animals or older, debilitated pets. The aims of fluid therapy are to keep the pet euvolaemic and well hydrated and to provide electrolyte supplementation, e.g. potassium and glucose, as required. Airway secretions are best expectorated if they are moist, and crystalloids are often provided at 40–60 ml/kg per day. Fluid rates should be provided to meet the metabolic needs of the patient. Excessive volumes of fluids and diuretics should be avoided.

Oxygen therapy: Oxygen supplementation is often required in pneumonia cases that are severe enough to require hospitalization. A pulse oximetry reading of 93% saturation or lower is considered indicative of severe hypoxaemia (P_aO_2 <60 mmHg) and the need for supplemental oxygen. If a patient has increased respiratory effort or rate despite a normal oximetry reading, supplemental oxygen is still warranted. This can be achieved by a variety of methods (see Chapter 1). Small animals benefit most from being housed in an oxygen cage, which is often able to deliver up to 60% O_2. Nasal oxygen is useful, especially in larger dogs, but is variably tolerated by patients. A facemask can be used in very calm or obtunded patients, or a mini oxygen cage can be fashioned by delivery of oxygen into an Elizabethan collar covered with clear plastic wrap. For very severe cases of respiratory failure due to pneumonia, endotracheal intubation with mechanical ventilation may be required. These patients unfortunately have a very guarded prognosis with survival rate of <25% being reported (Hopper *et al.*, 2007).

Airway therapy: Saline nebulization for 5–10 minutes three or four times daily, followed by coupage, can assist in the breakdown and expectoration of thick mucoid secretions. Severely distressed or vomiting animals may not tolerate coupage and it should be avoided in these cases or in patients that become stressed by the procedure. Aminoglycoside antibiotics can be delivered directly by nebulization and this is particularly beneficial in animals with persistent cough associated with bordetellosis.

Nutrition: Nutrition is an important consideration in animals with severe pneumonia. Young small-breed puppies will require glucose supplementation if anorexic, although usually the severe stage of the disease is short lived with appropriate treatment and the patient will begin to eat again. If an animal does not eat within a couple of days of commencing therapy, or if there are contraindications to oral feeding, such as megaoesophagus or severe gastrointestinal disease, other strategies have to be employed. Coax feeding or gentle syringe feeding may be possible in animals that can take food orally, but those with respiratory compromise must not be force-fed under any circumstances. Naso-oesophageal tubes or oesophageal tubes are useful if the animal can tolerate placement. If animals cannot be fed orally due to dysphagia or oesophageal disease, a gastric feeding tube (either surgically or endoscopically placed) is a good option. For animals that cannot tolerate enteral feeding, placement of a central line and total parenteral nutrition are indicated until they are able to take enteral feedings. (See the *BSAVA Manual of Canine and Feline Rehabilitation, Supportive and Palliative Care* for more details.)

Follow-up
Repeat thoracic radiographs are of limited benefit in the first few days of treatment because radiographic changes lag significantly behind clinical changes. However, radiography is useful to help determine whether antimicrobials can be discontinued in cases where clinical signs are improving 2–4 weeks after beginning therapy. Some puppies will have a lengthy course of disease, and an apparent reinfection may actually be a relapse from an infection that was treated for an inappropriate length of time.

Dogs should remain in hospital for treatment until they are no longer oxygen-dependent, are eating and drinking normally, and are afebrile. Treatment with antimicrobials at home should continue for a total of 2–6 weeks, and at least 1 week after complete resolution of clinical signs. Survival for pneumonia in young dogs (<1 year old) has been reported as approximately 90%. Survival in older animals with underlying disease will depend significantly on the veterinary surgeon's ability to control the underlying disease as well as the severity of the disease. Hospital-acquired infections typically respond well to therapy, provided that the correct antimicrobial is selected.

Atypical pneumonias

Most canine pneumonia is bacterial in origin, but other organisms may also result in pneumonia. These infections are typically distinguished from bacterial pneumonia by radiographic pattern, culture and cytological results.

Fungal pneumonia
Fungal pneumonias show a marked regional distribution. The UK is free of dimorphic fungal infections, but rare cases of disseminated aspergillosis or cryptococcosis may occur. An example of a disseminated fungal infection (blastomycosis) is shown in Figure 32.3c.

Mycobacterial pneumonia
This is a rare presentation in cats and dogs but is highly significant due to its zoonotic potential. The history is usually more chronic than with other pneumonias and may include weight loss and failure to thrive. Bassett Hounds are considered predisposed, as are Siamese cats. It is important to determine the species

of the mycobacterium, as *Mycobacterium tuberculosis* complex is more concerning than *M. avium*. Radiographic findings are variable but can include a nodular interstitial pattern, lung lobe consolidation, perihilar lymphadenopathy and pleural effusion. The organism may be identified by an acid-fast stain in a cytology preparation or via polymerase chain reaction (PCR). Owners and local public health officials should be informed of the diagnosis and the zoonotic potential of this disease, and the animal should not be returned to a house containing immunosuppressed people. Treatment involves a protracted course of antimicrobials, but many affected pets are euthanased.

Viral pneumonias
Viral pneumonias have occurred less commonly in dogs since the development of modern vaccinations. Distemper virus, a member of the paramyxovirus family, is associated with pneumonia, as well as gastrointestinal and neurological abnormalities. Affected dogs may also develop secondary bacterial infections. Other viruses, such as herpesvirus, adenovirus or parainfluenza virus, have also been recognized in canine pneumonia. Recently in the USA a mutation of the equine influenza virus H3N8 was reported to affect dogs (Yoon *et al.*, 2005). Since dogs do not have naturally occurring protective immunity, some infected dogs have had severe clinical disease, including death associated with secondary bacterial pneumonia.

Eosinophilic pneumonias
Eosinophilic bronchopneumopathy has been described in dogs and may occasionally be mistaken for bacterial pneumonia. Clinical signs of affected dogs include coughing, respiratory distress and lethargy. Substantial pulmonary infiltrates are usually observed on thoracic radiographs. Affected dogs often have a history of prior antibiotic therapy with little or no improvement. Cytological interpretation of respiratory samples demonstrates markedly increased numbers of eosinophils. Some dogs also have a high peripheral eosinophil count, but this is not required for the diagnosis. Investigation for a parasitic (heartworm or lungworm (Figure 32.5)) infection is warranted, depending upon regional predispositions,

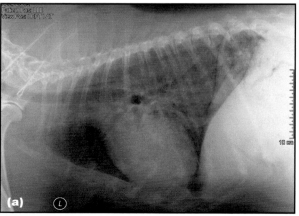

32.5 **(a)** Thoracic radiograph of a dog with eosinophilic pneumonia due to lungworm infection. (continues) ▶

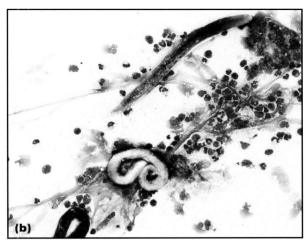

32.5 (continued) **(b)** Larvae identified in a transoral tracheal wash. Note additionally the presence of eosinophils. Wright's stain; original magnification X20. (Courtesy of P. Bain.)

and treatment with antiparasitic drugs results in gradual improvement. Idiopathic eosinophilic pneumonia requires long-term treatment with glucocorticoids.

Interstitial lung disease

Interstitial lung disease represents a diverse subset of pulmonary diseases that include abnormalities in the microscopic interstitium (the anatomical space between the basement membranes of the epithelial and endothelial cells) as well as the inflammatory and/or fibrotic processes that extend into the alveolar space, the bronchioles and bronchiolar lumen. Interstitial lung disease (ILD) is recognized uncommonly in veterinary medicine in comparison with human medicine. However, in the past decade or so a form of interstitial disease has been recognized in dogs, most commonly the West Highland White Terrier, and more recently in cats (Corcoran *et al.*, 1999; Cohn *et al.*, 2004).

Clinical signs

The most common signs in animals with ILD include cough, tachypnoea, exercise intolerance or overt respiratory distress. Due to the misperception that exercise intolerance is an accepted part of ageing, a lengthy course of disease may exist before veterinary care is sought. Physical examination is usually remarkable for pulmonary crackles. Occasionally, a loud S2 is present or other signs of pulmonary hypertension (see Chapter 28). Some dogs have concurrent mitral regurgitation, but sinus arrhythmia is common rather than a sinus tachycardia associated with heart failure. Weight loss is not common in dogs but may be found in cats.

Diagnosis

Diagnostic testing is often limited to thoracic radiographs, which document a heavy interstitial pattern, occasionally with right-sided cardiomegaly. In recent years, high-resolution computed tomography (HRCT) has evolved into the standard of care for evaluation

of patients with suspected interstitial disease (Figure 32.6). HRCT has a better correlation with physiological dysfunction than does thoracic radiography.

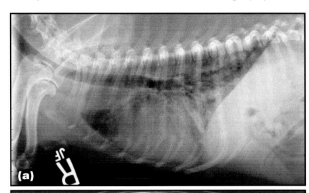

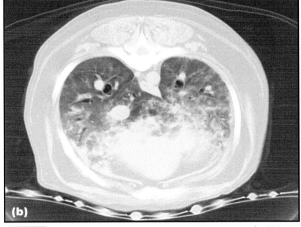

32.6 **(a)** Radiographic and **(b)** CT images of a West Highland White Terrier with pulmonary fibrosis.

Collection of arterial blood gases is often challenging in small animals with respiratory distress but, if performed, will document an increased A–a gradient and moderate to severe hypoxaemia. Bronchoscopy or BAL is unlikely to be helpful except for excluding other diseases. Open-lung biopsy is warranted to classify the disease, but is rarely performed in veterinary medicine due to inherent risks and also due to the current inability to treat patients better based upon histopathological findings.

Treatment

Treatment is limited to supportive care. A trial on a bronchodilator or prednisone therapy can be considered. The prognosis is guarded, with many dogs dying from progressive pulmonary failure within 12–18 months.

Cats

In cats with interstitial lung disease, histopathological findings are similar to the human condition of pulmonary fibrosis. In a recent report, approximately 25% of affected cats also had pulmonary neoplasia (Cohn *et al.*, 2004). Thus, if a cat with an obvious pulmonary mass on chest radiographs has respiratory effort disproportionate to the size of the mass, concurrent interstitial lung disease should be considered. The owners should be aware that the prognosis may be worse in such a situation.

References and further reading

Cohn LA, Norris CR, Hawkins EC *et al.* (2004) Identification and characterization of an idiopathic pulmonary fibrosis-like condition in cats. *Journal of Veterinary Internal Medicine* **18**, 632–641

Corcoran BM, Cobb M, Martin MW *et al.* (1999) Chronic pulmonary disease in West Highland White terriers. *Veterinary Record* **29**, 611–616

Fransson BA, Bagley RS, Gay JM *et al.* (2001) Pneumonia after intracranial surgery in dogs. *Veterinary Surgery* **30**, 432–439

Hopper K, Haskins SC, Kass PH *et al.* (2007) Indications, management, and outcome of long-term positive-pressure ventilation in dogs and cats: 148 cases (1990–2001). *Journal of the American Veterinary Medical Association* **230**, 64–75

MacPhail CM and Monnet E (2001) Outcome of and postoperative complications in dogs undergoing surgical treatment of laryngeal paralysis: 140 cases (1985–1998). *Journal of the American Veterinary Medical Association* **218**, 1949–1956

Radhakrishnan A, Drobatz KJ, Culp WT *et al.* (2007) Community-acquired infectious pneumonia in puppies: 65 cases (1993–2002). *Journal of the American Veterinary Medical Association* **230**, 1493–1497

Weese JS (2005) Methicillin-resistant *Staphylococcus aureus*: an emerging pathogen in small animals. *Journal of the American Animal Hospital Association* **41**, 150–157

Yoon KJ, Cooper VL, Schwartz KJ *et al.* (2005) Influenza virus infection in racing greyhounds. *Emerging Infectious Diseases* **12**, 1974–1976

33

Pleural and mediastinal disorders

Catriona M. MacPhail

Introduction

The thoracic or pleural cavity is the potential space between the lungs, mediastinum, diaphragm and thoracic wall. It is lined by the pleura, a serous membrane that is described by the particular structure that it covers. The visceral pleura covers the lungs, whilst the parietal pleura lines the rest of the thoracic cavity and is further classified as costal, diaphragmatic or mediastinal. The mediastinum is the central tissue partition of the thoracic cavity that separates the two hemithoraces. Controversy exists as to whether the mediastinum is a complete or a fenestrated structure; regardless of this, it is easily disrupted and a unilateral disease process typically affects the contralateral side. The mediastinum has anatomical boundaries of the thoracic inlet, diaphragm, thoracic spine and sternum; it encloses the heart, aorta, trachea, mainstem bronchi, oesophagus, thymus, thoracic duct, and phrenic and vagus nerves. Anatomically, the mediastinum is divided by the heart into cranial, middle and caudal portions.

Clinically and radiographically, the mediastinum is separated most commonly into ventral (cranial), central (medial) and dorsal compartments to help categorize mediastinal disease processes (Figure 33.1).

A small amount of transudative fluid is normally contained within the pleural space. The purpose of this fluid is to allow structures to slide freely during respiration. The production and absorption of this fluid is a continuous process controlled by Starling's forces. Pleural effusion develops when disease processes alter normal fluid dynamics, vascular permeability, lymphatic drainage or pleural surface area. Seven general types of pleural and mediastinal effusions, based on cytological characteristics, have been described (see Figure 8.7).

A retrospective study of pleural and mediastinal effusions in 81 dogs found the most common disease to be pyothorax, although 28 distinct disease processes were identified (Mellanby *et al.*, 2002). The pleural space and mediastinal compartments can also be abnormally occupied by air or by space-occupying masses.

Compartment	Anatomical structures	Mediastinal lesions
Ventral or cranial	Heart	Cardiomegaly; pericardial disease
	Ascending aorta	Aortic dilatation, neoplasia
	Cranial vena cava	Caval thrombosis, caval dilatation
	Thymus	Thymoma
	Lymphatic tissue	Lymphoma
	Miscellaneous	Mediastinal cysts; ectopic thyroid tissue; neoplasia
Central or medial	Trachea	Pneumomediastinum; mediastinitis
	Oesophagus	Megaoesophagus; oesophageal diverticulum
	Aortic arch	Heart base tumours
	Caudal vena cava	Caval thrombosis
	Main pulmonary arteries	Pulmonary artery dilatation
Dorsal	Descending aorta	Aortic dilatation
	Paravertebral tissues	Infiltrative or neoplastic disease

33.1 Mediastinal compartments with associated structures and diseases. (Data from Rogers and Walker, 1997).

Clinical signs

Animals with pleural disease typically present with rapid, shallow respirations indicative of a restrictive respiratory pattern due to fluid, tissue or air occupying the pleural space. Other clinical signs may include pyrexia, lethargy, anorexia and weight loss. The duration of clinical signs varies widely, as animals may present in acute distress or with insidious signs of chronicity.

Physical examination and thoracic auscultation will typically reveal muffled cardiac sounds. Thoracic percussion can be valuable in identifying pleural disease as the cause of respiratory distress. Percussion over normal lung fields results in a low-frequency vibration, while percussion over the heart, consolidated tissue, or fluid-filled pleural space causes a dulling of the vibration or hyporesonance. Systematic percussion of the thoracic cavity may identify a fluid line, giving the examiner a subjective assessment of the amount of fluid within the pleural space. Hyper-resonance in combination with diminished or absent respiratory sounds is highly suggestive of pneumothorax.

Pneumomediastinum as a sole event may have more subtle clinical signs, and many animals may be initially asymptomatic. Dogs and cats with space-occupying mediastinal masses can present with variable clinical signs, including respiratory difficulty, regurgitation, inappetence, coughing and exercise intolerance. Precaval syndrome can also occur with large cranial mediastinal masses. This is manifest by pitting oedema of the head, neck, thoracic inlet and forelimbs due to interference of venous return through the cranial vena cava.

Diagnostic approach

Thoracic radiography
Diagnostic evaluation of pleural and mediastinal disease starts with thoracic radiography.

- If the animal is stable, a full radiographic examination is performed, which includes right and left lateral recumbent views and a ventrodorsal (VD, if a small volume effusion) or dorsoventral (DV, if a large volume effusion) view.
- If the animal becomes stressed but can tolerate a sternal position, lateral views can be obtained with a horizontal beam technique in addition to the DV view.
- If an animal is severely compromised, it may be safer for the patient to confirm the presence of pleural fluid using ultrasonography, and thoracic radiographs should be delayed in favour of therapeutic thoracocentesis (see below).

Thoracic radiography should ultimately be performed to assess the degree and type of pleural disease, determine unilateral *versus* bilateral involvement and evaluate for intrathoracic masses. The appearance of pleural effusion on thoracic radiographs is dependent on the volume, character and distribution of the fluid. Minimal volume might be best seen on a VD view. Small amounts of fluid are best appreciated on a lateral thoracic view and appear as soft tissue opacities that form wedges between the sternum and interlobar fissures of the lungs. These wedges may coalesce to give a scalloped appearance to the lung borders. In addition, there is typically blunting of the costophrenic angles on the DV view. Large amounts of fluid result in classic Roentgen signs of pleural effusion as the cardiac silhouette and diaphragmatic border are obscured, the mediastinum is widened and lung lobes collapse (Figure 33.2). Collapsed lung fields demonstrate alveolar patterns, which may indicate atelectasis or infiltrative disease.

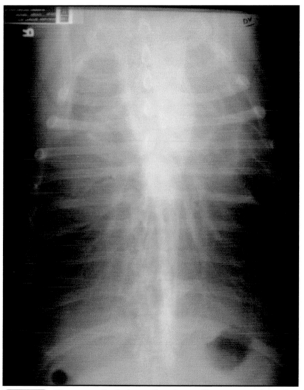

33.2 Dorsoventral view of a dog with severe pleural effusion. The cardiac silhouette is obscured, as is the border of the diaphragm. Lung lobes are retracted and there are multiple interlobar fissures.

The mediastinum on thoracic radiographs is identified by the large structures that lie within it (heart, trachea, caudal vena cava and aorta). Smaller mediastinal structures and the mediastinum itself are not typically visualized in the normal animal. The presence or absence of mediastinal disease is initially evaluated from the VD view. In the normal dog, the width of the mediastinum should be approximately twice the width of the spine, whilst a normal feline mediastinum should not be any wider than the sternum. Mediastinal masses or fluid in the cranial compartment cause widening of the mediastinum and elevation of the proximal thoracic trachea (Figure 33.3).

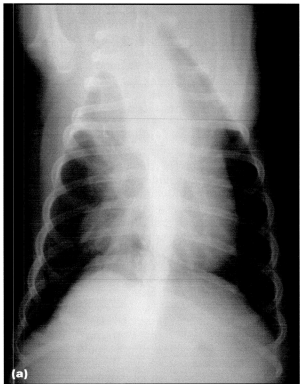

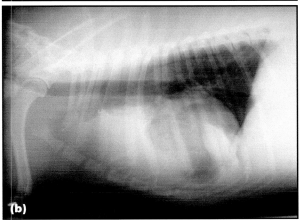

(a) Ventrodorsal and **(b)** lateral radiographs demonstrating widening of the cranial mediastinum with pleural effusion and pulmonary metastasis from a mediastinal thymoma.

Thoracocentesis

Needle aspiration of the pleural cavity can be both diagnostic and therapeutic. After initial sampling of the fluid for diagnostic evaluation, removal of as much of the fluid as possible will provide considerable relief to severely affected animals. As bilateral distribution of fluid and air is common, thoracocentesis should be performed on both sides of the animal. Typically a 20- or 22-gauge needle is used, although butterfly catheters or small over-the-needle catheters are also utilized. The needle should be attached to extension tubing, which is connected to a three-way stopcock and 60 ml syringe (Figure 33.4).

Thoracocentesis is most safely performed with the animal standing or in sternal recumbency. If pleural effusion is suspected, the needle is advanced

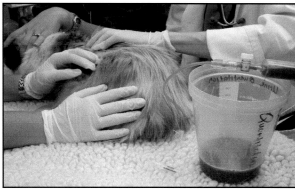

Cat with pyothorax undergoing therapeutic thoracocentesis.

into the pleural cavity at the level of the ventral third of the thorax, caudal to the 5th to 6th rib space to avoid injury to the heart. The needle should enter at an angle of 45 degrees, with the bevel facing the thoracic wall. For suspected pneumothorax, the needle is inserted cranial to the 8th to 10th ribs in the dorsal third of the thorax.

The needle is inserted slowly as an assistant aspirates with 5–10 ml of pressure. Retrieved fluid is evaluated cytologically and submitted for bacterial culture. Repeat needle thoracocentesis as a means of therapy is not recommended, as there is morbidity and risk associated with this technique and it is inefficient for complete thoracic drainage. If further drainage is indicated, placement of a thoracostomy tube is warranted (see below).

Ultrasonography

Thoracic ultrasonography may be indicated to identify causes of pleural effusion such as: pulmonary, pleural or mediastinal neoplasia; lung lobe consolidation with or without abscessation; diaphragmatic herniation; or lung lobe torsion. In one study, samples obtained by ultrasound-guided fine-needle aspiration were found to be diagnostic in 91% of cases (Reichle and Wisner, 2000). Thoracic ultrasonography can also be used to aid sample procurement when only a small amount of pleural fluid is present.

Advanced imaging

Advanced imaging, such as computed tomography (CT) or magnetic resonance imaging (MRI), can be beneficial in assessing mediastinal disease, determining the aetiology of pleural effusions, or locating the source of spontaneous pneumothorax. Identification of blebs or bullae by CT occurred in 75% of dogs that presented for spontaneous pneumothorax, compared with only 17% from thoracic radiographs (Au *et al.*, 2006), but atelectasis can obscure detection of lung pathology in some cases. Fine-needle aspiration or core biopsy of intrathoracic structures can also be performed under CT guidance (Zekes *et al.*, 2005).

Thoracotomy and thoracoscopy

Ultimately, exploration of the thoracic cavity may be required for diagnosis. Access to the thorax ranges from a simple keyhole intercostal approach, for focal lung and pleural biopsy, to a median sternotomy, for assessment of the entire pleural space.

Thoracoscopy has been proposed as an alternative diagnostic tool to determine the aetiology of pleural effusion (Kovak *et al.*, 2002). It is less invasive than thoracotomy and allows for excellent visualization of intrathoracic structures and sampling of abnormal tissues (lung, pleura, mediastinal tissue, lymph node).

Thoracostomy tube placement

Unilateral or bilateral thoracostomy tubes are placed to facilitate complete emptying of the thoracic cavity. The decision to place single or multiple tubes is based on the volume, distribution and character of the pleural fluid or extrapulmonary air. Sedation and local anaesthesia or general anaesthesia is usually required for tube placement (see Chapter 17).

Proper placement is through a skin incision in the dorsal third of the thoracic cavity at the level of the tenth to twelfth intercostal space. The tube is advanced through a generous subcutaneous tunnel from a caudodorsal to cranioventral direction, and enters the pleural cavity through the midthoracic level of the seventh or eighth intercostal space. Once the tube is secured, placement should be verified on thoracic radiographs.

Pleural drainage may be intermittent or continuous, depending on the volume of fluid initially retrieved and whether negative pressure can be established within the pleural cavity. The volume and character of the fluid should be closely monitored to aid decisions about tube removal. Complications of thoracostomy tubes include kinking, clogging, inadvertent removal and risk of ascending nosocomial infections.

Pneumothorax and pneumomediastinum

Pneumothorax is typically classified as traumatic, iatrogenic, or spontaneous.

- *Traumatic pneumothorax* primarily occurs from blunt force injury that suddenly increases intrathoracic pressure and ruptures pulmonary parenchyma. Less commonly, penetrating injury or fractured ribs will lacerate the lung, trachea, or bronchi. A *tension pneumothorax* develops when injured soft tissues on the thoracic wall or in the lung create a one-way valve that traps air in the pleural space. This is a **life-threatening emergency** as the increasing intrathoracic pressure severely compromises ventilation and venous return, quickly resulting in shock and then death.
- *Iatrogenic pneumothorax* may happen secondary to thoracocentesis, thoracostomy tube placement, or thoracic surgery.
- *Spontaneous pneumothorax* can occur due to a ruptured pulmonary bleb or bulla, leaking pulmonary tissue from neoplasia or abscess, and migrating foreign material.

Pneumomediastinum can occur alone or in conjunction with pneumothorax. Air most commonly enters the mediastinum as an extension of pneumothorax. Alternatively, pneumomediastinum occurs when air dissects through the thoracic inlet due to head or neck injury, or less commonly as an extension from the abdomen or retroperitoneal space following abdominal surgery, penetrating abdominal injuries, or rupture of a gas-filled viscus.

The degree of respiratory compromise resulting from pneumothorax depends on the amount of lung collapse and concurrent pulmonary injury. Pneumothorax is usually tolerated if there is less than 50% collapse and no other underlying injury or pulmonary pathology exists. However, pulmonary contusions often occur in concert with traumatic pneumothorax and a mild pneumothorax can cause significant respiratory compromise.

Diagnosis and treatment

Emergency thoracocentesis is performed on animals in respiratory distress with consistent clinical signs of pneumothorax prior to radiographic confirmation. Radiographs are performed when the animal is stable, to assess the degree of pneumothorax and the presence of concurrent injuries. Typical radiographic signs of pneumothorax on lateral views include elevation of the cardiac silhouette away from the sternum, visualization and retraction of visceral pleural margins away from the thoracic wall, and increased lung lobe opacity due to atelectasis (Figure 33.5). Pneumomediastinum is best identified from the lateral view, as free gas in the mediastinum allows for stark contrast with, and visualization of, intramediastinal structures (Figure 33.6).

The goal of treatment in traumatic pneumothorax is to remove extrapulmonary intrapleural air to allow re-expansion of the lungs. Mild traumatic pneumothorax with minimal respiratory compromise is often treated conservatively by observation alone while the animal resorbs pleural air. If the animal is in respiratory distress, or if a tension pneumothorax has been identified, thoracocentesis is indicated. Often only a single thoracocentesis is required, but thoracostomy

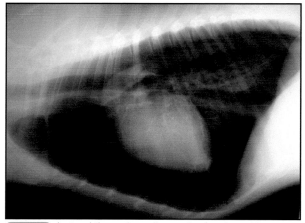

33.5 Lateral thoracic radiograph of a dog with moderate to severe pneumothorax, as demonstrated by the elevation of the cardiac silhouette from the sternum and retraction of the lung fields.

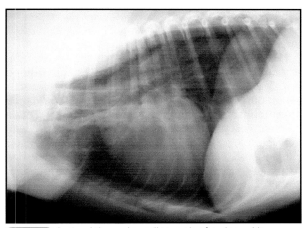

33.6 Lateral thoracic radiograph of a dog with pneumomediastinum. Tracts of air are seen within the mediastinum, outlining the trachea and enhancing visualization of the oesophagus and descending aorta. A mild pneumothorax is also present.

tube placement is indicated if air retrieval is continuous or if the animal requires multiple aspirations to alleviate clinical signs. Following chest tube placement, intermittent evacuation may be effective; however, continuous evacuation is preferred to permit complete lung expansion and to achieve contact between the visceral and parietal pleural surfaces. The thoracostomy tube is removed as soon as there is sufficient evidence that the pulmonary leak has sealed.

If the pneumothorax persists longer than 3–5 days, if the animal cannot be stabilized even with continuous evacuation, or if a large airway laceration is suspected due to the volume of air retrieved, thoracotomy is indicated to correct the source of air leakage. Early surgical intervention is advocated in cases of spontaneous pneumothorax, as it is associated with a lower recurrence and mortality rate than dogs managed conservatively (Puerto *et al.*, 2002) (Figure 33.7). If the location of the leak is not known, a median sternotomy is preferred to allow complete exploration of the thoracic cavity. However, the hilus and large airways are more accessible through an intercostal approach.

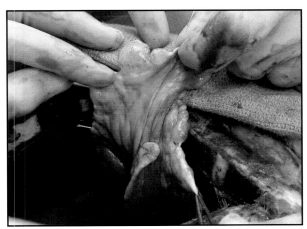

33.7 Intraoperative appearance of pulmonary blebs in a dog with severe spontaneous pneumothorax.

Prognosis

In general, if pneumothorax is readily identified and managed appropriately, and if concurrent life-threatening injuries are not present, treatment of traumatic pneumothorax is straightforward and carries a reasonable prognosis. Due to challenges in identifying the source, as well as controversy over treatment approaches, the prognosis for spontaneous pneumothorax is variable.

Pyothorax

The accumulation of septic exudate within the pleural cavity is commonly referred to as pyothorax. In dogs and cats the cause and source of infection are often unknown, which can make these cases difficult to manage.

Suspected and reported aetiologies in dogs include migrating foreign material, penetrating bite wounds, extension of bronchopneumonia, extension of discospondylitis, oesophageal perforation, parasitic migration, haematogenous spread or iatrogenic causes. Grass awns and other barbed plant material are the most commonly implicated migrating foreign bodies, and there is an association of pyothorax with young hunting dogs (Dementriou *et al.*, 2002). Causes identified in cats include extension of aspiration pneumonia, pulmonary abscess rupture, parasitic migration, foreign body penetration from the oesophagus or lung, or penetrating thoracic bite wounds. It is widely believed that the most common route of infection is through penetrating bite wounds from other cats (Waddell *et al.*, 2002). However, others have theorized that the most common source of infection is aspiration of normal oropharyngeal flora and colonization of the lower respiratory tract (Barrs *et al.*, 2005). Pyothorax then develops as an extension of infection from the lung into the pleural space.

Multiple bacterial organisms have been associated with pyothorax (Figure 33.8), but obligate anaerobes or a mixture of obligate anaerobes with facultative aerobic bacteria are most commonly isolated. *Pasteurella* spp. are the most common organisms found in cats with pyothorax, whilst dogs are infected with *Escherichia coli*, *Pasteurella* spp. and filamentous organisms such as *Actinomyces* spp. and *Nocardia* spp.

Escherichia coli
***Pasteurella* spp.**
***Actinomyces* spp.**
***Nocardia* spp.**
Bacteroides spp.
Fusobacterium spp.
Peptostreptococcus spp.
Clostridium spp.
Porphyromonas spp.
Prevotella spp.
Enterobacter spp.
Klebsiella spp.
Staphylococcus spp.
Streptococcus spp.

33.8 Organisms isolated in pyothorax. Those most commonly found are in **bold**.

Diagnosis

The diagnosis of pyothorax in companion animals is usually straightforward and made from a combination of historical and physical examination findings, thoracic radiograph evaluation and pleural fluid examination. The duration of clinical signs varies widely from days to months, and animals may present in acute distress or with more insidious signs of chronicity. A diagnosis of pyothorax is made when the pleural fluid is characterized as an exudate with degenerate neutrophils as the predominant cell type, and bacteria are identified cytologically.

Treatment

There are numerous options for case management, none of which is known to be optimal. At a minimum, systemic antimicrobial therapy and supportive care are indicated. Initial antimicrobial therapy should be broad-spectrum to address the possible multiple organisms that could be involved. No single agent can be recommended to address all possible infective organisms, but penicillins and penicillin derivatives are most commonly prescribed. Cefoxitin, enrofloxacin and trimethoprim/sulphonamide are also advocated as good empirical choices. Long-term treatment with antibiotics in the beta-lactam class is the treatment of choice for *Actinomyces* spp. Other drugs that are commonly effective include clindamycin and chloramphenicol. *Nocardia* spp. infections are not a common cause of pyothorax in dogs and cats, but, if diagnosed, long-term administration of sulphonamides may be indicated and, as with *Actinomyces* spp., treatment is prolonged.

Thoracic drainage can be provided through needle thoracocentesis, thoracostomy tube placement or thoracotomy. Although surgical intervention is aggressive, surgery is advantageous as it allows exploration of the thoracic cavity, possible identification and removal of an underlying cause, and thorough thoracic lavage. Thoracoscopy has also been mentioned as a less invasive alternative, although there are currently no veterinary studies that describe the use of this modality for pyothorax.

Prognosis

The prognosis for pyothorax is highly variable and the argument of medical *versus* surgical therapy has yet to be settled. Mortality rates vary, and animals may be euthanized without treatment due to poor prognosis, financial constraints or the potential for recurrence. The recurrence rate is variable but it is thought to be more of a concern for *Actinomyces* spp. or *Nocardia* spp. infections.

Haemothorax

Haemorrhagic pleural effusion occurs in approximately 10% of animals sustaining blunt or penetrating thoracic trauma. This is a result of lung laceration or injury to major vascular structures. Haemothorax may also occur due to erosion of large vessel walls secondary to local tumour invasion. Haemothorax can also occur with a coagulopathy, although pulmonary bleeding is usually more clinically significant than is accumulation of blood in the pleural space.

Haemorrhage due to lung lobe laceration is usually clinically insignificant because the haemorrhage is self-limiting. However, damage to large arteries or veins, particularly the intercostal vessels, can cause **significant life-threatening haemorrhage**. These animals will present in hypovolaemic shock with tachycardia, pale mucous membranes and decreased capillary refill time. Circulatory compromise precedes respiratory compromise from haemothorax, as ventilation impairment will not occur until 30 ml of blood per kilogram has accumulated in the pleural space.

Diagnosis

Auscultation of patients with severe haemothorax reveals muffled heart and lung sounds. A fluid–gas interface may be identified if concurrent pneumothorax is also present. Thoracocentesis is the diagnostic tool of choice as these animals are often too unstable to allow radiographic examination. Blood in the thoracic cavity is quickly defibrinated by the constant motion of the lungs and therefore will not clot after aspiration, although subacute massive haemorrhage may clot if the blood is accumulating too rapidly. The packed cell volume (PCV) of the aspirated fluid is typically equal to or above the animal's peripheral PCV.

Treatment

Small amounts of thoracic haemorrhage are typically clinically insignificant, but more substantial haemorrhage requires aggressive treatment. Systemic bleeding disorders should first be ruled out by assessing platelet number and function and performing coagulation tests. If these are normal, drainage of the pleural cavity is performed through thoracostomy tube placement; needle aspiration will not drain the area fast enough and the blood may clot in the needle if there is peracute haemorrhage. Volume replacement must also be instituted to address hypovolaemic shock. Transfusion is indicated if >20–30 ml of blood per kilogram is retrieved from the chest and is usually required if the PCV drops acutely below 20%.

If haemothorax is a result of trauma, autotransfusion is a reasonable treatment option, particularly if blood products are in short supply or are not readily available. There are several methods of autotransfusion, but the most appropriate in an emergency situation is direct aspiration and reinfusion. Blood is aspirated though intravenous tubing and three-way stopcock into a 60 ml syringe. The blood is then pushed into a blood collection bag and returned to the patient through a blood filter set. Complications of autotransfusion include haemolysis, coagulopathy and sepsis.

Exploratory thoracotomy is rarely indicated for haemothorax, because the source of haemorrhage is not typically located or the animal is too unstable to survive the procedure. However, if the animal is not responsive to replacement therapy or if intrathoracic blood loss is continuous, surgery may be the only remaining treatment option.

Chylothorax

Access of chyle to the pleural cavity occurs with disruption or obstruction of the thoracic duct. The thoracic duct runs from the cisterna chyli, through the aortic hiatus, with termination in the jugular veins, azygous vein and/or mediastinal lymph nodes. There are multiple proposed causes of chylothorax, including neoplasia (lymphoma, cranial mediastinal masses), trauma, caval thrombosis and cardiac disease (heartworm disease, right heart failure, pericardial disease, cardiomyopathy). However, often the cause is undetermined and those cases are deemed idiopathic.

Diagnosis

Animals can present in varying degrees of respiratory distress. Thoracic radiographs identify significant pleural effusion, and thoracocentesis will retrieve a pink-tinged white fluid (Figure 33.9). Chylothorax is diagnosed by comparison of pleural fluid and serum triglyceride and cholesterol levels, with triglyceride content being higher and cholesterol content lower in the pleural fluid. Lymphocytes are usually the predominant cell type, but if the chylothorax has been longstanding the fluid often has a suppurative component as well. The thorax should be drained as completely as possible to help identify any underlying cause. Thoracic radiography is repeated and echocardiography performed.

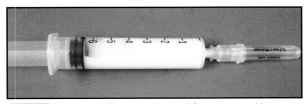

33.9 Chylous effusion obtained from a cat with a peritoneal–pericardial–diaphragmatic hernia.

Treatment

If an underlying cause is not identified, medical management consists of intermittent thoracic drainage, low-fat diet and use of benzopyrones (e.g. Rutin, 50–100 mg/kg orally q8h). The efficacy of benzopyrones in small animals is unknown.

Surgery is indicated when animals become refractory to medical management, although it should be considered earlier in cats due to the potential for the development of fibrosing pleuritis from longstanding effusion. Multiple surgical techniques for treatment of chylothorax have been described over the last 10–20 years.

- The cornerstone of surgical management is thoracic duct ligation, which is successful in approximately 60% of cases when used as a sole technique (Birchard *et al.*, 1998).
- Subtotal pericardiectomy has been advocated in conjunction with thoracic duct ligation with reported success in 10/10 dogs (Fossum *et al.*, 2004). It is unknown what role the pericardium plays in this disease process, but it has been

suggested that pericarditis, particularly constrictive pericarditis, can induce chylous effusion due to increases in central venous pressure and impairment of chylous return to the venous system. Alternatively, it is theorized that pericardial thickening is a secondary event that results from chronic irritation of longstanding chylous effusion.

- Omentalization of the thoracic cavity as a sole technique has been reported to be successful in isolated case reports.
- Thoracic duct ligation in combination with partial pericardiectomy using two right-sided intercosal thoracotomies was associated with a successful outline in 13 of 14 cases (Carobbi *et al.*, 2008).
- A combination of three techniques via median sternotomy (thoracic duct ligation, subtotal pericardiectomy, omentalization) has also been shown to have a good outcome in a small number of cases (Duerr and Monnet, 2007).
- Cisterna chyli ablation in combination with thoracic duct ligation has been investigated as a new form of therapy; a successful outcome was reported in 7/8 clinical cases (Hayashi *et al.*, 2005).
- Other surgical techniques include active or passive pleuroperitoneal shunting, mechanical pleurodesis and thoracic duct embolization, all of which have varying degrees of success.

Neoplastic effusion

In a study of canine pleural and mediastinal effusions, 27/81 dogs (33%) had an underlying neoplastic disease process, but neoplastic cells were identified in only three effusions (4%) (Mellanby *et al.*, 2002). Neoplastic effusions are identified by the presence of neoplastic cells on cytology and can be associated with metastatic disease, cranial mediastinal masses or mesothelioma.

Diagnosis

Mesothelioma is a rare tumour that originates from the serosal lining of body cavities. It manifests as diffuse nodular or multifocal masses that are highly effusive, and animals present with significant pleural, pericardial or peritoneal effusion. Diagnosis can be challenging, as mesothelial cells may proliferate under any condition associated with fluid accumulation, and malignant mesothelial cells are difficult to distinguish from reactive hypertrophied mesothelial cells. Therefore, definitive diagnosis requires tissue biopsy obtained by thoracoscopy or open thoracotomy.

Treatment and prognosis

No successful treatment for mesothelioma exists at this time. Partial pericardiectomy is a palliative option for animals with pericardial effusion, with or without adjunctive chemotherapy. Intracavitary cisplatin has been reported to be of palliative benefit in a few dogs, but it arrests tumour growth and decreases fluid production for only a limited time. As this tumour is uncommon, survival rates are difficult to determine. In general, the prognosis for mesothelioma is poor.

Mediastinal masses

Space-occupying lesions of the mediastinum include, but are not limited to, abscesses, granulomas, branchial cysts, lymphadenopathy and neoplasms. The most common tumours within the mediastinum are thymoma and lymphosarcoma. Ectopic thyroid carcinomas, chemodectomas and neuroendocrine or anaplastic carcinomas may also occur in this compartment.

Diagnosis

Differentiation between thymoma and lymphosarcoma can be challenging, as fine-needle aspiration of cranial mediastinal masses may yield populations of small lymphocytes in both disease processes. However, flow cytometry has recently been described as a useful tool for distinguishing thymoma, lymphoma and non-haematological malignancies (Lana et al., 2006).

Thymomas are tumours of the thymic epithelium that can occur in both dogs and cats. They are characterized based on behaviour as invasive or non-invasive. Non-invasive thymomas are well encapsulated, whilst invasive tumours invade local tissues and are more likely to be associated with pleural effusion. Aside from signs associated with a space-occupying cranial mediastinal mass or pleural effusion, up to 40% of dogs with thymomas have the paraneoplastic syndrome of myasthenia gravis characterized by muscle weakness and signs associated with megaoesophagus. Hypercalcaemia has been reported with thymomas, but is more commonly associated with thymic lymphoma. Advanced imaging is beneficial to help to determine the degree of local invasion and aid in assessment of resectability of the mass.

Treatment and prognosis

Surgical resection is the treatment of choice for thymomas. The approach to the thoracic cavity is based on the size and invasiveness of the mass. Large masses that involve other structures in the cranial thorax may require median sternotomy. Approximately 70% of thymomas are resectable, regardless of the size of the mass. In these circumstances, the long-term prognosis is good. Dogs with a resectable tumour without megaoesophagus have a reported 1-year survival rate of 83%, whilst cats have median survival of almost 2 years. Dogs and cats with non-resectable thymomas generally have a poor prognosis, although chemotherapy or radiation treatment may achieve a positive response in some cases.

References and further reading

Au JJ, Weisman DL, Stefanacci JD et al. (2006) Use of computed tomography for evaluation of lung lesions associated with spontaneous pneumothorax in dogs: 12 cases (1999–2002). Journal of the American Veterinary Medical Association **228**, 733–737

Barrs VR, Allan GS, Martin P et al. (2005) Feline pyothorax: a retrospective study of 27 cases in Australia. Journal of Feline Medicine and Surgery **7**, 211–222

Birchard SJ, Smeak DD and McLoughlin MA (1998) Treatment of idiopathic chylothorax in dogs and cats. Journal of the American Veterinary Medical Association **212**, 652–657

Carobbi B, White RAS and Romanelli G (2008) Treatment of idiopathic chylothorax in 14 dogs by ligation of the thoracic duct and partial pericardiectomy. Veterinary Record **163**, 743–745

Dementriou JL, Foale RD, Ladlow J et al. (2002) Canine and feline pyothorax; a retrospective study of 50 cases in the UK and Ireland. Journal of Small Animal Practice **43**, 388–394

Duerr F and Monnet E (2007) Long-term outcome associated with surgical treatment of idiopathic chylothorax in 10 dogs (1995–2005). Veterinary Surgery **35**, E6

Fossum TW, Merterns MM, Miller MW et al. (2004) Thoracic duct ligation and pericardiectomy for treatment of idiopathic chylothorax. Journal of Veterinary Internal Medicine **18**, 307–310

Hayashi K, Sicard G, Gellasch K et al. (2005) Cisterna chyli ablation with thoracic duct ligation for chylothorax: results in eight dogs. Veterinary Surgery **34**, 519–523

Kovak JR, Ludwig LL, Bergman PJ et al. (2002) Use of thoracoscopy to determine the etiology of pleural effusion in dogs and cats: 18 cases (1998–2001). Journal of the American Veterinary Medical Association **221**, 990–994

Lana S, Plaza S, Hampe K et al. (2006) Diagnosis of mediastinal masses in dogs by flow cytometry. Journal of Veterinary Internal Medicine **20**, 1161–1165

Mellanby RJ, Villiers E and Herrtage ME (2002) Canine pleural and mediastinal effusions: a retrospective study of 81 cases. Journal of Small Animal Practice **43**, 447–451

Puerto DA, Brockman DJ, Lundquist C et al. (2002) Surgical and nonsurgical management of and selected risk factors for spontaneous pneumothorax in dogs: 64 cases (1986–1999). Journal of the American Veterinary Medical Association **220**, 1670–1674

Reichle JK and Wisner ER (2000) Non-cardiac thoracic ultrasound in 75 feline and canine patients. Veterinary Radiology and Ultrasound **41**, 154–162

Rogers KS and Walker MA (1997) Disorders of the mediastinum. Compendium on Continuing Education for the Practicing Veterinarian **19**, 69–82

Waddell LS, Brady CA and Drobatz KJ (2002) Risk factors, prognostic indicators, and outcome of pyothorax in cats: 80 cases (1986–1999). Journal of the American Veterinary Medical Association **221**, 819–824

Zekes LJ, Crawford JT and O'Brien RT (2005) Computed tomography-guided fine-needle aspirate and tissue-core biopsy of intrathoracic lesions in thirty dogs and cats. Veterinary Radiology and Ultrasound **46**, 200–204

Drug formulary

The doses here are primarily from the recommendations given within this Manual. For those drugs without recommended doses within chapters, doses are derived from published sources (including the *BSAVA Small Animal Formulary*), data sheet recommendations and personal experience.

Drug	Doses (dogs)	Doses (cats)	Comments
N–Acetylcysteine	50–70 mg/kg (capsules) orally q6–12h (not to exceed 600 mg q8h) 50–70 mg/kg i.v. slowly q6h		**Must give diluted if i.v. (5% solution)**
Amiloride	Combined with hydrochlorothiazide as 2.5 mg A + 25 mg H, or 5 mg A + 50 mg H. Calculate dose for hydrochlorothiazide		
Amiodarone	10 mg/kg orally q12h for 7–14 days *or* 10–15 mg/kg orally q24h for 7–14 days *then* 5–7.5 mg/kg orally q24h 4–8 mg/kg i.v. over 10–15 min **Do not exceed 10 mg/kg/h**		Expect severe hypersensitivity reaction with current commercially available formulation administered i.v.
Amlodipine	0.1–0.4 mg/kg orally q24h Start at low dose and titrate upwards to effect	0.625–1.25 mg/cat orally q24h Start at low dose and titrate upwards to effect	Do not exceed 0.4 mg/kg q24h Monitor blood pressure **Do not use if hypotensive**
Aspirin	0.5–10 mg/kg orally q24h	5–75 mg/kg orally q72h	
Atenolol	0.2–1.5 mg/kg orally q12–24h Some dogs will tolerate doses of 2 mg/kg q12h if no myocardial failure present	0.5–3 mg/kg orally q12–24h Doses of 6.25–12.5 mg/cat orally q12–24h are often given for efficacy and convenience	
Atropine	0.02–0.04 mg/kg i.v. 0.02–0.04 mg/kg i.m., s.c. q6–8h		Transient bradyarrhythmias often occur, especially with low doses i.v.
Benazepril	0.25–0.5 mg/kg orally q24h	0.5–1 mg/kg orally q24h	
Bromhexine	2 mg/kg orally q12h 3–15 mg/dog i.m. q12h	1 mg/kg orally q24h 3 mg/cat i.m. q24h	
Butorphanol	Antitussive: 0.2 –1 mg/kg orally q6–12h; 0.05–0.1 mg/kg i.v., i.m., s.c. q6–8h Sedation: 0.1– 0.3 mg/kg i.v., i.m., s.c. q2–6h	Sedation: 0.1–0.3 mg/kg i.v., i.m., s.c. q2–6h	Can combine with acepromazine (0.01–0.05 mg/kg) for greater sedation
Carvedilol	0.05–0.4 mg/kg orally q12–24h Start at low dose and titrate upwards over several weeks. Some dogs tolerate doses up to 1.5 mg/kg q12h if no myocardial failure present		
Clopidogrel	3–4 mg/kg orally q24h *or* 10 mg/kg orally (loading dose) followed by 1–2 mg/kg orally q24h	18.75 mg/cat orally q24h	
Codeine	0.2–2 mg/kg orally q12h		

Drug	Doses (dogs)	Doses (cats)	Comments
Dalteparin	100–150 IU/kg s.c. q8h	100–180 IU/kg s.c. q6–24h	
Dexamethasone	0.1–0.5 mg/kg i.v., i.m., s.c. q12–24h		
Digitoxin	0.015–0.03 mg/kg orally q8h	**Do not use in cats**	
Digoxin	3–5 µg/kg orally q12h (lean bodyweight) **Do not exceed 0.25 mg/dog q12h, or 0.1875 mg q12h in Dobermanns** **Decrease dose by 10% for elixir** 0.1–0.15 mg/m² orally q12h (BSA calculated from lean bodyweight)	7–10 µg/kg (0.03125 mg/cat) orally q48h **Decrease dose by 10% for elixir**	Few, if any, indications for i.v. dosing
Diltiazem	0.1–0.25 mg/kg i.v. over 1–2 min (repeat q5–15min up to 0.75 mg/kg) 2–6 µg/kg/h i.v. infusion 0.5–2 mg/kg orally q8h (loading dose: 0.5 mg/kg, then 0.25 mg/kg q1h up to 2 mg/kg)	0.05–0.2 mg/kg i.v. over 2–3 min (repeat q5–15min up to 0.5 mg/kg) 2–6 µg/kg/h i.v. infusion 1.5–2.5 mg/kg orally q8h (7.5–15 mg/cat q8h) Oral sustained release preparation: 30–60 mg/cat q24h	
Dobutamine	2–15 µg/kg/min i.v. infusion for up to 48–72 hours	0.5–2 µg/kg/min i.v. infusion for up to 48 hours (higher doses may be tolerated in some cats)	**Monitor ECG for arrhythmias** **May cause seizures in cats**
Dopamine	2–10 µg/kg/min i.v. infusion		**Monitor ECG for arrhythmias**
Enalapril	0.5 mg/kg orally q12–24h	0.25–0.5 mg/kg orally q12–24h	
Enoxaparin	0.8 mg/kg s.c. q6h	1.25 mg/kg s.c. q6h	
Esmolol	50–500 µg/kg i.v. over 5 min 25–200 µg/kg/min i.v. infusion		
Etamiphylline	10–33 mg/kg orally, i.m., s.c. q8h Suggested dosing based on *bodyweight* (data sheet): *3–10 kg*: 100 mg/dog orally q8h; 70–140 mg/dog i.m., s.c. q8h *10–30 kg*: 100–300 mg/dog 100 mg/dog orally q8h; 140–420 mg/dog i.m., s.c. q8h *>30 kg*: 300–400 mg/dog 100 mg/dog orally q8h; 420–700 mg/dog i.m., s.c. q8h	100 mg/cat orally q8h 70–140 mg/cat i.m., s.c. q8h	
Flecainide	1–5 mg/kg orally q8–12h		Dose used experimentally to convert atrial fibrillation potentiated by vagal tone
Fluticasone	<20 kg bodyweight: 110–125 µg via metered dose inhaler q12h >20 kg bodyweight: 220–250 µg via metered dose inhaler q12h	110–125 µg via metered dose inhaler q12h or 220–250 µg via metered dose inhaler q24h	
Furosemide	1–6 mg/kg orally, s.c., i.m., i.v. q1–24h 0.2–0.5 mg/kg/h i.v. infusion Typical dose for mild to moderate congestive heart failure: 1–2 mg/kg orally q12h		Doses >10–15 mg/kg/day usually have no further clinical benefit
Glyceryl trinitrate	6–50 mm of 2% w/w ointment percutaneously q6–8h	3–6 mm of 2% w/w ointment percutaneously q6–8h	**Wear gloves to administer**
Glycopyrrolate	5–10 µg/kg i.m., i.v. 10–20 µg/kg s.c. 8–12h		

Drug	Doses (dogs)	Doses (cats)	Comments
Heparin sodium	Arterial thromboembolism: 300–500 IU/kg i.v. (loading dose), *then* 100–300 IU/kg s.c. q6–8h Thromboprophylaxis: 70 IU/kg s.c. q8–12h		
Hydralazine	0.5–3 mg/kg orally q12h Start at low dose and titrate upwards to effect	2.5–5 mg/cat orally q12h Start at low dose and titrate upwards to effect	**Monitor blood pressure** **Do not use if hypotensive**
Hydrochlorothiazide	0.5–4 mg/kg orally q12h		
Hydrocodone	0.22 mg/kg orally q6–12h		
Imidapril	0.25 mg/kg orally q24h	0.5 mg/kg orally q24h	Dose in cats used experimentally without adverse effects
Isoproterenol	0.01 µg/kg i.m., s.c. q4–6h 0.01–0.1 µg/kg/min i.v. infusion		
Levosimendan	0.05 mg/kg orally q12h		Dose from unpublished data
Lidocaine	2 mg/kg i.v. over 1–2 min (repeat in 2 mg/kg boluses up to 8 mg/kg in 10 min) *or* 0.8 mg/kg/min i.v.infusion (up to 8 mg/kg) 25–100 µg/kg/min i.v. infusion (after bolus dose) 4 mg/kg i.m. (takes 10–15 min for effect in humans and lasts 90 min)	0.25–0.75 mg/kg i.v. over 2–3 min (repeat in 0.25–0.5 mg/kg boluses up to 2 mg/kg in 10 min) 10–40 µg/kg/min i.v. infusion (after bolus dose)	Intravenous infusion to be given *after* successful bolus therapy; otherwise takes up to 6 hours to reach steady state concentration
Magnesium sulphate	0.15–0.3 mEq/kg i.v. (20–40 mg/kg) over 5–10 min (emergency loading dose) 0.75–1 mEq/kg/day i.v. infusion (replacement dose) 1–2 mEq/kg orally q24h		
Metoprolol	0.2–1 mg/kg orally q8–12h Start at low dose and titrate upwards over several weeks	2–15 mg/cat orally q8–12h Start at low dose and titrate upwards over several weeks	
Mexiletine	4–8 mg/kg orally q8–12h 3.5 mg/kg i.v. over 2–3 min		Intravenous dose from experimental and anecdoctal data; dose with food
Nitroprusside	1–5 µg/kg/min i.v. infusion Start at 1–2 µg/kg/min and titrate upwards to effect		**Monitor blood pressure** **Do not use if hypotensive**
Phenoxybenzamine	0.25–2.5 mg/kg orally q12h Start at 0.25 mg/kg and titrate upwards to effect		Monitor blood pressure **Do not use if hypotensive**
Pimobendan	0.1–0.3 mg/kg orally q12h	0.625–1.25 mg/cat orally q12h	Dose in cats from anecdoctal data; dose at least 1h before food
Prazosin	0.5–2 mg/dog orally q8–12h Start at low dose and titrate upwards to effect	0.25–1 mg/cat orally q8–12h Start at low dose and titrate upwards to effect	**Monitor blood pressure** **Do not use if hypotensive**
Prednisolone	0.5–1 mg/kg orally q12h for 3–10 days; *then taper dose* every 10–14 days based on continued clinical response For eosinophilic lung disease, higher doses and longer courses may be required	1–2 mg/kg orally q12h for 3–10 days; *then* 1 mg/kg orally q24h for 10–20 days if good clinical response; *then* 0.5 mg/kg q24h maintenance therapy	
Procainamide	6–10 mg/kg i.v. over 2–3 min 25–50 µg/kg/min i.v. infusion (after bolus dose) 8–20 mg/kg i.m. q4–6h 8–20 mg/kg orally q6h (sustained release: q8h)	1–2 mg/kg i.v. over 3–5 min 10–20 µg/kg/min i.v. infusion (after bolus dose) 3–8 mg/kg i.m. q6–8h (up to 20 mg/kg) 3–8 mg/kg orally q6–8h (up to 20 mg/kg)	

Drug	Doses (dogs)	Doses (cats)	Comments
Propantheline	0.25–0.5 mg/kg orally q8–12h (up to 2 mg/kg q8h) Suggested dosing based on *bodyweight*: *<5kg*: 3.75 mg/dog q8–12h; *5–10 kg*: 7.5 mg/dog q8–12h; *10–25 kg*: 15 mg/dog q8–12h; *25 kg*: 30 mg/dog q8–12h	7.5 mg/cat orally q48–72h	Gastrointestinal side effects may limit higher doses
Propranolol	0.02–0.08 mg/kg i.v. over 5 min 0.1–1 mg/kg orally q8h Some dogs will tolerate doses of 0.3 mg/kg i.v. or 1.5 mg/kg orally if no myocardial failure present	0.02–0.06 mg/kg i.v. over 5 min 0.4–1.2 mg/kg (2.5–5 mg/cat) orally q8h Some cats will tolerate doses of 0.1 mg/kg i.v. or 10 mg/cat orally if no myocardial failure present	
Quinidine gluconate	6–20 mg/kg i.m. q6–8h (loading dose 14–20 mg/kg)	6–16 mg/kg i.m. q8h	
Quinidine sulphate	6–20 mg/kg orally q6h (sustained release: q8h)	6–16 mg/kg orally q8h	
Ramipril	0.125–0.25 mg/kg orally q24h	0.125–0.5 mg/kg orally q24h	Dose in cats used experimentally without adverse effects
Rutin	50–100 mg/kg orally q8h	250 mg/cat orally q12h	
Salbutamol	20–50 µg/kg orally q8–12h	90 µg via metered dose inhaler as needed	
Sildenafil	0.5–3 mg/kg orally q8–24h		
Sotalol	1–3 mg/kg orally (up to 5 mg/kg) q12h 1 mg/kg i.v. over 3–5 min; repeat to effect	10–20 mg/cat orally (up to 30 mg/cat) q12h 1 mg/kg i.v. over 3–5 min; repeat to effect	Intravenous and cat doses from anecdoctal data
Spironolactone	1–2 mg/kg orally q12–24h		Dose with food
Tadalafil	1 mg/kg orally q24h		
Terbutaline	5–10 µg/kg i.m., s.c. q4h 0.625–5 mg/dog orally q8–12h	5–15 µg/kg i.m., s.c. q4h 0.625–1.25 mg/cat orally q8–12h	
Theophylline	10–20 mg/kg orally q12–24h	15–19 mg/kg orally q24h	
Torasemide	0.2 mg/kg orally q12–24h		Administer at one tenth of furosemide dose
Verapamil	0.05 mg/kg i.v. over 5 min (repeat 0.025 mg/kg q5min up to 0.15 mg/kg) 0.5–2 mg/kg orally q8h	0.025 mg/kg i.v. over 5 min (repeat q5min up 0.15 mg/kg) 0.5–1 mg/kg orally q8h	

Conversion tables

Biochemistry

	SI unit	Conversion	Non-SI unit
Alanine aminotransferase	IU / l	x 1	IU / l
Albumin	g / l	x 0.1	g / dl
Alkaline phosphatase	IU / l	x 1	IU / l
Aspartate aminotransferase	IU / l	x 1	IU / l
Bilirubin	µmol / l	x 0.0584	mg / dl
Calcium	mmol / l	x 4	mg / dl
Carbon dioxide (total)	mmol / l	x 1	mEq / l
Cholesterol	mmol / l	x 38.61	mg / dl
Chloride	mmol / l	x 1	mEq / l
Cortisol	nmol / l	x 0.362	ng / ml
Creatine kinase	IU / l	x 1	IU / l
Creatinine	µmol / l	x 0.0113	mg / dl
Glucose	mmol / l	x 18.02	mg / dl
Insulin	pmol / l	x 0.1394	µIU / ml
Iron	µmol / l	x 5.587	µg / dl
Magnesium	mmol / l	x 2	mEq / l
Phosphorus	mmol / l	x 3.1	mg / dl
Potassium	mmol / l	x 1	mEq / l
Sodium	mmol / l	x 1	mEq / l
Total protein	g / l	x 0.1	g / dl
Thyroxine (T4) (free)	pmol / l	x 0.0775	ng / dl
Thyroxine (T4) (total)	nmol / l	x 0.0775	µg / dl
Tri-iodothyronine (T3)	nmol / l	x 65.1	ng / dl
Triglycerides	mmol / l	x 88.5	mg / dl
Urea	mmol / l	x 2.8	mg of urea nitrogen / dl

Temperature

	SI unit	Conversion	Conventional unit
	° C	(x 9/5) + 32	° F

Haematology

	SI unit	Conversion	Non-SI unit
Red blood cell count	10^{12} / l	x 1	10^6 / µl
Haemoglobin	g / l	x 0.1	g / dl
MCH	pg / cell	x 1	pg / cell
MCHC	g / l	x 0.1	g / dl
MCV	fl	x 1	$µm^3$
Platelet count	10^9 / l	x 1	10^3 / µl
White blood cell count	10^9 / l	x 1	10^3 / µl

Hypodermic needles

	Metric	Non-metric
External diameter	0.8 mm	21 G
	0.6 mm	23 G
	0.5 mm	25 G
	0.4 mm	27 G
Needle length	12 mm	$^1/_2$ inch
	16 mm	$^5/_8$ inch
	25 mm	1 inch
	30 mm	$1^1/_4$ inch
	40 mm	$1^1/_2$ inch

Suture material sizes

Metric	USP
0.1	11/0
0.2	10/0
0.3	9/0
0.4	8/0
0.5	7/0
0.7	6/0
1	5/0
1.5	4/0
2	3/0
3	2/0
3.5	0
4	1
5	2
6	3

Index

Index